ETHNOVETERINARY MEDICINE

INDIGENOUS KNOWLEDGE AND DEVELOPMENT SERIES

Series Editors

Professor David Brokensha, University of Cape Town
Alfonso Peter Castro, Syracuse University
Professor L. Jan Slikkerveer, University of Leiden

Other titles in the *Indigenous Knowledge and Development Series:*

Facing Kirinyaga: A social history of forest commons in southern Mount Kenya
Alfonso Peter Castro

The Cultural Dimension of Development: Indigenous knowledge systems
L. Jan Slikkerveer, D. Michael Warren and David Brokensha

Ethnoveterinary Research and Development
Edited by Constance M. McCorkle, Evelyn Mathias and
Tjaart W. Schillhorn van Veen

Indigenous Organizations and Development
Peter Blunt and D. Michael Warren

*Hungry for Hope: On the cultural and communicative
dimensions of development in highland Ecuador*
Carmen Hess

Intercropping and the Scientific Basis of Traditional Agriculture
Donald Innis

*Jurema's Children in the Forest of Spirits:
Healing and ritual among two Brazilian indigenous groups*
Clarice Novaes Da Mota

*Nature is Culture: Indigenous knowledge and socio-cultural
aspects of trees and forests in non-European cultures*
Edited by Klaus Seeland

Hometown Associations: Indigenous knowledge and development in Nigeria
Rex Honey and Stanley Okafor

*Biological and Cultural Diversity: The role of indigenous
agricultural experimentation in development*
Edited by Gordon D. Prain, Sam Fujisaka and Michael D. Warren

The Roots of Change: Human behaviour and agricultural evolution in Mali
Brent M. Simpson

Indigenous Knowledge Development in Bangladesh: Present and future
Edited by Paul Sillitoe

Ethnoveterinary Medicine

*An annotated bibliography of
community animal healthcare*

MARINA MARTIN, EVELYN MATHIAS
AND CONSTANCE M. McCORKLE

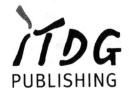

ITDG
PUBLISHING

Published by ITDG Publishing
103–105 Southampton Row, London WC1B 4HL, UK
www.itdgpublishing.org.uk

Cover photograph: by kind permission of Dr Ilse Köhler-Rollefson

First published in 2001

ISBN 1 85339 522 6

This book only describes the existing literature in ethnoveterinary medicine.
No recommendations are made or should be implied as to the use or otherwise
of the treatments described in this book.

The authors and publisher assume no responsibility for and make no warranty
with respect to the results of using the treatments described in this book. The
authors and publisher accept no liability for any damage or loss whatsoever
resulting from the use of or reliance on any information contained in this book.

A catalogue record for this book is available from the British Library.
ITDG Publishing is the publishing arm of the Intermediate Technology
Development Group. Our mission is to build the skills and capacity of people in
developing countries through the dissemination of information in all forms, enabling
them to improve the quality of their lives and that of future generations.

VETAID, Pentlands Science Park, Bush EH 26 0PZ, Scotland, UK
Tel. 44 131 445 6241, Fax. 44 131 445 6242, e-mail: mail@vetaid.org
www.vetaid.org

Typeset by J&L Composition Ltd, Filey, North Yorkshire
Printed in Great Britain by SRP, Exeter

Contents

About the Authors   vi

Foreword   vii

Acknowledgements   ix

Acronyms   xi

Introduction to the Bibliography   1

Annex to the Introduction   30

The Bibliography Abstracts   37

Index   563

About the authors

Marina Martin, BSc (Hons), MSc. With degrees in Applied Animal Biology from the University of Wales and in Tropical Animal Production and Health from the University of Edinburgh, Martin has conducted ethnoveterinary research in Nigeria and Tanzania. Currently, she is employed by VETAID, a livestock development NGO based in Scotland (e-mail marina@vetaid.org).

Evelyn Mathias, MS, Dr med vet. A veterinarian with a degree in international development from the USA, Dr Mathias has worked for more than 10 years in Ethiopia, Indonesia, Kenya, the Philippines, Tanzania, Thailand and Tunisia in research, training, networking, project management and evaluation. Her specialties are ethnoveterinary medicine, animal healthcare provision, gender and livestock development, and the use of participatory approaches and indigenous knowledge in rural development. Presently, she works out of Germany as a freelance consultant (e-mail evelynmathias@netcologne.de).

Constance M. McCorkle, MA, MA, PhD. The 'mother' of the field of ethno-veterinary medicine, Dr McCorkle is an agricultural anthropologist, cultural ecologist and linguist, with graduate degrees all from Stanford University. Her main areas of expertise lie in livestock sociology, local knowledge systems, environment, gender, rural development, and monitoring and evaluation. McCorkle is a former professor of Rural Sociology and has been director of various international development programmes for USAID. Currently she is based in Washington DC as an independent consultant (e-mail mccorkle@boo.net).

Foreword

FOR MILLENNIA, PEOPLE have used home-grown veterinary skills and techniques to keep their animals healthy. But only during the last decade have people's local knowledge and skills received much scientific attention, under the rubric of 'ethnoveterinary medicine' (EVM). This development is largely due to the efforts of Drs Evelyn Mathias and Constance McCorkle who compiled and published much of the then-existing literature on EVM in a 1989 bibliography.

Today, ethnoveterinary medicine is a growing field that brings together a synergistic mix of researchers and practitioners. They include not only veterinarians, anthropologists and folk practitioners but also sociologists, linguists, historians, ethnobotanists, animal and range scientists, foresters, development workers, some medical doctors and the occasional quack. The quality of work in EVM varies. Some is anecdotal, and some is well-documented; some is proven, and much is simply taken on faith. In the aggregate, however, ethnoveterinary studies provide useful insights into animal (and also often human) healthcare and, equally useful, into how animals and their diseases are perceived and managed in different societies.

In other words, ethnoveterinary R&D encompasses social as well as biomedical sciences. It also interlinks science and ethnoscience, i.e. bodies of local (or indigenous or traditional) knowledge. It is not simply another topic in the broadening arena of non-conventional animal medicine. Rather, it relaunches veterinary medicine in a more holistic perspective. This perspective was lost in many Western societies, where for the past 50 years veterinarians were taught that disease is purely a structural or physiological dysfunction. Whether in animals or humans, however, ordinary people see health and illness as far more comprehensive issues, often involving religion, environment, intra- and inter-species social relations, and more. This bibliography offers a wealth of both new and old knowledge of community animal healthcare rarely ever found in Western textbooks of the late 20th century.

The recognition of people's own knowledge and skills embodied in the following pages may renew appreciation not only among veterinarians but also among stockraisers and healthcare practitioners in poor rural regions for the value of their own veterinary and husbandry savvy under prevailing conditions. Animal health does not always or necessarily have to depend on manufactured, exogenous medicines.

Indeed, EVM is one of the few fields of study where scientists and 'folks', North and South are equal partners. If anything, researchers, stockraisers and traditional practitioners in developing countries are 'first among equals' when it comes to contributing to the field. Generally, Southern cultures and environments appear to harbour richer troves of ethnoveterinary knowledge and resources than do Northern ones, where reductionist science has been wiping out other forms of 'knowing' and threatening the natural environment. But this trend is changing as interest grows in more comprehensive medical options than just a pill or a shot.

The fact that this bibliography is published in hard-copy at a time when the worldwide web of the Internet has come to the fore is a tribute to the publisher, who appears to recognize that such documents should be accessible to a wider public than just the 'electronicized'. Especially in developing countries, both social and biomedical scientists should find the volume a stimulating source of research ideas. Ethnoveterinary R&D does not (yet) require sophisticated equipment or fancy theories; it can and should be studied *in situ* under real-world conditions. Many of the abstracts in this volume demonstrate that careful field observations can advance scientific learning as much as can many laboratory experiments – and often in a more illuminating and culturally acceptable setting. The volume may also help local veterinary practitioners to gain greater validation of and status for their craft.

    History has repeatedly shown that much can be learned from diversity, whether it be sociocultural, biological, or merely differing opinion. Few bibliographies in the social or biological sciences provide a global view of diversity in the way this one does. The loss of such varied 'knowledges' would be a loss to all humankind. It is hoped that this volume will encourage further field study, sharing, and education in local/indigenous/traditional knowledge generally, be it from the North or the South, the East or the West.

June 2000
Tjaart W. Schillhorn van Veen, DVM and PhD
The World Bank[1]

Note

[1]Formerly, Professor of Veterinary Parasitology at Michigan State University, East Lansing, Michigan, USA; and, before that, at Ahmadu Belo University, Zaria, Nigeria.

Acknowledgements

VERY SPECIAL THANKS are due the late Dr D. Michael Warren, an anthropologist and the former Director of CIKARD (Center for Indigenous Knowledge for Agriculture and Rural Development) at Iowa State University. He provided the original stimulus to the idea of an annotated bibliography on ethnoveterinary medicine. This idea was made a reality by further professional encouragement plus financial and in-kind support from the SR-CRSP Sociology Project at the University of Missouri-Columbia, which at the time was headed by rural sociologist Dr Michael F. Nolan.

Major financial support for the preparation and publication of the present volume came from a mix of governmental, non-governmental and private-enterprise sources: most notably, the Animal Health Programme of the Natural Resources Research Department within the UK's Department for International Development (DFID); an affiliate of the larger European network of Vétérinaires Sans Frontières, the British NGO VETAID, which forms part of the Moredun Group of animal health research institutes in Scotland; and CMC Consulting, a small US firm specializing in international development and operated by the volume's third author.

Above all, however, the authors would like to acknowledge the scores of colleagues from all around the world who so graciously contributed of their own and others' writings and insights on ethnoveterinary medicine (EVM) to the present bibliography and its 1989 predecessor. Without their collaboration, quite simply this extensive compilation of sources would have been impossible. Particular thanks are due the following individuals for assistance above and beyond the call of duty: Dr Hernando Bazalar of Peru's Instituto Veterinario de Investigaciones Tropicales y de Altura, who marshalled a team of student veterinarians to search out recondite Spanish-language literature; Dr Denis Fielding, a lecturer in the Centre for Tropical Veterinary Medicine at Edinburgh University's Royal (Dick) School of Veterinary Studies, who introduced the first author to the other two (perhaps to her later chagrin); and veterinarian and policy analyst Dr Tjaart W. Schillhorn van Veen of the World Bank, who graciously consented to write a foreword to the present volume.

The authors would also like to recognize a number of dedicated librarians who, across the years and sometimes with only the most fragmentary reference information in any of half a dozen languages, have rooted out the often-fugitive and widely scattered documents on which the bibliography is based. They are: Trenton Boyd, Head of the Veterinary Medical Library at the University of Missouri-Columbia; Gerard McKiernan, former Coordinator of the CIKARD Documentation Center; and the delightful Moredun Research Institute librarians, Diane Donaldson and Heather Edgar.

Of course, various family members of the authors did not escape this monolithic undertaking unscathed. For their patience with proofreading and editing, we are grateful to the parents of the volume's first author, Elizabeth and Peter Martin; and for both critical and conceptual inputs, to the second author's spouse, Dr Paul Mundy.

Acronyms

ACCOMPLISH	Action Committee for the Promotion of Local Initiative in Self-Help
ACIAR	Australian Centre for International Agricultural Research
AFPRO	Action for Food Production
ASEAN	Association for South East Asian Nations
b.w.	Bodyweight
BAHA	Barefoot animal health assistants
CAHW	Community animal health worker
CBO	Community-based organization (local)
CBPP	Contagious bovine pleuropneumonia
CCPP	Contagious caprine pleuropneumonia
CEDECUM	Private Center for the Development of Rural and Urban Bordering Residents
CEPIA	Centro de Proyectos Integrales a Base de Alpaca de Juliaca
CNS	Central nervous system
CTA	Centre Technique de Coopération Agricole et Rurale
CTVM	Centre for Tropical Veterinary Medicine
CUSO	Canadian University Service Overseas
DFID	Department for International Development
ECF	East Coast Fever
ECHO	European Community Humanitarian Office
ED50	Experimental dose at which 50% of test animals are cured
epg	Eggs per gram of faeces
ER&D	Ethnoveterinary research and development
EVK	Ethnoveterinary knowledge
EVM	Ethnoveterinary medicine
FAO	Food and Agriculture Organization of the United Nations
FMD	Foot and mouth disease
g	Gram(s)
GO	Government organization
GTZ	Deutsche Gesellschaft für Technishe Zusammenarbeit
ha	Hectare(s)
HPI	Heifer Project International
i.m.	Intramuscular
ICAR	Indian Council of Agricultural Research
IEI	Instituto de Estudios Indígenas
IIED	International Institute for Environment and Development
IIRR	International Institute of Rural Reconstruction
ILCA	International Livestock Centre for Africa
ILEIA	Information Centre for Low External Input Agriculture
ILRAD	International Laboratory for Research on Animal Diseases
ILRI	International Livestock Research Institute
INIANSREDEF	Indonesia International Animal Science Research and Development Foundation
IPM	Integrated pest management

ITDG	Intermediate Technology Development Group
kg	Kilogram(s)
km	Kilometre(s)
l	Litre(s)
lbs	Pounds of weight
LD50	Lethal dose at which 50% of test animals show CNS signs or death
M	Molar(s)
mg	Milligram(s)
ml	Millilitre(s)
ND	Newcastle disease
NGO	Non-governmental organization (regional or national)
NVV	Nam Vazhi Velanmai Network
ODI	Overseas Development Institute
OFRD	On Farm Research Division
OIE	Office Internationale des Epizooties
ORSTOM	l'Office de la Recherche Scientifique et Technique Outre-Mer
OXFAM	Oxford Committee for Famine Relief
PPEA	Proyecto Piloto de Ecosistemas Andinos
PPR	Peste des petits ruminants
PRA	Participatory rural appraisal
PRATEC	Proyecto Andino de Tecnologías Campesinas
PRELUDE	Programme de Recherche et de Laison Universitaries pour le Developpement
PVO	Private voluntary organization (international)
R&D	Research and development
RRA	Rapid rural appraisal
SEVA	Sustainable Agriculture & Environmental Voluntary Action
sp., spp.	Species (singular, plural)
SR-CRSP	Small Ruminant Collaborative Research Support Program
SRISTI	Society for Research and Initiatives for Sustainable Technologies and Institutions
UK	United Kingdom
UNACH	Universidad Autónoma de Chiapas, México
UNICEF	United Nations International Children's Emergency Fund
US	United States of America
v/w	Volume by weight
VBKVK	Krishi Vigyan Kendram Badgaon
VSF	Vétérinaires Sans Frontières
WWII	World War II

Introduction to the Bibliography1

Constance M. McCorkle, Marina Martin and Evelyn Mathias

ALL OVER THE WORLD, people who keep livestock have developed their own ideas and techniques of doctoring and healthfully managing their animals. But until recently, scientists took little notice of such on-farm or at-home veterinary savvy. Only in about 1980 did they and development projects and organizations begin to pay serious attention to community approaches to livestock healthcare and related management practices. This interest was kindled by the realization that conventional, formal-sector resources and high-cost 'high-tech' interventions had proven inadequate for sustainably meeting the basic animal healthcare needs of a great many of the world's stockraisers (for a summary of such findings and arguments, see McCorkle 1995: 55).

Thus, science and development began to acknowledge the utility of building on and working with traditional and community animal healthcare and husbandry resources. Some of the earliest studies in this vein for Africa, Asia and Latin America were, respectively, Sollod and Knight 1983, FAO 1980 and McCorkle 1982. Later, the term 'ethnoveterinary research and development' (ER&D) was coined as a label for the systematic study of community animal healthcare and its development applications (McCorkle 1986). ER&D can be defined as:

> The holistic, interdisciplinary study of local knowledge and its associated skills, practices, beliefs, practitioners, and social structures pertaining to the healthcare and healthful husbandry of food, work, and other income-producing animals, always with an eye to practical development applications within livestock production and livelihood systems, and with the ultimate goal of increasing human well-being via increased benefits from stockraising (McCorkle 1995: 53).

In 1989, the first annotated bibliography on the subject appeared (Mathias-Mundy and McCorkle 1989). After its publication, worldwide interest in ethnoveterinary medicine (EVM) surged, and so did the number of formal publications and graduate theses on the topic. Today, many more journal articles and, indeed, entire monographs and books about EVM are available. Examples of the latter are Bizimana 1994b, IIRR 1994, ITDG and IIRR 1996, Matzigkeit 1990, McCorkle et al. 1996, and Wanyama 1997. The 1990s also witnessed the first regional and international conferences devoted to EVM. These yielded published abstracts and/or proceedings on the subject for Africa (Kasonia and Ansay 1994), Europe (Pieroni 1999), India (Mathias et al. 1999a), and the world (Mathias et al. 1999a&b). In addition, major international journals have since devoted whole issues to the subject (e.g. OIE 1994). Further, national governments and universities have begun to institute extension units and research centres on EVM (cf. McCorkle et al. 1999 for examples).

Nevertheless, much ER&D still emerges in non-formal forms, notably as reports and working papers from development projects and organizations. Increasingly, these and other sources are available electronically, in a new sort of fugitive or grey literature. But whether published or unpublished, hard-copy or electronic, information on

EVM is widely dispersed. Consequently, for professionals who work outside universities and large government agencies or who lack modern communication technologies, it is often very difficult to identify and access.

This bibliography is designed to make a basic body of EVM information readily and compactly accessible to researchers and development workers, via a publishing house with a solid international marketing network focused on development. It offers 1240 abstracts, spanning perhaps some 1260 documents (some abstracts review more than one document). This figure includes nearly all the 261 abstracts from the first bibliography, itself a fugitive publication. Box 1 briefly characterizes some of the present bibliography's key content.

Box 1: Overview of the bibliography

The bibliography's 1240 abstracts cover 118 countries: 39 in Africa, 32 in Asia, 25 in Europe, 19 in the Americas and 3 in Australasia. The percentage distribution of abstracts across continents roughly parallels this country count. Recorded in the following pages are ethnoveterinary knowledge, skills, beliefs, and both empirical and medico-religious practices from 160 named ethnic groups (apart from nationalities) for some 200 health problems of 25 livestock species.

This last figure includes 23 and 22 breeds of cattle and sheep, respectively. In addition to other familiar farm animals like pigs, goats, horses, donkeys, mules, rabbits and all manner of poultry, the bibliography encompasses 'exotic' stock such as elephant, reindeer, yak, buffalo, guinea pigs and both Old and New World camelids. Whether as work or companion animals, dogs and cats are also well-represented. Further noted are traditional healthcare and husbandry measures in apiculture and aquaculture. No such information was found for other micro-livestock, however (e.g. silkworms, snails, frogs).

In terms of *materia medica*, reference is made to: 765 plant species or genera (as counted by Latin and English names) with reported medicinal, nutritional, or toxic effects on livestock; more than 35 animal-based medicinal products; some 45 minerals or inorganic compounds; and a galaxy of sometimes-surprising foods, beverages, and household items employed in EVM. When it comes to preparing and administering traditional medicines and other treatments, the EVM literature documents every mode known in human ethnomedicine, plus a few that are not. Also recorded are some of the ethnodiagnostic techniques that guide treatment choice, whether the latter be medicinal, surgical, physical/mechanical, magico-religious, or a combination thereof.

Too numerous and complex to count are people's environmentally sensitive herding, housing, husbandry and breeding practices, many aimed at preventing disease in the first place. Of particular interest are natural biological controls on disease that stock-raisers exercise. The bibliography further highlights the existence of over 100 named or recognized types of local and alternative practitioners who regularly treat animals in their societies.

The wide variety of sources and topics represented in this volume provides a good indication of where to look for more information on EVM, both now and in the future. A signal addition to this updated and greatly expanded bibliography is Annex 1's catalogue of e-mail and internet resources by which, as of mid-2000, professionals interested in EVM can be contacted and new information in the field can be identified, searched, or obtained.

Materials, methods, and terminologies

Materials collection
Sources for the bibliographic materials collected can be summarized as follows: scholarly books and monographs; scientific and development journals of many different disciplines and organizations from all around the world; student theses and dissertations; manuals, guides, and kits generated by bi- and multilateral, governmental, and especially private-voluntary and non-governmental organizations (PVOs, NGOs) active in international development; newsletters and bulletins of all sorts; both published and unpublished research and project reports; other bibliographies; conference proceedings or presentation abstracts; and personal communications (letters, e-mails, and exchanges at conferences, seminars and workshops).

The 1989 predecessor to the present volume was based mainly on materials gathered through professional contacts and announcements in development-oriented journals and newsletters to solicit articles, conference papers, manuscripts and field notes on the subject. Only limited library searches were conducted. Consequently, many of the 261 entries in the 1989 bibliography consisted of unpublished reports and other fugitive literature. For the present bibliography, collection methods relied more heavily on computerized searches of library and other databases. These included widely available documentation systems like AGRIS and CABI, as well as more sectoral- or topic-specific databases like the library holdings of the International Livestock Centre for Africa in Ethiopia. Other website databases or internet sources tapped in for preparation of the bibliography are noted in Annex 1.

Whatever the search mechanism, the following fields were targeted as most likely to yield information on EVM in applied, development contexts: veterinary medicine, animal husbandry, anthropology, ethnobotany, and to a lesser extent range management, forage agronomy and agroforestry. No systematic search of the vast literature on pharmacology, phytochemistry or chemistry was made, e.g. as of *Chemical Abstracts or Medicinal and Aromatic Plant Abstracts*. However, a number of items from such sources were included in the bibliography thanks to the collaboration of a library-science research project on ethnoveterinary botanicals that drew upon the DIALOG information services and its 300 online databases (Zeutzius 1990).

Materials selection
Because of the huge amount of potentially relevant literature, this volume was perforce selective. It focuses on documents containing specific information on community animal healthcare concepts, practices and practitioners. However, also included are a few items that provide background or context for better understanding, studying or applying EVM. A few examples are: modern advances in 'probiotics' for livestock, which appear to parallel ancient wisdom about medication through nutrition (Gilling and Ponting n.d.); Martin's (1996) study of rapid rural appraisal methodologies for eliciting ethnoveterinary information; and Yilma's (1989) work on vaccines grounded in ethnoveterinary precedents.

Conversely, some related yet tangential subjects from the 1989 bibliography have been largely eliminated here. They include, for example: breeds and breeding except where there is a health-related outcome, intent or risk; social epidemiology; paraveterinary healthcare programmes; and intersectoral healthcare delivery. But again, any document on such subjects that also noted specific EVM concepts, practices, etc. *is* abstracted. Likewise for any materials that mention local veterinary specialists and their skills.

Pharmacological, pharmacognostic and phytochemical studies of plants used in EVM abound. However, the overwhelming majority deal with the plants' applications in human medicine. Such studies are referenced here only if they met at least one of the following criteria: the plant materials were tested in an animal species they could be used to treat, as versus only in laboratory animals; or the study's findings were clearly applicable to animal health problems. Defined as animal self-medication or self-treatment, the fascinating field of autoveterinary medicine is not covered, in that no human intervention is involved.[2] On the other hand, when works on EVM discuss or draw parallels with practices in human ethnomedicine, these *are* noted in order to point up the 'one medicine', human+animal orientation of so many healthcare systems (Mathias 1998, Schillhorn van Veen 1998) plus the potentials for EVM to contribute to human medicine.

In tandem with scientists, across the past 20 years Northern publics have become increasingly interested in traditional or 'alternative' medicine for animals and humans alike. Alternatives include acupuncture, herbalism, homeopathy, physical therapy (including massage and hydrotherapy), chiropractic (bone manipulation) and nutraceuticals. Technically speaking, whether such alternatives can be considered EVM depends on their historical origin and depth of integration within a given culture. Like Western/Northern veterinary medicine, medical traditions such as veterinary acupuncture in China or Ayurvedic herbalism in India began as folk medicine but have since been codified and institutionalized in formal educational curricula in their regions of origin. Homeopathy took a rather different evolutionary path, but it shares many principles and *materia medica* with traditional treatments around the world. A vast literature on all the foregoing alternatives exists. But the present volume abstracts only a smattering of it, mainly by way of providing background or comparative information. The bibliography's principal focus is on ethnoveterinary knowledge and techniques employed in everyday life at the farm/camp or community level, regardless of their genesis or parallels in one or another medical system.

The bibliography also prioritizes twentieth century literature. Nevertheless, some historical texts and latter-day studies on earlier EVM are included, for several reasons. Such texts may reveal the centuries-long persistence of certain EVM concepts and practices and/or their intercontinental distribution. This information can tag simple or cheap healthcare techniques of yore that perhaps deserve a second look at their appropriateness for some communities' situation today. Likewise for discredited practices and beliefs that may well warrant re-evaluation in light of modern scientific discoveries. Also, older writings and studies on EVM may recapture lost yet valuable ethnoveterinary therapies (e.g. Minja n.d.) and diagnostic techniques (e.g. Veena 1997). Furthermore, such texts sometimes constitute the only accessible source of EVM information for a given area. Until very recently, this was the case for inner Mongolia, for instance (see the various publications by Meserve). Finally, at the very least, they can stimulate a people's renewed awareness of and pride in their rich ethnoscientific heritage.

That said, most of the materials reviewed date from after 1989. To bring closure to the bibliographic work, a cut-off date of 31 December 1998 was set for items' inclusion in this volume. Some exceptions were made to this rule, mainly for documents resulting from conferences held specifically on the subject of EVM, if the documents were available by mid-1999. The authors felt it important to include this material as representative of state-of-the-art thinking in the field. Their hope is that a new generation will shoulder the task of chronicling the explosion of EVM literature since 1998. In the process, perhaps these chroniclers will bring to bear new information and dissemination technologies that will make this emerging corpus of data even more widely accessible, appreciated, and above all, critically analysed and usefully applied.

Annotation methods

Once the present three-person team of annotator-authors was assembled, work began with design of a minimum dataset, as it were, of information to be extracted from each document selected for annotation. Box 2 outlines the components of this dataset.

Box 2: Minimum data sought in abstracting

o The countries and ethnicities of the peoples whose animal healthcare practices and beliefs are described in the document.
o The general type of livestock production system involved (pastoralism, agro-pastoralism, mixed farming).
o The animal species for which treatments are presented.
o The existence, native-language titles, and skills of traditional livestock healers.
o In the case of survey- or interview-based studies, respondent numbers and break-downs by biosocial groups (e.g. women/men, elders/youth, clan or caste) or professions (farmers or herders, healers or ordinary stockraisers, traders and storekeepers, students and teachers, or extensionists, veterinarians, developers, scientists, etc.).
o Relatedly, the differential distribution of ethnoveterinary knowledge, skills and tasks across such groups and professions.
o Local disease classifications and other taxonomies.
o The Latin/scientific equivalents for local plant and livestock-disease names.
o A precise count or at least a close estimate of all medicinal, nutritional, toxic, etc. plant species mentioned.
o Some indication of non-plant materials in the ethnopharmacopoeia.
o Common prescription types (mono/poly) and modes of preparation and administration.
o As complete as possible details of preparation, administration and outcome (including medico-religious aspects) for treatments selected for illustrative annotation.
o Health-related husbandry operations.
o Stockraisers', veterinarians' or other authorities' estimation of treatment effectiveness.
o Likewise for the stockraiser rationale (e.g. medical, religious, economic) behind a given treatment or practice.

Of course, all the dataset information available in a given document could rarely be fit into an annotation; and doubtless the three authors' differing disciplinary backgrounds biased selection of the information and examples to be included. On the other hand, hardly ever was all the desired dataset information present in a document. This was especially true for 'abstracts of abstracts', i.e. where the source was another annotated bibliography or the abstract of a conference paper that was unavailable for firsthand review. Thus, annotations occasionally include the bracketed comment '[unspecified]', or a parenthesized question mark (?) following a local plant or disease name for which the source document gave no Latin or scientific equivalent.[3]

Also note that, because much EVM literature is fugitive, sometimes full reference information was lacking in book extracts and third- and fourth-generation photocopies that reached the authors via professional networks. Finally, translation responsibilities were assigned as follows: Martin shared responsibility with McCorkle for annotating French-language documents; Mathias handled all references in Bahasa Indonesian and German; and McCorkle abstracted all publications in Italian, Portuguese and Spanish. Gracious colleagues kindly assisted with other languages.

Terminologies

It is helpful to define a few of the terms frequently encountered in the EVM literature. One is 'ethnomedicine', i.e. the whole of a people's popular-culture concepts, beliefs and practices as these pertain to healthcare for both animals and humans. 'Traditional' merely denotes popular-culture concepts, beliefs and practices that a society has held and used for some time, regardless of their place, time or culture of origin. But particularly in historically non-literate societies, it is not easy to distinguish traditional elements from relatively recent adoptions or from truly 'indigenous' knowledge and techniques, i.e. those elaborated *de novo* by the society using them today. The literature tends incorrectly to employ these two words interchangeably. Where detailed historical records are lacking, 'local' is usually the best characterization of a particular human group's pool of EVM knowledge and practice – as, say, among Fulani pastoralists of the African Sahel or Amish farmers of North America.

In addition to magical and medico-religious 'medicines', local traditions of healthcare may employ either or both allopathic and homeopathic prescriptions. These two terms denote whether the medical agents used to treat a disease are intended to produce different (allopathic) or similar (homeopathic) effects from/to the disease's. Allopathic medicines are the norm in 'modern', 'conventional', 'orthodox' and 'Western' medicine. These four terms reference veterinary knowledge, practice and drugs as sanctioned by modern-day scientific authorities and as taught in the vast majority of veterinary colleges and universities.

'Western' medicine is contraposed to medical traditions within non-European-derived and/or little-industrialized societies. Among other features, it is noted for its heavy reliance on commercially produced, synthetic pharmaceuticals. As discussed earlier, some non-Western medical traditions are as highly formalized as Western medicine. Others at least had the benefit of a writing system and/or a recognized profession of healer-husbandmen – as in Sri Lankans' 400-year-old palm-leaf records of veterinary treatments and their still-existing cadre of traditional specialists. But most non-Western systems have perforce relied only on oral tradition, on a congeries of healer types (next section), and on 'natural' medicaments.

'Southern' is the latest and most politically correct word to designate what previously were called non-industrialized, Third World, or developing countries and areas. In this new usage, 'the North' replaces the terms 'industrialized', 'First World', and 'developed'. This admittedly imperfect distinction is meant to be a more value-neutral one that identifies societal and national groups more by climatic zone (tropical versus temperate). Finally, two other terms merit brief definition. One is techno-blending, i.e. the merging of endogenous and exogenous or folk and scientific know-how to achieve a better problem solution than could either knowledge base alone. The second is paraveterinarian or 'paravet', a sort of barefoot doctor for animals.[4]

By and large, however, the annotations simply follow the terminology used in the document being abstracted. In this way, readers gain a flavour of the times, cultures and biases of the materials reviewed. Moreover, it would have been an overwhelming and ultimately fruitless task to try to systematize the foregoing terminologies in over a thousand documents written across three centuries (1797 to 1998). In any case, terminologies are bound to change in future.

That said, some basic vocabulary *was* standardized, so readers can efficiently search the index for topics of interest to them. For instance, from among 'donkey', 'burro', and 'jackass', the first was selected as the preferred term for indexing; and it should thus appear at least once in any abstract referring to this species. Likewise for certain ethnoveterinary techniques (such as 'bloodletting' for 'venipuncture' or 'phlebotomy' and other forms of medical bleeding) and oft-cited ethnicities (e.g. English 'Fulani' for the French 'Peul' and other specialized names for Pulaar-speaking groups). In addition, ethnic-group spellings were systematized – e.g. Twareg instead of Touareg, Baggara for Baqqara, and Quechua in place of Kechwa, Keshwa or Q'iswa.

In the same spirit, plant names and orthographies were checked and standardized according to the following, authoritative sources: Mabberley 1997; Wrobel and Creber 1996; and various websites and databases mounted by leading botanical gardens and university groups (consult Annex 1).[5] Similarly, scientific names for live-stock diseases were made to conform with SNOMED International (Cote et al. 1993).

The nature of ethnoveterinary medicine

What is EVM?
As documented throughout this bibliography, most stockraising peoples control detailed knowledge about their animals' health problems. With or without the benefit of writing, down through time communities have compiled this knowledge through astute clinical, ethological and ecological observations, deliberate experimentation, trial and error, and practical necropsy.

As a result, long-time stockraising communities have elaborated extensive disease taxonomies, genealogies and sophisticated vocabularies for animal anatomy, physiology, reproduction and phenotypes. Producers can usually tell when an animal is ill and can describe the disease's symptoms (behavioural as well as physical), sometimes in chronic and acute forms and with prodromes and post-mortem signs. Knowledge of the latter typically derives from practical necropsy during butchering (usually by men) and from observations during the cleaning and cooking of organs and flesh (usually by women). Other common kinds of EVM knowledge about a given disease may include its cause and contagiousness; the species, ages and sexes of animals most affected; the season of the year when it typically strikes; the movements and distribution of the relevant vectors or pathogens (sometimes perceived as evil spirits, winds, etc.); the advisability of attempting a cure as opposed to simply selling or slaughtering the affected animal; and the times and places of past and present outbreaks or epidemics.

Pastoralists and agropastoralists are also keenly aware of the location of vital minerals, clean water, healthy forage, medicinal plants and so forth. Indeed, observations like the following are found throughout the EVM literature.

'[they] know perfectly the virtues and noxiousness of the vegetation in their
region . . . are capable of designating almost all the plants . . . by their common
name and of indicating their usages . . . ultimately attaining a remarkable level
of knowledge about the properties of the vegetation' (Kerharo and Adam 1964:
392, on Fulani and Toucouleur pastoralists of Senegal).

To decide on and implement appropriate medical action, people draw upon all
such knowledge plus a wide array of skills, techniques, cultural beliefs, and both
animal and human resources. These can be roughly categorized as discussed below.

Diagnostic techniques.   The first step in any medical intervention is detection
and diagnosis of the health problem. Stockraisers and local healers employ many
conventional methods of diagnosis, such as palpation, percussion, taking the pulse,
feeling for fever, pinching the skin, and of course visual observation of patent
clinical signs. In lieu of laboratories, microscopes, chemical reagents, and
'cowside' test kits, other ethnodiagnostic techniques include: smelling an ailing
animal's breath, urine or dung; tasting its milk; listening to its respiration and
vocalizations; and remarking subtle changes in its behaviour – feed and water
intake, stance, gait, excitement or lethargy, social interaction, etc.
   In a sort of applied epidemiology, people may also review the patient's recent
travels vis-à-vis contact with others' animals or with wildlife, disease outbreaks,
areas known to be heavily infested with pests or poisonous plants, polluted water
points, etc. Further, ethnodiagnosis typically takes into account seasonal or exceptional weather conditions. It may also consider patient medical history and gene-
alogy and, especially for supernaturally-attributed ills, the master's emotional
state, recent social or religious transgressions in the community, and so forth.

Materia medica.   By far the most-studied element of EVM is veterinary ethnopharmacopoeia, especially botanicals. Indeed, the great majority of the documents
reviewed note the medicinal use of plant materials. Table 1 displays a sampling of
references that catalogue 10 or more such plants; several record literally hundreds.
Also represented in these catalogues are toxic flora, which are a source of livestock
poisoning problems but also of some of the most powerful ethnopharmaceuticals.
Because pharmaco*therapies* figure so prominently in writings to date, and because
plant-based materials play a role in so many therapeutic interventions, EVM is
often wrongly equated solely with herbal remedies. But plant materials are also
employed prophylactically and promotively. And many other items of non-plant
origin are used in all three treatment types.
   For instance, ingredients of animal origin play a prominent role in all ethnopharmacopoeia. Commonly used are butter, fat, honey, cobwebs and dung, all of
which are widely employed in wound dressings; meat, bonemeal and marrow,
which may be fed as energizers; urine, saliva, scabs, pus and organ tissue from diseased animals, from which home-made vaccines are fashioned; cud from a healthy
animal, to improve a sick animal's rumen and gut ecology; and as prescription or
carrier ingredients, milk, ghee, blood, marrow, gall, tallow, eggs and eggshells,
beeswax, sea- and snail-shells, snakeskin, termite leavings, insects, body parts and
carcasses of reptiles and other animals – to name but a few. Of course, minerals
such as salt, phosphorus and copper are vital for good nutrition and health (see
section on herding strategies). These and other inorganic materials also loom large
in ethnopharmacopoeia, e.g. alum, ammonia, clay, ferrous or copper sulphate,

Table 1. A sampling of documents listing plants used in EVM[a]

Author	Country	Number of plant species mentioned
Abbas 1997	Sudan	23
Abu-Rabia 1983	Israel	35
Ake-Assi and Keck 1994	Ivory Coast	81
Andriamanga-Rahaga 1994	Madagascar	18
Baerts and Lehman 1993	Sub-Saharan Africa	158
Bailey and Danin 1981	Israel	36
Baïracli-Levy 1973	Worldwide	203
Balagizi and Ntumba 1994	Zaire	45
Bizimana 1994b	Africa	1000
Bizimana and Schrecke 1995	West Africa	30+
Bollig 1992	Kenya	25
Brisebarre 1985b, 1988b	France	15, 26
Chavunduka 1976	Africa	53
Cihoyoka Mowali 1994	Zaire	44
Coly 1994	Senegal	14
Cueva-Abena 1996	Philippines	15
CUSO 1987	Thailand	30
Dayrit 1990	Philippines	40
DENR/IIRR/FF 1990	Philippines	43
Djarwaningsih and Uji 1992	Indonesia (Java)	44
Dy 1989	Philippines	40
Evans 1910	Burma	300
FAO 1980	Asia	49
FAO 1984a	India	250
FAO 1984b, 1991c	Nepal	142, 156
FAO 1984c	Thailand	146
FAO 1991b	Indonesia	106
FAO 1991d	Sri Lanka	240
FAO 1992	Philippines	87
Fehrmann 1993	Philippines	120
Fernández 1988	Peru	10
Fernandez Jr. n.d.	Philippines	160
Gourlet 1979	France	150
HPI/India 1995	India	50
Ihiga et al. n.d.	Kenya	31
IIRR 1994	Asia	200
IIRR/DENR/FF 1992	Southeast Asia	12
Issar 1981	India	16
ITDG and IIRR 1996	Kenya	115
Jain and Tarafder 1970	India	76
Jean 1984	France	42
Joshi 1979	Nepal	37
Kasonia and Yamalo 1994	Zaire	19
Kerharo and Adam 1964	Senegal	12
Konate et al. 1994	Burkina Faso	15
Lans 1996	Trinidad and Tobago	76
Loculan 1985	Philippines (urban)	45
Loculan and Mateo 1986	Philippines	45
Maliki 1981	Niger	70
Manandhar 1989, 1991, 1992a	Nepal	35, 95, 45
Martin 1996	Nigeria	40

Table 1. Continued

Author	Country	Number of plant species mentioned
Maryanto and Astuti 1992	Indonesia	24
Ma'sum 1990	Indonesia (Java)	108
Mathias-Mundy 1991, et al. 1992	Indonesia (Java)	50, 44
Mbarubukeye 1994	Rwanda	25
Minja 1994	Tanzania	103
Mishra et al. 1996	India	20
Moscoso 1953	Peru	10
Namada 1997	Kenya	17
Noerdjito 1985	Indonesia (Java)	151
Novaretti and Lemordant 1990	France	136
Nwude and Ibrahim 1980	Nigeria	92
Padua 1989	Philippines	116
Pal 1980	India	20
Pierre 1994	Haiti	35
Piyadasa 1994	Sri Lanka	250
Rangnekar n.d.	India	37
Reddy and Sudarsanam 1987	India	57
Sangat-Roemantyo and Riswan 1991	Indonesia	23
SEARCA 1989	Philippines	116
Sebastian and Shandari 1984	India	16
Sharma and Singh 1989	India	18
Sikarwar et al. 1994	India	31
Singh 1987	India	15
Singh and Kolih 1956	India	30
Soukup n.d.	Peru	10+
Toigbe 1978	Benin, Senegal	146
Toyang et al. 1995	Cameroon	14
Vega 1994	Philippines	45
Wahua and Oji 1987	Nigeria	40
Wahyuni et al. 1991	Indonesia	46
Wickens 1980	Africa	28
Wynn and Kirk-Smith 1998[b]	Europe and US	35
Zuberi 1999	Bangladesh	16

[a] Documents listed here are those that use Latin or unequivocal English (e.g. 'rice') names in their plant lists, although they may give local nomenclatures as well. Documents that cite only local names are not included in this table. And again, this is only a sampling. Not all documents with 10 or more plant names are represented in the table.
[b] The list refers to plants used in aromatherapy.

quicklime, saltpetre, silver, sulphur, zinc, numerous petroleum products, and soap, detergent and bleach.

In addition, innumerable items of human food and drink may be used in therapeutic, prophylactic or promotive treatments. Some that stand out in the literature are: cooking oils, vinegar, molasses/treacle; alcoholic and carbonated beverages; special feedings of grains, greens and meat broths or boluses of meat. Such human consumables seem particularly popular for problems of livestock fertility, libido, pregnancy, lactation, appetite, energy, digestion, excretion and poisoning. Finally, it should be noted that most ethnopharmacopoeia today pragmatically incorporate at least some Western-commercial drugs.

Modes of preparation and administration for *materia medica*. In EVM, *materia medica* are prepared in all the same ways as for human ethnomedicines. The ingredients may be used whole and fresh, or they may entail only selected plant parts and require various combinations of crushing, pounding, drying, powdering, boiling, hot or cold infusing, fermenting, burning to ashes, human chewing, and so forth. The resulting medicaments are administered in many ways, whether externally (topically) or internally.

Topical administration typically involves unguents, pomades, poultices, plasters, pastes, salves, powders, washes, etc., applied much the same as in human medicine. An exception is the inclusion of powdered medicaments in animals' dust baths (for ectoparasitism). Another popular external mode of administration in EVM consists of adorning or piercing animals with prophylactic and therapeutic objects such as coloured ribbons and yarns, fetishes, amulets and necklaces or neck-pouches of medicinal or religious items. Just one practical example is home-made 'flea collars' of kerosene-soaked neckerchiefs.

For internal administration, the oral route is the most frequent. This usually means drenching, i.e. force-feeding liquids; but the *materia medica* may instead be fed directly, placed on the tongue or mixed into animals' food, drink or mineral supplements. Also prevalent is intranasal administration of liquids, drops, powders and snuffs or medicinal steam or smoke. The latter inhalation therapies are particularly popular for respiratory ailments. Somewhat related is fumigation. This consists of lighting smoky fires of medicinal woods, herbs and other items near the patient. Yet another 'intranasal' option is to hang up bouquets, bags or pots of often-odoriferous medicinal plants and other items – as do British farmers, Ethiopian pastoralists, French shepherds and New Guinea pig-raisers, among others. For eye ailments, the intraocular mode is universally favoured. Drops, powders or masticated materials may be dripped, blown or spat into the eye, or the eye may be bathed. Similar preparations can be introduced intra-aurally for ear problems. Indeed, EVM treatments make use of all orifices. Thus, both anal and vaginal suppositories plus enemas and douches are attested in the literature.

Likewise for surgical administration, in which an incision or flap is made in the skin for insertion of *materia medica*, such as a bit of medicinal root. EVM also features vaccinations, employing age-old variolation techniques and other methods such as autogenous immunization. Around the world, people have invented crude vaccines for poxes and a surprising number of other livestock diseases. Along with injection, vaccination that breaks the skin is technically a part of surgery. However, stockraisers also have indirect methods of immunization, through controlled exposure of healthy animals to infected ones. Injection of traditional medicines using a hollow reed or straw is attested in species and countries as disparate as ruminants (China, Europe, Mexico, Tanzania, South Africa), poultry (Mexico) and elephant (Burma).

Surgical operations. An overview of general surgery in EVM reveals the following: trocarization and rumenotomy, e.g. to release gases or to extract plastic bags ingested by livestock; debriding, cauterizing or otherwise sterilizing, and then suturing wounds; amputation, including tail-docking, ear-cropping and -notching, de-horning, hoof-paring, snipping off infected teats and penises, and clipping

queen bees' wings; lancing or excising abscesses, boils and tumours; slitting the
nostrils of racing animals; bloodletting, performed in various ways (venipuncture,
scarification, incision); and in China and elsewhere, acupuncture. Somewhat more
specialized procedures are: cutting away cataracts; extracting the brain cysts of
coenurosis; in crop-bound poultry, slicing open, clearing, and then stitching closed
the crop; for nasal bots, trephining and curettage of the sinuses; and for he-camels
with urinary blockages, catheterization with a reed. More complicated internal
operations are also reported, such as successful abdominal surgery on gored animals.

Perhaps one of the most impressive and universal of ethnosurgical skills is bonesetting. Particularly famed are African and Near Eastern bonesetters, who are often
consulted in preference to conventional orthopaedicians. For compound fractures
in livestock, African bonesetters have been reliably reported to do successful bone
grafts. Healers, midwives and ordinary stockraisers in many cultures successfully
perform numerous obstetric operations: episiotomy, embryotomy, foetotomy and
Caesarean section; surgical correction of uterine prolapse or retained placenta;
removal of persistent *corpus luteum*; vaginal or uterine debriding to promote
fertility; and conversely, spaying.

The most common ethnoveterinary surgery is probably castration. It takes both
open and bloodless forms, depending on the culture and species. Open castration
usually consists of surgically removing the testes or severing the spermatic cord. In
parts of Africa, Australia, Europe and the US, the latter operation was/is effected
by stockraisers' biting through the cord. Bloodless castration techniques consist of:
crushing the spermatic cord using wooden blocks, stones, hammers, iron bars or
other blunt instruments; for elephant, rapidly rubbing crossed sticks together;
destroying the testes and/or the spermatic cord by inserting a red-hot needle or
skewer; relatedly, cauterizing the testes of young animals; or tying off or banding
the testes until they wither from lack of blood flow. Mauritanian Fulani have a
'temporary' castration method for sheep and goats. In this procedure, the testes are
lodged under a slit in the abdominal skin until mating time, when they are let down
again.

There are still other, more-or-less invasive EVM techniques. One is firing
(including moxibustion), used worldwide to treat sprains. Indeed, firing, branding
and cauterization are administered for myriad ills almost everywhere. Treatment
involves caustic agents or flammable materials, smouldering sticks or coals, or
stones, potshards, and metal implements heated to varying temperatures and then
applied to stipulated anatomical sites for different conditions and, at least in Africa,
often with stipulated branding designs. Cauterization is of course a universal disinfectant and bloodstopping technique. An unusual but effective application is
footrot treatments in which gunpowder or petrol is sprinkled on the afflicted hoof
and then briefly ignited, as French and Brazilian stockraisers respectively do.
Occasionally, cauterization is also applied internally, as when Basuto of South
Africa place a heated stone in a barren cow's vagina to stop the discharge of oestral
fluids.

Finally, ethnodentistry operations should not be forgotten, such as sharpening
dulled teeth, filing down overgrown ones, pulling rotted ones and clipping piglets'
milkteeth. Also, it should be noted that surgery is often accompanied pre- and -post
by special hygienic as well as ethnopharmaceutical and medico-religious measures.

Hydro/physical/mechanical techniques. Whether in Africa, Asia, or elsewhere,
as natural 'dips' to remove parasites, people make sure their stock take regular

wallows, river runs, sea or dust baths, and in some areas day-long sun baths. Animals with sprains, lameness, or castration wounds may be made to stand for long periods in cold or fast-flowing water. Moist compresses are applied for these and many other conditions. Holy water blessed by a priest has many uses in Catholic countries, while Amerindians in North America set great store by steam and sweat baths, to which they subject their dogs as well as themselves.

Everywhere, massage is given to alleviate aches, pains and stiffness. Exercise is another common and multi-purpose ethnoveterinary technique. Both Amerindians and Mongols emphasize exercising their horses in order to work out stiffness and pain, build resistance to stress and disease, or increase the cleansing flow of blood after castration or snakebite. Such disparate groups as British farmers and Nepali animal doctors recommend 'a ruddy good gallop' (in the formers' words) to relieve bloat. Ayurveda and other EVM traditions underscore the importance of stretches, runs and walks for limbering up racing or working animals and stimulating healthy blood flow. In Indonesian Borneo, duck-raisers believe exercise is so important in warding against disease that they place exercise equipment in their ducklings' cages. In like vein, European authorities on holistic medicine advise placing logs and brush piles in goat pastures. The opposite of exercise, enforced rest, is of course a standard treatment for lame, post-operative, post-partum and otherwise weakened or stressed animals.

A plethora of mechanical techniques centre on the problem of ruminant bloat. The patient may be variously strapped, bound, gagged, flogged, sat upon or suspended over a cliff (e.g. Germany, Mexico, Mongolia). For instance, German farmers fill the animal's mouth with its own dung and gag it with a rope while working a rubber tube around in its anus. Lozi of Zambia manually extract the dung of bloated cattle. Javanese content themselves with shoving a papaya stalk up the anus. One Mexican remedy is to place a bitter twig in the patient's mouth in order to stimulate salivation and mastication and, with them, gas release.

Other mechanical techniques include: in Africa and Israel, manually removing or burning off ticks; in Bhutan and India, extracting aquatic leeches in the throat and sinuses via clever ploys to entice the leeches partway out; also in India, clipping cattle's coats to combat lice; in Bolivia, tying a stone to a retained placenta, so that gravity slowly pulls the placenta free; and worldwide, a variety of 'birth control' devices. The latter include: a cloth, felt, or leather apron tied over the genitalia, as practised among East Africa's Maasai and Somali pastoralists, Kazakstanis and Mongols in Asia, and Navajo Indians in the US; a string tied so as to deviate the penis or a sheath affixed over the penis (Africa); and for she-camels, a stone inserted in the uterus.

Environmental controls.   These can be defined as steps taken to modify animals' immediate environment to make it safer, healthier or more productive. Traps may be set, poisoned baits laid and hunts organized to destroy disease-bearing pests and predators of livestock. Rangelands may be burned or otherwise cleared to foster regrowth of more nutritious forages. Grazing grounds, village environs, and animal quarters may be periodically burned over, grubbed or mucked out, fumigated or treated with traditional insecticides and disinfectants. Pest-repellent plants may be cultivated or botanical and other preparations sprinkled, strewn or burned in and around such areas.

For instance, Andean stockraisers may spread quicklime or creosote in their corrals to cleanse them of disease-bearing pests and pathogens. Nigerians plant tobacco around their farmyards and poultry coops to repel snakes. For the same reason, Zimbabweans sprinkle a cold infusion of *Annona senegalensis* root in their hen runs. People in Trinidad and Tobago dust their chickens' nests and litter with neem and other pesticidal leaves to combat ectoparasites. Fulani in Benin do like-wise with cassava leaves, and also periodically burn over poultry runs with petrol or straw. Ugandans and Andeans respectively burn marigold bushes and old tyres around their animal pens to drive off flies and other pests. Indeed, setting smudge fires (often of medicinal materials) near resting animals to repel swarming insects is a popular practice generally. Also, natural pesticides may be placed in streams and ponds to destroy snails and leeches, as Quechua Indians of Peru and nomadic Gujjars of India respectively do with sacks of the alkaloid-laden grain of *Lupinus mutabilis* and crushed *Bauhinia vehlii* plants.

Meanwhile, humans and companion species may police all these areas for encroaching populations of pests and predators. Indeed, animal domesticates are often deployed as biological controls in EVM. Pigs and dogs clean up ordure and garbage in and around livestock quarters. Dogs also guard against predators that threaten injury to livestock or their masters. Cats patrol corrals, barns and homes to hold down populations of rodents that transmit both animal and human diseases. Poultry are widely valued as exterminators of insects that annoy and infest both livestock and people. In fact, Bedouin consider this is one of the main reasons for keeping poultry. In Asia, family fowl daily 'disinfect' water buffalo of ecto-parasites; the buffalo even lie down and lift their legs so the birds can peck at para-sites clinging to the axilla and britch. Also in parts of Asia, people release ducks into pastures and streams for the birds to gobble up disease-bearing pests before other livestock are turned out to graze or drink.

Herding and related strategies. Primarily, these involve mixing, separating or moving stock so as to diminish their exposure to danger and disease. In mixed grazing, different species are herded together because one (sometimes less-valuable or wild) species 'grazes down' the disease agents specific to another, or dilutes them via competition for intermediate hosts. Further, one species may sound the alarm or help protect its other-species herdmates when predators approach. Of course, since different species thrive on different forages, mixed grazing also makes maximal use of available graze and browse. To judge by the worldwide distribution of mixed grazing, herders consciously or unconsciously appreciate many of these benefits. In the Andes, for instance, sheep, llama and cattle are often herded together. In Kenya, Maasai cattle graze amidst zebra. Similarly, Kirghizstanis intermingle sheep and horses. Russians run ruminants and geese together on humid floodplains (the favourite haunt of the snails that host liverfluke larvae), and in the US West, sheep flocks now include llama to warn of and ward against coyotes and cougars.

Quarantine of stock exposed to or infected by contagious diseases is common-place, as a way of moving disease away from animals, so to speak. Conversely, animals can be moved away from the disease – as when pastoralists take pains to skirt localities where epidemics rage and/or where animals have died of deadly plagues like anthrax or blackquarter (people may also fence off or post warning markers in such areas). Whenever possible, seasonal migrations are organized so as to avoid places and ecological conditions where hosts and vectors of disease proliferate – as Saami reindeer herders do to evade devastating fly worry. Likewise for areas heavily colonized by toxic plants. An alternative is aversion training to dissuade stock from eating tempting but poisonous forages, as Tibetans do to keep their equines and yak from consuming aconite (a type of wolfsbane) or as Peruvians train their horses to dislike locoweed (*Astragalus* spp.).

Practised by communities as far-flung as the Andes and Atlas mountains and the Siani, seasonal and multi-year systems of reserve and rotational pastures represent another disease avoidance technique. These systems allow the build-up of pathogens to subside and/or they break parasitic life-cycles for want of hosts, before pastures are grazed again. In addition, many stockraising people time grazing and watering to accord with hours of the day and night when pests are least active or accessible to livestock.

Of course, herd movements are also made to furnish stock with sufficient and healthy forage, minerals and water, because well-nourished and -watered animals are more resistant to disease. In virtually all rangestock systems, herds are regularly or aperiodically driven to salt licks, pastures with salty soils or vegetation, salty wells and so forth. Likewise for newly fertilized fields (to prevent aphosphorosis) or rangelands with green browse and plants rich in vitamin A (to prevent night blindness). In a contrary strategy to mixed grazing, sometimes herds may be temporarily subdivided by species in order to drive them to micro-ecozones where special medicinal forages or those best suited to each species are most plentiful.

When it is not feasible to bring animals to key nutrients, the nutrients may be brought to them. No matter what, producers endeavour to provide supplemental feeds when they deem it necessary for forestalling deficiency and other diseases. To this end, native New Guinea swineherds feed their pigs a certain powdered rock mixed with cooked yam. Once a year, Senegalese Fulani convene in large kin and ceremonial groups to regale their livestock with ditch-fulls of a special seasonal 'dish' featuring natron (hydrated sodium carbonate), salt, grains and greens. To avert copper deficiency – known variously as enzootic ataxia, pine, swayback and 'licking disease', in which animals eat the proverbial washing off the line – European farmers invented the trick of feeding their ruminants a copper penny. In yet another strategy, special classes of livestock may be sharply confined for extra disease protection and feeding – as in Islamic communities' staking or penning their feast rams close by the house, or as in Cameroonians' and Malagasy systems of 'pit beef' production.

Management of animal genetics.   The outcome of centuries of both natural and anthropogenic selection, local breeds may appear less productive than so-called high-yielding breeds introduced from elsewhere. But unlike Northern-style intensive stockraising regimes, most Southern animal husbandry is not aimed at maximizing production of one or maybe two animal products. Rather it seeks to optimize and secure the uninterrupted output of the plural livestock goods and services upon which family and community well-being and cultural survival hinge (McCorkle, 1996). In fact, when viability, maintenance requirements and input costs are calculated vis-à-vis liveweight gains and other, multiple product-output values, local breeds often turn out to be just as, or even more, productive than alien ones (e.g. Fredrick and Osborne 1977, Rege 1998).

Indeed, local breeds or crossbreds may be the *only* ones capable of surviving, producing reasonably well, and thus meeting imperative economic, nutritional, social and unique cultural needs under the harsh ecological and management conditions in which most of the globe's livestock is raised. Just a few examples represented in the bibliography from among literally thousands (Scherf 1995) of hardy local breeds or strains are the following. Scotland's North Ronaldsday sheep thrive on a diet of the local seaweed. Yakut horses of Siberia tolerate temperatures as low as −70°C. Sichuanese have developed a purebred dairy yak that produces well at altitudes inimical to other breeds or species. Specialized strains of riding, racing, draft, meat, dairy and dual-purpose (meat+ milk) camels bred by desert tribes of Africa and Asia make human habitation of these arid lands possible. And feisty local varieties of chickens in Nigeria fight off snakes to protect their chicks.

Besides being adapted to local biophysical conditions, many native or natural-ized breeds are also uniquely adapted to local disease challenges. Throughout West Africa, for instance, the many dwarf races of cattle, sheep and goats resist such diseases as trypanosomosis, streptothricosis, heartwater and gastrointestinal para-sitism. Fulani have engineered a cross between the dwarf N'Dama cattle of West Africa's rainforests and their own Sahelian breed (the famous Fulani White or *Bunaji*), thus adding some of the former's resistances to the latter's so Fulani can exploit multiple ecozones. Many East African cattle breeds can survive and thrive despite heavy tick burdens and the endemic East Coast Fever (ECF) the ticks trans-mit. Texas Longhorn cattle are relatively immune to tick fever and screwworm, while Indonesian Thin Tail sheep boast a major gene for resistance to the tropical liver fluke. And the mongrel *chusca* or *criolla* chickens of the Andes are resistant to all but one of the diseases that regularly wipe out exotic poultry in the region.

To develop and maintain such hardy breeds, producers have devised an amazing array of often highly ingenious husbandry and other mechanisms in addition to the various medicinal, surgical, and mechanical controls on breeding discussed earlier. Where fencing or pastoral labour are available, a common husbandry strategy is to divide and re-group herds or flocks by sex, age and reproductive desirability, thus making for more selective mating. Further, such groupings can prevent premature first- or re-breeding and can shape the seasonality of parturition so that young are born when disease challenge is low, feed supplies for dams are high, and weather is mild.

Other ways to manipulate the gene pool are judicious culls and fresh breedstock. For accessing the latter, many socio-economic and socio-organizational mecha-nisms exist. Whenever Fulani migrate into a new area, for instance, they always buy some local bulls and rams (even if different breeds from their own) in order to enhance their herds' adaptation to local pathogens and other conditions. Besides outright cash purchase, other ways to obtain 'new blood' include sharing, borrow-ing and renting studs, often according to generations-old cultural mores and social relationships; temporarily boarding animals out to other families with more desir-able breedstock; pooling different households' herds across the grazing day; relatedly, sneaking stock into (or conversely, avoiding) other's herds; and targeted rustling. At the same time, to keep carefully-nurtured gene pools intact, social or religious rules may taboo the sale or exchange of prime breedstock to other-culture outsiders.

Medico-religious acts.   Interventions grounded in religious and other beliefs about health are frequently intertwined with empirical healthcare action. From an emic (cultural insider's) point of view, these are just another part of veterinary treatment and good husbandry. Yet the mixing of supernatural and natural is one of the major reasons for outsiders' denigration of local healthcare systems. Scientists and devel-opers are prone to view medico-religious beliefs as dangerous superstitions to be eradicated – even though these same scientists and developers may perceive no such contradictions when they themselves light votive candles in church, or hold masses, and offer up prayers for ailing loved ones.

In fact, medico-religious beliefs sometimes dictate actions that help to restore or at least improve health. A few examples attested in the literature are: feeding salt, bread or grain that has been blessed by a priest or monk to an ailing or infertile animal or as a promotive technique; sheltering stock from 'evil' winds, which may induce hypothermia or transmit airborne pathogens; and keeping stock away from the haunts of 'evil spirits,' which often turn out to be places where disease-bearing pests abound or the spores of deadly contagious diseases linger. As these practices illustrate, sometimes perfectly sensible interventions are merely couched in a supernatural idiom.

Other widespread medico-religious acts include singing, chanting, praying, reading Koranic verses, dancing over the ailing animal, painting or otherwise adorning the patient, ritual flogging or stroking, and holding ceremonies with health ends in view. Scientific data on the benefits of similar actions in both human and livestock healthcare are only now emerging. For example, recent research has demonstrated that soothing music enhances milk production – although from ancient times, European milkmaids have known that singing and talking to their cows facilitate milk letdown. The Northern media regularly report new findings about the benefits of intra- and inter-species social interaction for promoting healing of both physiological and psychosomatic ills.[6] Stroking a pet has been shown to calm both the animal and its master and to lower and regularize their heartrates; and light blows and massaging/stroking are standard techniques in modern physical therapy for humans and animals alike. Meanwhile, research in both anthropology and veterinary medicine has found that livestock-oriented rituals, ceremonies and proverbs sometimes encode healthcare and husbandry information in their acts and incantations, thereby helping practitioners make diagnoses, recall complex prescriptions, share EVM knowledge amongst themselves, and pass it on to new generations (or inquisitive researchers).

Moreover, one cannot help but wonder: when a given sort of medico-religious act shows up all around the world, might not it have some practical effect? One case attested in the bibliography is adorning stock with brightly coloured (usually red-spectrum) ribbons, yarns, cloths and paints to ward against harm and evil. Some references suggest that these and other accoutrements like bells and flashing metal bits may work to confound or dissuade predators. In short, there may be more to be learned from medico-religious beliefs and practices before discounting them, especially if they have been used for centuries in many different parts of the globe.

Other practices.   A wealth of other practices to promote livestock survival and safe and healthy production and reproduction surround the birthing/hatching and rearing of young stock, and the harvesting or handling of animal products like milk, eggs and fibre. For instance, many poultry-raising peoples of Asia and Africa demonstrate tremendous technical savvy when it comes to both intra- and inter-species incubation, including for semi-wild species like guineafowl. Wherever dairy products are a dietary staple, the arts of fostering young animals and prolonging lactation appear to be highly developed, as evidenced in numerous ingenious stratagems grounded in a profound knowledge of animal reproduction and ethology. Shearing without seriously wounding the animal is an art too, especially if all one has to hand is a shard of glass or a tin-can lid.

Also implied in EVM are steps taken to prevent inter-species transmission of disease, i.e. zoonoses. These may entail special hygiene and care in, for example, handling, operating on, slaughtering, or butchering diseased stock; preparation of foodstuffs from sick animals; or disposal of diseased carcasses. Finally, prompt sale or slaughter must not be overlooked as common and valid medical responses to livestock health problems.

Tools and technologies.   To implement their various healthcare interventions, people have recourse to many kinds of tools and technologies. These range from such simple items as soda-pop bottles for drenching, thorns for immunizations, and hollow reeds or quills for injections; through the various castration tools described earlier; to special-purpose surgical instruments, needles and suture materials for delicate operations. Still other equipment noted in the bibliography are: moccasins and sandals to cushion tender or wounded feet; leather blinkers to protect the eyes from fly worry; muzzles to keep stock from munching on poisonous plants; nose-sticks on weanlings and udder guards on their dams, to force weaning; whips, ropes, belts, hobbles, etc. to control or restrain patients and apply pressure or traction treatments; a panoply of dressing, splinting and casting/plastering materials; blankets, sacks, nosebags, blankets and old dresses to administer smoke or steam treatments, give special feeds, warm young stock, keep off pests, etc.; and as noted earlier, various contraceptive devices. Nor is this to mention whatever paraphernalia are involved in medico-religious acts and the 'other practices' discussed above.

Also implicated in EVM are housing and handling structures and practices that are closely adapted to different species' strength, behaviours and disease suscepti-bilities, to the local ecology (temperature, humidity, predators), and to socio-economic (e.g. pervasive rustling) and even medico-religious considerations. To illustrate how such structures and practices may impinge on animal health and safety, most Indonesians keep their goats in stilted sheds with slatted floors and feed them wilted cut-and-carry fodder. As a result, these stock have much lower endoparasite burdens than do free-range goats. In hot climates, horizontal beehives like the African long-hive are the norm because they dissipate heat better than ver-tical ones; conversely, Ethiopian highlanders plaster their hives with cattle dung as insulation against the cold. Borneo duck-raisers are almost obsessive about the cleanliness of their birds' cages, food and water for preventing disease. African pastoralists take care to clean and rotate corral- and camp-sites to ward against the build-up of parasites and pathogens. African pastoralists also take great pride in their ability to handle animals safely, noting that outsiders – like many veterinary field staff – may injure animals (and themselves) out of ignorance of how to call, calm, guide, throw and tie stock properly. Andean stockraisers usually corral their sheep separately from their cattle and camelids because the latter can easily injure or crush the former. Also, as a stronger and taller species, their llama require sturdier and higher stone or adobe walls to prevent escape and to block the evil winds and eyes believed to sicken livestock.

Human resources.   An all-too-often forgotten part of EVM is the human beings who develop and become expert in applying EVM interventions. While ordinary stockraisers know and perform many basic healthcare and husbandry tasks, other procedures require more specialized attention. Hence the existence of professional practitioners in nearly all ethnomedical systems. Such individuals include pastoralists in general, exceptionally knowledgeable farmers, and above all, recognized local and sometimes also regionally renowned healer-specialists (Table 2).

Table 2. Practitioners that treat livestock

Practitioner title[a]	Practice[b]	Groups/countries/areas[b]	Also treat humans[c]
Acupuncturist	Acupuncture	China, Europe, US	Y
Animal doctor	General	Central Asia, France, Raika in India, Tibet	Y
Animal trainer	Training	US	N
Anti-*mangkukulam*	Exorcism	Philippines	X
Apeth	Toxicology	Sudan	Y
Arbularyo, herbolario, herbalista	Herbalism	Philippines	Y
Aromatherapist	Aromatherapy	US	N
Atet	General, surgery, obstetrics, herbalism	Dinka and Nuer in Sudan	Y
Attar	Herbalism	Arabs in Near East	Y
Awalag, awwalag	Obstetrics	Ethiopia	Y
Bakuro	Equine medicine	Japan	X
Bany bith, 'spearmaster'	Removal of terminal animals, ritual healing	Sudan	X
Barefoot doctor	Herbalism and acupuncture	China	Y
Bharud	Surgery, acupuncture, firing	India	X
Bhopa	Spirit medium	India	X
Bileejo	Anti-sorcery	Senegal	X
Blacksmith	General horse medicine	Belgium, England, France	X
Bokaddo, bokao	Unspecified	Cameroon, Niger	X
Bonesetter	Orthopaedics	Africa, France, India, Mexico, Near East	Y
Bori	Charms, talismans, herbalism	A cult in Cameroon and Niger	X
Breeder	Breeding	Raika in India, Fulani in Niger	NA
Buddhist monk	Herbalism and spiritism	Thailand, Tibet	Y
Camel castrator	Castration	Samburu, Turkana in Kenya	NA
Camel healer	General camel medicine	India, Kenya	X
Camel scarifier	Scarification	Bouzou and Twareg in Cameroon and Niger	NA
Camel surgeon	Surgery	Sudan	N
Castrator	Castration	Bolivia, Bantu in Kenya, Amerinds in North America, Mongolia, Latuka in Sudan	NA
Catholic priest	Blessings of stock and medico-religious items	France, Mexico, Peru	Y
Chachamim, Jewish priest	Unspecified (lit. 'bearers of knowledge')	Near East	Y
Chatib	Amulets and tokens	Arabs in Near East	Y
Chires	Reproduction and chronic ailments in camels	Kenya	N
Chiropractor	Chiropractic	Europe, China, US	Y
Christian spiritualist	Spiritual and ritual healing, prayer	India, Trinidad and Tobago	Y
Curandero, curandera	Herbalism and other	Mexico, Philippines, Venezuela	Y
Dairyman-priest	Husbandry, hygiene, ritual	Toda in India	N
Debtera, dabtara	Coptic 'church chanting' over medico-religious items	Ethiopia	Y
Derwish	General	Arabs in Near East	Y
Deshi	General	India	Y
Dhami	Massage, exercise, Ayurveda, Unani, Sidha, homeopathy	Nepal	Y

Table 2. Continued

Practitioner title[a]	Practice[b]	Groups/countries/areas[b]	Also treat humans[c]
Diviner	Divination	Kenya, Rwanda	X
Dokotoro n'ai	General (lit. 'cow doctor')	Burkina Faso	NA
Emorong	Divination	Turkana in Kenya	X
Empirical healer	Herbalism and other	France	X
Firer	Firing for mange	India	NA
Gannduße	Unusual or complex livestock ills	Senegal	X
Garso	Direction of group herd movements	Benin	NA
Gawali	Surgery, acupuncture, firing, witchcraft	India	X
Ghuni, guni	General	India	X
Griot	Unspecified	A caste in Cameroon and Niger	X
Hakuraku	Equine medicine	Japan	X
Herbalist	Herbalism	Bolivia, China, Ethiopia, Europe, India, Kenya, Mexico, Peru, Rwanda, Tanzania, Trinidad and Tobago, UK, US	Y
Hindu priest	Prayer and spiritual healing	India	Y
Holyman	Unspecified	Bangladesh	Y
Homeopathist	Homeopathy	Europe, US	Y
Horse castrator	Castration	Amerinds of North America	NA
Horse doctor	Equine medicine	Amerinds of North America	NA
Huihua yachac	General (lit. 'knower of animals')	Ecuador	NA
Izangoma	Divination	Zulu in South Africa	X
Izinyanga	Herbalism	Zulu in South Africa	X
Jhankrie	Herbalism and faith healing	Nepal	Y
Kallicha	Spiritism	Ethiopia	Y
Kaviraj	Herbalism	Bangladesh	N
Kohanim, Jewish priest	Unspecified	Near East	Y
Laibon	General	Maasai in Kenya	Y
Laibon	Divination	Samburu in Kenya	Y
Layer-on of hands	Touch and incantation	France	X
Leert	Surgery, orthopaedics, obstetrics	Dinka and Nuer in Sudan	X
Lha-rje	Lay Ayurvedic medicine, prayer	Tibet	N
Malam, Islamic priest	Medico-religious acts	Chad, Nigeria	Y
Mambonog	'Witchdoctoring' and sacrifice	Philippines	X
Masseur	Massage	Trinidad and Tobago	X
Medicineman/woman	General and ritual healing	Amerinds of North America	X
Medjabar	Orthopaedics	Arabs in Near East	Y
Midwife	Obstetrics	China, Mexico	Y
Miot	Herbalism	Kenya	X
Mugaa, muganga	General	Kenya	Y
Nati vaidhya	Orthopaedics, dermatology, wound care, firing	India	X
Ñeeñduße	Unusual or complex livestock ills	Senegal	X
Obeahman	Herbalism and magic	Trinidad and Tobago	Y
Obstetrician	Obstetrics	Kikuyu in Kenya	X
Ocak	Firing and modern vaccination	Turkey	Y
Ojha	Ayurvedic medicine and medico-religious techniques	India	X

Table 2. Continued

Practitioner title[a]	Practice[b]	Groups/countries/areas[b]	Also treat humans[c]
Pasu vaidyulu	Herbalism	India	X
Paq'o	Ritual healing	Bolivia, Peru	Y
Physical therapist	Massage, exercise, acupressure	Japan, US	X
Pichas, pinchasi	Ayurvedic, Unani, Sidha, homeopathy	Nepal	Y
Prayerman	Prayer	Mexico	Y
Qallacha	Coptic 'church chanting' over medico-religious items	Ethiopia	X
Ran wal	Herbalism	Dinka in Sudan	X
Sacoyagan	General	Somalia	X
Seb-lalamro	Surgery, obstetrics, firing, vivisection (lit. 'men of knowledge')	Beni-Amer in Eritrea and Sudan	X
Shaman	Medico-religious acts	Amerinds in North America, Tibet	X
Siana	Herbalism	Pakistan	X
Sngag	Herbalism, prayer, exorcism, amulets, fetishes	Tibet	Y
Sorcerer	Unspecified	Ethiopia, France, Rwanda	Y
Sorcier-guérisseur	Unspecified	France	X
Spirit medium	Channeling herbal knowledge	Kenya	X
Tenkuwai	Fortune telling	Ethiopia	Y
Tharakar	Herbalism and stock-brokering	India	X
Vaccinator	Modern vaccinations	Cameroon, Kenya, Sudan, Uganda	N
Vaid	Variable – general, or specializations by species, obstetrics or firing	India	Y
Vaidhya	Herbalism	Nepal	Y
Vein-puller	Unspecified	India, Trinidad and Tobago	X
Witchdoctor	Unspecified	Mundari in Sudan	X
Woghesha, wagesha	Orthopaedics, bonesetting	Ethiopia	Y

[a] The table lists native- or English-language terms as cited in abstracts but excludes conventional veterinary practitioners.

[b] This information is drawn mainly from the abstracts, but in some cases it is supplemented from the authors' own professional knowledge and firsthand field experiences.

[c] Key: Y = yes, at least some practitioners in some of the groups/countries/areas indicated also practice on humans; N = no, they do not treat humans; X = not specified in abstract; NA = not applicable.

As Table 2 suggests, many societies do not parse healers and their services by humans versus animal patients, as Northerners do for physicians versus veterinarians. Rather, community practitioners often minister to both. But, different types of healers may be called upon depending upon the diagnosis and thus the treatment indicated.

Likewise, patient species, age or class sometimes dictates choice of specialist. For instance, castration is a more delicate operation in some species than others. It may thus call for a species-specific expert in this procedure. Certain livestock tasks and treatments may be culturally designated as the purview of one gender, clan, caste, etc. For example many societies give women primary responsibility for the basic healthcare of young stock and poultry; thus women are the experts on these animals' common ills in such societies. In others, a single clan may control the secret to curing one type of disease. In general, biosocial groups assigned the job of daily milking tend to know more about ailments affecting lactation, milk letdown, and milk quality. An interesting suggestion in the literature is that women may have greater or at least different knowledge from men when it comes to endoparasitism because women normally do the cleaning and cooking of the meat and internal organs of slaughtered stock. Also, where women or men gather or process certain medicinal botanicals, one gender or another may have special knowledge of the plants distribution, preparation and effects.

A critical look at EVM

Similarities and differences in 'EVMs'

As outlined above, EVM is comprised of many components. Needless to say, any one EVM tradition – even a single community's – is shaped by numerous local, historical, legal and other factors, as suggested in Box 3 (for greater discussion see Mathias and McCorkle 1996).

Box 3: Factors that shape EVM systems

o   The local biophysical environment and the natural resources therein (plants, minerals, water, etc.).
o   Production system and mix of animal species.
o   Associated lifeways and social organization (e.g. settled or nomadic, gendered and other divisions of EVM knowledge, skill and labour).
o   Religious beliefs and cultural concepts of the human-animal bond.
o   Purposes for keeping different animal species, and the relative economic, nutritional, spiritual and other values assigned to them and their products.
o   Relatedly, stockraisers' relationship to markets and money economies.
o   Characteristics of endogenous versus exogenous veterinary and husbandry technologies, breeds, practitioners, etc. in terms of their availability, perceived and actual efficacy or quality, cost, ease of application, cultural acceptability, and so forth.
o   National laws and policies, which may influence many of the foregoing characteristics.
o   'Status thinking', which typically privileges conventional over ethnomedicine.

As a result of such interacting variables, EVM concepts and treatments differ widely across societies and even within a single community according to members' gender, age, education, caste and so forth. Indeed, the variation in 'EVMs' is far greater than that represented in the present bibliography. For one thing, the 1240+ references abstracted here still leave many peoples and parts of the world undocumented. For another, even the lengthiest abstract can capture only a portion of the information contained in any substantial study of EVM.

Despite these caveats, some broad similarities and commonalities are evident across ethnoveterinary traditions. While *materia medica* may be constrained by biophysical environment, wherever they can be gathered, cultivated, or otherwise obtained, certain multi-purpose medicinal plants turn up time and time again in numerous ethnopharmacopoeia. A few examples are species of aloe, cassia, citrus, garlic, tobacco and solanum. Likewise for vital minerals and elements of so-called 'dirty pharmacy' (mud, dung, urine, soot, ash, etc.). Modes of preparation and administration of ethnopharmaceuticals are much the same worldwide, although there are identifiable cultural preferences for some modes over others. General surgery is understandably similar everywhere; and only a limited number of castration techniques are found across cultures. Branding/firing, bloodletting and fumigation are practised by a majority of peoples. Fundamental principles of herding, feeding and breeding are also widely shared, especially in rangestock systems.

In view of such overlaps and congruencies, some authors suggest there may be a common core of EVM, echoing the greater universality of conventional veterinary medicine. To investigate this issue, the present bibliography could provide a helpful starting point. For one thing, it could facilitate analysis of commonalities in medicinal botanicals. As various authors remark, when a given treatment's ingredients are discovered to have the same or similar ethnomedical applications among distinct and distant peoples, it constitutes a good candidate for more in-depth study and possible scientific validation. Conversely, if treatments and ingredients are deployed differently, there may be opportunity to transfer their applications from one people to another. The foregoing possibilities are especially promising where local opinion of treatment efficacy is uniformly high.

Limitations and potentials of EVM[7]

As with any body of medicine, EVM has its strengths and weaknesses. Much of it makes sound scientific sense in that it involves some of the same pharmaceutical ingredients and interventions as conventional veterinary medicine and animal science. Even seemingly bizarre EVM techniques sometimes make sense – as when Fulani of Niger place fresh goat's liver in the eyes of cattle with night blindness from vitamin A deficiency. This is an 'insightful' treatment since the liver is the main body depot for vitamin A, and browsers like goats have higher hepatic levels of the vitamin than other species (Stem 1996).

A number of ethnoveterinary treatments have been scientifically tested and proven to work (to date, most testing appears to have centred on plant-based treatments for parasitism and skin conditions). At least for ethnopharmaceuticals, this should come as little surprise. As much as 25% of modern chemotherapies derive from substances or molecular models of plant origin; and plants used in traditional medicine are 2 to 5 times more likely to test out as pharmacologically active than any random sample of plants (Attiso 1983, Plotkin and Famolare 1983). Some examples of proven EVM treatments are found in: Auró and López 1988, Avila et al. 1985a&b, Jiménez et al. 1983 and 1985, Sánchez V. n.d., various publications by Bazalar and colleagues, Bennet-Jenkins and Bryant 1996, Caballero Osorio 1984a&b, deMaar n.d.-a&b, Iskandar et al. 1983, Mursof 1990, Puyvelde 1994, Sapre 1999b, Satrija et al. 1995, Thakur et al. 1992, Thompson et al. 1978, and Yuan-Chang 1978.

Of course, studies have also found that while some EVM treatments are effective against the problem they are intended to address, others are not (e.g. Fernandez 1990 and 1999, Sharma et al. 1967, Valenciano et al. 1980); that a given treatment can be scientifically recommended for some livestock species but not others (e.g. Bogdan et al. 1990); and that some treatments do not appear to work at all (e.g. Jost et al. 1996). Moreover, whether they work or not, some EVM interventions may have negative side effects. In fairness, however, these largely mirror the same problems that beleaguer conventional medicine, e.g.: secondary infections from poor practitioner hygiene or contaminated *materia medica* or equipment; dosage miscalculations; on occasion, perforce recourse to toxic treatments; inadequate treatment follow-through or post-operative care; and sheer malpractice.

Other EVM interventions may be deleterious to the patient in and of themselves, however. A few examples are: withholding water from diarrhoeal patients and colostrum from neonates; indiscriminate bloodletting; excessive or misguided firing (e.g. New Guineans's singeing off their pigs' bristles to eradicate lice or Zambians' burning around and inside the anus to halt diarrhoea); doctoring dermatological or ectoparasitic conditions with harsh or poisonous items like spent engine oil, kerosene, battery acid, DDT and mercury-based compounds; and treating ocular disorders with highly abrasive materials.

When it comes to ethnopharmaceuticals, these may be limited in other ways. The requisite materials may not always be available year-round or in all areas. The levels of pharmacologically active ingredients in botanicals can vary greatly according to the season, site, maturity, etc. at which plants are collected plus other factors. Further, crude botanicals may not work as rapidly or thoroughly as more concentrated or synthetic modern drugs. Thus, traditional medicines may avail little for acute and peracute infectious conditions, epidemics, diseases and dangerous zoonoses (e.g. anthrax, blackquarter, haemorrhagic septicaemia, pneumonia, rabies, rinderpest). Finally, stockraisers sometimes complain about the time it takes to obtain and prepare traditional medicines. Likewise for administration, insofar as remedies based on crude botanicals can make for bulky dosages. However, stockraisers level similar complaints at commercial drugs wherever: drug import and distribution systems are haphazard; unscrupulous vendors are wont to sell expired or adulterated products; producers must undertake lengthy, difficult, or costly travel to buy drugs; and large numbers of animals must be treated quickly.

In any case, EVM for infectious disease should not be dismissed out-of-hand. Even if home remedies do not always attack pathogenic agents directly, they may at least enhance animal nutrition, assuage painful or debilitating symptoms, or stimulate positive physiological responses (immunogenic, haematogenic, cardiogenic, etc.). This is probably especially true for polyprescriptions. Indeed, proponents of herbal medicine argue that one of its greatest strengths is precisely such polyvalency, as opposed to synthetic drugs' reliance on only a few active ingredients and effects.

Especially where conventional treatments are inadequate, unsafe or uneconomical, EVM might offer some alternatives. A case in point is trypanosomosis, a disease caused by various species of blood parasites that, in livestock, are vectored mainly by biting flies. Unfortunately, the majority of trypanocides currently on the market are highly toxic to stock; they are also very expensive – indeed, some are no longer manufactured for lack of paying customers; and the haemoparasite has become resistant to most of the remainder (e.g. Dwivedi 1999, Köhler-Rollefson 1996b). By comparison, it can be more difficult for pests and pathogens to develop resistance to herbal medicines because the crude botanicals used in ethnomedicine are generally more biochemically complex than synthetics.[8] Botanicals also tend to be cheaper than commercial drugs. In short, it is conceivable that, with concerted scientific research, new, more lasting, and more affordable drugs for some diseases could be found among home remedies.

To take another example, for ectoparasitism conventional veterinary medicine recommends intensive dipping, dusting or spraying with powerful chemical insecticides. Not only do such poisons induce chemoresistance, but also they have been known to sicken stockraisers who handle them; to poison drinking-water supplies used by humans, livestock, and wildlife alike; to kill wildlife like birds that feed on the ectoparasites of treated stock; and to leave toxic residues in food products. Moreover, World Bank and other studies have calculated that the cost of chemical dips, dusts and sprays frequently far outstrips the economic benefits to be gained from them (e.g. Haan and Bekure 1991). By comparison, people's herbal insecticides and certainly their mechanical and managerial pest-control and -avoidance strategies are probably much less toxic, biostable, bioaccumulative (both in the body and in the environment) and expensive. Although these inter-ventions may be less effective than modern agrotoxins in terms of pest kill-rates, they may be well be *more* effective in cost/benefit terms, especially when asso-ciated human-health and environmental costs are factored in.

As preceding sections and the foregoing examples should hint, one of the most promising aspects of EVM lies in integrated disease management or 'IDM' pack-ages. These take a combination approach to preventing and/or curing a given health problem, and they may greatly diminish the need for expensive store-bought prod-ucts. A good example is, again, trypanosomosis. Fulani attack this problem with a defensive IDM armoury consisting of: clearing away brush and burning over rangelands to destroy fly habitat; avoiding heavily fly-infested grazing grounds or using them only when fly populations are at seasonal lows; if stock must enter such areas, then washing them with a home-made fly repellent beforehand; moving, grazing, and watering stock by night, when flies are less active; staking out the resting herd in small groups around smudge fires; above all, breeding for trypano-tolerance; and subjecting special animals to an additional conditioning or 'season-ing' procedure designed to build extra immunity. To take another example, for anoestrous sows, Chinese pig-raisers combine acupuncture with a variety of management changes that provide the patients more exercise plus increased contact with the boar and other sows. This IDM package cures 80% of the afflicted sows so that pricey commercial hormones need be purchased only for the remain-ing 20%. Scientific study and refinement of such IDM packages could well make for major savings on the costs and dangers of commercial pesticides and drugs for many common livestock health problems. To date, however, very little IDM research has been undertaken.

In sum, certainly for ordinary, chronic, and non-epidemic diseases and for every-day healthcare and husbandry, EVM has much to offer. As the bibliography attests, it is often adequate for problems like pests and parasitism, skin diseases, wounds and fractures, strains and sprains, reproductive disorders, nutritional deficiencies, mild diarrhoeas, plant poisoning and snakebite, and more. Indeed, some authors think that selected EVM treatments in these domains may be *more* effective than available commercial ones (e.g. Arowolo and Awoyele 1982, Avila et al. 1985a, Bayer and Waters-Bayer 1991, Legbagah 1983, Ndamukung et al. 1987, Peña et al. 1988, Toigbe 1978). There is little doubt that EVM can contribute to an integrated traditional+modern approach to basic animal healthcare, especially since the economic importance of epidemic diseases has declined relative to production-oriented ailments (e.g. FAO 1991a, Haan and Bekure 1991). The challenge is to find which ethnoveterinary interventions are beneficial and appropriate in which contexts.

Responding to this challenge opens the way to discovery of 'new' remedies for inexpensive national commercialization, recuperation of forgotten ones, or novel cross-species applications. In Rwanda, for example, discovery of an excellent traditional scabicide for cattle led to its reformulation and national commercialization for human as well as animal use (Puyvelde 1994). In Peru, an effective vermifuge based on seeds of the giant South American squash was recuperated from its human ethnomedical prescription and re-applied to ruminants (McCorkle and Bazalar 1996). In Mexico, scientists adapted a local herbal fungicide for humans to one for tilapia (Auró and Sumano 1988) and in India, a fish farmer invented an entirely new aquaculture application from an indigenous neem-leaf+turmeric treatment for smallpox (Ganapathi 1995).

Experiences like the foregoing can increase public awareness of the value of natural medicinal resources and local knowledge about them that, in turn, can promote maintenance of biological and cultural diversity. Recognition and validation of EVM can also help create new employment and income opportunities in, for example, medicinal plant production and processing, product development and sales, and integrated traditional+modern practitioner services. In the last regard, empirically-oriented community practitioners represent a valuable human resource for recruitment and training as, or of, other healthcare workers like paravets or intersectoral healthcare workers who can attend both human and animal patients (Agriculture and Human Values, 1998).

Other potentials for enhanced healthcare services to communities lie in an increased appreciation and informed application of people's veterinary knowledge base. For example, producers often prioritize animal health problems differently from veterinarians and livestock developers. Learning about such differences can sharpen veterinary services' focus on local needs. Also important is an understanding of local disease classifications, if only to avoid gross misunderstandings between stockraisers and veterinary field staff. To illustrate, coastal Kenyans have two terms for the tick-borne disease of theileriosis (ECF) to denote its occurrence in young versus adult cattle. If extensionists are ignorant of this distinction and advertise a dipping campaign as being for only one of the two terms, then coastal Kenyans would present only their calves or only their adult cattle (Delehanty 1996).

Taking into account such subtle conceptual and terminological distinctions as the foregoing, epidemiological surveillance can also profit from local veterinary information (ibid.). Drawing upon healers' and stockraisers' awareness of disease incidence and spread and involving them in reporting outbreaks can help cut costs and improve the quantity, quality and timeliness of epidemiological intelligence and related disease-control programmes (e.g. Sollod and Stem 1991). Finally, since EVM relies primarily on local materials, practices, tools, technologies, and usually same-culture healers who are often stockraisers themselves, it is generally more familiar, user-friendly, and culturally comfortable than alien drugs and techniques or outside practitioners. Recourse to valid EVM alternatives thus could obviate some of the problems reported in the literature concerning stockraisers' and healers' misusing and abusing potent modern drugs out of unfamiliarity with them.

The study and application of EVM offers still other, less tangible potentials and advantages. While engendering greater respect and understanding among scientists, developers, and extensionists for their clients' healthcare and husbandry expertise and needs, work in EVM can also: vouchsafe producers a renewed respect for their own veterinary know-how; reinvigorate socio-organizational structures that promote animal health and well-being; reinforce empirical practitioners' status; and empower communities to take greater control of their own livestock and other development needs and agendas. In consequence of all the foregoing plus the increased producer participation implicit in good ethno-veterinary R&D, better development planning and implementation, policymaking and institution-building may result across a number of sectors (next section) pertaining to community services and livelihoods.

Putting EVM to work

During the last decade, efforts to promote the hands-on use of EVM have clearly increased, as signalled by several trends. One is the proliferation of workshops and training seminars as well as conferences aimed at identifying and disseminating EVM information and integrating it with conventional healthcare approaches (see Mathias et al. 1999a for a listing). Paralleling that trend is the recent publication of training and information manuals for livestock development workers (Cueva-Abena 1996, Jones 1997, Köhler-Rollefson et al. 2001), practical reference works (Brightwell et al. 1998, Forse 1999), and even policy-analysis texts (Peeling in progress) that recommend local/traditional as well as conventional veterinary options. Still more telling is the growing number of field projects on EVM around the world (again, see Mathias et al. 1999a for a mapped listing). Finally, between the 1989 bibliography and now, many more studies have emerged that present quantitative data drawn from field surveys and clinical or on-farm trials.

Still and all, EVM is not yet an integral part of livestock development, where its incorporation would widen all producers' healthcare and husbandry options. Indeed, in a preliminary study of the 472 annotations from the present bibliography that were completed as of October 1997, Mathias and Perezgrovas (1999) found that 42% consisted merely of lists of remedies or medicinal plants or of general and historical descriptions of EVM systems and practices. Only 12.5% were based on applied research aimed at analysing local-level veterinary needs and resources or addressing specific R&D questions. Far more of the latter types of studies are needed, plus validation, education, training, information dissemination and networking initiatives along the following lines.

Technical validation. Especially wanted are studies to validate or invalidate ethnoveterinary understandings and treatments. Different degrees of validation are possible.

- o Critical review of the literature on: e.g. a given treatment's botanical components; their phytochemical and laboratory effects *in vitro* and *in vivo* in human as well as veterinary medicine; the geographical distribution of the treatment's use; observer testimony as to its effectiveness; and so forth.
- o Systematic surveys of community users' experiences with and opinion about the treatment.
- o *In vitro* and *in vivo* laboratory tests of the treatment.
- o Clinical trials on-station or in experimental herds kept at the field level, using the target livestock species.
- o Participatory clinical trials on-farm, involving the target livestock species under normal community management regimes.
- o Once validated and disseminated, subsequent monitoring of the treatment's use and effects as systematically reported by stockraisers and both traditional and modern practitioners.

Ideally, these different levels should be interlinked in order to arrive efficiently at the most reliable results possible. In reality, however, field trials have been the exception rather than the rule. In part this is because it is difficult to hold research conditions constant enough to control and account for the multitude of intervening variables that characterize such 'natural laboratories'.

Also difficult is designing scientifically sound methods to test local interventions accurately. Orthodox drug-testing methods, for instance, normally capture only very specific and short-term effects. Nor are they geared to deal with modes of preparation and administration such as chewing and spitting the *materia medica* or – given the artificial historical divide between veterinary versus animal science in the North – IDM packages. Yet as discussed earlier, ethnopharmaceuticals and IDM may exert more delayed, generalized, or additive effects than do conventional approaches. This means that a great deal more research and perhaps also new research methodologies will be required in order to definitively validate/invalidate many EVM interventions.

Sociocultural, socio-economic and environmental validation.   Aside from more hard data and field trials, another pre-requisite for putting EVM to work is greater and more direct stockraiser involvement in ER&D. Local technical knowledge typically is grounded in complex cultural logics that are alien to outsiders (e.g. Hess 1994). Thus, from the outset, any R&D initiative must involve the people who hold the local knowledge as co-researchers and co-developers. Their participation is also imperative because local knowledge is usually unwritten and unevenly distributed across biosocial groups and communities. Without close producer collaboration in identifying key livestock health problems and feasible ethno-veterinary, techno-blended, or conventional solutions, livestock development initiatives risk imposing inappropriate measures and services (for useful discussions and examples of participatory tools in livestock development, see Catley 1999, IIED 1994, and Waters-Bayer and Bayer 1994).

Economic and environmental as well as technical and sociocultural considerations must be also be taken into account in putting EVM to work. To assist stockraisers in making wise healthcare and husbandry choices, it is essential to understand the complex trade-offs between costs and benefits among all possible options in terms of their effects both on producers' pocketbooks and on the bio-physical environment.

Education/training, dissemination and networking.   Of course, all the foregoing R&D is wasted unless the resulting information is built into mainstream education and training and widely disseminated in such a way that communities can actually use it. One way of extending valid EVM and techno-blended options is to teach them in rural schools, using local-language booklets such as those described by Bonfiglioli et al. (1996) and VETAID (in progress). This is a win-win strategy, because it also addresses the acute lack of life-relevant course material in rural schools around the world. In addition, training in the conduct and findings of ER&D needs to be folded into university courses on veterinary medicine and animal science in both the North and the South (Fielding 1999). Similarly, valid EVM alternatives must be incorporated into training for any veterinary or para-medical extensionists, as some projects are already doing (e.g. Adolph-LaRoche and Linquist-LaRoche 1993, Blakeway et al. 1999, John 1999, Nuwanyakpa 1992).

Actually or potentially instrumental in all the tasks discussed here are many different kinds of organizations (McCorkle et al. 1999). They include United Nations units like FAO and WHO; universities and research centres of all sorts; government livestock and extension agencies; PVOs, NGOs, and grassroots organizations; producer associations like dairy co-operatives or stockmen's federations; and private-sector entities such as pharmaceutical houses and for-profit consulting firms that respectively specialize in natural medicines and livestock development. Other groups on this list include botanical and zoological gardens, wildlife reserves (some of the latter two now use EVM treatments), rare-breeds societies, and the multitude of professional organizations for Ayurvedic medicine, holistic veterinary medicine, veterinary acupuncture, veterinary homeopathy, and so forth. Neither should national associations of local medical/veterinary practitioners be forgotten. There is strong evidence that training local healers in the use of some modern medicines and techniques as well as validated local ones can dramatically increase healthcare coverage for humans and animals alike. To make a real impact, linkages among all such players are essential. Modern information technologies such as electronic mailing lists, e-mail conferences, and the internet have already become important tools in this regard (Annex 1).[9]

What next?

The wealth of publications, conferences/seminars, and organizations already dealing with EVM signals a clear and growing consensus that the field promises help for stockraisers who have little, no, or declining access to conventional animal healthcare and inputs in their efforts to feed themselves and the world's burgeoning human population. Lessons from field studies and development projects show that it is both socio-economically and scientifically imperative to draw upon the rich storehouse of local knowledge (of which ethnoveterinary medicine is but one small part) and its human bearers and practitioners if any real progress is to be made in meeting the basic livelihood needs of the new millenium's billions.

The timing for putting EVM to work is favourable. For one thing, there are some salubrious trends in research and development circles to build bridges across different perspectives and groups that heretofore have been poorly interfaced, e.g.: North and South; the social and the biological/technical sciences; science and religion; certainly, research, development, and extension; conventional and alternative medicine; agriculture and education; and womens' as well as mens' participation in and benefits from R&D. For another thing, international development thinking and action currently emphasize decentralizing healthcare and other services, minimizing people's and nations' dependency on external inputs, and maximizing the use of local knowledge, skills and resources. At the same time, thanks to the new information age, there is a concurrent trend toward greater global sharing of knowledge of all sorts.[9] This bibliography is one example of such.

Now is the time to move ahead from merely writing about, and annotating writings about, EVM publications to putting this rich local-knowledge resource to practical development work in the communities who gave it birth.

Annex to the Introduction: internet resources

Mailing Lists

The Ethnoveterinary Mailing List
Launched in June 1999, the Ethnoveterinary Mailing List is open to anyone interested in the study and application of EVM. Hosted by the Netherlands' Centre on International Research and Advisory Networks (CIRAN) of Nuffic (Netherlands Organization for International Cooperation in Higher Education), the list is supervised by an international team of moderators from Africa, Asia, Europe, and Latin and North America. Only in its second year of existence, the list has already brought together some 200 scientists, developers and policy analysts interested in EVM. To subscribe, send a blank e-mail message to the following address: join-EVM@lyris.nuffic.nl.

The Phytomedica Mailing List
This worldwide discussion list on medicinal plants and traditional medicine provides an open forum for information exchange on issues relating to policies, practices and utilization of medicinal and aromatic plants, phytotherapy and natural/traditional medicine and healing. It also displays relevant announcements of: new publications and websites; opportunities for jobs, grants, volunteer work, internships, etc.; upcoming meetings, seminars, etc. To subscribe, send a blank e-mail message to the following address: phytomedica-subscribe@egroups.com.

Websites relevant to ethnoveterinary medicine

http://csf.colorado.edu/
SRISTI is an NGO that works to strengthen the creativity of grassroots inventors, innovators and eco-entrepreneurs engaged in conserving biodiversity and developing environmentally friendly solutions to local problems. SRISTI produces the *Honey Bee Newsletter*, which is liberally referenced in the present bibliography.

http://netvet.wustl.edu/
Ken Boschert, a veterinarian at Washington University's Division of Comparative Medicine, operates this website. It focuses on veterinary medicine (alternative as well as conventional) and related fields. The site features comprehensive lists of related organizations and websites, plus a 'World Wide Web Virtual Library of Veterinary Medicine'.

http://www.angelfire.com/de/lpp
The League for Pastoral Peoples (LPP) is an advocacy and support NGO for pastoralists who depend on common-property resources. Together with its Indian partner organization Lokhit Pashu-Palak Sansthan, LPP runs a camel project in Rajasthan

that integrates both Western and local methods of animal healthcare. The site describes a number of projects that involve working with local veterinary knowledge.

http://www.assisiacupunctureltd.com
This website is operated by Ann-si Li, a veterinarian who combines allopathy with alternative veterinary medicine in her small-animal practice. The site gives information about veterinary acupuncture and traditional Chinese medicine.

http://www.geocities.com/TheTropics/Cove/1003
Hosted by DevArt, this website offers non-copyrighted line drawings for use in development publications. Offerings include pictures of livestock and stockraisers.

http://www.netcologne.de/~nc-mundypa/workshop.htm
Designed and managed by development communication specialist Paul Mundy, this site describes a participatory 'writeshop' process that can be used to produce rapid and inexpensive but professionally packaged development information and extension materials. A companion website (http://www.netcologne.de/~nc-mundypa/publications.htm) describes two manuals on EVM and a third on recording and using local knowledge, all of which were generated through this process.

http://www.nuffic.nl/ciran/ikdm
Located in the Netherlands, CIRAN (Centre for International Research and Advisory Networks) aims to improve the exchange of information within the International Indigenous Knowledge Network. CIRAN produces the *Indigenous Knowledge and Development Monitor*. Available online at the above address, the *Monitor* often includes articles on EVM and reviews of books pertaining to EVM topics.

http://www.public.iastate.edu/~anthr_info/cikard/
The Center for Indigenous Knowledge for Agriculture and Rural Development (CIKARD) maintains this website out of Iowa State University in Ames, Iowa, USA. Established in October 1987, CIKARD focuses on preserving and applying the local knowledge of rural peoples worldwide and on facilitating participatory and sustainable approaches to development. The CIKARD site contains a facility for searching an extensive database of abstracts on EVM.

http://www.vetaid.org
An affiliate of Vétérinaires Sans Frontières, VETAID is a British NGO that works with local organizations in under-privileged countries to prevent suffering and hunger through improved stockraising thanks to improved animal healthcare. The website gives information about VETAID projects and publications, including reports, EVM-oriented theses from the University of Edinburgh's Centre for Tropical Veterinary Medecine, and other documents on EVM.

http://www.vetwork.org.uk
A British NGO, Vetwork promotes participatory livestock development. The website presents information and contact addresses relating to community-based animal healthcare. In addition, it contains the abstracts and proceedings of the international conference on ethnoveterinary medicine held in Pune, India, in

November 1997 (cf. Mathias et al. 1998 and 1999), plus the proceedings of a related international conference on integrated approaches to animal healthcare, also held in India (cf. Mathias et al. eds. 1999).

http://www.worldbank.org/html/afr/ik
The World Bank's Indigenous Knowledge Initiative hosts this website. The initiative seeks to help WB partners learn more about local knowledge and technology in the WB's client countries, the better to adapt global knowledge to local conditions and design activities that meet country-specific needs.

Websites related to ethnobotany and plant databases

http://pc4.sisc.ucl.ac.be/prelude.html
This is the website of the PRELUDE network (Programme for REsearch and Link between Universities for DEvelopment), which endeavours to interconnect researchers from both university and non-university and Northern and Southern backgrounds in a spirit of co-development partnership. The site includes a large database on African medicinal plants for both humans and livestock.

http://www.ag.uiuc.edu/~ffh/napra.html
Operated by the Natural Products Alert Project (NAPRALERT) at the Department of Pharmacognosy and Pharmacology, College of Pharmacy, University of Illinois, USA, this website offers a computerized database on the chemistry and pharmacology of natural medicinal materials. The database is available for a fee from the Scientific and Technical Information Network (http: //www.lights.com/hytelnet/ fee/fee023.html).

http://www.ansci.cornell.edu/plants/medicinal
Established by the Animal Science Department of Cornell University in the USA, this site focuses on medicinal plants for livestock and discusses topics such as their safety and efficacy.

http://www.cieer.org/directory.html
Hosted by the Centre for International Ethnomedical Education and Research, the Ethnobotanical Resource Directory of this site features bibliographies, databases, publications, online courses, research projects, a web directory and more pertaining to medicinal plants.

http://www.herbaria.harvard.edu/data/gray/
The Gray Card Index Database at this Harvard University Herbaria website catalogues over 325 000 citations of names of New World vascular plants.

http://www.mobot.org/search.html
The VAST (VAScular Tropicos) nomenclature databases can be accessed at this Missouri Botanical Garden website. The databases contain a wealth of botanical and bibliographic data collected over the last 12 years by staff, students and visitors of the MBG, as well as information gathered by several cooperative and other projects and institutions.

http://www.netcologne.de/~nc-pieronan2
Ethnopharmacologist Andrea Pieroni built this website about natural foods and herbs, medicinal plants, and their use by different peoples. The site also offers information on publications and conferences of possible interest to EVM researchers.

http://www.rbgkew.org.uk/ceb/sepasal/internet/
Operated by the Royal Botanic Gardens in Kew, UK, this website features a database derived from the Survey of Economic Plants for Arid and Semi-Arid Lands (SEPASAL). The database contains information on more than 6200 useful tropical and subtropical dryland species, excluding major crops.

http://www.rz.uni-duesseldorf.de/WWW/GA/Welcome.html
This is the website of the Society for Medicinal Plant Research. The site links to other pages of interest, such as the Phytochemical Society of Europe and the Society for Economic Botany.

References to the Introduction

Agriculture and Human Values. 1988. Special issue: Interfaces between Human and Animal Medicine 15(2): Pp. 105–151.

Attiso, Michel A. 1983. Pharmacology and phytotherapy. In: Robert H. Bannermann, John Burton and Ch'en Wen-Chieh (eds). *Traditional Medicine and Health Coverage.* World Health Organization, Geneva, Switzerland. Pp. 194–206.

Bodeker, G. C. 1994. Traditional health knowledge and public policy. *Nature and Resources* 30(2): 5–16.

Brightwell, R., J. Kamanga and R. Dransfield. 1998. *Key Livestock Diseases of Dryland Kenya.* KEPADA, Nairobi, Kenya.

Catley, Andy. 1999. *Methods on the Move: A Review of Veterinary Uses of Participatory Approaches and Methods Focussing on Experiences in Dryland Africa.* IIED, London, UK.

Cote, R.A., D.J. Rothwell, R.S. Beckett, et al. 1993. *SNOMED International, the Systematized Nomenclature of Human and Veterinary Medicine* (3rd edition). College of American Pathologists, Northfield, Illinois, US.

Etkin, Nina L. 1990. Ethnopharmacology: Biological and behavioral perspectives in the study of indigenous medicines. In: T. M. Johnson and C. F. Sargent (eds). *Medical Anthropology: Contemporary Theory and Method.* Praeger Publishers, New York, US. Pp. 149–158.

Forse, Bill. 1999. *Where There Is No Vet.* Macmillan Press, Ltd. with Oxfam and CTA, London, UK.

IIED. 1994. *RRA Notes: Special Issue on Livestock.* No. 20. IIED, London, UK.

Jones, Peta. 1997. *Donkeys for Development.* Animal Traction Network For Eastern and Southern Africa (ATNESA) and Institute for Agricultural Engineering, Agricultural Research Council of South Africa, Pretoria, South Africa.

Köhler-Rollefson, Ilse, Paul Mundy and Evelyn Mathias. 2001. *A Field Manual of Camel Diseases: Traditional and Modern Health Care for the Dromedary.* ITDG Publishing, London, UK.

Haan, Cornelis de and Solomon Bekure. 1991. *Animal Health Services in Sub-Saharan Africa: Initial Experiences with Alternative Approaches.* The World Bank, Washington DC, US.

Mabberley, D.J. 1997. *The Plant-Book: A Portable Dictionary of the Vascular Plants* (second edition). Cambridge University Press, Cambridge, UK.

Mathias, Evelyn, Denis Fielding and Marina Martin (eds). 1999a. *Integrated Approach for Animal Health Care: Proceedings of an International Seminar Held at Calicut, Kerala, India, 4–6 February 1999. Volume 1: Abstracts.* Malabar Regional Co-operative Milk Producers' Union, Ltd, Kodhikode, Kerala, India. 20 pp.

Mathias, E., D.V. Rangnekar and C.M. McCorkle (eds). 1999b. *Ethnoveterinary Medicine: Alternatives for Livestock Development. Proceedings of an International Conference held in Pune, India, on November 4–6, 1997. Volume 1: Selected Papers.* BAIF Development Research Foundation, Pune, India.

McCorkle, Constance M. 1996. The roles of animals in cultural, social and agroeconomic systems. In V.U. James (ed.). *Sustainable Development in Third World Countries: Applied and Theoretical Perspectives.* Greenwood Publishing, Westport, Connecticut, US. Pp. 25–43.

McCorkle, Constance M. and Evelyn Mathias. 1996. Paraveterinary healthcare programs: A global overview. In: Karl-Hans Zessin (ed.). *Livestock Production and Diseases in the Tropics: Livestock Production and Human Welfare. Proceedings of the VIII International*

Conference of Institutions of Tropical Veterinary Medicine held from 25 to 29 September, 1995 in Berlin, Germany. Deutsche Stiftung für internationale Entwicklung, and Zentralstelle für Ernährung und Ladwirtschafts, Eurasburg, Germany. Pp. 544–549.

McCorkle, Constance M., Evelyn Mathias and Tjaart W. Schillhorn van Veen (eds). 1996. *Ethnoveterinary Research & Development*. Intermediate Technology Publications, London, UK.

OIE (ed.). 1994. *Revue Scientifique et Technique de l'Office International des Épizooties*. Volume 13, Issue 2, entitled 'Anciennes Méthodes de Prophylaxie des Maladies Animales – Early Methods of Animal Disease Control – Los Antiguos Métodos de Profilaxis de las Enfermedades Animales. OIE, Paris, France.

Peeling, Dil (ed.). In progress. *Community-based Animal Health Workers: Threat or Opportunity?* (working title). Livestock in Development, Somerset, UK.

Pieroni, Andrea (ed.). 1999. *Herbs, Humans and Animals/Erbe, Uomini e Bestie: Proceedings of the International Seminar, Coreglia (Tuscany), Italy 8–9 May 1999/Atti del Seminario Internazionale, Coreglia (Toscana), Italia 8–9 Maggio 1999*. e^{x}periences Verlag, Köln, Germany.

Plotkin, M. and L. Famolare (eds). 1983. *Sustainable Harvest and Marketing of Rain Forest Products*. Island Press for Conservation International, Covelo, California and Washington DC, US.

Scherf, Beate D. (ed.). 1995. *World Watch List of Domestic Animal Diversity*. Second edition. FAO, Rome, Italy.

VETAID. In progress. Ethnoveterinary knowledge practised by the Maasai in Simanjiro District of Northern Tanzania. VETAID, Arusha, Tanzania.

Waters-Bayer, Ann and Wolfgang Bayer. 1994. Planning with pastoralists: PRA and more. A review of methods focused on Africa. Working Paper. GTZ, Eschborn, Germany.

Wrobel, M. and G. Creber. 1996. *Elsevier's Dictionary of Plant Names*. Elsevier Science Publishing Co., London, UK and New York, US.

Notes to the Introduction

1. Except for the publications noted in the reference list at the end of this introductory chapter, all others cited in this introduction can be found among the annotations themselves. For references to particular EVM *materia medica*, treatments, beliefs, etc. described in the section on 'The Nature of Ethnoveterinary Medicine', readers should consult the index.

2. A number of abstracts in the bibliography do note that people may well observe such behaviour in both wild and domestic animals and then mimic or build on it in their ethnomedicine. For instance, there are reports of people compounding medicines for both livestock and humans out of the plants they observe sick animals to seek out; and herders are known to drive stock to pastures rich in such plants.

3. Other bracketed comments indicate technical or editorial observations on the part of the volume's three author-annotators. Otherwise, the authors endeavoured to annotate each entry impartially, though occasionally this proved difficult in view of some documents' dramatic content.

4. In veterinary circles, 'paravet' commonly denotes a person who has received some limited formal or vocational training in selected aspects of conventional animal healthcare and who then delivers basic services in a local area. When such paraprofessionals are salaried government or clinic workers, they are often known as 'veterinary auxiliaries'. However, as NGOs have taken over the lead in mounting rural veterinary delivery programmes, new and more participatory, grassroots, and self-sustaining ideas about paravets and their training have come into being (cf. McCorkle and Mathias 1995).

5. When discrepancies between a text and these authorities were detected, if the original document's spelling of the plant name could be matched unequivocably to a correct spelling in these authoritative sources, then the former was changed to concur with the latter. If a plant name could *not* be matched to any entry in these sources, then it was left as spelled in the document.

6. Veterinarians, wildlife specialists, zookeepers, ethological researchers and scientists who experiment on animals all report that mammals, at least, also suffer from psychosomatic ills and social isolation (e.g. deMaar 1992).

7. For much more thorough on-going discussions of the following and still other limitations and potentials, consult Mathias et al. 1996 and McCorkle 1995.

8. As just noted, the latter typically rely on only one or a few active ingredients. But the former are relatively unpurified and, especially in the case of polyprescriptions, thus incorporate untold numbers of phytochemicals, which can increase the adaptive challenge to pathogenic organisms. For further discussion of these and related points, consult e.g. Bodeker 1994, Etkin 1990 and Ibrahim 1996.

9. This trend is accompanied by vexing issues of intellectual property rights and differential access to modern information technology such as the internet. But these issues lie beyond the scope of this introduction.

The Bibliography Abstracts

Aaker, Jerry (ed.). 1994. *Livestock for a Small Earth: The Role of Animals in a Just and Sustainable World.* Seven Locks Press for HPI, Washington DC, USA. 111 pp.

This collection of essays seeks to share lessons learned in the course of HPI's 50 years of livestock development work worldwide. Observations of ethnoveterinary interest include the following. There is a profound threat of loss of EVK despite EVK's indisputable importance given that the use of imported or costly veterinary inputs 'cannot be viewed as sustainable' (p. 22). HPI projects in several countries have thus emphasized the importance of traditional methods of animal healthcare. Indeed, this PVO's Community Animal Health Volunteers Project in the Philippines now relies mainly on local remedies, coupled with preventive practices. Also noted is the common use of poultry as biological controls on disease-bearing pests. In some places, like the Dominican Republic, small ruminants are likewise deployed as living herbicides. If only by judicious culling, stockraisers consciously select stock to promote genotypic characteristics such as disease- and drought-tolerance, strength, good mothering abilities, tameness, and, in pastoral systems, ability to walk long distances. On the other hand, there is an alarming loss of genetic biodiversity in domesticated animals. HPI has found this to be the case, e.g., for water buffalo in the Philippines and llama and alpaca in the Andes of South America, due to increasing pressures from cash-based economies that force farmers' to sell off some of their best animals and keep inferior stock for breeding. The book thus sounds a clarion call for 'serious attention to genetic diversity of livestock breeds before another valuable resource is lost forever' (p. 23).

Abadome, François. 1998. 'Ethnovet and vet. medicine are complementary' says Dr Abadome. *La Voix du Paysan English* 35: 15.

A veterinarian, Dr Abadome is an adviser to the HPI-sponsored Ethnoveterinary Council of Bui District, Cameroon. In this interview, he describes the Council's structure and functions. Some of the latter include verifying farmers' reports of local disease treatments and training people in community-based animal healthcare. Also discussed are some of the advantages and disadvantages of home remedies, along with Council plans for self-sustainability via: marketing some of the medicinal plants it has worked with but that are not available in all areas; preparing and selling manuals on EVK; and applying for grants.

Abbas, Babiker. 1997. *Ethnoveterinary Practices of Camel Pastoralists in Butana, North-eastern Sudan.* DHP Publications Series No. 4. Dryland Husbandry Project and OSSREA (Organization for Social Science Research in Eastern and Southern Africa), Addis Ababa, Ethiopia. 55 pp.

Between 1992 and 1996, the EVK of 15 well-known healers and 56 herders in the deserts of northeastern Sudan was studied as part of the Dryland Husbandry

Project, implemented by the University of Khartoum's Institute of Environmental Studies. Ethnic or linguistic groups represented included, Beni-Amer, Bishariin, Hadendewa, Lehwee, Rashaida, Shukria and Tibdawet. The study results are presented in two sections, divided by healers versus herders. Among the former (all male), seven treated humans as well as livestock (camels, cattle, equines, sheep), with most of these polyvalent practitioners coming from nomadic or transhumant tribes; eight dealt with both surgical and medical problems, while the other seven specialized in one or the other. Along with a number of younger male colleagues, the healers identified several women with 'outstanding reputations' in EVM; but these individuals could not be located for interviews. Healers in the sample had been practising EVM for between 5 and 50 years each, indicating that they begin their work at an early age and continue to gain experience throughout their lives. In rank order of importance, they cited their sources of EVK as apprenticeship with a male relative, a non-family clan member, or a former non-clan employer, or as simply personal initiative, observation and trial-and-error. Most of the older men had apprenticed with a relative, while younger men predominated in the personal initiative category. All affirmed that they continue to add to their knowledge through exchanges with other healers from near and far. All are usually paid for their services in cash or kind (clothes, coffee, sugar, occasionally a young animal); most also own herds and/or cultivate seasonal plots. All make outpatient calls for immobile patients. Healers' surgical interventions centre on reproductive problems, musculoskeletal disorders, chronic abdominal pain, abscesses and non-specific or unyielding conditions. Successful obstetric operations include: manual relief of dystocia, for which healers describe numerous well-known presentations; occasional caesarian sections, especially if twins justify the risk to the dam; embryotomy of dead foetuses, performed with a short bent knife and sometimes with antiseptic soap; and uterine prolapse, for which the procedures are the same as in Western veterinary medicine. For infertility in large animals, the vagina (equines) or uterus (bovines) may be debrided using a short, curved, dull knife to gently abrade the area until the blood runs clean; then salt water is applied and the vulva is held closed for half an hour. Castration is performed traditionally in one of two ways. For camels and cattle, the testicles are stretched across a thick log and then the spermatic cord is crushed just above the scrotal sac by a blow from a blunt iron rod. For lambs, a string is tightly tied around the scrotum head and the animal is tethered for 4 to 5 days, after which the string is removed. Nowadays, a few healers and herders also own and use burdizzos. Musculoskeletal interventions centre on sprains, fractures and lameness, for all of which healers demonstrate great diagnostic expertise. An 'open plaster' (*gabira*) of a damp grass mesh that later dries is applied to support sprained areas. A *gabira* of small sticks laced together and flattened on one side is assembled precisely over the point of line of a fracture. A certain type of congenital lameness in camels, related to tendon flexion, receives an acupuncture-style treatment in which a hot needle is inserted between the tendon and the muscle or bone attachment at the suspected site of the problem for 5 to 10 minutes; alternatively, a thong of leather or sinew may be inserted. When the scar tissue heals, it increases the tension on the tendon. Other kinds of musculoskeletal conditions are treated by cauterization (e.g. acute arthritis, bog-spavin, bent-neck, hygroma, lumbago). Indeed, cauterization is a multi-purpose technique. It is used for, e.g. removal of broken or injured horns, hoof trimming, radical treatment of abscesses, and pathologies linked to specific organs according to named and known cautery points. 'Ripe cautery' is the most common type of cauterization; it is administered with a glowing-hot iron rod, until the skin turns white [also see Agab 1998]. Healers' medical interventions involve mainly botanicals, both wild and cultivated. In addition to local plant materials, these include imports from India and more humid parts of Africa. Other ingredients such as soil, honey, urine, hair, salt, camphor, coffeebeans, sesame oil, meat broths, animal fats and some commercial products (e.g. acaricides, anthelmintics) are also used. An illustrative listing of 23 plants and their scores of associated treatments for humans as well as livestock is given, along with comments on their veterinary effectiveness as reported by healers, observed or applied by the author himself, and attested in the literature. To take just one example, *Acacia nilotica* pods are used to good effect in numerous ways: prepared as a powerful astringent; in a decocted drench of whole pods for diarrhoea; as an external powder for fevers, measles, and purulent and especially fistulous wounds (the latter attested by the author); as a fumigant and/or a gargle against coryza, rhinitis and sore throat; in a polyprescription paste for chronic arthritis and sciatica; and occasionally as an anthelmintic drench. Healers are also aware of botanicals' side effects and thus may also give antidotes with some. An example is strong black tea administered to counterbalance overpurgation from a taeniacidal broth of *Cassia senna* leaves. An interesting new application for an old remedy involves a drench of ground wild okra (*Hibiscus trionium*) fruits mixed in small amounts of warm water. Traditionally given as a mild laxative and for rainy-season bloat, this okra drench is now also prescribed to help expel the plastic bags that even pastoral livestock are increasingly ingesting. A summary finding of interest is that no healers in the sample felt threatened by Western medicine because, they said, demand for their skills was on the rise in the face of the high prices and the unavailability of Western surgical or medical services in the deserts. The second section of this report outlines herders' EVM. Before consulting a healer, almost invariably herders first try to treat their animals themselves. They have a meticulous, organ- and often species-specific system of disease diagnosis, the nomenclature for which is detailed in Annex 5. This system signals an appreciable knowledge of anatomy, which herders say they study at necropsy; during necropsy, they also definitively diagnose certain diseases so as to add to their pre-mortem diagnostic abilities for the next occurrences. Herders can also detail the progression of many diseases – for example, the weakness, anaemia, watery eyes, inappetence, and finally, unique urinary odour of trypanosomosis in camels. There is less know-how about a syndrome of unidentified and non-system-specific symptoms they call *haboub* 'wind'. While they have fair obstetric skills, they leave cauter- ization to the healers (who, interestingly, are less keen on it than herders). Herders are also less botanically astute than healers, generally turning first to antibiotics for most livestock health problems, even though they sometimes inad- vertently kill their own animals with faulty or unsterile injections. But they are expert in all aspects of pasture flora, including toxic plants. And they excel in tra- ditional vaccinations for FMD, CBPP and CCPP, although sometimes they mistake haemorrhagic septicaemia for the latter two diseases. Other disease control measures they take are: herd movements to avoid threats of trypanoso- mosis, babesiosis, theileriosis and footrot; prompt quarantine of animals within a herd, and avoidance of other herds, with contagious conditions such as mange, ecthyma, pox, pneumonia, and abortions; at night, quartering camels on a bare rise, where insects and snakes are few; not turning stock out to pasture before the dew has dried; regularly shearing young camels to discourage lice and tick infestation;

and standing camels in the salty water of the Red Sea for several hours while also pouring the sea water over them to rid them of ticks (a technique the author observed to be effective) and to ward against mange. Pastoralists take special nutritional measures, such as: confining camels with night blindness to fields of *Calotropis* spp.; during the dry season, grazing pastures rich in certain trees, and collecting their fruits and pods to feed to lactating and pregnant females and the principal riding camel; and for young racing camels, continual muzzling except for watering and hand-feeding on special diets of sorghum, dates, butter, sesame seed, salt, acacia leaves and pods, and green grasses. However, they restrict neonate camels' colostrum intake, in the belief that too much colostrum can cause fatal gastroenteritis. The desert pastoralists keep close tabs on animal ancestries, particularly for camels, whom they often speak of as human. They check all their camels' health daily. Some concluding observations are that: healers and herders exchange EVK freely; healers' wide range of skills reveals a huge potential for EVM, which is a dynamic and growing craft; however, certain botanicals are becoming nearly as difficult to obtain as Western medicines; healers and herders alike stand helpless in the face of some diseases – which may explain some of the over-reliance on firing; and, understandably in an arid environment, there is considerable room for improvement in surgical hygiene. Finally, the author offers a wide range of recommendations. One is further study, under controlled experimental conditions, of some widely-used botanicals for which there is little pharmacological literature. Relatedly, more cross-cultural comparisons of pastoral practices should be made. The author also advocates establishing an EVM branch in every provincial Veterinary Department, to register and interact with healers as local extensionists. Healers could benefit from targeted and accredited paravet training in certain arenas, and older healers could serve in turn as trainers for younger entrants to the profession. In this regard, the author mentions three 1– to 2–month sessions jointly mounted by a number of NGOs and projects to train 75 young men as paravets.

Abebe, Dawit and Ahadu Ayehu. 1993. Veterinary practices and medicines. In: *Medicinal Plants and Enigmatic Health Practices in Northern Ethiopia.* Editor and publication information unavailable. Pp. 419–431.

This book chapter lists indigenous Ethiopian treatments for improving dairy products and livestock reproduction. Prescriptions are given for 16 categories of ailments in cattle, sheep, goats, horses and mules. These include eye diseases, emaciation, saddle sores, wounds, colic, trypanosomosis, anthrax, scabies, hyena or snake bites, and several unidentified and/or locally-named conditions. Treatments may involve both natural and supernatural elements, plant, animal and mineral *materia medica.* To stimulate cattle breeding, for example, 21 cotton seeds are placed in a cattle horn along with the tongue of a black sheep and 64 river pebbles. The horn is carried clockwise three times around the cattle pen and then buried at the entrance. In addition to some 60 plant species identified by their Latin names, other items in the Ethiopian ethnoveterinary pharmacopoeia include: salt, soot, cow's urine, the excrement and bone marrow of wild and/or domestic animals, pot shards, butter, lentil bread, and food grains. Modes of administration span: eye, ear and nose drops; hanging 'bouquets'; powders and poultices; oral, topical and anal applications of infusions and rubs; and livestock fumigation plus a traditional beehive fumigation technique intended to accelerate bee reproduction.

Abu-Rabia, Aref. 1983. ***Folk Medicine among the Bedouin Tribes in the Negev.*** Social Studies Center, The Jakob Blaustein Institute for Desert Research, Ben-Gurion University of the Negev, Sede Boqer Campus, Israel. 30 pp.

This report deals mainly with human ethnomedicine. It lists 35 medicinal plants and 17 medicines made from animal products. However, the author mentions that the Bedouin hang amulets with combinations of letters, words, symbols, numbers or Koranic verses on their horses, cows, female camels, sheep and other animals in order to protect them from the evil eye. The same amulets are also used for humans (pp. 4–5).

Abu-Rabia, A. 1994. ***The Negev Bedouin and Livestock Rearing: Social, Economic and Political Aspects.*** Berg Mediterannean Series, Oxford, Massachusetts and Providence, Rhode Island, USA. 139 pp.

In making and implementing stockraising decisions, modern-day Bedouin in Israel's Negev desert must take into account not only the biophysical ecology but also the equally rocky socio-political landscape. Among other subjects, this book focuses on how Bedouin struggle with bureaucratic privilege, corruption, and red-tape in order to access vital feeds and forages for their sheep, goats, donkeys, horses, camels and poultry. The author documents the great lengths and expense to which Bedouin may have to go in nourishing, watering, dividing and sheltering their herds now that they are prohibited from ranging freely. During much of the year, stockraisers may have to purchase and truck-in tons of feed, which then must be carefully measured, mixed and doled out in varying formulae according to different ages and species of stock, the season, and any available grazes and browses. Ration ingredients include bran, whole and crushed barley, vetch hay, wheat chaff and straw, and in the case of one innovator, 20-ton loads of rejected oranges, grapefruits, and their peelings, which he purchases semi-illicitly from a distant packing house. An example of specialized rations is one-month-old lambs' hand-feedings of compressed barley – known as 'training them to eat' – so as to fatten them from an early age. Indeed, newborn lambs are given exceptional attention, including their own pens to protect them from predation, the elements, the evil eye of envious neighbours and trampling to death by other stock. Older lambs and kids are also penned separately, as they form the *rabayitt* herd, which is destined for special feeding and slaughter. Weanlings may be put in yet another pen; alternatively, households may temporarily exchange lambs to effect weaning. Nowadays Bedouin may supplement their lambs with veterinarian-recommended commercial vitamins and minerals (notably E and selenium); and they must see to legally required immunizations. For all stock, care must be taken not to over-feed such rich items as barley and vetch since, say Bedouin, doing so can cause constipation, diarrhoea, disease, female infertility and other problems. When diarrhoea is detected in a few animals, they are immediately quarantined in a separate pen while the remainder of the flock is grazed on natural forages for a while. Whenever possible, of course, stockraisers seek out pasture and field grazing, whether from their own or others' holdings. Access to the latter is negotiated via complex, delicate and often extra-legal contracts with authorities. Such resources span failed barley fields, post-harvest stubble grazing and gleaning, fallow fields that have re-sprouted grain left from earlier years, and recondite hillsides and gulches (*wadi*). Under the traditional *hima* system, in the past Bedouin set aside certain rangelands as dry-season or drought reserves; in still other areas, grazing was prohibited in order to maintain flowers and other plants as food for bees and wildlife, thus ensuring supplies of honey and bushmeat for humans. These sensitive centuries-old and multi-year reserve systems are evidence that 'Bedouin learned about guarding natural resources long before scientists comprehended the principles of pasture management' (p. 53). International agencies have instituted some efforts (e.g. in Oman) to re-establish *hima*-like systems. Other observations of ethnoveterinary and husbandry relevance include the following. Stockraisers separately pen pregnant ewes for whom birth is imminent. Relatedly, Bedouin recognize a progression of more than a dozen pre-parturient signs. People also ensure that a neonate suckles immediately so that it will receive colostrum and so that – via smelling, licking and suckling – its dam will accept it. At the same time, all other lambs and kids are removed from the area, leaving only one newborn's scent for the dam to detect. Special *tawrim* measures are taken for a ewe or doe who rejects her young. She is tethered and fed separately on delicacies like bread while a human helps the neonate to suckle. People may also frighten her into nursing by beating on tin cans or setting the dogs on her. At cisterns and wells, sheep are watered in small groups in turns in order to prevent crowding and pushing that can result in animals (and children) falling in and drowning. Gender roles in stockraising are mentioned briefly (p. 60 ff.), along with Bedouin women's independent ownership of poultry.

ACIAR. 1996a. Duck droppings combat liver fluke. *ACIAR Newsletter* 29 (Feb-Aug): 10–11.

This article illustrates the value of ecologically sensitive and integrated disease management, here via mixed-species stockraising. In Indonesia, a study of fasciolosis in cattle and buffalo discovered that local ducks are parasitized by *Echinostoma revolutum* flukes. *Echinostoma revolutum* competes for the same intermediate snail host as the bovine liver fluke *Fasciola gigantica*. In fact, *E. revolutum* is more aggressive than *F. gigantica*. The former consumes the latter and thus breaks the liver fluke's cycle. Cattle and buffalo are thereby protected from fasciolosis. Moreover, they cannot be parasitized by the duck's fluke.

ACIAR. 1996b. Sustainable parasite control. *ACIAR Newsletter* 29 (Feb-Aug): 13.

This brief review of discussions at a workshop on sustainable parasite control summarizes the workshop's conclusion that sustainable disease control systems merit much greater R&D attention. Elements of such systems can include breeding (e.g. for helminth resistance) and devising grazing and mixed-species management systems for parasite control.

Adamou, Laoualy. 1990. Funktionen und Entwicklungsmöglichkeiten der Tierhaltung im Sahel. In: Horst S.H. Seifert, Paul L.G. Vlek and H.-J. Weidelt (eds). *Tierhaltung im Sahel. Symposium 26–27 Oktober 1989.* Göttinger Beiträge zur Land-und Forstwirtschaft in den Tropen und Subtropen, Heft 51. Forschungs- und Studienzentrum der Agrar- und Forstwissenschaften der Tropen und Subtropen, Georg-August-Universität Göttingen, Germany. Pp. 123–139.

Entitled 'Functions and Development Possibilities of Animal Production in the Sahel', this chapter notes that although nomadic pastoralists and agropastoralists keep livestock mainly for food, the formers' animals also have important social functions while the latters' serve a capital-investment function. Thus, developers need to consider different groups' varying animal-production goals. Also, developers can build upon traditional pastoralist institutions geared to help households survive in the face of herd loss. An example is the practice of *jokkereji*, i.e. lending female animals to households who have lost their own herds and allowing the recipients to keep the milk. In *habannaji*, recipients are also allowed to keep the first three offspring from the borrowed stock in order to start rebuilding their herds. Because animals may be lent across communities or between pastoralists and agropastoralists, these practices can help integrate different groups in a region. Also, nomads can work as herders for other groups. Conceivably, *habannaji*-like arrangements could even act as the basis for a national livestock credit system. The author discusses this and other survival options for both nomads and agropastoralists.

Adeyemi, I.G. 1998. Profile of ethnoveterinary care of livestock in southwestern Nigeria. In: E. Mathias, D.V. Rangnekar and C.M. McCorkle, with M. Martin (eds). *Ethnoveterinary Medicine: Alternatives for Livestock Development – Proceedings of an International Conference Held in Pune, India, 4–6 November 1997. Volume 2: Abstracts.* BAIF Development Research Foundation, Pune, India. P. 1.

In southwestern Nigeria, small-scale livestock production prevails and farmers are amenable to ethnoveterinary care because their system is based on low inputs and outputs. In rural areas ethnoveterinary care is the norm, while peri-urban and urban stockraisers additionally use modern veterinary medicine. Also, in some serious cases (e.g. livestock dysentery), animals are treated with modern drugs designed for human ailments with similar symptoms. Because of the high cost of commercial drugs plus scarce foreign exchange, however, the proportion of stockraisers relying on EVM has been increasing recently. Yet most indigenous treatments for livestock are curative rather than preventive. This report discusses the efficacy, acceptability, affordability and modifications of ethnoveterinary treatments along with their implications for rural livestock development and public health in the region.

Adjid, R.M.A. 1990. *Survey of Traditional Medicine Use for Sheep Health Problems by OPP Farmers in the Bogor District of West Java.* SR-CRSP Working Paper No. 118. Balai Penelitian Ternak, Pusat Penelitian dan Pengembangan Peternakan, Bogor, Indonesia. 12 pp.

An earlier study of traditional medicines for chicken health problems in Indonesia suggested the need for a similar study of small ruminants. This working paper reports on a survey, using a checklist of 18 sheep and goat health problems, among farmers of West Java. It found that traditional medicines existed for all the sheep problems listed. Moreover, 100% of informants employed ethnoveterinary treatments for myiasis and diarrhoea; 94% for poor lactation; 82% for lice; 76% for endoparasites, poisoning and scabies; 65% for tympany and parturient paresis; 47% for dam's refusal to be milked; 41% for orf; and 35% for pink eye. Other ailments for which 17% to 29% of respondents employed traditional medicines were: abscesses, coughs, mastitis, infertility and low libido. Farmers indicated they found their ethnomedicines generally efficacious, with no side effects. They obtained their ethnoveterinary information from their own ideas, their parents and other farmers. The author believes that formal study of these ethnomedicines is warranted, so as to encourage their broader use.

Adolph, David, Stephen Blakeway and B.J. Linquist. 1996. *Ethno-veterinary Knowledge of the Dinka and Nuer in Southern Sudan: A Study for the UNICEF Operation Lifeline Sudan Southern Sector Livestock Programme, December 1996.* UNICEF, Nairobi, Kenya. 57 pp.

Commissioned by UNICEF/Operation Lifeline Sudan (OLS) for the Livestock Section of its Household Food Security Programme, this is a study of EVK among Dinka and Nuer in southern Sudan. Both Dinka and Nuer have a large vocabulary of animal health terms and identify a wide range of animal health problems. A high level of knowledge is distributed unevenly through both societies: the authors note that there is a much higher level of knowledge in settled and agricultural groups. Both groups use with confidence a number of plant medicines, although the Dinka use a wider variety of plants. Both also practise successfully a number of surgical procedures. There are Dinka and Nuer specialists (*atet* and *leert* respectively) whose assistance is sought for setting bones, cutting lumps, dystocias (including foetotomy) and castration. These specialists are also often more knowledgeable than most about the medicinal use of plants.

Adolph-LaRoche, David and B.J. Linquist-LaRoche. 1993. *Marsabit Project Annual Review.* In-house report. ITDG, Marsabit, Kenya. 13 pp.

In the Marsabit District of Kenya's Northern Frontier, ITDG assists Gabbra pastoralists of the Galbo clan with their livestock and other development needs. A major undertaking in the veterinary arena has been to establish a clan drugstore and to train store operators and mobile paravets in the use of commercial drugs. Various EVK activities are also under way or consideration. For example, ethnoveterinary information is being collected and computerized, and plans are being laid to test confidently used traditional treatments such as dewormers and mange remedies, with the goal of including them in training packages. Plantings of medicinal trees in the drugstore plot are also being considered.

Agab, H. 1998a. Traditional treatment methods of camels in eastern Sudan with emphasis on firing. *Journal of Camel Practice and Research* 5(1): 161–164.

Sudan boasts one of the largest camel populations in the world. There, nomadic and semi-nomadic tribes like the Bawadra, Lahawiyin, Rashaida, Rufa and Shukria keep alive an age-old camel culture. These unique animals in turn keep the tribes alive thanks to camels' numerous products (meat, milk, hides, wool) and services (riding, racing, portage, traction for cropping, oil milling and water lifting). In the Butana desert of eastern Sudan, however, disease and a corresponding lack of formal veterinary care are major constraints to camel production and productivity. The most common and feared diseases are trypanosomosis, mange, *haboub* syndrome (a musculoskeletal stiffness of the neck region), internal parasitism, streptothrichosis, contagious skin necrosis, mastitis, camel pox, and in calves, diarrhoea. Another problem for herders is the lack of adequate veterinary services. Butana stockraisers perforce rely mainly on themselves and on local healers when it comes to camel healthcare. Indeed, a survey of Butana herders and healers found that recourse to healers is on the rise in the face of the high price and inaccessibility of Western veterinary medicine in this desolate region. Botanicals constitute the major weapons in healers' arsenal against camel diseases, as illustrated here in a table of 23 plant species used for some 25 different health effects. However, the most common traditional treatment for a host of camel ills is firing/cauterization. It is particularly recommended for lameness and other musculoskeletal disorders, for which firing seems to be more successful than modern chemotherapies. Firing is normally performed by pressing red-hot iron bars of 1 to 3 cm in diameter against the skin for 20 to 60 seconds until the skin turns white. There are multiple methods of firing – in points, lines, crosses and rings. Although different tribes use different ones for the same disease, there is some agreement on the preferred method for certain diseases. An example is ring firing for contagious skin necrosis. Cauterization treatments can be divided not only by method but also by whether their target is system- versus organ-specific. For the latter, there are well-known and recognized cautery sites, which correspond to the organ(s) assumed to be involved in the pathological process. The ethnotheory behind firing appears to relate to the counter-irritant principle, in which chronic intractable inflammatory conditions are converted to the acute stage. However, Sudanese pastoralists also apply firing as a last resort and on an experimental basis when they are confronted with new or undiagnosed conditions. Since the brands left behind by firing are often indicative of chronic intractable ills, oft-treated animals are hard to sell to breeders or to traders except for slaughter.

Agab, H. 1998b. Traditional treatment methods of camels in Sudan. In: E. Mathias, D.V. Rangnekar and C.M. McCorkle, with M. Martin (eds). ***Ethnoveterinary Medicine: Alternatives for Livestock Development – Proceedings of an International Conference Held in Pune, India, 4–6 November 1997. Volume 2: Abstracts***. BAIF Development Research Foundation, Pune, India. P. 1.

This conference paper re-caps much of the same information as Agab 1998a.

Agaceta, L.M., P.U. Dumag, J.A. Batalos, N.B. Escandor and F.C. Bandiola. 1980. Study on the control of snail vectors of fascioliasis: Molluscicidal activity of some indigenous plants. Paper presented to the 17th PSAS Annual Convention. PICC, Manila, Philippines.

In the Philippines, the intermediate snail host of liverfluke disease is *Lymnaea auricularia rubiginosa*. Indigenous plants with molluscicidal potential were evaluated as possible alternatives to chemical molluscicides. Of 150 plants screened, seven were found to have strong potential: *Croton tiglium* L., *Entada phaseolides* M., *Nicotiana tabacum* L., *Coryza balsamifera* L., *Citrus mitis* B., *Jatropha curcas* L. and *Menispermum coculus* L. Screening was conducted in three stages. In Stage I, the selected plants were pulverized and tested by immersing them with the snails. In Stage II, the seven plants listed above were subjected to further tests: for molluscicidal activity, effect on *Lymnaea* eggs and young, photosensitivity, and toxicity for fish. Stage III consisted of small-scale field trials of *C. tiglium, E. phaseolides* and *N. tabacum* in rice paddies. Laboratory tests showed that molluscicidal activity increased with concentration of plant matter and time of exposure. As a result, snail eggs failed to develop to young snails. The three plants tested under field conditions followed the same trends as in the laboratory.

Aguilar C., Abigail. 1988. Antecedentes históricos y contexto sociocultural de la herbolaria: Rutas a seguir para el conocimiento de las plantas medicinales. In: Luz Lozano Nathal and Gerardo López Buendía (coordinators). *Memorias: Primera Jornada sobre Herbolaria Medicinal en Veterinaria.* Universidad Nacional Autónoma de México, Facultad de Medicina Veterinaria y Zootecnia, Coordinación de Educación Continua, México DF. Pp. 4–7.

This abstract of a presentation in the above-referenced conference outlines the historical antecedents and sociocultural context of herbalism in Mexico and suggests methods for their study, beginning with the examination of pre-Hispanic murals and early chronicles, medical and botanical treatises. The author describes four stages in the development of the scholarly study of Mexico's ethnobotany. She concludes with a list of five ways to gather information on the subject: bibliographic research, studies of medicinal plants available in marketplaces, regional and national surveys of such plants' use, ethnobotanical field studies and herbarium collections.

Aguilar Contreras, Abigail. 1991. Sistematización de la Información sobre Medicina Tradicional Mexicana. In: Abigail Aguilar Contreras and Miguel Angel Martínez Alfaro (eds). *III Jornada sobre Herbolaria Medicinal en Medicina Veterinaria: Parte 2 – Curso de Etnobotánica para Veterinarios.* Universidad Nacional Autónoma de México, Facultad de Medicina Veterinaria y Zootecnia, División de Educación Continua y Departamento de Fisiología y Farmacología Veterinaria, México DF, México. Pp. 77–88.

An overview of the study of traditional/popular medicine in Mexico, this article pays attention to animal as well as human ethnomedicine. For instance, the section on traditional practitioners mentions not only the usual ones for humans (curers, herbalists, bonesetters, layers-on-of-hands, prayermen, midwives, housewives) but also traditional veterinary healers. Discussion of ethno-anatomy and ethno-physiology, of 'cultural' or supernatural versus organic or natural diseases, of categories of users of ethnomedicine, and of treatment types systematically touches on traditional concepts and practices as applied to animals as well as humans.

Aguilar C., Abigail, Miguel Angel Martínez A., Arturo Argueta V., José Antonio Dorantes and Heberto Esparza. 1988. Mesa redonda: Perspectivas de la herbolaria medicinal en la medicina veterinaria. In: Luz Lozano Nathal and Gerardo López Buendía (coordinators). *Memorias: Primera Jornada sobre Herbolaria Medicinal en Veterinaria.* Universidad Nacional Autónoma de México, Facultad de Medicina Veterinaria y Zootecnia, Coordinación de Educación Continua, México DF. Pp. 178–189.

Several recurrent themes characterize these roundtable remarks, which concluded the above-referenced conference: the many points of contact between human and animal ethnomedicine; the need for a conscious respect for the empirical acumen of rural producers, and recognition of the wealth of knowledge that veterinary science can reap from them; the implications for academic programmes and future career possibilities in veterinary medicine of a commitment to serving rural smallholders through ethnoveterinary research and development, versus serving only medium- and large-scale enterprises through costly, 'high-tech' solutions to animal health problems; the need for Mexico to free itself of intellectual and economic dependency upon other nations; a caution not to forget the primary importance of prevention over curing; and perhaps above all, the immediate need for concerted interdisciplinary action in ethnoveterinary research, development and extension.

Agyemang, K., R.H. Dwinger, D.A. Little and G.J. Rowlands. 1997. *Village N'Dama Cattle Production in West Africa: Six Years of Research in the Gambia.* ILRI and International Trypanotolerance Centre, Nairobi, Kenya and Banjul, The Gambia. 131 pp.

The socioeconomic portion of this longitudinal study of N'Dama production in Gambia surveyed a random but wealth-stratified sample of 75 Mandinka and Fulani farmers from 16 districts as to their livestock feeding practices. Findings revealed that 93% of farmers raised groundnuts and fed the hay to their livestock; and of the 15% who pressed some of their groundnuts for oil, almost all used the residue for livestock feed. Forty-two percent cut and carried annual legumes (especially *Alysicarpus* spp.) from the bush, and 44% fed millet and sorghum grain, mainly to equines used for crop cultivation during the rainy season. Oxen were supplemented just prior to and during cultivation, but other cattle rarely received supplements. Those that did were mainly weaners, older pregnant cows or sick animals that farmers felt could not stand the seasonal migration to better pastures. Among small ruminants, mainly only rams destined for slaughter at the Moslem festival of Tabaski received supplements. The authors discuss how efforts at increased supplementation, especially of cattle, might be blocked by current herding arrangements. For instance, Mandinka who hire Fulani herders would receive only a portion of the productivity benefits of increased supplementation since herders take most of the milk from their employers' animals in payment for their herding services. And with less secure land tenure and an already-significant income from milk, Fulani farmers might not be interested in crop strategies designed to yield more fodder.

Ahmed, Saleem and Michael Grainge. 1986. Potential of the neem tree (*Azadirachta indica*) for pest control and rural development. *Economic Botany* 40(2): 201–209.

Neem is cited in Ayurvedic medicine and is found in numerous countries of Africa and Asia. Various plant parts of the neem tree have been found effective in controlling many economically important crop pests. Neem also figures in a wide range of human ethnomedicines, such as anthelmintics, astringents, diuretics, etc. It has additional applications for animals. For example, neem seedcake is used as a nitrification inhibitor in livestock feed. Moreover, the incorporation of 20% neem cake into sheep diets results in higher growth rates. In addition, recent experiments on dogs revealed that aqueous extracts of neem leaves can lower blood pressure and increase respiration rates.

Ajayi, Femi. 1990. How to raise better poultry: Violet chicks and other tips. *African Farmer* 5(Nov): 52–53.

This article gives four farmer-to-farmer tips for poultry production based on Nigerian ethnoveterinary knowledge. One farmer recommends dyeing chickens with gentian violet or any bright natural, non-toxic colouring agent to ward off birds of prey. He also plants tobacco around his chickens' roaming range because, he says, the smell keeps soldier ants and snakes away. Another farmer shares his success at treating Newcastle disease by dosing the birds with a concentrated solution of potassium permanaganate. He reports that this low-cost and readily available chemical produces a 50% survival rate. This figure is not insignificant for a disease that is normally 100% fatal. Finally, a guinea-fowl farmer offers husbandry tips for increasing laying rates by removing eggs from the clutch. The extra eggs may then be incubated by local chickens.

Akabwai, D., T. Leyland and C. Stem. 1999. Provision of sustainable animal health delivery systems, which incorporate traditional livestock knowledge, to marginalised pastoralist areas. In: E. Mathias, D.V. Rangnekar and C.M. McCorkle, with M. Martin (eds). *Ethnoveterinary Medicine: Alternatives for Livestock Development – Proceedings of an International Conference Held in Pune, India, 4–6 November 1997. Volume 1: Selected Papers.* BAIF Development Research Foundation, Pune, India. Pp. 171–184.

This paper describes special characteristics of marginalized pastoralist areas in sub-Saharan Africa that make it difficult for government veterinary services to deliver Western-style clinical and vaccination services to such areas. Also discussed are herders' perceived needs, existing veterinary knowledge, and current access to formal-sector animal healthcare. Examples are drawn from project work with pastoralist communities in Kenya's Turkana District, Ethiopia's Afar region, Southern Sudan, Cameroon's Northwest Province, Chad's Salamat region, and Uganda's Karamoja District. The paper describes a 'privatized pastoral veterinary practice' approach to establishing a sustainable delivery system that incorporates local perceptions and knowledge, local organizational structures, and national or local government. Advances in this methodology are based on actual project work carried out in marginalized pastoralist areas. The paper also discusses alternative approaches and factors that have guided this work, and its different phases of implementation, highlighting some of the most common problems encountered plus issues that must be addressed in order to ensure that privatized pastoral veterinary practices are both attainable and sustainable. Specific attention is paid to how to stimulate the long-term incorporation of EVK into delivery systems. This is achieved in two phases. The first centres on identifying local healers, learning about their veterinary techniques in general, and re-building community confidence in their EVK. The second phase focuses on detailed investigation of ethnoveterinary treatments and then promotion of the most useful and cost-effective remedies.

Akabwai, D.M.O., J.C. Mariner, J. Toyang, A. Berhano, Sali Django and T. Osire. 1994. Ethnoveterinary knowledge: A basis for community based animal health work in pastoral areas. *The Kenya Veterinarian* 18(2): 520.

Preparatory to mounting a community-based vaccination programme against rinderpest, a survey of EVK among 20 Fulani, 40 Karamajong and 20 Afar pastoralists in Africa was conducted. Results revealed that all three groups can clearly describe the diseases affecting their herds. Moreover, 'These descriptions often correspond with the western notions but are profoundly richer'. This lexicon is presented here, along with available laboratory confirmations. The survey also indicated the existence of traditional remedies [not reported here] to combat live-stock diseases. Overall, pastoralists ranked rinderpest as their most troublesome veterinary problem.

Ake-Assi, Yolande and Gérard Keck. 1994. Pharmacopée traditionnelle vétéri-naire. In: Kakule Kasonia and Michel Ansay (eds). *Métissages en Santé Animale de Madagascar à Haïti: Actes du Séminaire d'Ethnopharmacopée Vétérinaire 'KAGALA', un Partage de Savoirs Burkina-Faso, Ouagadougou, 15–22 Avril 1993.* Presses Universitaires de Namur, Namur, Belgium. Pp. 213–217.

A survey of ethnoveterinary medicines in Ivory Coast yielded 111 prescriptions involving 81 plant species. The mono- and poly-prescriptions were prepared in several ways: pulverization, decoction, or reduction to ashes. Also recorded was the widespread use of charms, mystical incantations and talismans to protect, promote or cure animal ills. The authors point out that there are different ways to consider and categorize traditional medicines' efficacy besides just scientific veri-fication. One is the sheer extent of popular knowledge about and use of a treatment; i.e. some efficacy is likely for remedies that are widely known and used. Another consideration is short- versus long-term efficacy, as reflected in temporary allevia-tion of symptoms versus complete cure or operational success. They note that the latter outcomes are most common for problems like snakebite, ectoparasitosis and dystocia. In concluding, the authors note several common problems linked to the study of plant-based ethnomedicines: the difficulties of plant collection and identi-fication; the alarming destruction of tropical forests and hence the disappearance of valuable medicinal plants; and healers' and stockraisers' failure to specify or standardize dosages and expiry dates for traditional medicines. In addition to increased research efforts in general, they urge: organization of a research network on African medicinal plants; preservation of medicinal plant biodiversity; and the construction of pilot units to produce botanicals.

Akingboye, K.A. 1997a. Ethnobotany in animal care. *ILEIA Newsletter* 13(2): 21.

This thumbnail sketch of Fulani (Bororo) EVK encapsulates some of the informa-tion presented in Akingboye 1997b and in a longer publication by the same author, entitled 'The Significance of Ethnobotany in Animal Care' (1977), available from the University of Ibadan's Department of Veterinary Public Health and Preventive Medicine, Ibadan, Nigeria. Here, the author notes that Fulani gauge the potency and effectiveness of their home remedies by reference to improvements in patients' feed intake, carcass size and quality, body weight and milk yields.

Akingboye, K.A. 1997b. The use of ethnobotany in animal care. Unpublished manuscript. Department of Veterinary Public Health and Preventive Medicine, University of Ibadan, Ibadan, Nigeria. 8 pp.

University of Ibadan fieldwork has documented a wealth of ethnoveterinary botan-icals among Fulani (Bororo) herdsmen of northeastern Nigeria. Seeds, roots, leaves, barks, tubers and fruits are gathered for processing. They serve to combat skin diseases, wounds, colds and reduced appetite in herd animals. Examples of commonly used plant species are: baobab (*Adansonia digitata*) against diarrhoea, skin disorders and CBPP; ginger (*Zingiber officinale*) as a laxative, appetiser and eructative (antibloat); garlic (*Allium sativum*) as an anthelmintic and general antidote [to poisoning]; eggplant (*Solanum incanum*) for intestinal anomalies; African locust beans (*Parkia filicoidea*) for skin infections, wounds and worms; also for worms, onion; tobacco (*Nicotiana tabacum*) against myiasis, hoof infections and ectoparasites; and neem (*Azadirachta indica*) as an insect repellent. Preparation techniques span grinding, soaking in water, crushing out juice, boiling alone or with other ingredients like salt, honey, eggs and camphor, or sometimes simply feeding the whole plant. Farmers describe the efficacy of these ethnomedicines by reference to improved animal health and production as reflected in such variables as feed intake, carcass size and quality, body weight, vigour, conceptual and birth rates, and lactation. The author argues that greater recourse to herders' ethnopharmacopoeia can have bonuses for environmental conservation and the sustainable use and management of Africa's many natural resources.

Alarco de Zadra, Adriana. 1988. *PERU el Libro de las Plantas Mágicas: Compendio de Farmacopea Popular.* Gráfica Bellido for CONCYTEC (Consejo Nacional de Ciencia y Tecnología), Lima, Perú. 152 pp.

Drawing upon numerous publications, this compendium of the folk pharmacopoeia of Peru lists 333 plants used in ethnomedicine both contemporaneously and historically. Each listing gives the botanical identification of the plant plus its multiple folk names, a physical and historical description, and a summary of its uses. In only four listings are ethnoveterinary applications mentioned. *Catagua* (*Hura crepitans* L.) and *chilca* (*Eupatorium amygdalinum* Lam and *E. ligustrinum*) serve as purgatives for herd animals. *Matico* (*Piper angustifolium* R & P and *P. elongatum*) is employed as an infusion to cleanse wounds and then, as a powder, to poultice them. *Maycha* (*Senecio pseudotites* Griseb and *S. vulgaris*) works as a vermifuge. Wild tomato (*Physalis alkekengi*) is used to treat unidentified diseases in small livestock and poultry.

Alders, R.G., S.J. Mudenda and J.C. Katongo. 1992. Preliminary investigations into the control of Newcastle disease in village chickens in Zambia. In: John Young (ed.). *A Report on a Village Animal Health Care Workshop – Volume II: The Case Studies.* ITDG, Rugby, UK. Pp. 151–160.

A nationwide survey of 412 village poultry farmers in Zambia was undertaken in order to determine whether people would be interested in purchasing a vaccine for Newcastle disease (ND), and how such a vaccine could best be designed so as to fit into farmers' current poultry production practices and goals. The survey included the question 'What traditional medicines do you use?' In total, respondents named 19 local plants whose pounded leaves, stalks or, more rarely, roots or bark they administer in chickens' drinking water. Most of these plants are in fact employed to treat Newcastle disease (ND). This was hardly a surprising finding, given that government-sponsored vaccinations against ND had been suspended since 1978. Survey results also revealed that: 85% of farmers enclose their birds at night; 50% already use either traditional or modern medicines, generally in the drinking water; 95% are interested in buying an ND vaccine; and the amount they are willing to pay would be sufficient to cover vaccine production costs. Based on all these ethnoveterinary, husbandry and socioeconomic findings, researchers concluded that a thermostable vaccine administered in birds' drinking water would be the most acceptable and technologically appropriate ND immunization option for Zambian poultry raisers.

Ali, Talib M. 1991. Training nomadic 'barefoot vets'. *ILEIA Newsletter* Oct (3): 26–27.

FAO supported a programme of paraveterinary services that included training male Somali nomads as mobile animal health auxiliaries (NAHAs) and females, elders and children as settlement livestock carers (SLCs). Chosen by their co-villagers, NAHAs were instructed in routine prevention and cure of common livestock diseases, mainly for camels, sheep and goats. In addition to standard Western-veterinary topics and techniques, NAHA training included the use of herbal remedies. SLCs received training in one or two simple techniques, such as how to castrate small ruminants using an elastrator and rubber rings as an alternative to traditional castration, which entails passing red-hot skewers through the testes or hammering the testes with blocks of wood. Hoof trimming is traditionally performed by chopping with an axe. In general, Somali nomads are receptive to new practices and especially modern drugs. However, the programme encouraged NAHAs to use traditional herbal treatments when commercial drugs were unavailable, and it provided advice on these treatments' application.

Allan, William. 1965. *The African Husbandman.* Barnes and Noble, New York, USA.

Page 304 mentions that the Turkana bleed camels and that the Maasai pierce the vessels above the eyes when collecting blood from their sheep.

Altschul, Siri von Reis. 1975. *Drugs and Foods from Little-Known Plants: Notes in Harvard University Herbaria.* Harvard University Press, Cambridge, Massachusetts.

In parts of North America, *Eysenhardtia texana* was placed in the drinking water of poultry as a general disease prophylaxis. Notes from Harvard's herbaria also mention eight other plants of traditional veterinary use.

Amachi Fernández, Felipe Santiago. 1986. *Prácticas Sanitarias en la Ganadería Campesina: El Caso Moxolahuac, Puebla.* Thesis, Desarrollo Rural, Colegio de Postgraduados, Institución de Enseñanza e Investigación en Ciencias Agrícolas, Centro de Estudios del Desarrollo Rural, Chapingo, México. 257 pp.

This thesis in rural development describes and evaluates smallholder stock raising in the community of Santa Cruz de Moxolahuac in Puebla State, Mexico, with a focus on evaluating the management of animal health. Traditional veterinary practice primarily relies on: plant substances; minerals, salts, clays and commercial carbonates; petroleum derivatives; beverages like coffee, *pulque* and *tequila*; and, in some cases, massages, cold baths and exercise. Varying according to species (bovine, equine, caprine, porcine, canine, avian), the thesis details ethnoveterinary treatments for: wounds, bites, saddle or harness sores; endo- and ectoparasitism;

bloat, colics and other digestive disorders; diarrhoeas and respiratory ailments; and castration wounds and reproductive problems. Stockowners' use of commercial drugs and vaccines is also noted. While the author observes that many ethno-therapies are at least partially or potentially effective, he feels that peasants' overall management of animal health and hygiene is inadequate in that problems often go untreated, are treated belatedly, or are misdiagnosed. Above all, stockowners focus on curing when instead they should give more attention to prevention, about which they apparently know little. In large part, the author attributes these problems to the inadequacy of government extension programmes.

Ambekar, V.W. 1998. Pests also pollinate: When does an insect become a pest? *Honey Bee* 9(1): 11–12.

An astute traditional grazing strategy in India benefits not only animal nutrition (and thus health) but also soil quality and crop yields . It consists of systematically driving 40 to 50 sheep slowly across fields planted with Bengal gram about a week after the fields have been irrigated. The animals' trampling areates the soil and mixes in their manure. Moreover, as scientists have demonstrated, sheep's nibbling of young shoot tips helps overcome apical dominance, thereby promoting lateral branching of the gram and increasing fruit production. In fact, this practice can increase crop yields by 15 to 30 quintals per hectare.

Anderson, Myrdene. 1978. *Saami Ethnoecology: Resource Management in Norwegian Lappland.* PhD dissertation, Anthropology, Yale University, New Haven, Connecticut, USA. *Ca.* 850 pp.

This three-volume study of reindeer-herding among sedentary Saami Lapps in northern Norway is based on nearly five years of fieldwork. The author investigated the social organization, folk knowledge and physiographic factors that affect the relationship between the Saami and their physical environment. She examined how these people's knowledge is structured and changes. Pages 708–727 of volume 3, appendix 3, deal especially with reindeer management, including their parasites and diseases. [Annotation based on abstract and table of contents.]

Anderson, Myrdene. 1996. The interpenetration of endogenous and exogenous in Saami reindeer raising. In: Constance M. McCorkle, Evelyn Mathias and Tjaart W. Schillhorn van Veen (eds). *Ethnoveterinary Research & Development.* Intermediate Technology Publications, London, UK. Pp. 91–102.

About 6000 or 10% of the Saami [Lapp] people of Finland, Norway, Sweden and a part of the former USSR depend upon reindeer for a living. They manage half a million head under an extensive, migratory production system. Although Saami reindeer-raising methods have been exogenously regulated to some extent for several centuries, folk husbandry and healthcare beliefs and practices remained largely unchanged until World War II, when government intensified its control over, and medical-model veterinary research on, reindeer-raising. Even though no veterinarians were available at the local level, along with other factors including the Chernobyl explosion of 1986, this new government activism affected traditional practices both positively and negatively, depending upon one's ethnic and market point of view. The result was a syncretism of endogenous and exogenous, traditional and modern stockraising methods. Still today, all aspects of reindeer raising are accompanied by offerings, rituals and magic performed by shamans and ordinary herders to ensure herd health, well-being, and protection from predators. But other things have changed. For example, until WWII, Saami simply followed reindeer on their normal migratory routes, as though the animals were herding the people, rather than vice versa! Only occasionally was it necessary to manoeuvre the herd a bit to direct it to richer forage or away from other herds [and possible disease]. But migration routes were changed or broken by new political boundaries; by the usurpation of traditional grazing grounds for cultivation, recreation, tourism, military activities and infrastructures like roads, snowmobile routes and power plants; and after Chernobyl, by forbidden contaminated areas. Now herders must sometimes truck or ferry animals and hay to distant, approved grazing lands. This makes for less forage all around; greater concentrations of animals, which may favour disease outbreaks; young reindeer who no longer know their own way to seasonal forage; and thus harder and less remunerative work for herders. In terms of herd composition and breeding, Saami traditionally exercised no control other than to cull aged, sick, infertile, lame or special animals (e.g. white ones for making Saami's requisite white-hide wedding costumes). With today's shrinking forage resources, however, herders half-heartedly follow extension recommendations to keep only 5% of male calves as studs, castrating and training the others as draught animals or slaughtering them. 'Half-hearted' because some animals manage to breed before this point, and large herds are a point of prestige and economic security for Saami. Castration techniques have changed from the traditional biting off of the testes with the teeth to the government-mandated use of castration tongs. Likewise slaughter – traditionally a quick knife stab to the neck – now must be preceded by stunning. Nor can Saami now choose when and where to slaughter, if they wish to sell the meat; slaughter must be performed under government supervision [and taxation]. On the other hand, since Chernobyl, demand for reindeer meat and milk has plummeted, leaving Saami themselves to eat excessive quantities of the most contaminated products. A perhaps salubrious government move has been the restriction of ear-notching to the summer months, when surgical complications are less likely. But government also prohibited the harvesting of antler velvet from live animals, even though the market will not accept velvet from shed antlers. The result was greatly diminished herder incomes, due to lower production not only of velvet but also of meat, given that reindeer slaughtered at the time of velvet growth in the spring are so emaciated from the winter. Traditionally, Saami ethnoveterinary efforts centred on trained or pet geldings, because reindeer ethology provided good controls on the larger herd's main health problem of parasitoses: especially warble flies, but also mosquitoes, gnats and midges; and endoparasites of the lungs, brain, intestines, muscles and particularly liver. Reindeer naturally avoid fly-infested areas; when they cannot, they head into the wind, move to smoky areas, or in the absence of wind or smoke, scatter. Reindeer migrations also kept the animals away from the areas most heavily infested with the snail hosts of liver flukes (although Saami management of herd dogs involved in parasite life cycles left much to be desired). But natural escape from such problems is no longer an option, as grazing grounds have shrunk and herd movements have been increasingly confined. Modern medicine tried to fill the gap, with organophosphate treatments for warbles and ivermectin inoculation for flukes. But such measures have so far proved haphazard and overly costly in the face of reaching and handling thousands of head of only semi-tame migratory animals – not to mention the dangers of overdosing, chemoresistance, and environmental damage. Except for trying to direct herds to better forage, both traditionally and today Saami take little trouble with nutrition. When natural forage is scarce, modern Saami may set out mineral blocks and provide supplements; but reindeer do not tolerate sudden changes in feed. Finally, Saami have been beset by the new and frightening animal health and nutrition problem of nuclear fallout, to which neither herders nor government scientists have found fully satisfactory solutions. The Chernobyl incident marked an historic threat to Saami reindeer raising and livelihoods. But it also brought herders, veterinarians and scientists into greater contact, with the result that researchers and government have become better attuned to grassroot needs for appropriate and feasible healthcare and policy interventions, such as: stocking and culling strategies that serve sociocultural as well as economic ends; practical, safe and cost-effective parasite control strategies; and local-level ensilage methods to offset critical forage bottlenecks.

Andriamanga-Rahaga, Norosoa. 1994. Résultats préliminaires sur l'étude de l'efficacité d'une plante anti-parasitaire Malgache. In: Kakule Kasonia and Michel Ansay (eds). ***Métissages en Santé Animale de Madagascar à Haïti: Actes du Séminaire d'Ethnopharmacopée Vétérinaire 'KAGALA', un Partage de Savoirs Burkina-Faso, Ouagadougou, 15–22 Avril 1993.*** Presses Universitaires de Namur, Namur, Belgium. Pp. 243–252.

A list of 18 plant species used in traditional treatments for endoparasites in Madagascar was collected from stockraising families there. A bibliographic and extent-of-use review narrowed this list to 13 promising species. After pharmacological screening of the 13, *Pittosporum* sp. was selected for anthelmintic trials in livestock. These were conducted by the author, a scientist in Madagascar's Department of Zootechnical and Veterinary Research, with help from the National Centre of Pharmaceutical Research. Naturally infected sheep kept under extensive management were utilized. The dried and powdered plant bark was prepared in two ways for oral administration to the trial animals: decoction and infusion. Both preparations were successful in that they produced a diarrhoea which completely evacuated the *Moniezia* eggs, although other parasites (*Strongyles, Coccidies* and *Trichuris*) were noted in the autopsies. The Department now recommends these preparations to farmers for combatting *Moniezia* infestations in their sheep. At a broader level, the author notes the cost-effectiveness and general appropriateness of this testing approach in contrast, on the one hand, to the long, drawn-out and very expensive 'perfectionist method' used in modern pharmaceutical research and, on the other hand, the 'dangerous and simplistic method' (p. 244) of trial-and-error employed by amateur local healers. The approach taken 'can satisfy our [Madagascar's] immediate needs with an acceptable guarantee' (ibid.).

Aniyere, Fatimé. 1994. Ethno-pharmacopée vétérinaire: Vue du Tchad. In: Kakule Kasonia and Michel Ansay (eds). ***Métissages en Santé Animale de Madagascar à Haïti: Actes du Séminaire d'Ethnopharmacopée Vétérinaire 'KAGALA', un Partage de Savoirs Burkina-Faso, Ouagadougou, 15–22 Avril 1993.*** Presses Universitaires de Namur, Namur, Belgium. Pp. 224–228.

In this published collection of papers from the first Africa-wide conference to be held on EVM, this chapter reports on 22 plants used by Chadian Fulani in treating nearly as many livestock diseases. For example, poultry are cured of ectoparasites by placing a few tobacco leaves under the birds' nests. *Citrullus colocynthis* or *Coccinia grandis* is placed in birds' drinking water to cure them of 'green diarrhoea'. An unguent of roasted, powdered locust beans (*Parkia biglobosa*) in groundnut oil relieves dermatophilosis. Respiratory conditions are treated by throwing *Combretum glutinosum* leaves on the fire, for animals to breathe the smoke. Wounds in all animals are disinfected with urine, and may also be dressed with fresh *Calotropis procera* leaves. Various treatments for endoparasites are described. After castration, bulls are given a glass of unsweetened, strong green tea and sheep get half a glass [although the reason for this practice is not recounted].

Anjaria, J.V. 1986. Indigenous drug research – a brief review. Paper presented to the In-Service Training Course of Veterinary Surgeons in Traditional Veterinary Medicine. Veterinary Research Institute, Gannoruwa, Peradeniya, Sri Lanka, October 1986. 21 pp.

The first part of this paper deals with *Leptadenia reticulata*, a herb that stimulates milk production in cows and egg production in hens (see Anjaria 1988). The second part consists of an extensive review of research from India and other Asian countries on indigenous drugs used in folk veterinary medicine. The review includes galactagogues; drugs against reproductive, respiratory and digestive disorders; antifertility drugs; anthelmintics; coagulants; drugs against urinary calculosis; anti-cancer drugs; drugs with analgesic, antirheumatic and anti-inflammatory effects; and antifungal and antiseptic drugs.

Anjaria, J.V. 1987. ***Traditional (Indigenous) Veterinary Medicine Project (Ayurvedic Veterinary Medicine).*** Final report, SL-ADB Livestock Development Project. Veterinary Research Institute, Gannoruwa, Peradeniya, Sri Lanka.

In Sri Lanka, Ayurvedic medicine has long been used to treat horses, elephants and other animals. Presently, about 2000 traditional veterinary physicians are listed with the Ministry of Indigenous Drugs. From January 1986 to January 1987, a project on Ayurvedic veterinary medicine was implemented by the Ministry of Rural Industrial Development with a loan from the Asian Development Bank. The project included the following activities: collection and documentation of information on Ayurvedic drugs for livestock; a survey on ethnoveterinary beliefs and practices in ten districts; investigations and laboratory research on the efficacy of treatments; promotion of the use of indigenous drugs at the production, distribution and user levels; recommendations for the commercialization of manufacturing indigenous drugs; and training of local staff to continue the project after its termination.

Anjaria, Jayvir. 1988. Herbs in therapy of milk and reproductive disorders. *AYU* June: 16–30.

Leptadenia reticulata, a creeper, is mentioned in the ancient Atharva Veda as a tonic, a galactagogue and a remedy for several ailments. The author describes the nomenclature and botanical features of this plant and reviews some chemical and pharmacological investigations. Powdered *Leptadenia* given on 12 consecutive days increases the milk yield in Hariana cows, Murrah buffaloes, Bikaneri sheep, Barbari goats and Gir cows. *Leptadenia* also increases egg production in hens and shows oestrogenic activity in rats and mice.

Anjaria, Jayvir V. 1996. Ethnoveterinary pharmacology in India: Past, present and future. In: Constance M. McCorkle, Evelyn Mathias and Tjaart W. Schillhorn van Veen (eds). ***Ethnoveterinary Research & Development.*** Intermediate Technology Publications, London, UK. Pp. 137–147.

Throughout Asia, modern and traditional medicine exist side-by-side; but there has been an upsurge of interest in the latter, including herbal and other treatments for livestock. This chapter briefly overviews three ancient Indian ethnoveterinary traditions: Ayurveda, Siddha and Unani-Tibb. Then, it presents a sampling of contemporary research on veterinary pharmaceuticals and techniques derived from these ethnomedical systems. A number of such treatments enjoy widespread use either in traditional formulations or as trademarked herbal drugs manufactured by some 80 pharmaceutical houses in India and sold both nationally and internationally. Examples of the latter include drugs for easing milk let-down, stimulating calf growth, increasing yields of milk and eggs, inducing heat, correcting reproductive and urinary disorders in male animals, treating gastrointestinal (including helminth) problems, and combating ectoparasitoses, bacterial infections and inflammations. A highlight of the chapter is its referencing of the scientific research behind the scores of Indian medicinal plants thus employed. The chapter concludes with a discussion of future potentials and problems in creating an even stronger and rural-based but global-oriented industry in ethnoveterinary drugs. Issues addressed include: cost and quality control in herbal drug manufacture; protection and local management of the habitats from which the raw plant materials are collected; rural and national job creation based on ethnoveterinary drug production, sales and clinics; export earnings projections; and the need for more complete and sustained scientific study of ethnoveterinary pharmaceuticals.

Anjaria, J. 1997. Grass-'shoots' man. ***Undhyoo*** 13: page number unavailable.

This short article reports the results of the author's work with SRISTI to create a live herbarium, a specimen collection, a display, a technical database, and a corresponding illustrated catalogue of 250 plants used by poor farmers of India in their ethnoveterinary treatments. [See also Anjaria et al. 1997.]

Anjaria, Jayvir. 1998. Ethnoveterinary research and development (ER&D) in south Asia – An overview. In: E. Mathias, D.V. Rangnekar and C.M. McCorkle, with M. Martin (eds). ***Ethnoveterinary Medicine: Alternatives for Livestock Development – Proceedings of an International Conference Held in Pune, India, 4–6 November 1997. Volume 2: Abstracts.*** BAIF Development Research Foundation, Pune, India. Pp. 2–3.

Traditional veterinary practices have been known in Asia for thousands of years. India, Graeco-Arabia and China have been home to ancient centres of EVM. Some major traditional veterinary medical systems and practices of global importance have been influenced by the Ayurveda, Siddha and Unani-Tibb systems, Chinese barefoot practitioners, acupuncture and herbal folklore. Research on medicinal plants is an important facet of biomedical research. Considerable literature on veterinary herbal drug research has been generated, spanning basic research, pharmacological studies, and clinical trials conducted to systematize and validate ethnoveterinary practices and folklore claims with the goal of applying findings to animal treatment and production. The current state of such studies needs to be surveyed Asia-wide, as many of the same ethnoveterinary practices are known to be used in several Asian countries (especially Bangladesh, Cambodia, China, India, Indonesia, Laos, Malaysia, Myanmar, Nepal, Pakistan, Philippines, Sri Lanka and Thailand). The paper provides an overview of the past, present and future of ER&D in south Asia.

Anjaria, Jayvir, Minoo Parabia, Gauri Bhatt and Ripal Khamar. 1997. *Nature Heals: A Glossary of Selected Medicinal Plants of India.* SRISTI, Indian Institute of Management, Vastrapur, Ahmedabad, India. 50 pp.

This booklet lists approximately 245 plants found in India that are used in human and animal medicine. Listings are arranged in alphabetical order by Latin plant name. For each plant, the booklet presents a line drawing, regional synonyms, the plant parts used, and their constituents, actions and applications. The booklet concludes with references and indices of the plants' local and Latin names.

Anne, HRH the Princess Royal. 1996. Foreword. In: Peter Fry (ed.). *Vetaid Book of Veterinary Anecdotes.* Vetaid, Edinburgh, UK. P. i.

In her foreword to this volume of anecdotes by UK veterinarians practising in Britain and worldwide, Her Royal Highness the Princess Royal comments on a trip she made to Somalia, during which she visited veterinarians working on a project to vaccinate camels and goats. As President of Save the Children Fund (SCF), the Princess noted that veterinarians apparently enjoyed much greater success in delivering vaccinations to livestock than did SCF's human-medical personnel in vaccinating women and children. [Also see Schwabe 1998.] Thus she suggests that veterinarians could be of considerable help in SCF's Extended Programme of Immunisation for women and children who accompany animals to the livestock vaccination points, instead of obliging people to go to separate clinics or meeting places [i.e. intersectoral healthcare delivery].

Anonymous. 1991. Ipil-ipil as dewormer for goats. *Sustainable Agriculture* 3(1): 23.

Ipil-ipil (*Leucaena leucocephala*) is found throughout much of the tropical and subtropical world, where it has a multitude of uses as wood, forage, windbreaks, fertilizer, dye and more. Smallholder goat raisers have discovered that a drench of a paste of 50 to 100 young ipil-ipil seeds in 5 to 8 oz of water makes an excellent dewormer. The drench produces a laxative effect sufficient to kill or expel *Ascaris lumbricoides* and other stomach worms.

Anonymous. 1996. A clove a day can keep piggy OK. *Appropriate Technology* 23(3): 31.

Researchers in Switzerland have been experimenting with swine diets to find out whether the large quantities of antibiotics they are fed are really necessary. One group of test animals was put on an additive-free diet; another group was given its normal quota of antibiotics; and a third was fed garlic supplements. This last group suffered the least from common ailments, and had lower mortality rates than the two other groups. However, it did not put on weight as fast as the antibiotic-fed pigs.

Ansay, Michel and Kakule Kasonia. 1994. Enrichir les savoirs traditionnels. In: Kakule Kasonia and Michel Ansay (eds). *Métissages en Santé Animale de Madagascar à Haïti: Actes du Séminaire d'Ethnopharmacopée Vétérinaire 'KAGALA', un Partage de Savoirs Burkina-Faso, Ouagadougou, 15–22 Avril 1993.* Presses Universitaires de Namur, Namur, Belgium. Pp. 22–28.

This foreword introduces the published proceedings from the first pan-African conference to be held on EVK. The authors note that everywhere, including in Europe, there are many different bodies of local knowledge and ways of knowing, including traditional and modern ones. Exchange among them can have mutually enriching effects. The goal of this first conference on EVK in Africa was to begin to promote such exchange for EVK and to build a network to promote and continue it, using all possible means. Three adjunct conference objectives were: first of all, to rescue fast-disappearing EVK, using a standardized collection technique and disseminating the findings as widely as possible; second, to explore methods and principles for validating EVK; and third, to offer to stockraisers – and to promote renewed recognition and 'valuation' of – ethnoveterinary treatments that have been verified, standardized, and possibly enriched in ways that are of immediate assistance to local healers and stockraisers. Further, all such treatments should meet the criteria of the '4 A's': availability, accessibility, acceptability and adaptability. Also discussed in the introduction are different 'stakeholders' interests in or reservations about EVM. Stakeholders include developers, environmentalists, scientists, and of course livestock healers and producers. Particular emphasis is given to the importance of including healers in all ER&D, as 'Each healer is a whole pharmacy' (p. 26). The authors also recommend the method of total extracts, or 'totum', for verifying identifiable pharmacological effects of ethnomedicines. Beyond this, they raise many provocative questions and research and implementation challenges for stakeholders to consider. For example: Is there such a thing as a universal, or even ethnic, ethnopharmacopoeia? If so, how might these be defined, e.g. botanically or therapeutically? Is therapeutic as well as pharmacological verification of ethnoveterinary treatments always necessary? And, on the basis of what criteria should one choose which ethnomedicines – and which among sometimes multiple variations on a given prescription – to subject to verification? What mechanisms can be put in place to ensure that the fruits of ER&D are returned to healers and stockraisers versus, for example, First World scientists, pharmaceutical companies and animal owners? In conclusion, the authors state that EVM cannot be exempt from assessments of efficacy and safety as well as 'necessity'. Thus, it should be subjected to fair comparison with Western veterinary medicine in these regards. But the larger goal is a 'progressive independence in veterinary inputs' such that each culture can safely 'drink at its own well' of EVK (p. 27).

ANTHRA. 1998. Farmers' perception of ethnoveterinary medicine. In: E. Mathias, D.V. Rangnekar and C.M. McCorkle, with M. Martin (eds). *Ethnoveterinary Medicine: Alternatives for Livestock Development – Proceedings of an International Conference Held in Pune, India, 4–6 November 1997. Volume 2: Abstracts.* BAIF Development Research Foundation, Pune, India. Pp. 4–5.

ANTHRA (an Indian women's veterinary NGO) surveyed over 400 farm families from approximately 54 villages in India's Andhra Pradesh and Maharashtra States on their perceptions of EVM. The aim was to study the relevance and relative importance of local systems of animal healthcare across different regions. Almost all interviewees had used ethnoveterinary treatments at some time. Specific treatments were identified for some 60 diseases of livestock, including horses and poultry. Farmers said they use EVM mainly because: modern veterinary doctors and facilities are not available near their villages or, if available, charge enormous fees; commercial drugs (including vaccinations) do not always work, and sometimes they create new and even more severe health problems, e.g. when wrongly selected or administered or when unclean injection needles are used; and ethnoveterinary medicines resulted in more permanent cures. EVK and its use differed greatly across and within regions, and also by gender and age within a community. For example, women preferred traditional medicines; and they were more knowledgeable than men about such remedies for routine diseases, care of young or pregnant and lactating animals and poultry. Traditional stockraisers like the Dhangars were more knowledgeable about surgical conditions like fractures and snake bite. Younger members of the community had neither the knowledge nor the experience to practice EVM effectively. Although a distinct preference for EVM was noted overall, many interviewees expressed increasing difficulty in practising it, due to: the growing scarcity of medicinal plants; the time required to prepare ethnomedicines; the lack of traditional cures for emerging diseases like enterotoxaemia in cattle; excessive use of agricultural chemicals, such that stock do not respond to treatments; and confusion between superstitious beliefs (*bhoot vaidya*) and ethnoveterinary treatments. Most farmers expressed a desire to learn more about the proper use and application of ethnoveterinary practices as these were economically, socially and culturally more acceptable for marginalized communities. Farmers also suggested some ways to disseminate EVK.

ANTHRA Team. 1999. Community-based research on local knowledge systems: The ANTHRA project on ethnoveterinary research. In: E. Mathias, D.V. Rangnekar and C.M. McCorkle, with M. Martin (eds). *Ethnoveterinary Medicine: Alternatives for Livestock Development – Proceedings of an International Conference Held in Pune, India, 4–6 November 1997. Volume 1: Selected Papers.* BAIF Development Research Foundation, Pune, India. Pp. 13–18.

Since May 1996, ANTHRA has been involved in an extensive research project on traditional veterinary and husbandry practices in rural communities of India, with an emphasis on gender issues and the role of women in stockraising. The project's overall goal is to understand and integrate useful EVM, and its practitioners, into on-going livestock development programmes. To understand differences across agroecozones, this research is being undertaken in six regions of Andhra Pradesh and Maharashtra. The study also notes differences in practices across communities, castes and livestock species. A key feature of this effort is training community-based researchers and fieldworkers to document local knowledge pertaining to animal healthcare, nutrition, breeding, local production systems and product markets. Documentation techniques include written records, case histories, PRAs, photography and herbaria. Information from the different regions is shared with the communities through audiovisual aids presented at village *yatras* and fairs. Local experts in livestock healthcare have greatly aided the documentation process with their unique insights, and ANTHRA is now compiling a healers' directory. While documentation has been precise, it has also been slow, as fieldworkers are new to keeping records and time schedules for this kind of task. Nevertheless, this overall approach has had several advantages. For one, trainees are present in their villages throughout the year; thus documentation reflects seasonal variations. For another, people are more willing to talk and share information with someone they know and recognize; and language barriers do not exist. Relatedly, the process evokes a lot of local interest, stimulating debate among local communities about their problems. Local-level documentation also contributes to the beginnings of a community register to safeguard local rights to local knowledge and prevent its appropriation for ends that do not benefit the source community. The project has also helped younger members of the community to appreciate their legacy of biodiverse environmental resources, and how these can be used to strengthen rural livelihoods. The same documentalist fieldworkers have also been trained in primary animal healthcare; this means that someone is on-the-spot to address emergencies such as outbreaks of a livestock disease. Overall, having local fieldworkers has helped win acceptance of the study, the programme, and ANTHRA as an organization.

Apantaku, Samson O. 1998. Indigenous knowledge and uses of forest plant products for controlling crop pests in Ogun State (Nigeria). *Indigenous Knowledge and Development Monitor* 6(1): 27.

In describing a number of botanicals used to combat crop pests in Nigeria, this article also mentions Nigerians' preventive practice of planting tobacco in and around the farmyard and poultry coops in order to repel snakes from people and livestock. The author notes that, based on testing to date, about 65% of such biological controls prove to be effective. Wherever the agroecology permits, such environmentally friendly and inexpensive controls should be incorporated into extension packages to benefit wider groups of resource-poor farmers.

Araujo, F.P. , C.W. Schwabe, J.C. Sawyer and W.G. Davis. 1975. Hydatid disease transmission in California: A study of the Basque connection. *American Journal of Epidemiology* 102(4): 291–302.

Basque shepherds from Spain and France practise transhumant sheep husbandry in California. This study examined the impact of these shepherds' husbandry practices on the incidence of hydatidosis in both sheep and people. The disease is caused by infestations of the tapeworm *Echinococcus granulosus*. Most of the shepherds interviewed were unaware of this parasite's existence and of its transmission via dog faeces. They classified all sheep diseases characterized by weight loss simply as *errezelatu*. Hydatidosis often falls in this category, and thus has no special name in the Basque language. Transmission of the disease is promoted by dogs eating the meat of infected sheep then defaecating in the pastures, where sheep can become re-infected by consuming egg-infested faeces or water. Indeed, it was found that the shepherds' dogs subsisted almost entirely on dead sheep, many of which had expired from hydatidosis. This case offers an example of a serious lack in local knowledge of disease transmission.

Arévalo T., Francisco and Hernando Bazalar R. 1986. Ensayo de la eficacia contra Fasciola hepatica de la shepita y alcachofa en ovinos altoandinos naturalmente infectados. Paper presented to the Vth Congreso sobre Agricultural Andina, Puno, Perú. Pp. 111–118.

This is an early, partial version of a much expanded and refined chapter on the subject in Bazalar and McCorkle 1989.

Arévalo, Francisco and Hernando Bazalar. 1989a. Eficacia antihelmíntica de la semilla de zapallo. In: Hernando Bazalar and Constance M. McCorkle (eds). *Estudios Etnoveterinarios en Comunidades Altoandinas del Perú.* Lluvia Editores, Lima, Perú. Pp. 111–118.

Stomach and gut worms are a perennial problem worldwide. People of highland Peru have long employed the seeds of the giant squash *Cucurbita maxima* Duch to alleviate such problems in both humans and animals. This chapter reports the results of SR-CRSP on-farm participatory trials to test the effectiveness of a suspension of ground squash seeds against six species of gastrointestinal worms commonly found in *criollo* sheep. Necropsies revealed high parasite mortality rates ranging between 78% and 80% for the species studied. Faecal egg counts showed reductions of 74% and 80% in parasite loads on days 7 and 14 post-treatment; for controls, these figures were only 14% and 5%. The authors note that equivalent commercial drugs cost approximately US $0.20 per animal, whereas the squash seeds have very little market value. As in other chapters in this volume, they also emphasize the fact that such locally-inspired remedies are much easier for peasant stockowners to understand and access. They also allow villagers more control over product quality because they need not rely on the unscrupulous merchants of an oppressive, superordinate ethnic group who often foist off out-of-date or contra-indicated drugs on their peasant clients.

Arévalo, Francisco and Hernando Bazalar. 1989b. Eficacia de la alcachofa y jaya-shipita contra alicuya (Fasciola hepatica). In: Hernando Bazalar and Constance M. McCorkle (eds). *Estudios Etnoveterinarios en Comunidades Altoandinas del Perú.* Lluvia Editores, Lima, Perú. Pp. 99–108.

This chapter reports the success of participatory on-farm experiments conducted by the SR-CRSP in a Peruvian peasant community to test the efficacy of two indigenous Andean treatments for ovine liver fluke. These consisted of drenching with an infusion of an as yet unidentified highland plant known as *jaya-shipita* in mineral oil, or with a decoction of fresh artichoke leaves (*Cynara scolymus*) with oil and salt. Post-treatment necropsies showed that both preparations are highly effective against adult flukes, with mortality rates of 84% and 89%, respectively. Faecal egg counts were also significantly reduced, averaging a drop of 67.5% and 71% respectively at days 7 and 14 after treatment; for the control group, this figure ranged between only 13% and 20%. Also, there were measurable weight gains in the treated group. Further research is indicated on the precise dosage and frequency of treatments and on more rapid and convenient ways to apply them. In contrasting these indigenous treatments with comparable commercial products, the authors note that the latter are less labour-intensive but much more expensive and of uncertain supply.

Argueta Villamar, Arturo. 1988. Medicina popular, animales de traspatio y etno-zoología en México. In: Luz Lozano Nathal and Gerardo López Buendía (co-ordinators). *Memorias: Primera Jornada sobre Herbolaria Medicinal en Veterinaria.* Universidad Nacional Autónoma de México, Facultad de Medicina Veterinaria y Zootecnia, Coordinación de Educación Continua, México DF. Pp. 164–177.

This essay presents a brief overview of the position of animal domesticates in Mexico's history and reviews several key works in Mexican ethnoveterinary and ethnozoological research [see Esquivel 1982, and Rangel and Ortiz 1985] along with McCorkle's 1986 introductory article. The author concludes with a plea for animal health and husbandry systems that are truly appropriate to rural Mexican peoples and ecologies, rather than unworkable alien technologies that increase dependency.

Arowolo, R.O. and M.A. Awoyele. 1982. Traditional methods of veterinary practice in south western Nigeria. *Proceedings of the Workshop on Traditional African Medicine, March 1982 at the University of Ibadan, Ibadan, Nigeria.* Pp. 11–13.

The authors distributed questionnaires about traditional veterinary practices to students and staff of institutions in Ibadan, civil servants, farmers, traders, drivers, tailors, carpenters and goat and sheep sellers. A total of 184 people was question-naired or personally interviewed. Only 29 of the 184 had absolutely no comment on traditonal treatments. From the other 155, a list of prescriptions was compiled, divided into three categories by animal species: sheep and goats, dogs and cats, and fowl. For each category, several diseases are listed, each with more than one pre-scription for its prevention or cure. Examples of *materia medica* included cobwebs, kola nuts, oranges, palm oil and soap. For PPR or goat catarrhal fever, two orally-administered prescriptions are noted: a mixture of ground alligator-pepper and locally brewed gin; and a decoction of *Vernonia amygdalina* leaves mixed with palm wine. The survey findings show that farmers can correctly diagnose a number of livestock diseases and effectively treat them using local ingredients. Some informants reported that certain traditional preparations were even more effective than veterinarians' treatments.

Asad, Talal. 1964. Seasonal movements of the Kababish Arabs of northern Kordofan. *Sudan Notes and Records* 45: 48–58.

Sudan's Kababish pastoralists herd camels, sheep and goats, and keep cattle, donkeys, horses, dogs and chickens. Kababish do not buy animals for breeding purposes; rather, they borrow them to improve strains. During the sheep breeding season, shepherds have to assist most rams to cover the fat-tailed ewes. Lambing also demands human assistance. At the start of the rainy season, Kababish migrate to new pastures, leaving the reserve pastures (*damar*) that have been intensively grazed during the dry season – and where disease pathogens may have built up – to recover. During the migration, information about the state of water and grazing ahead is always obtained. Towards the end of the rainy season, Kababish congre-gate at water points with their herds. They weigh several health-related factors in choosing where to camp. For example, large bodies of water ensure a more plenti-ful and prolonged supply of water for livestock, but they foul more quickly, thus increasing disease risk; also, such areas are more quickly overgrazed and experience a more rapid buildup of pathogens in grazing grounds.

Ashdown, Stephen and John Smith. 1999. Community-based animal healthcare and ethnoveterinary medicine in Sudan. In: E. Mathias, D.V. Rangnekar and C.M. McCorkle, with M. Martin (eds). ***Ethnoveterinary Medicine: Alternatives for Livestock Development – Proceedings of an International Conference Held in Pune, India, 4–6 November 1997. Volume 1: Selected Papers.*** BAIF Development Research Foundation, Pune, India. Pp. 19–24.

Since 1984, Operation Lifeline Sudan (OLS) has provided emergency veterinary relief to stockraisers in Sudan. Operated by a variety of NGOs and a small UNICEF team, the programme has established a CBAH system throughout most of southern Sudan in rebel-held areas and, to a lesser extent, in inaccessible government-controlled regions of the north. CBAH services are founded on training community members, thereby affirming their own skills and knowledge of disease while enhancing their ability to use modern medicines safely and effectively. OLS studies, initiated in 1996, on the extent of herbal medicines and other traditional practices in southern Sudan revealed considerable knowledge and use of herbs throughout the project area. For example, Arab tribes of southern Darfur are particularly skilled in the use of complex herbal remedies, which they often purchase in preference to modern drugs available in local pharmacies. This paper compares findings from the 1996 studies with information gathered later on herbal medicine for both animals and humans in the north. In conjunction with his training in herbal medicine and work with alternative veterinary medicine in the UK, the author concludes that – when combined with nutritional, husbandry and environmental improvements – non-conventional veterinary practices can provide high-quality animal healthcare. Thus it is important for developers in places like Sudan to understand and incorporate traditional health practices into new delivery systems. This will be of benefit not only to resource-poor pastoral peoples but also to the human and animal health sectors in richer nations, where new ideas and medicines to improve health services are also being sought.

Ashton, Hugh. 1952. ***The Basuto.*** Oxford University Press, for the International African Institute, London, UK.

The Basuto of South Africa are pastoralists who herd cattle, sheep, horses and donkeys. Chapter 9 of the above-referenced volume discusses Basuto animal husbandry, seasonal transhumance patterns and veterinary lore. Castration is described, as are remedies for fractures, impotence, diarrhoea and horse bots. Fractures are splinted, and the bone near the break is injected with an unspecified medicine through a hollow reed. To cure impotence in bulls, the animals are made to jump their kraal wall while a herdboy sings to them. If this fails, the bull is stabbed above the anus with a stiff grass smeared with the medicine *motsoso*, and the tail is rubbed with more of the medicine. A form of cattle sterilization consists of thrusting a heated stone into the vagina of a barren cow. This cauterizes the *os cervix* and thus prevents the discharge of oestral fluid. The procedure makes the cow suitable as a traction animal. A general protective medicine called *kubetso* is sprinkled on glowing coals placed in the kraal to fumigate cattle. There are also protective medicines for specific dangers; for example, hunters may 'vaccinate' their dogs against snake bite. To prevent supernaturally caused diseases, accidents and general bad luck with livestock, medicine is placed at kraal entrances, especially if sorcery is suspected. Flocks and herds may also be 'vaccinated' against lightning, predators and sorcery in the same way that Basuto vaccinate themselves at the beginning of each year.

Atkinson, V.T., W. Dickson and W.H. Harbaugh *et al* (eds). 1942. *Special Report on Diseases of Cattle*. US Government Printing Office, Washington DC. 507 pp.

Among other things, this US government report notes a variety of on-farm measures that, as of the first half of the 20th century, American cattlemen themselves were using themselves to ensure herd health. The first chapter outlines modes of treatment administration. Next discussed are diseases of the digestive organs. Puncture of the rumen [presumably to relieve bloat] is mentioned. The section on poisoning addresses toxins in feedstuffs and toxic range plants of North America. Therapies involved changing the patient's feed and liberally dosing with purgatives such as castor oil, linseed oil or Epsom salts. A coal-oil drench was sometimes given for endoparasites, although coal oil is toxic in large quantities. Other home treatments for endoparasites included mild stimulants such as aromatic spirits of ammonia, soft feeds and mucilaginous drinks. Concerning ectoparasites, lice were removed using a brush or cloth to cover the body with a thin, even coating of any of the following: kerosene mixed with lard, petrol, nicotine and coal-tar/creosote dips. Ear ticks were prevented for a month by injecting a mixture of pine tar and cottonseed oil into the ears with a syringe. A heart condition successfully treated by stockraisers is the pericarditis often associated with pneumonia, pleurisy, rheumatism and other constitutional diseases. The ailing animal was kept in a quiet, comfortable place, free from excitement and wrapped in warm blankets; its legs were rubbed to restore circulation and then snugly bandaged; and it was given nutritious but moderate quantities of feed. Cattle with catarrh [a headcold] were housed in well-ventilated and hygienic quarters, warmly blanketed, and given hot medicated inhalations and sometimes also a drench of Epsom salts via a stomach tube. A commonly recommended treatment for encephalitis (inflammation of the brain) was bloodletting, performed by drawing off a gallon [4.4 l] of blood from the jugular of an average-sized animal. Thereafter, the animal could be given an enema of warm water mixed with common salt or soapsuds, provided with drinking water *ad libitum*, and allowed no feed other than bran slops in small quantities, or cut-and-carried grass, if in season. Animals with diarrhoea from haemoglobin-urea (also known as 'redwater') were drenched with olive or linseed oil, and sometimes also given an enema of a heaping teaspoonful of table salt in approximately 1 l of warm water. Some of the instruments used in difficult labour are diagrammed, including embryotomes – long, short, straight and curved knives used to cut away parts of a dead or unwanted foetus so it can be extracted from the uterus. In dystocia, cords were used to pull out the foetus by the legs or head if necessary. To staunch bleeding of the navel in newborn calves, the navel was cauterized with alum, copper or a red-hot iron rod. After injuries sustained in calving, cows were injected intra-uterine with a mild antiseptic solution and warm salt water, and then fed iron sulphate and ground ginger. A mustard poultice on the right flank cured metritis. Bone brittleness was avoided by supplying mineral-rich feeds such as beans, cowpea, alfalfa, clover, oats, cottonseed meal, wheat bran or bonemeal mixed with salt to increase its palatability. Fractures were treated with padded wooden splints; thereafter, the patient was kept as quiet as possible and given feeds that kept the bowels working smoothly. The chapter on surgical operations describes techniques of dehorning, tracheotomy, rumenotomy, castration, spaying, and treatment of wounds and abscesses. Tumours such as lipomas [a cluster of fat cells] were removed by ligature or excision with a knife. Goitre called for giving iodine, completely changing the diet, and regularly exercising the animal in the open air. Snake-bite swellings were bathed with ammonia water and frequently thereafter with hot water. Boils were covered with camphor oil twice or thrice daily or poulticed in order to 'ripen' them before popping the boils and draining the pus. Feeds such as linseed meal, bran, ground oats and clean hay cured the seborrhoea, dandruff, or scurf that afflicts cattle wintered indoors. Foot problems such as soreness were treated with rest and wet-clay poultices. Animals with an inflamed cornea were put in a darkened stable, and their eyes washed with a solution of silver nitrate; they were also fed green feed and a sodium sulphate solution, sometimes along with a tonic of iron sulphate, gentian and ginger. Ear lacerations (often from dog bites) were treated by fastening the torn edges of the ear with silver wire, catgut or strong linen thread and then dressing the tear with pine tar. A priority in infectious diseases is, of course, disinfection. Commonly used disinfectants were quicklime, chlorinated lime, carbolic acid, mercury compounds, formaldehyde, cresol and lye (sodium hydroxide).

Attfield, Harlan H.D. 1990. *Raising Chickens and Ducks.* VITA (Volunteers in Technical Assistance) Publications Services, Arlington, Virginia, USA. 140 pp.

One chapter in this volume (pp. 73–86) describes a techno-blended adaptation of the ancient Chinese rice-husk incubation system used for centuries throughout much of southeast Asia to produce ducklings. The slightly modified and updated system described is still labour-intensive, but it requires few and inexpensive inputs and it can yield large numbers of ducklings for market. Besides fertilized eggs, materials needed are housing, bamboo mats and cylinders, wood and bamboo boxes, rice husks, cloth and a kerosene stove and lamp. The eggs are washed, marked with a date in pen, bundled in cloth, and heated in the sun or safely above the kerosene stove. The bundles are placed in the bamboo cylinders between bags of heated rice husk. The eggs are turned every morning and evening for 4 days, after which they are candled and the infertile ones discarded. New eggs may be added to the bundles. The husk is reheated every time the eggs are turned. By the 14th day, the eggs themselves generate sufficient heat. On the 17th day they are transferred to the incubation bed, which consists of a flat mat insulated with rice husk. There, the eggs are turned four times a day. On day 26, the first batch should begin to crack their shells. Two days later the ducklings will have hatched.

Aubert, Ivonne. 1988. Antecedentes históricos de algunas plantas medicinales utilizadas como antidiarréticos en animales domésticos. In: Luz Lozano Nathal and Gerardo López Buendía (coordinators). *Memorias: Primera Jornada sobre Herbolaria Medicinal en Veterinaria.* Universidad Nacional Autónoma de México, Facultad de Medicina Veterinaria y Zootecnia, Coordinación de Educación Continua, México DF. Pp. 12–22.

This paper presents the results of bibliographic research on ten plants reported as effective antidiarrhoeal agents in both Old and New World ethnoveterinary pharmacopoeia. For each plant, the author gives the scientific name, synonyms, a brief physical description, historical background, and information about its administration and use with different animal species. The ten plants are: *Acacia catechu*,

Anthemis nobilis, *Castanea vulgaris* (chestnut), *Ceratonia siliqua* (*algarrobo*), *Hordeum vulgare* (barley), *Lythrum salicaria*, *Oryza sativa* (rice), *Papaver somniferum* (poppy), *Polygonum bistorta* and *Quercus robur ilex* (holm oak).

Auró Angulo, Ana and Héctor Sumano López. 1988. Uso de la manzanilla (*Helenium quadridentatum*) para el tratamiento de la saprolegniasis (*Saprolegnia* spp.) en tilapias (*Tylapia mossambica*): Estudio comparativo con la acriflavina. In: Luz Lozano Nathal and Gerardo López Buendía (coordinators). ***Memorias: Primera Jornada sobre Herbolaria Medicinal en Veterinaria.*** Universidad Nacional Autónoma de México, Facultad de Medicina Veterinaria y Zootecnia, Coordinación de Educación Continua, México DF. Pp. 90–95.

Manzanilla is a popular item in Latin American ethnopharmacopoeia that contains natural fungicides. This study compares the efficacy of a *manzanilla* extract with acriflavin, the orthodox but very expensive treatment of choice to combat the constant problem of saprolegniasis in fish farms. Preliminary findings indicate that the *manzanilla* treatment is statistically as effective as acriflavin. The authors believe that, with further research, *manzanilla* extracts could prove *more* effective than such costly commercial products.

Ávila Cazorla, Edgar, Victor Bustinza Choque and Salustio Jiménez. 1985a. Estracto [sic] etanólico del tarwi (*Lupinus mutabilis*) en el tratamiento de la sarna de alpacas. In: Victor Bustinza Ch. et al. (eds). ***Proyecto Piel de Alpaca: Informe Final.*** Universidad Nacional del Altiplano (UNA), Instituto de Investigaciones para el Desarrollo Social del Altiplano (IIDSA), Convenio UNA-NUFFIC, Puno, Perú. Pp. 85–89.

Because of the high cost of commercial pharmaceuticals and of dipping structures, community-level producers in the Andes turn to their indigenous technologies to control ectoparasitism in their herd animals. This chapter describes research on the effectiveness of using *tarwi* to treat ectoparasites in sheep [see also Avila Cazorla et al. 1985b, Jiménez et al. 1983, PRATEC 1988b, Sánchez n.d., and Tillman 1983]. The method tested was modified by scientists from an indigenous practice. One group of mange-ridden alpaca were topically treated with an ethanol extract of *tarwi*; another group of the same number were treated with a spray of the extract. Results revealed that while both treatments were effective, the spray was much faster-acting. It reduced the parasite count to zero by day 5 of the treatment program, whereas the topical applications did not reach this figure until the experiment's end, at day 30. Comparing their results with those of other studies on commercial products, the authors find that the *tarwi* extract is a more effective ectoparasiticide for alpaca. They attribute this to the nine alkaloids and the nicotiana found in *tarwi*, and the fact that these elements have multiple beneficial effects (cardiotonic, anti-inflammatory and disinfectant).

Avila Cazorla, Edgar, Victor Bustinza and Rómulo Sapana. 1985b. Alternativas de tratamiento de la sarna de alpacas. In: Victor Bustinza Ch. et al. (eds). ***Proyecto Piel de Alpaca: Informe Final.*** Universidad Nacional del Altiplano (UNA), Instituto de Investigaciones para el Desarrollo Social del Altiplano (IIDSA), Convenio UNA-NUFFIC, Puno, Perú. Pp. 90–98.

The alpaca is the greatest source of wealth for the high-Andean producer. But this wealth is threatened by *sarna*, a highly contagious ectoparasitic mange that causes terrific economic losses. Control of this disease through standard commercial products has proved disappointing. This chapter evaluates seven such products vis-a-vis two treatments with *tarwi* compounds based on indigenous therapies for *sarna*. *Tarwi* is an indigenous food plant of the high Andes [see also Avila Cazorla et al. 1985a, Jiménez et al. 1983, PRATEC 1988b, Sánchez n.d., and Tillman 1983]. A total of 150 infected alpaca divided into nine groups were treated, each with a different therapy. The authors conclude that the *tarwi* treatments – some of which are readily prepared at home – constitute a cost-effective alternative to purchased pharmaceuticals, particularly since none of the human food value of *tarwi* is lost in extracting the ectoparasiticide. They further note that, unlike equivalent commercial products, the *tarwi* compounds are entirely non-toxic. However, they warn that in cases of severe infestation, of the nine therapies tested, only three (all commercial drugs) were 100% successful. They also note that the effectiveness of several of these therapies in part depends upon management practices – whether, as in large-scale alpaca enterprises, the animals are sheared annually; or whether, as in community-level production systems, they are sheared only once every 2 to 3 years, thus making early detection of infestation difficult.

Ba, Abou Sidi. 1982. *L'Art Vétérinaire des Pasteurs Sahéliens.* Environnement Africain: Cahiers d'Étude du Milieu et d'Aménagement du Territoire. Série Études et Recherches No. 73–82 (July 1982). ENDA, Dakar, Senegal. 98 pp.

Based on interviews and observations in 18 villages and 30 camps, this report details animal husbandry and veterinary arts among the Fulani in southern Mauritania and the bordering areas of Mali and Senegal. It also gives background information on climate, ecology, culture and how Fulani interpret their environment, plus the meaning of cattle in Fulani life. The author discusses the herders' knowledge of the reproductive physiology of their livestock; their criteria for selection of sires; breeding, obstetrical practices and calf rearing; and milk and meat production. He presents the clinical symptoms, treatments and possible Western diagnoses for some 72 disease conditions and lists medicinal, poisonous and lactogenic plants. This study shows that the Fulani have detailed knowledge of the reproductive physiology and diseases of their animals. Their ethnoveterinary treatments and practices include herbal medicines and other remedies, cauterization, bloodletting, obstetrical manipulations, castration, surgical methods and indigenous techniques of vaccination against CBPP.

Ba, Abou Sidi. 1984. *L'Art Vétérinaire en Milieu Traditionnel Africain.* Imprimerie Express Tirages for Agence de Coopération Culturelle et Technique, Paris, France. 136 pp.

This is a slightly revised version of Ba 1982. Both publications are based on the author's doctoral dissertation in veterinary medicine.

Bâ, A.S. 1994a. L'art vétérinaire et la pharmacopée traditionelle en Afrique sahélienne. *Revue Scientifique et Technique de l'Office International des Épizooties* 13(2): 373–396.

This article describes traditional Fulani pharmaceuticals for livestock, including seven toxic and five medicinal plants plus more than 50 locally named and recognized pathologies common to cattle, small ruminants, horses, camels and poultry.

The pathologies are classed by: infectious diseases; abscesses, tumours, wounds and other traumas; nutritional conditions; and species-specific ailments. Where known and relevant, for each ill the author describes: the clinical and post-mortem signs and the modes of transmission Fulani recognize; the corresponding therapies and prophylaxes, and herders' estimation of their effectiveness; and any special measures taken in handling the carcasses or meat of diseased animals. To take one example, a horse suffering from pasteurellosis with nasal symptoms is given a smoke treatment that involves burning paper in a grain-milling mortar over which the animal's muzzle is positioned; alternatively, the patient's nosebag may be filled with the buds and leaves of freshly pounded *Boscia senegalensis*. After a few minutes of inhaling the smoke or aroma, the horse's sinuses should clear.

Ba, Abou Sidi. 1994b. L'ethnomédecine vétérinaire africaine. In: Kakule Kasonia and Michel Ansay (eds). *Métissages en Santé Animale de Madagascar à Haïti: Actes du Séminaire d'Ethnopharmacopée Vétérinaire 'KAGALA', un Partage de Savoirs Burkina-Faso, Ouagadougou, 15–22 Avril 1993.* Presses Universitaires de Namur, Namur, Belgium. Pp. 41–56.

Part I of this chapter discusses and illustrates (mainly from present-day Fulani) the general components of African EVM and muses about its origins, including healers' and stockraisers' trial-and-error plus their empirical observation of animal foraging behaviour in their search for ethnoveterinary medicines. In the last regard, of particular note are certain plants (*Andropogon gayanus*, *Commelina forskalei*, *Ipomoea cairica*) that, via observation of lactating females' grazing them, herders saw could increase the quality and quantity of ruminant milk production. Also described are various indigenous vaccinations. Part II turns to an analysis of the current state of EVM in Africa, as it co-exists with an at-first colonially-imposed modern veterinary medicine. While the latter clearly has brought some benefits to stockraisers who can access and afford it, modern medicine has also raised some new problems, such as: the denigration of often-valuable EVK; the misuse of modern medicine in the hands of people unfamiliar with it; and relatedly, the spectre of chemoresistance. Overall, however, the author opines that the two medical traditions can, and should, be complementary. Part III turns to the future and limits of ethnomedicine for both humans and livestock in Africa. Here are noted the many advantages of ethnomedicine, such as its familiarity and hence general safety, ease of preparation and use, low or no cost, accessibility and free circulation (in contrast to a dangerous contraband traffic in commercial drugs). Disadvantages include: lack of standardization in preparation and posology; little understanding of how traditional and modern medicines may interact when both are administered to a single patient; and lack of formal recognition and support for, and sometimes even government criminalization of, EVM. In conclusion, the author offers an action agenda for addressing some of these disadvantages, including e.g.: consciousness-raising and official recognition of the value of EVM and its practitioners; participatory action research that involves practitioners and transfers research skills to them; and increased protection and/or cultivation of medicinal plants.

Ba, Abou Sidi. 1994c. Recommandations. In: Kakule Kasonia and Michel Ansay (eds). *Métissages en Santé Animale de Madagascar à Haïti: Actes du Séminaire d'Ethnopharmacopée Vétérinaire 'KAGALA', un Partage de Savoirs Burkina-Faso, Ouagadougou, 15–22 Avril 1993.* Presses Universitaires de Namur, Namur, Belgium. Pp. 41–56.

Four kinds of recommendations are made in this conclusion to the proceedings of the first conference on EVM in Africa. First are recommendations directed to conference participants themselves. These centre on widely disseminating information about the conference's outcomes and on creating and supporting national-level networks of EVM 'cells'. For such cells as already exist, greater interdisciplinarity in membership and action is recommended, along with the elaboration of concrete EVK research, training, extension and consciousness-raising projects, including the establishment of national databanks on EVM and national reference herbaria for ethnoveterinary botanicals. Also noted is the need for: better strategy formulation, structural organization, publication and outreach efforts, and so forth within such cells; and their obligation to do more to support the profession of traditional healers and to encourage people to cultivate medicinal plants. To the larger, Africa-wide EVK network, recommendations include, e.g.: building an Africa-wide databank on the subject, and making it readily available to all national cells; coordinating and communicating about and among all the cells; seeking donor funding for projects. To African governments, conference participants recommend: creation of official R&D units focused on EVM; provision of financial, material and other kinds of support to the national cells; elaboration of legislation to encourage and support EVM and its practitioners; and utilization of the mass media to disseminate EVK.

Baekbo, Poul and Knut Nielsen. 1994. Immunization of pregnant sows by feeding faeces from piglets with diarrhea: Attempt to prevent diarrhea in suckling pigs. *Swine Updates* Jan: 8–9.

Based on a total of 2247 litters born across 2 years, this study investigated the possibility of preventing diarrhoea in suckling piglets by feeding sows in late pregnancy with faeces from other piglets with diarrhoea. This procedure may be regarded as a form of autogeneous oral vaccination with prevailing pathogens that induces colostral immunity. Although no statistically significant differences emerged between test and control groups of sows and gilts along a number of parameters relating to diarrhoea, there was a 'remarkable' (p. 9) tendency to more live-born pigs in the test group. Also, the incidence of diarrhoea did not increase in the test group, nor were any gastrointestinal disorders recorded in this group. [Also see Ellefson 1993.]

Baerts, Martine and Jean Lehmann, with Salvator Ntore. 1989. Deuxième partie: Médecine vétérinaire traditionnelle dans la région des crêtes Zaire-Nil au Burundi. In: M. Baerts and J. Lehmann (eds). *Guérisseurs et Plantes Médicinales dans la Région des Crêtes Zaire-Nil au Burundi. Annales Sciences Economiques du Musée Royal de l'Afrique Centrale* 18: 57–125.

This report focuses on plants used in EVM as identified during a larger study of Burundian medicinal plants generally. First, methods of data collection and of healer-informant selection are detailed, along with the content of the questionnaire that was administered. The latter spanned: names of healer and translator; place and date of interview; plant name in Kirundi, with scientific name to be added later; plant part(s) utilized; their preparation (ground, decoction, infusion, maceration, juice, unguent, powder, ash); mode of administration (bath, drink, cataplasm or compress, friction, fumigation, instillation, wash, scarification); symptoms treated and Kirundi disease name; treatment effects; whether the plant is used alone or in a polyprescription; and accompanying rites, ceremonies or incantations. The remainder of the document presents the findings, organized in three parts: a list of the plants identified, ordered by family and with accompanying lexical, preparation, etc. information; a lexicon of primary disease names and synonyms, as per healers' descriptions; and a summary of current practices, including mention of surgical and obstetric techniques as well as herbal medicines. Some concluding observations of interest are as follow. The ten most frequently mentioned diseases – and thus those which healers treat most often – fall into three types: ECF, which is the only microbial problem healers attempt to cure but which appears to constitute 20% of their caseloads; parasite-, serpent- and insect-related ills (e.g. diarrhoea, snakebite, worms); and reproductive ailments (e.g. retained placenta, vaginal prolapse, agalactia, refusal to nurse). If one discounts diseases unique to livestock (like ECF), then nearly 30% of all ethnoveterinary prescriptions cited are also used for humans. There is much greater consistency across healers in their use of traditional veterinary, versus human, medicines. The authors hypothesize that this may be because many more medicaments are brought to bear in Burundian ethnomedicine for humans in order to treat numerous psychosomatic ills, to which Burundians do not consider animals subject. Overall, many more health problems were cited for humans (96) than for livestock (37). The authors also feel that fewer magical elements and 'family secrets' are involved in Burundian veterinary, as versus human, medicine. Also in contrast to human ethnomedicine, the origin of veterinary treatments can be more readily distinguished as having come from pastoral versus horticultural groups, with the former contributing the majority of such treatments, perhaps as a result of ancient migrations. In any case, taken together, these considerations suggest the existence of a recognizable body of Burundian EVM, whereas the same cannot be said for Burundian medicine for humans.

Baerts, Martine and Jean Lehmann. 1991. Plantes medicinales vétérinaires de la region des crêtes Zaire Nil au Burundi. *Annales Sciences Economiques du Musée Royale de l'Afrique Centrale* 21. 134 pp.

See Baerts and Lehmann, 1989.

Baerts, Martine and Jean Lehmann. 1993. L'utilisation de quelques plantes médicinales au Burundi. *Annales Sciences Economiques du Musée Royal de l'Afrique Centrale* 23. 158 pp.

A 5-year-long survey of 129 healers (27 of livestock) in Burundi resulted in the collection of 5696 medicinal plants (791 for ethnoveterinary purposes) employed in 2729 recipes for curing, preventing or exorcising 136 symptoms of human (96) and livestock (40) ills. The plants fell into a total of 499 species from 107 families. For veterinary medicine these figures were 158 and 55, respectively. This report highlights the plants and prescriptions most frequently identified in the course of the survey, as these can be considered truly representative of a coherent tradition of 'popular medicine' for people or livestock. The discussion is organized in five parts: the survey framework; the healers; diseases in Burundi; medicinal plants there; and analysis of results. Cattle are the focus of the ethnoveterinary information, as the authors consider them the most traditional livestock species in Burundi. The main health problem of all stock, however, appeared to be malnutrition. It in turn lays the animals open to numerous other ailments, especially parasitoses. For cattle, reproductive health is another major concern. Kirundi names for 36 livestock ailments are given, along with their literal translations in French. This is followed by coded tables of the plants used to treat the 36 conditions, plus data on the number of times healers mentioned a given plant overall and in a given plant+ailment combination. Overall, research revealed a much higher correlation in plant+ailment usage in traditional veterinary as versus human medicine (50% versus 28%). Also, EVK was found to be more widely shared amongst healers than human ethnomedical information.

Baerts, Martine and Jean Lehmann. 1994a. Analyse des résultats d'une enquête ethnobotanique menée auprès de tradipraticiens Burundais. In: Kakule Kasonia and Michel Ansay (eds). *Metissages en Santé Animale de Madagascar a Haïti: Actes du Séminaire d'Ethnopharmacopée Vétérinaire 'KAGALA', un Partage de Savoirs Burkina-Faso, Ouagadougou, 15–22 Avril 1993.* Presses Universitaires de Namur, Namur, Belgium. Pp. 89–98.

This conference contribution relates the results of an ethnobotanical survey conducted by botanists in the high plateaus of the Zaire-Nile region of Burundi. The authors interviewed 131 traditional healers (104 for human, and 27 for animal, ethnomedicine) and collected 5696 plant samples representing 503 different species. The main research question was: Are there phytotherapeutic methods common to Burundian healers in general? A positive response might suggest that, as a clue to treatment efficacy researchers should pay particular attention to medicines known to large numbers of healers and uniformly used by them to treat the same conditions. It would also suggest that, despite the lack of schools or conferences on traditional medicine, healers nevertheless have ways of exchanging and sharing ethnomedical knowledge. Statistical analysis of the survey results found that, for 93% of the plants collected, there was no greater-than-chance correlation across practitioners of human ethnomedicine in the plants' use. For ethnoveterinary medicine, however, fairly strong correlations were found. These findings led the authors to question their hypothesis that frequency of plant use necessarily has implications for efficacy. Rather, they conclude that, for human ethnomedicine in Burundi, there are 'private' or 'secret' (the 93%) versus 'public' or 'popular' (the remaining 7%) domains. In contrast, Burundian EVM represents a more coherent body of knowledge, possibly due to the lesser role of magic and psychology in its practice.

Baerts, Martine and Jean Lehmann. 1994b. Quelques plantes médicinales en usage au Burundi et en Afrique sub-Saharienne. In: Kakule Kasonia and Michel Ansay (eds). *Métissages en Santé Animale de Madagascar à Haïti: Actes du Séminaire d'Ethnopharmacopée Vétérinaire 'KAGALA', un Partage de Savoirs Burkina-Faso, Ouagadougou, 15–22 Avril 1993.* Presses Universitaires de Namur, Namur, Belgium. pp. 231–241.

This chapter elaborates on the findings of the Burundian ethnobotanical survey reported in Baerts and Lehmann 1994a. For livestock health problems, the survey details 13 categories, each with a list of plants said to be helpful in curing them. Every plant is assigned a percentage according to its frequency of citation in the survey. For example, *Lantana trifolia* L. – a popular multi-purpose plant – is scored at 29% because it was mentioned in 29 out of 100 interviews. There was a marked consensus across interviewees as to which plants were used for treating animals, but the same was not true for human ethnomedicine, due to the more 'private' or proprietary nature of such information. At least in part, the authors attribute this distinction to the importance of healers supposedly imbued with supernatural powers who mainly treat human disorders believed to result from supernatural [psychosomatic?] phenomena. But animal ailments are dealt with by community-based ethnoveterinary specialists (often themselves herders) who practise on both animals and humans. The most renowned such specialists may become wealthy as a result of their ministrations. Although the authors overview human ethnomedical data from a total of 15 African countries, they do not do likewise for EVM because of the dearth of bibliographic references. However, they offer a table of some 20 plant species used for treating various livestock ills by country or region in Sub-Saharan Africa. An interesting finding from Rwanda is that, without exception, the disease and plant names collected there were all of exogenous, Bantu origin. Further study of such nomenclatures would illuminate the origins of ethnomedical practices for both animals and humans in much of sub-Saharan Africa.

Baerts, Martine, Jean Lehmann, Michel Ansay and Kakule Kasonia. 1996. *A Few Medicinal Plants Used in Traditional Veterinary Medicine: A Data Bank.* Louvain University Press, Belgium. 154 pp.

This book is a print-out of the PRELUDE database on traditional veterinary medicine. As of 1996, the database contained over 5000 plant-based prescriptions for livestock disorders, with each plant listed by family. Reference(s) in which a plant is cited are given, along with the country, livestock disorders (more than 200) and animal species in which it is used. The database is geared to serve researchers, veterinarians, agricultural and veterinary instructors, and any other groups interested in obtaining information on African plant medicines. It can now be accessed on the Internet at http://pc4.sisc.ucl.ac.be/prelude.html. [See also Castillo and Ansay 1998.]

Bagga, M.S. 1967. *A Study of Calf-rearing Practices and Problems in Villages of Hissar District.* MS thesis, Haryana Agricultural University, Hissar, India.

Unavailable for review.

Bah, Mohamed Sidi. 1983. *Observations on Disease Problems and Traditional Remedies Relating to the Use of Work Oxen in the Karina Area.* Report on a pilot study of preparation for the research project 'The health and management of N'Dama cattle in Sierra Leone, with special reference to the use of work oxen in village conditions'. Sierra Leone Work Oxen Project, Private Mail Bag 766, Freetown, Sierra Leone. 12 pp.

Work oxen have been used since 1928 in Karina and Warridale in Sierra Leone. Farmers see diseases as one of the biggest constraints to ox traction. The author reviews farmers' descriptions of livestock diseases and their cures. Small red flies are a great threat to oxen and cattle. Farmers combat the flies by setting smudge fires in the sheds and by rubbing kerosene and other substances on the animals. They control ticks by piercing them with a needle or a blade. The author discusses intestinal problems, wounds and accidents, exhaustion, blood diseases, feeding practices, mortality in livestock and taboos and beliefs relating to livestock management.

Bailey, C. and A. Danin. 1981. Bedouin plant utilization in Sinai and the Negev. *Economic Botany* 35(2): 145–162.

This article reports on a 6-year survey (1968–1974) of Bedouin usage of plants in their environment, i.e. the Sinai and Negev deserts. All the plants listed in the article were attested by at least three informants and were also collected by the authors. They note that 'there is no species of plant in the desert that is not eaten by at least one of the animals that the bedouin raises' (p. 147). Moreover, Bedouin know precisely which species are poisonous, and which most palatable, at different seasons and stages of plant growth to each type of livestock they keep (goats, camels, donkeys). To treat intestinal parasites, Bedouin drive their stock at least once yearly onto pastures with salty and sour plants, of which they identify 27 species. In fact, many of these 'sour' plants contain large quantities of organic acids, which may be helpful against parasites. In addition to these 27, Bedouin employ another nine species in ethnoveterinary medicines for the eight most common ills of their herds. Some examples are: the irritating sap of *Anabasis syriaca*, applied to mangy areas; chewn bark of *Tamarix nilotica* spat into a camel's scratched or sore eye; a concoction of salt and ground *Thymelaea hirsuta* leaves placed in a she-camel's vagina to encourage conception; a hot plaster of ground *Retama raetam* branches and green leaves for leg sprains and fractures. For general aches and pains in camels, *Ochradenus baccatus* plants are burned in a 0.5 m-deep hole over which the blanketed patient is made to lie for 24 hours.

Balagizi, Karhagomba and Kayembe Ntumba. 1994. Plantes utilisées dans le traitement des helminthoses gastro-intestinales des petits ruminants dans le groupement d'Irhambi-Katana (Region du Bushi, Est du Zaïre). *Lettre du Sous-réseau PRELUDE: Santé, Productions Animales et Environnement* 6: 2–6.

Zaire is experiencing a shift away from cattle to small ruminant and poultry production. But small ruminants suffer greatly from gastrointestinal worms, for which farmers are unable to access or afford costly modern pharmaceuticals. Perhaps alternatives are to be found in traditional botanicals already known and used by rural people. Thus the authors – both scientists in the Veterinary Entomology Laboratory of Zaire's Centre for Research in the Natural Sciences – interviewed 350 stockraisers and traditional healers in one part of Zaire on this subject in 1991. Interviewees identified 45 plant species of 24 families that they employed to treat stomach and gut worms. Leaves and roots were the most-used plant parts, employed fresh or ground/pounded and macerated in water, then administered orally. A review of the pharmacological literature suggests that many, if not the majority, of the 45 species have principles that act as vermifuges and vermicides.

Baharani, Mahamat Saleh. 1989. *Compte Rendu de l'Enquête sur la Santé Animale de Base et le Travail des Auxiliaires dans le Projet 'Isthirak' [sic].* In-house report. Oxfam, N'Djaména, Chad. 12 pp.

This document reports the results of an interim impact survey of the Ishtirak Project's paravet programme in Chad. In passing, it notes that herders there ascribe many diseases to the annual rainy season. Also noted is the local practice of regularly giving natron to small ruminants in order to fatten them and promote milk production. But strangely, Chadians do not give natron to their cattle.

Bairacli-Levy, Juliette de. 1954. *The Complete Herbal Book for the Dog.* Faber and Faber, London, UK.

Above all else, canine health depends upon good diet. This book highlights the author's own system of Natural Rearing for producing generations of disease-free dogs. The basic principles behind the system are giving mainly raw foods and meat, alternating with periods of fasting, according to animal age and climatic conditions. Raw bones are also important for jaw exercise and tooth development. For diseases in general, a liquid fast of water or honeyed water coupled with daily herbal purges is recommended. More specific treatments presented in the chapter reviewed here are given for distemper, encephalitis, hysteria, pneumonia, diarrhoea, gastritis, eczema and other skin ailments, canker, eye problems, abscesses, worms, jaundice, lice and fleas, sore pads, and for puppies, milk rash, ingestion of foreign bodies, vomiting and stomach swelling. Treatments involve various combinations of feeding and watering regimes, drenches, enemas, poultices, hot herbal compresses, warm jacketing, and – in the case of skin diseases and ectoparasites – herbal and soap- or alcohol-based lotions, powders and baths, plus complete fumigation of all collars, leads, grooming equipment, kennels, runs, etc. Bathing in the sea is also mentioned for removing lice and fleas. For pad problems, leather booties (shoe-like pouches) containing curing herbs are tied on the feet. [Abstract based on synopsis in Baracli-Levy 1973, Chapter 9, pp. 265–294.]

Bairacli-Levy, Juliette de. 1973 [1952]. *Herbal Handbook for Farm and Stable.* Faber and Faber, London, UK. 320 pp.

Herbal alternatives have 'brought new hope to farmers and horse owners, disillusioned by the failure of chemical therapy to safeguard and restore health' (unpaginated). This third, updated edition of a herbal handbook for the most common ailments of cattle, sheep, goats, horses, donkeys, poultry (chickens, ducks, geese, turkeys, pigeons), sheepdogs [see Baracli-Levy 1954], and bees sets out not only 'cures . . . fully proved, . . . entirely safe and comparatively inexpensive' (ibid.) but also, and especially, preventive nutritional and other measures for use by stockowners worldwide. Taking a whole-body rather than just a symptomatic approach and excluding all poisonous plants for internal applications, the book draws on contemporary EVM from Algeria, Britain, France, Germany, Greece, Israel, Mexico, Morocco, Portugal and Spain based on the author's own observations, discussions and veterinary practice in many of these countries and with gypsy herbalists. In passing, the author remarks on the curious fact that, in her world travels, she rarely met any women herbalists. Chapter 1's introduction bemoans the 'over-commercialization of the earth and the creatures . . . domesticated' (p. 1) due to the power of advertisement, a tendency for the modern veterinarian to operate as 'a mere vendor of the products of the vast and powerful chemical and serum manufacturers' (p. 10) along with 'modern farmers' trusting attitude to orthodox veterinary medicine' (p. 31) of which they understand little, plus 'the error of over-domestication of animals, with its consequent artificial rearing methods and medical treatments' (p. 1) that themselves undermine animal health. After discussing the dangers of DDT, in a telling anecdote the author recounts how a large chemical firm cautioned that its deworming drug passes into the milk of dairy animals, changing the milk's colour and taste; the firm thus instructed farmers to drench only half their cows at a time but to mix together the milk from the whole herd so that consumers would not notice the worm medicine! In contrast, internally-administered herbal medicines can be used not only to promote the health of milk- and egg-producing animals but also to manipulate the flavour, colour and health-giving properties of these products to the active benefit and tastes of consumers. The book's Chapter 2 describes when and how to gather, prepare, store and calculate dosages of plant remedies, noting that often the best way to administer herbs is prophylactically, simply by planting them in pastures and hedgerows where farm animals graze. Hedgerows are particularly favourable localities because they also create habitat for many wild bird, insect and other wild species while also enriching the soil and blocking erosion. The author opines that exact dosages are not important in herbal medicine, given that dosage is uncontrolled when animals instinctively self-medicate. Chapter 3 lists 203 *materia medica botanica* alphabetically by the common English names along with their Latin names and general veterinary uses, the latter in perhaps some 600 recipes here and throughout the text. These materials span every possible plant part and type, most notably including seaweed. Also figuring in prescriptions are: honey, molasses, treacle; vinegar, wine and port, brandy, beer, ale; milk, buttermilk, butter, eggs and eggwhite; flour, brown and white sugar, salt, fat, cooking and salad oils; waste engine oil, turpentine, paraffin, borax, soda, charcoal, ashes, soot, Epsom and Glauber's salts; beeswax, spider webs, slugs; coldcream; and any of the commercialized natural remedies produced by the English firm N.R. Products. In addition, Chapter 3 lists plants according to 12 vital minerals that they provide to livestock. Also noted here and elsewhere are tips on making clean, nutritious hay and on maintaining hygiene in pastures, farm buildings and coops. For example, worm-infested pastures can be cleansed by deworming and removing the stock and then spreading the land with lime or soot, or planting it with garlic or a thick crop of mustard, the latter of which is then ploughed under green. The remaining chapters are organized by species and health problem. Each problem's common English name, background information, symptoms and treatments are systematically detailed. Symptoms cited often include particular patterns of bleating, lowing, bellowing, grunting and panting, as well as other kinds of behavioural signs. Besides plant medicines, many treatments involve other *materia* and methods. For instance, massage accompanies many external applications. To cure mastitic sheep, English farmers apply warm packs of cow dung to the udder; if pressed for time, however, the farmers simply cut off the infected teat. For braxy, an old English Highlander prophylaxy is to dose sheep with pig dung. Turks give lambs a big draught of olive oil and powdered charcoal to remove obstructing wool balls in the digestive tract; to prevent the problem in the first place, however, ewes' udder-area should be shaved before lambing. Everywhere except in very cold weather, treatment of ovine skin disorders logically begins with immediate clipping of the wool, followed by a wide variety of treatments. For advanced milk fever in ruminants, the now-centuries-old technique of inflating the udder with air is effective. For pneumonia in cattle, a plaster of fresh cow dung on the chest is recommended. Worldwide, bloat in cattle is commonly relieved by puncturing the abdomen.

Mexican peasants, however, may drive a bloated animal up a steep mountain crag and hold it on ropes in a near-perpendicular position there, so as to induce anal release of gases. In Germany, an effective, one-hour-only cure is to gag the bloated animal with a rope and fill its mouth with its own fresh dung – both of which promote vigorous chewing and oral expulsion of gases; meanwhile, any handy type of rubber tubing is inserted in the anus and worked about to release additional gases. To prevent some of the most common causes of bloat, English farmers have long known not to turn animals out on dew- or frost-ridden grass and to control feed intake and give herbal and hay digestives during the spring change-over in diet. Rubbing waste oil on horses' hides to prevent horse-flies from laying their eggs is an effective treatment known in places as far-flung as Israel, Mexico and Spain. Equally important for preventing fly strike and worry is not to cut horses' manes and tails. One treatment for sprained tendons in horses is to bandage the limb with a paste of whitewash and warm cow dung. Jets of water or cold compresses remedy swollen legs in horses. For a dislocated shoulder, in England the horse is led into a deep pool or river, where it strikes into a swimstroke that rapidly corrects the dislocation; the animal is then left to stand in the river for a bit, so the cool water can reduce the resultant inflammation. A sampling of Arab remedies for poisonous insect bites is external application of raw onions, of the acidic juice of unripe tomatoes, or of ammonia extracted from camel dung. Also noted are some basic dentistry operations for horses. For all herd animals, retained placenta can be remedied by drenching the patient with its own colostrum. After setting, padding, splinting and bandaging a fracture using soft mosses, boughs and old clothes, the limb is stood in a bucket of cold water thrice daily. Noteworthy in the extensive chapter on poultry are: providing for roosts, shade and runs; furnishing dust-bath areas with Derris powder, coal or coke cinders, etc. added to the bath; keeping clean, dry, insect-free poultry houses by treating woodwork with a blow-lamp and creosote, liming the runs, and fumigating yearly with cayenne pepper; ensuring grit in the diet from, e.g. oyster shells, old mortar, chalk, crushed eggshells; and keeping clutches moist during dry spells. A simple surgical operation for crop-bound birds is to cut open the crop and remove its contents, sprinkle the crop walls with a teaspoon of black pepper, and then sew up the incision with an ordinary needle and strong thread. A French method for preserving eggs for up to two years is to varnish them with warm olive oil and beeswax and then store the eggs small-end-down in airtight containers filled with bran and/or charcoal powder. Cold and hot, herbal or merely water-moistened compresses figure in a great many treatments for all species, as does absolute or liquid fasting of the patient for a few days. The vast majority of the treatments the author urges consist of chained poly-prescriptions, usually combining an internal with an external intervention, plus dietary and often rest or exercise recommendations – with certain treatments timed according to phases of the moon. Only rarely is surgery or slaughter advised, when herbal remedies may be non-existent or are impractical for all but prize animals. The instruments required for all the treatments described are few and simple: tweezers, knives, a drenching horn, perhaps a hoof clipper; cotton wool or swabs, and maybe a stiff brush for applying medicaments; coarse sacking or cloth bags for straining herbal preparations or for tying medicaments around hooves, udders and muzzles; brown paper or old sweaters, socks and sheets for positioning or applying poultices, plasters and compresses; and for warmth-giving treatments, blankets, rugs and heated bricks. Every possible route of administration is noted, frequently including douches, enemas and inhalations of smoke or steam (the latter with a 'steam bag' around the nose). For prevention of disease in all non-insect species, the value of clean drinking water and exercise cannot be overemphasized. Especially for kids, it is recommended to place 'exercise equipment' in their pastures, in the form of logs or piles of branches for them to leap. The benefits of massage, friendly speech, and traditional European milkmaid's singing while milking are noted for stimulating easy milk flow. Finally, a chapter on beekeeping opines that the best thing is simply to leave bees alone, short of whitewashing the hive, using a Queen excluder to keep larvae out of the hive's upper stories, occasionally feeding a syrup of sage honey, and planting herb gardens and orchards for bee food.

Bamba, M., D. Kouakou, M. Quattara and M. Camara. 1992. L'aviculture villageoise dans le centre de la Côte-d'Ivoire: Contexte traditionnel et proposition d'amélioration. In: G. Tacher and L. Letenneur (eds). *Proceedings of the Seventh International Conference of Institutions of Tropical Veterinary Medicine, Yamoussoukro, Ivory Coast: Volume I.* Pp. 275–279.

In discussing traditional poultry-raising practices in Ivory Coast, this conference paper mentions that people put ashes in birds' dust-bath sites to help combat ectoparasites. Also noted are variations in poultry housing. Shelters may consist of a mobile cage of woven bamboo, a simple structure of beaten earth, or a coop constructed of locally available materials. All serve the purpose for which they are designed, which is to foil predators. The authors further remark poultry's many roles in Ivorian life – as sacrifical animals, feast food, gifts, dowry and income-generators.

Bandophadhyaya, Subhash. 1995. Perception of young scientists: Why doesn't learning from people continue? Part II. *Honey Bee* 6(4): 5.

This article reports on four ethnoveterinary practices that, as a young Indian scientist, the author observed during field visits. To delay sexual maturity in heifers, farmers feed them oil cakes. To improve conception rates, cows are fed germinated gram, which is a rich source of energy, vitamins and minerals. Jackfruit leaves mixed with mustard oil are fed for retained placenta; scientists suggest that the alkaloids in the leaves may act on the uterus. Mustard oil is also fed for bloat, which it may help relieve by changing the viscosity of the gastrointestinal contents.

Bantugan, S.C., S.B. Singzon, A.P. Obusa and E. M. Tabada Jr. 1989. Indigenous health practices and breeding management of carabao. *Farm and Resource Management Institute Information Service Newsletter* 3(1): 11–13.

In the Philippines, carabao (water buffalo) are used for draught work. In this article, two farmers impart their prescriptions for diarrhoea, deworming and *pasmo*. They give a decocted drench of *Hyptis suaveolens* for diarrhoea. To deworm 2–3-month-old calves, a drench of 40 ml of coconut milk mixed with one egg from a native chicken is given. *Pasmo* is a disorder caused by overwork and characterized by weakness, boils and diarrhoea. It can be cured by a combination of therapies consisting of drenching with a bottle of human urine every morning, allowing the buffalo to wallow and rest for 3 months, and feeding it a handful of salt every other day. The farmers also offer advice on the management of carabao reproduction. For example, during dry or hot weather, buffalo should be allowed to

wallow in cool water before service so that the sperm and ova will be cooler and
thus more 'vigorous'.

Barfield, Thomas J. 1981. *The Central Asian Arabs of Afghanistan: Pastoral
Nomadism in Transition.* University of Texas Press, Austin, Texas, USA. 182 pp.

This ethnography documents the shift of Arab sheep pastoralists in Afghanistan
from a subsistence to a cash economy. Chapter 2 focuses on aspects of animal
husbandry, including flock composition, mortality and other losses, age and sex
taxonomies, control of breeding, milking patterns, marketing decisions, migratory
movements, access to pasture, salt feeding, shearing, ear-marking, slaughter and
rustling. Little is said of veterinary practices, other than to note the many deaths of
lambs from bloat, parasitic flies and other diseases; the complete lack of access to
commercial remedies; and stockowners' general fatalism (*kismet*) with regard to
flock losses.

Barth, Frederik. 1975. *Ritual and Knowledge among the Baktaman of New
Guinea.* Yale University Press, New Haven, Connecticut, USA. 292 pp.

In this monograph on the Baktaman of New Guinea, the chapter 'Ecology and
Subsistence' has a brief section on domestic animals (pp. 34–37). Pigs receive
sweet potatoes as feed supplements. To enhance the pigs' growth and the formation
of fat, a white earth is dried, crushed, wrapped in leaves and then hung over the
pigs' sleeping area. This earth is also rubbed over the back and flanks of each pig.
Chapter 15 of this book deals with human ethnomedicine.

Baumann, Maximilian P.O. 1990. *The Nomadic Animal Health System (NAHA-
System) in Pastoral Areas of Central Somalia and its Usefulness in
Epidemiological Surveillance.* Thesis, Master of Preventive Veterinary
Medicine, University of California, Davis, California, USA. 130 pp.

Attempts to design and implement a baseline disease survey in pastoral areas of
central Somalia underscored the difficulties of incorporating and precisely meas-
uring endogenous and exogenous variables influencing livestock management and
production. The solution, says the author, is a truly multidisciplinary approach.
Specifically, 'veterinary anthropology' could improve the analysis of disease
patterns and subsequent prevention and control strategies by inter-linking
household-level animal-production data and socio-anthropological findings with
veterinary data, and vice versa. In surveying caprine diseases for his thesis, the
author took note of some traditional Somali methods of treatment and control. For
CCPP, for instance, herders avoid areas where others' infected goats are grazing;
and in their own herds, they promptly separate the sick goats and graze them far
from the other animals. Other preventive measures range all the way from readings
from the Koran to homemade CCPP vaccinations. Stockraisers considered the
latter to be quite effective. It is performed by rubbing or surgically inserting tissue
from CCPP lung lesions into an incision between the eyes and nostrils of the
healthy goat. No extensive wounds following upon this operation were noted by
project staff, as reported for similar bovine vaccinations elsewhere in Africa. Many
herders also knew that goats who recover naturally from [certain strains of] CCPP
have lifelong immunity. Herders further observed that the incidence of CCPP

generally rises during droughts, as people are forced to move hungry herds into areas they would otherwise have avoided as harbouring the disease. For contagious ecthyma, herders cauterize around the goat's head, with variable success. Also noted is the existence of traditional Somali healers (*sacoyagan*) who attend livestock, and the NAHA project's encouragement of their recruitment as auxiliaries. The author comments that NAHAs' pride in their newly acquired Western-veterinary skills may have constrained their reports of EVK.

Baumann, M.O., Ahmad M. Hassan and Hgai A. Nuux. 1989. *Livestock Disease Surveillance Information through the Nomadic Animal Health Auxiliary System (NAHA – System) in Hiraan and Galgaduud Regions of the Central Rangelands of Somalia. Part I: Sheep and Goats.* Technical Project Report No. 20. Central Rangelands Development Project – Veterinary Component. GTZ and Ministry of Livestock, Forestry and Range, Beledweyne, Somalia. 28 pp.

In mounting a NAHA disease surveillance system in Somalia, the Central Rangelands Development Project ran into a nomenclature problem. Local people and NAHAs may apply the same Somali word for a single disease to a disease syndrome and/or to gross symptoms. Conversely, they may use one of several words that correspond to a single English-language gloss for a health condition: for example, *dhicis* and *dhisow* for abortion in small ruminants, or *cadho* and *canbaar* for mange in these species. Moreover, these terms may vary across speakers of the same language in contiguous, and sometimes even the same, villages. And sometimes, people lack any term at all to correspond with the Western identification of a given disease. To illustrate, across seven villages of a single Somali district, only two shared the same term for one disease tentatively identified as chlamydiosis in sheep and goats; a third village had a different term; a fourth had yet another word, but it applied only to goats; and the remaining three villages had no term at all for this ill. The project therefore endeavoured to set up semantic correspondence tables for each district in which it worked, based on NAHAs' oral reports of the symptoms they observed and their postmortem findings. Even so, some disease terms still defied translation.

Baumann, M.P.O. and K.H. Zessin. 1992. Productivity and health of camels (*Camelus dromedarius*) in Somalia: Associations with trypanosomosis and brucellosis. *Tropical Animal Health and Production* 24: 145–156.

Somalia has one of the world's largest dromedary populations – about 5.3 million. This study in central Somalia of 33 nomadic pastoralist herds, comprising a total of 1039 camels, found that traditional practices of keeping herds in the bush and away from rivers reduced contact between herds and thus diminished the risk of trypanosomosis (*T. evansi*) and brucellosis. These and other husbandry practices, individually and in combination with other factors such as pastoralists' attention to micro-ecological conditions, may explain most of the variation found in camel herd health and production in Somalia.

Bayemi, P.H. 1998. Laboratory trials on the efficacy of indigenous acaricides on *Boophilus decoloratus* in Cameroon. In: E. Mathias, D.V. Rangnekar, and C.M. McCorkle, with M. Martin (eds). *Ethnoveterinary Medicine: Alternatives for Livestock Development – Proceedings of an International Conference Held in*

Pune, India, 4–6 November 1997. Volume 2: Abstracts. BAIF Development
Research Foundation, Pune, India. P. 6.

The efficacy of two indigenous acaricides, *Euphorbia cameroonica* (*kerenahi*) and
Psorospermum guineensis (*sawoiki*), on female *Boophilus decoloratus* ticks was
evaluated in laboratory tests. *Kerenahi* sap was tested in four formulations: pure,
mixed with water, and at 4% and 8% concentrations with palm oil. *Sawoiki* sediment was tested at 2%, 4% and 6% concentrations in palm oil. Ticks were
immersed in the plant preparations for 3 minutes. Palm oil alone killed ticks, with
a 59% death rate on day 6 compared to a 50% death rate at day 15 for controls
($P < 1\%$). *Kerenahi* in a concentration of 4% and 8% in oil and the 6% *sawoiki*
preparation each killed as many ticks as Tigal, a commercial acaricide. The lethal
effect of *kerenahi* was quicker than that of *sawoiki*: 97% versus only 8% of ticks,
respectively, died by day 7. Also, *kerenahi* in palm oil prevented ticks' egg-laying.
Sawoiki and Tigal reduced the egg-laying period and rate while all acaricides prevented hatching. Results suggest that the traditional acaricides were efficient in
killing ticks and preventing ticks' normal reproduction.

Bayer, Wolfgang. 1989. Low-demand animals for low-input systems. *ILEIA
Newsletter* 5(4): 14–15.

Indigenous livestock breeds are generally well-adapted to their local environments
due both to natural selection and to human interventions in breeding. In Nigerian
pastoral systems, animals are bred for multiple functions: milk, meat and draught.
They must also be capable of walking long distances and surviving on very low
inputs. Animals are also bred for resistance to diseases such as heartwater.
Stockraisers in central Nigeria experimented with crossbreeding their trypanotolerant cattle with larger and more productive breeds from northern Nigeria in
order to increase milk yields. But the cross-breed requires greater inputs in terms
of feed, water and shelter as well as veterinary inputs.

Bayer, Wolfgang. 1990a. Behavioural compensation for limited grazing time by
herded cattle in central Nigeria. *Applied Animal Behaviour Science* 27: 9–19.

This study of Fulani herding strategies for their indigenous Bunaji breed of cattle
in central Nigeria debunks the theory that pastoral and smallholder corralling of
animals at night – versus more intensive systems' 24-hour paddocking – may
impair animal nutrition and health. Of particular interest are five findings. First,
aided by their white hair (which reflects solar radiation) and dark skin (which
limits penetration of the remaining radiation), the Fulani-bred Bunaji are able to
graze under higher ambient temperatures than any race of European origin, who
instead shift much of their grazing into the night hours during Nigeria's hottest
season. Second, thanks to anthropogenically enforced deferral of rest and rumination to the evening, pastoral and smallholder herds spend just as much time across
24 hours in overall grazing as do paddocked, or even wild, ruminants. Third,
despite the fact that pastoralist and smallholder herds do more walking and thus
less grazing than paddocked stock, the close personal supervision the herded
animals receive allows them to take advantage of more diverse, and often richer,
grazing sites such as: hedgerows or field borders; fallow fields, whether singly or
even in the midst of cultivated ones; and crop residues, often even before fields

have been fully harvested. Fourth, herders' lopping of trees makes more diverse and nutritious browse available to the animals year-round, but especially during the lean, dry season. Fifth, during the late wet season, herders purposely restrict grazing to an average of only 7 hours, versus a maximum of 10 hours at other times of the year. This strategy decreases worm and other infestations from grazing dew-ridden forage. When combined with the fact of plant cropping in the area, all of these herding strategies add up to a maximization of overall land use and forage resources.

Bayer, Wolfgang. 1990b. Use of native browse by Fulani cattle in central Nigeria. *Agroforestry Systems* 12: 217–228.

Studies of stockraisers' exploitation of naturally occurring browse in Africa have concentrated on arid and semi-arid areas, where browse forms a visibly important part of domesticated ruminants' diet. But local uses of non-cultivated browse for cattle in the humid and subhumid savannas have been largely ignored, despite the fact that during the late dry season cattle spend almost 30% of their monthly feeding time browsing rather than grazing. Thus, even in more humid zones, browse is critical to cattle survival. This study demonstrates the correspondingly extensive knowledge of browse held by Fulani pastoralists in central Nigeria, where interviewees identified 39 browse species and ranked each one by its impor-tance in cattle nutrition [and thus animal health]. Their rankings reflected not only the plants' relative abundance but also Fulani's profound knowledge of each species' relative nutritive value, as independently evaluated in scientific experi-ments. Fulani know-how in this regard is probably even greater than reported, because interviewees were reluctant to mention their use of trees protected by law and custom. On the other hand, informants cited several species heretofore over-looked by scientists. The author also notes interview difficulties due to the same vernacular name being applied to different plant species in the multilingual (Fulani and Hausa) study area.

Bayer, Wolfgang and Junaidu A. Maina. 1984. Seasonal pattern of tick load in Bunaji cattle in the subhumid zone of Nigeria. *Veterinary Parasitology* 15: 301–307.

In Nigeria, the only tick-borne disease of importance for the indigenous, Fulani-bred Bunaji cattle is heartwater, transmitted mainly by *Amblyomma variegatum* (Pulaar *koti*). But heartwater is most prevalent in places with high livestock con-centrations, such as government farms; and even there, Bunaji show considerable resistance. In contrast, exotic cattle are highly susceptible to this and other tick-borne diseases in Africa, including anaplasmosis and babesiosis, as well as dermatophilosis, which ticks may be involved in triggering. Whether for indige-nous or exotic breeds, however, regular, year-round tick control with an acaricide is not practical nor desirable for multiple reasons: the costs of acaricides on such a scale is prohibitive; dipping infrastructure is also expensive, or non-existent; ticks can develop resistance to a particular acaricide; and creation of a temporarily disease-free environment may reduce pre-immunity to the disease. In Nigeria, Fulani herders manually remove ticks from the entire body of all their cattle twice a week during the November-March dry season and thrice weekly during the April-October wet season. Needless to say, this is a laborious chore. Nor do herders achieve 100% removal, particularly of the smaller species such as *Boophilus*,

Hyalomma and *Rhipicephalus* spp. Fulani lump these smaller ticks together under the name *miri*, and note that they are less harmful than *koti*. Indeed, research suggests that zebu cattle are naturally more resistant to the small ticks. This study reports on a 12–month on-station trial mounted according to traditional pastoral practices and using only natural pastures. The goal was to determine whether the drudgery of manual tick removal could be relieved by strategic weekly sprayings of acaricide applied only during the two months of the year when Bunaji tick loads peak. However, findings revealed that hand spraying offered no labour savings over manual removal. Moreover, the traditional technique was more flexible and safer because no special preparation of chemicals or restraint of animals is required. Manual removal could be performed at any convenient time, often in conjunction with other daily livestock chores such as milking. Moreover, sprays posed additional difficulties, e.g. in ensuring: regular availability of the chemicals, water, spray equipment and spare parts; herder knowledge of equipment maintenance and repair needs; and safety in acaricide handling. The only possible advantage of the spraying regime lay in a somewhat more thorough removal of all kinds of ticks, and thus perhaps prevention of dermatophilosis at a lower cost than an in-any-case infeasible regime of year-round spraying. But even so, the authors conclude that the practice does not merit extension to pastoralists.

Bayer, Wolfgang and Ann Waters-Bayer. 1991. Relations between cropping and livestock husbandry in traditional landuse systems in tropical Africa. In: A. Bittner et al. (eds). ***Animal Research and Development: A Biannual Collection of Recent German Contributions Concerning Development through Animal Research.*** Institut für Wissenschaftliche Zusammenarbeit, Tübingen, Germany. Pp. 57–69.

Interactions between cropping and stockraising, farmers and herders in Africa are longstanding, complex and predominantly positive. Ways in which cropping works to the benefit of animal nutrition and health include the following. Considerable energy and nutrients are transferred to livestock via crop residues. Clearing land for crop production creates an open landscape in which it is easier and safer to herd animals than in the natural woodland savanna. Also, grass yields on fallow fields are higher than on natural savanna. Furthermore, clearing destroys habitats for tstetse flies, which transmit trypanosomosis, and thus reduces health risks for animals. Indeed, clearing has been found considerably more effective in controlling tsetse flies than chemical spraying. In Africa, however, clearing is only partial; many tree species are left on the land, where they serve as sites for beekeeping and provide critical dry-season browse for ruminants. Also during the dry season, burning-over of croplands stimulates green growth of grasses and shrubs, thus improving forage quality. At the same time, burning reduces the population of disease-bearing ticks and other pests. The benefits of stockraising for cropping are equally great. The authors argue that all such complex interactions must be fully understood before attempts are made to change traditional livelihood systems.

Bayoumi, M.S. 1966. Discussion of Mr. Gillespie's paper. ***Sudan Journal of Veterinary Science and Animal Husbandry*** 7(2): 24–25.

This article discusses the reasons for nomadism among the Baggara and Fung tribes of central Sudan. Their nomadism in fact consists of a seasonal migration designed to respond to a number of health- and nutrition-related needs. In high-rainfall areas, for example, fly worry may be so great that herds cannot graze, and so must move on. The vegetation, nutritive value and carrying capacity of pastures are other important factors in nomads' decision to move to, stay in, or leave a particular area.

Bazalar Ramírez, Hernando and Francisco Arévalo Tello. 1985. Informe del proyecto: Ensayo de la eficacia del utashayli contra *Melophagus ovinus* en ovinos altoandinos naturalemente infestados. Paper presented to LAPA, Huancayo, Perú. 6 pp.

This paper is an early, partial version of a much expanded and refined chapter on the subject in Bazalar et al. 1989.

Bazalar, Hernando, Enma Nunez, Edgar Olivera and Genaro Yarupaitan. 1992. Ethnoveterinarian research in the highlands of central Peru. In: John Young (ed.). *A Report on a Village Animal Health Care Workshop – Volume II: The Case Studies.* ITDG, Rugby, UK. Pp. 71–75.

Between 1983 and 1990, a community-based component of the multinational SR-CRSP operated among Andean peasants of central Peru. One of this component's R&D thrusts was EVK, conducted in conjunction with a national veterinary research institute. While many disciplines were involved, anthropologists and veterinarians led the way with two basic types of studies: descriptive and comparative household studies to understand local systems of animal health management; and identification of local veterinary remedies. The latter were further investigated with the active participation of stockraisers in on-farm trials on local sheep. This paper mentions trials on six such plant-based remedies, in each case using sheep treated with the herbal medicine, sheep treated with a commercial product, and untreated control groups. Two of these remedies were a tobacco-leaf wash for keds and a pumpkin-seed drench for gastrointestinal parasites, which proved 94% and (against adult worms) 79% effective, respectively. [For greater detail, see McCorkle and Bazalar 1996.] Other remedies tested were: also for gastrointestinal worms, an extract of *Chenopodium ambrosioides* L. leaves (69% effective against adults); a decoction of *Lupinus mutabilis* as a wash against ectoparasites (91% effective); for fasciolosis, a decoction of *Columellia obovata* (91% effective against adult flukes) or the macerated whole plant of *Gentianella thyrsoidea* (79%). All six plants are readily available in the region. The foregoing results were further evaluated in monthly inspections of two sheep flocks across two years, at the end of which the treated flocks showed an increase in production of 15% over untreated ones. From these data, a recommended calendar of treatments by seasonal estimates of parasite burdens was developed. The calendar also included modern medicines (notably, injections) where appropriate. A total of 70 paravets from 35 communities were then trained in all these treatments, as per the calendar.

Bazalar Ramírez, Hernando, Edgar Olivera Hurtado and Enma Nuñez Muñoz. 1998. *Uso de Plantas en el Control de Fasciola hepática en la Sierra Central del Perú.* Programa Colaborativo de Investigación ILEIA-GIAREC, Huancayo, Peru. 56 pp.

This report details nearly two decades of ER&D on liverfluke disease (distomatosis) in sheep and cattle of the central sierra of Peru. Work that began with the SR-CRSP in 1980 [see earlier articles by Bazalar and colleagues] has been continued, expanded, and now widely disseminated to farmers by the Ethnoveterinary Medicine Project of a new collaborative research program. This program brings together an international PVO (ILEIA), a regional agroecological research group (GIAREC), and two sub-regional NGOs (GINCAE and Yanapai in the Cajamarca and Huancayo areas, respectively), with semi-formal backstopping from a national veterinary research institute. Work proceeded in several phases: early descriptive efforts, in which a wide variety of ethnoveterinary beliefs and treatments were broadly documented; diagnostic, in which communities' current healthcare and management practices were investigated, along with their views on what are the key animal health problems; validation, in which on-station and participatory on-farm trials in pilot communities were mounted to test possible EVM solutions to these key problems; beginning in the late 1980s, extension of findings to farmers in larger groups of communities in the pilot area via additional participatory trials of a multi-locational validation+dissemination nature; subsequently, contractual agreements with farmer organizations and NGOs in larger and also new areas for mass extension; and throughout the later phases, collection of farmer feedback on trial treatments and, in new areas, of fresh EVK for possible future R&D. In the latter regard, as R&D moved from Huancayo to Cajamarca and, most recently, to Huancavelica Departments, in each case a new folk flukicide based on yet another plant species was recorded. Three ethnobotanical treatments for distomatosis have now been extensively tested, and corresponding dosage and agroecological recommendations formulated. They consist of drenches prepared from: decocted leaves of the mid-altitude ($\approx$3000 to 4000 m) shrub *Columellia obovata*; macerated and decocted whole plants of *Gentianella thyrsoidea*, a lake species identified from EVK in new, higher-altitude areas (> 4000 m); and decocted *Cynara scolymus* (artichoke) leaves. In brief, depending upon plant availability by agroecozone, the authors (who are also the lead scientists on this ER&D effort) recommend the use of one or the other of the first two preparations according to calendars formulated for each agroecozone, based on the zone's particular precipitation patterns, seasonal shifts, parasite life cycle and habitat concentration, etc. The *C. obovata* prescription has a kill rate of 80% for both adult and juvenile flukes while *G. thyrsoidea* kills 75% of adults. Although the artichoke drench has no lethal effect on the parasite, it does promote expulsion of adult flukes, and it has various hepatoprotective properties. Thus it is recommended as an adjunct treatment. Research revealed no adverse effects whatsoever from preparing or administering these ethnomedicines or from eating the milk and meat of treated animals. These botanicals appeared to be entirely safe for livestock, their human handlers and consumers, and the beneficial coprophagous insects that hold down fluke populations naturally. Moreover, sierran farmers have no difficulty in diagnosing distomatosis; they identify it by its characteristic submandibular oedema (Spanish 'water bags') and other clinical signs. So no problems of flukicide misapplication arose. The economic advantages of the ethnomedicines were patent. Where the plant materials can be freely gathered, these home remedies are 116% cheaper than any commercial flukicides commonly sold in the sierra. Even if the materials must be bought in the marketplace (where they are usually readily available), farmers in communities where the plants do not grow say it is still far more cost-effective for them to purchase and prepare the materials rather than to pay for more powerful, but vastly more expensive, commercial flukicides. If the zonally appropriate calendrical regime is followed, dosing with a botanical flukicide plus the artichoke drench reportedly can increase small producers' sheep production by 15%. Summing up, the authors confidently recommend the validated fluke treatments as part of regular preventive animal healthcare for sierran sheep and cattle. But for acute cases of distomatosis, farmers are advised to buy a commercial product that kills flukes at the immature juvenile stage (i.e. 1 week of age). Other observations of interest from this longitudinal ER&D effort include the following. Initial descriptive work on EVK may reveal many local variations on prescriptions. For example, seven different *C. obovata* recipes were recorded. These varied by mode (ground, macerated or steeped, as well as decocted) and time (ranging between 24 hours and 15 days) of preparation as well as by people's choice of an adjunct ingredient (salt or copper sulphate or eggs or lemon or hot chilli peppers or nothing). As an entrée into communities, EVM Project researchers found that a good strategy was to respond to community interest in human, as well as livestock, health matters. An example was people's desire to learn how to give injections to humans (and also animals). At a broader level, the authors observe that ethnomedicines validated for use with certain species may well be amenable to subsequent re-formulation for other species. For instance, it should be possible to re-tool the ethnoflukicides described here so as to increase guinea-pig production and perhaps also to advance repopulation of the central sierra with the indigenous camelids. All these species are very susceptible to flukes. (As few as three flukes can kill a guinea pig.) Another observation is that this EVM work – which was carried out mainly with women farmers – has greatly increased women's status and decision-making power in the pilot communities. Finally, the authors opine that, as a rule of thumb, ethnoveterinary medicines – which are a prime example of low-external-input and thus sustainable agricultural technology – are most appropriate for 'communities with mixed production systems that give priority to autoconsumption' (p. 3).

Bazalar, Hernando, Juan Zurita and Francisco Arévalo. 1989. Eficacia del utashayli contra la falsa garrapata (*Melophagus ovinus*). In: Hernando Bazalar and Constance M. McCorkle (eds). ***Estudios Etnoveterinarios en Comunidades Altoandinas del Perú.*** Lluvia Editores, Lima, Perú. Pp. 87–95.

Because of inflation running in the thousands of percent per year, many highland Peruvian peasants can no longer afford the commercial sheep-dip products for which they abandoned their indigenous treatments. This chapter describes the SR-CRSP's rescue of an old Andean technology for combating ectoparasitism in herd animals, based upon a wild tobacco known as *utashayli* (*Nicotiana paniculata* L.). Through both laboratory analysis and controlled but participatory on-farm trials, this remedy was modified and strengthened to serve as a highly effective dip against *Melophagus ovinus*. Indeed, stockowners found it even more powerful than the commercial products they had previously used. Data reveal that a regime of *utashayli* dips reduced *Melophagus* loads to nearly zero by day 18, and maintained this level until the end of the study at day 60, with parasite mortality rates varying between 97% and 93% during this period – in sharp contrast to the control animals. For this regime to be sustainable, however, systems to protect, maintain or even cultivate the sylvan plant on which it is based must be investigated and put in place.

Bedi, S.J. 1978. Ethnobotany of the Ratan Mahal Hills, Gujarat, India. *Supplement to Economic Botany* 32: 279–284.

This article reports on the ethnomedical use of 73 plant species from 41 families among India's Bhil hill tribes, based on the author's 21 trips between 1960 and 1967 to the Vindhya and Satpura Mountains. Only one mention is made of plants used in animal ethnomedicine, however. To wit, the leaves of *Mirabilis jalapa* L. are administered in their food to chickens in order to ensure regular egg-laying. The author also notes the use of *Albizia odoratissima* L. as a fish poison.

Beerling, Marie-Louise E.J. 1986. *Acquisition and Alienation of Cattle in the Traditional Rural Economy of Western Province, Zambia.* Department of Veterinary and Tsetse Control Service, Ministry of Agriculture and Water Development, Western Province, P. O. Box 910034, Mongu, Zambia. 140 pp.

This report focuses on how cattle ownership changes in the traditional rural economy of Western Province in Zambia. It discusses: gifts, rewards and payments involving cattle; inheritance; bride-price; ceremonies, celebrations and rituals; fines and damages; herding arrangements; natural herd increases and declines; purchase, disposal and slaughter; and rustling. Chapter 8 (pp. 88–95) briefly describes the selection of cows and bulls for breeding, traditional methods of fertility manipulation and disease control and management. The author mentions that, traditionally, animals are castrated just before they are to cross cold water.

Beerling, Marie-Louise. 1987. *Ten Thousand Kraals: Cattle and Ownership in Western Province.* Animal Disease Control Project Western Province, P.O. Box 910034, Mongu, Zambia. *Ca.* 60 pp.

This is a slightly revised and updated version of Beerling 1986. When it comes to healthcare and related husbandry decisioning like castration or slaughter of sick animals, it is important to remember that – because of many and complex ownership rights vested in cattle and equally complex social arrangements for cattle share- or contract-herding – the 'herder' may not be empowered to make such decisions unilaterally. Livestock developers and extensionists often do not realise that 'when visiting one herd and talking to one man . . . [they are] in fact dealing with several smaller herds belonging to many different owners . . . [who] may live far away' (p. 53). The author explains that what developers may see as 'traditionalism' and resistance to change in a herder is in fact responsible and 'rational reasoning' with regard to making choices about spending money and effort on such things as commercial drugs without first consulting owners' wishes.

Beerling, Marie-Louise and Mwenda Mwambwa Mumbuna. 1988. *Farmers' Perceptions of Constraints: Findings of a Short Survey among Contact Farmers with Special Reference to Fertility and Calf Mortality (draft).* Livestock Development Project, Department of Veterinary and Tsetse Control Services, Mongu, Zambia. *Ca.* 50 pp.

This draft report of constraints to cattle production among Lozi of Zambia's Western Province also provides a list of traditional treatments for 11 different disorders of cattle. Approximately 60 treatments are listed, most of them plant-based.

However, the use of dung and engine oil for treating wounds and infections is noted. Eye infections are treated by cauterizing the area around the eye. To relieve bloat in calves, Lozi manually extract dung from the animals. Ticks are mostly removed by hand, but another treatment is to make animals cross a river several times. Diarrhoea may be treated in 12 different ways. Non-botanical examples include drenching calves with the powdered shards of clay pots in water, or cauterizing the anus.

Bel, Andréine and Bernard Bel. 1998. Medical power: The place of 'holistic' indigenous health systems in the global model of 'scientific' medicine (case studies in Europe and India). In: E. Mathias, D.V. Rangnekar and C.M. McCorkle, with M. Martin (eds). ***Ethnoveterinary Medicine: Alternatives for Livestock Development – Proceedings of an International Conference Held in Pune, India, 4–6 November 1997. Volume 2: Abstracts.*** BAIF Development Research Foundation, Pune, India. Pp. 7–8.

This paper addresses the social, religious and political power systems that under-lie repressive or supportive actions towards research into traditional health systems. The argument is substantiated by two on-going project case studies. The first deals with the traditional *amchi* medical system in Ladakh, Kashmir vis-à-vis Tibetan medicine as practised in Tibet and in Indian refugee settlements. The second project is documenting practices among traditional midwives in rural India. At the individual level, social prejudice is accountable for misleading concepts about the efficacy of various healing techniques. Following market trends, patients and naturopaths tend to overlook or discard simple remedies such as water, clay or physiotherapy. At the policy level, the authors note how the establishment of scientific-medical authority can erase many popular health practices – as happened in 16th-century Europe. In the early 20th century the allopathic system consoli-dated its position as the unique and universal medical science. But recent work questions the relevance of experimental procedures on which this claim is based. Consequently, even some traditional medical systems (e.g. Ayurveda) now attempt to present themselves as a 'rational' science. The authors differentially define: holistic conceptions of health advocated by WHO; alternative medicine; 'New Age' quacks; and the Japanese-inspired *seitai* approach, which is based on accu-rate observation of natural healing processes. The latter advocates breaking free from therapy, disclosing personal experience in situations of acute disease and child delivery and revealing 'hidden knowledge', i.e. domains of expertise that are never elicited because they are restricted to specific communities whose voices do not count. An example is the knowledge of traditional midwives in rural India. Social and gender prejudice can drive this expertise into oblivion. The authors con-clude by urging a multidisciplinary scientific approach that emphasizes personal experience and commitment, and takes account of epistemological as well as tech-nical aspects of research into human or animal health and healing. In other words, 'The scientist's mind should also be there, on the dissection table'.

Bell, Charles Alfred. 1928. ***The People of Tibet.*** Clarendon Press, Oxford, UK.

Bell observed that a donkey in north Sikkim suffering from aconite poisoning was treated by slitting off the tips of its ears and pricking its hind-quarters. He also reports that people of the Chumbi Valley protected their ponies, mules, donkeys and yaks against aconite (a type of wolfsbane) poisoning by rubbing its boiled leaves over the animal's mouth and nostrils. Because this treatment irritates the sensitive buccal and nasal membranes, the animals become thus conditioned against eating the plant in the future (pp. 23–24).

Belsare, V.P. , S.K. Raval and P.R. Patel. 1998. Importance of indigenous knowledge of animal husbandry for development. In: E. Mathias, D.V. Rangnekar and C.M. McCorkle, with M. Martin (eds). *Ethnoveterinary Medicine: Alternatives for Livestock Development – Proceedings of an International Conference Held in Pune, India, 4–6 November 1997. Volume 2: Abstracts.* BAIF Development Research Foundation, Pune, India. Pp. 8.

Since the domestication of animals, the life of the people in Bharat, India, has been inextricably linked with their livestock and they have developed much knowledge in animal husbandry. In recent years, emphasis has shifted towards modern science in the maintenance and development of livestock. However, many technologies generated centuries ago are still in use; and some of these are demonstrably economic and sustainable. Present-day technology generation and transfer should therefore build on such indigenous knowledge. For this, it is necessary to identify promising local technologies and practices that can be integrated with scientific knowledge for even greater efficient and economic management of livestock. This paper discusses: documenting traditional animal husbandry practices for different species; identifying the scientific bases for the practices documented; and blending or modifying traditional wisdom with the help of scientific knowledge to improve its efficacy and livestock productivity.

Bene, Zsuzsanna. 1961. Die Schafzucht und die Verarbeitung der Schafmilch auf dem Gebiet des Cserehat (Nordostungarn). In: László Földe (ed.). *Viehzucht und Hirtenleben in Ostmitteleuropa: Ethnographische Studien.* Akadémiai Kiadó, Verlag der Ungarischen Akademie der Wissenschaften, Budapest, Hungary. Pp. 559–579.

Shepherds in northeast Hungary knew when one of their sheep was sick and how to treat it. To prevent liver flukes, they avoided muddy, humid pastures. For hoof wounds and footrot, the herders applied copper vitriol and other remedies. Coenurosis, caused by a parasite that encysts itself in the brain, was treated by opening the skull of the afflicted animal and surgically removing the cysts. The herders used their teeth to castrate bucks and disinfected the castration wounds with wood ash.

Bennet-Jenkins, E. and C. Bryant. 1996. Novel anthelmintics. *International Journal of Parasitology* 26: 937–947.

Tests to validate the ethnoveterinary use of *Eucalyptus grandis* leaves against gastrointestinal parasites of livestock were conducted on feral goats. Autopsy revealed 91% fewer *Haemonchus contortus* in the treatment as compared to the control group, with $p < 0.05$. [Abstract based on a citation in Fielding 1998.]

Benoit, Michel. 1979. *Le Chemin des Peul du Boobola: Contribution à l'Ecologie du Pastoralisme en Afrique des Savanes.* Travaux et documents de l'O.R.S.T.O.M. No. 101. ORSTOM, Paris, France.

Entitled 'The Path of the Peul [Fulani] of Boobola', this volume offers a chapter on sleeping sickness that describes how modern vaccination of cattle for trypanosomosis has been integrated into the veterinary customs of Fulani pastoralists in Upper Volta [now Burkina Faso]. The author also notes that Fulani's judicious seasonal movement of cattle constitutes an effective empirical method of disease control (pp. 50–52). But he stresses the term 'empirical', in that Fulani do not directly connect the fly vector of trypanosomosis with the sickness itself, even though they clearly recognize the symptoms of trypanosomosis.

Bensa, A. 1978. *Les Saints Guérisseurs du Perche-Gouët.* Institut d'Ethnologie, Paris, France. 301 pp.

Unavailable for review. However, according to Brisebarre 1985a, see especially Part 3, pp. 203–247.

Bentz, Kelly. 1994. Animal health practices in Noakhali – An ethnoveterinary study. Mennonite Central Committee Agricultural Programs, Dhaka, Bangladesh. *Station and Farming Systems Research Results* 20: 133–144.

This abbreviated version of Bentz's original report describes a survey conducted among 33 households in Noakhali, Bangladesh. Producers generally treat livestock diseases themselves; but if they require outside services, 24% turn to traditional veterinary practitioners, 15% to religious healers or holy men, 24% to government veterinarians, 18% to paravets, and 18% to other sources. The paper also provides prescriptions for the control of crop pests.

Berg, Hans van den. 1985. *Diccionario Religioso Aymara.* Talleres Gráficos del CETA [Centro de Estudios Teológicos de la Amazonia] with IDEA [Instituto de Estudios Aymaras], Iquitos, Perú. 280 pp.

This volume summarizes, in dictionary form, the ideological concepts and vocabulary of the Aymara Indians of Bolivia and Peru. It notes many supernatural aspects of ethnoveterinary belief and practice. For example, a bell and/or a fetish bundle is hung about the necks of young animals, who are believed to be especially susceptible to evil spirits' that can enter them, thereby causing disease and even death. Various amulets and figurines are used in rituals to ward against diseases, lightning, predators and evil spirits or to guarantee flock reproductivity, health and pastoral luck. Numerous other items serve similar functions, like dried wildcat carcasses and animal foetuses. Omens are used to prognosticate herd well-being. Also, certain beneficent spirits are believed to protect herds.

Bernatzik, Hugo Adolf. 1947. *Akha und Meau, Probleme der angewandten Voelkerkunde in Hinterindien.* Wagner'sche Universitaetsbuch-druckerei, Innsbruck, Austria.

Pages 500–501 of this ethnography briefly describe how Meau stockowners in Thailand castrate their domestic animals. With cattle, they clamp the scrotum between sticks and smash it with a cudgel. On pigs, dogs, horses and poultry, they use open surgery.

Bernus, Edmond. 1979a. L'arbre et le nomade. *Journal d'Agriculture Traditionelle et de Botanique Appliquée* 26(2): 103–127.

This article describes Twareg and Fulani nomads' use of many types of Sahelian trees and bushes. Of ethnoveterinary note is the application of dried, pounded *Maerua crassifolia* bark to saddle sores on camels. *Boscia senegalensis* has multiple uses. Along with the millet and the bark of *M. crassifolia*, its green fruit is pounded into a poultice for camel sores. *Boscia senegalensis* leaves are dried, pounded, boiled, then mixed with cow milk and administered orally to camels with stomach pain. Feverish camels are cured by an aqueous drench of the pounded leaves and salt. Animals weakened by trypanosomosis are given the leaves mixed with ewe's urine and tobacco.

Bernus, Edmond. 1979b. Le contrôle du milieu naturel et du troupeau par les éleveurs touaregs sahéliens. In: L'Équipe Écologie et Anthropologie des Sociétés Pastorales (eds). *Pastoral Production and Society/Production Pastorale et Société.* Proceedings of the International Meeting on Nomadic Pastoralism/Actes du Colloque International sur le Pastoralisme Nomade, Paris, 1–3 December 1976. Cambridge University Press and Editions de la Maison des Sciences de l'Homme, Cambridge, UK, and Paris, France. Pp. 67–74.

In describing Twareg pastoralists' natural resource use patterns, this chapter mentions how their nomadic movements are in part dictated by herds' need for periodic 'salt cures'. Designed to combat night blindness and internal parasites (among other conditions), such cures are effected through watering stock at highly mineralized wells and grazing them in regions with salty soils. The author also notes that the Twareg practice a sophisticated crossbreeding among their camels and 'very elaborate techniques of veterinary curing' (p. 71). Controlled breeding among small livestock is achieved in part by tying the penis to the scrotum or by hobbling the males. Castration is performed either by surgery or by hammering the testicles, depending upon the season and the age and type of animal. The first method is considered to increase the animal's overall size and hence is primarily used with camels and horses; the second, supposed to fatten, is used with sheep and goats. However, during the rainy season, the first method is not used due to the danger of infection. The author also mentions Twareg efforts toward genetic improvement of hunting dogs.

Bernus, Edmond. 1981. *Touaregs Nigériens: Unité Culturelle et Diversité Régionale d'un Peuple Pasteur.* Memoires ORSTOM No. 94. ORSTOM, Paris. 508 pp.

Twareg pastoralists of Niger keep mixed herds of sheep, goats, cattle, horses, donkeys, and especially camels. This *magnum opus* on every aspect of Twareg history and life includes one section on Twareg veterinary medicine (p. 190 ff.). Although capable of great feats, camels are in fact fragile animals when it comes to their health, says the author. Gastrointestinal upsets and diarrhoeas can be triggered in camels by myriad causes: drinking 'rotten' water; ingesting too much salty water or forage all at once or without being accustomed to it; likewise for certain pasture plants, especially at certain times of the year. Depending on the aetiology, treatments span, e.g.: running the animal to purge it; and especially for bloody diarrhoea, drenching with a decoction of pounded *Boscia senegalensis* leaves in water and cow's milk. A drench of the same leaves in salted water serves as a febrifuge. Wounds are plastered with a mixture of charcoal and chewn tobacco or one of the green fruits of *B. senegalensis*, millet, and *Maerua crassifolia* tree bark. A suite of remedies exist for wounds, blows, swellings, etc. of the foot, limbs, and ears in camels – from different varieties of firing, through scarification, and lancing. For congestion, camels are bled from the jugular vein. For sinusitis, pus-filled areas are scarified to expel the pus, then the incisions are cauterized and dressed with butter. 'Craziness' is treated by bleeding the tips of the ears, firing the temples, or scarifying the head. 'Calluses' on the eyes are surgically removed with a blade, and then dusted with powdered tobacco. Mange lesions are bandaged over with an elaborately cooked concoction of *Commiphora africana* gum and *Balanites aegyptiaca* fruit pits or with a sort of 'tar' cooked from another set of ingredients. An alternate mange application is made from charred bonemeal, camel hair from a hide about to be tanned, ash from *Cymbopogon proximus* or millet stalks, all in a decoction of *B. senegalensis*, which is left to rest for a week. The mixture is then applied to the mangey areas after they have been scraped clean of hair. Mangey goats are similarly treated with pounded *Calotropis procera* roots macerated in water overnight and then mixed with butter. Anthrax in cattle is treated by an intranasal drench of red clay in ewe's milk and by topical application of the milk froth to inflamed areas. Small ruminants with anthrax are scarified on the ears, nose and tail tip until the blood flows freely. The treatment for trypanosomosis is complex: the camel is fed roasted and pounded jackal meat or ostrich intestines, followed the next day by an intranasal drench of a strained infusion of pounded tobacco and *B. senegalensis* leaves steeped overnight in ewe's urine. Cooked and pounded meat is also a sometimes-effective antidote for *Ipomoea asarifolia* poisoning. Twareg know no cure for poisoning from *Chrozophora brocchiana* or for broncho-pneumonia in camels, nor for anthrax in cattle. For footrot in cattle and small ruminants, the feet and tongue are annointed with a paste of, respectively, sorghum and *M. crassifolia* fruits. Alternative treatments for small ruminants are firing and a plaster of crushed *Acacia nilotica* pods. 'Crazy' cattle are branded about the head. Sore or infected udders are spread with an ointment made from burnt, crushed *Acacia ehrenbergiana* root bark mixed into butter. When cattle become bloated from eating wild sorghum and other problem plants, they may be force-fed water and run until they vomit or their abdomen may be punctured. Besides poisonous plants, herders recognize several galactogenic species, including *Blepharis linariifolia* and especially *I. verticillata*. Today, Twareg use modern vaccines for rinderpest and haemorrhagic septicaemia instead of their traditional crude vaccines made from diseased lung-tissue surgically inserted, respectively, in the ear and forehead. Poxes and pneumonias in small ruminants are treated simply by feeding salty earth and branding the rump, respectively. For donkeys and horses with colds, one end of a dry *C. procera* branch is lit and the other end is stuck in one of the patient's nostrils, thus forcing the animal to inhale the smoke. Other equine cold remedies consist of pouring salty water or, alternatively, pounded *B. senegalensis* leaves in ewe's urine, down the nostrils. Syphilis-like sores on donkeys are incised to release the pus and blood, and then cauterized. Constipated horses and horses with intestinal parasites are fed purging boluses of pounded *M. crassifolia* leaves mixed with a little millet for palatability. A fast-acting laxative for horses consists of inserting *B. senegalensis* leaves into the anus. Many other remedies for unidentified ills in all species are described, along

with the many ways in which Twareg systematically search out and feed salt and
other nutrients to their herds. For example, salt is often mixed with termite earth or
herbs like *Bauhinia reticulata* and the ubiquitous *B. senegalensis*. When it comes
to breeds and breeding, Twareg keep two basic strains of camel: one mainly for
milk and one for transport. Herders assist camels in both mating and birthing. In
the latter, they blow into a newborn's nostrils to stimulate breathing, and they make
sure it suckles colostrum. She-camels that do not conceive after several matings are
treated for infertility by putting salt in their vaginas. If a camel-calf is stillborn or
dies shortly after birth, to keep the dam in milk the herder blindfolds her, smears
the placenta on another calf, lays it before the dam, and removes the blindfold. If
an older camel or cattle calf dies, its skin is tied over a foster calf and sprinkled
with salt until the dam accepts it as her own. If no foster camel is available, the skin
is placed on a straw dummy – a ruse that herders say rarely works, however. If both
these methods fail, a complex, three-day deception is essayed with a foster calf. It
entails blindfolding her; blocking her sense of smell by cutting her nose so that it
bleeds; and closing her anus with a grass mesh. When the anus is opened, faeces
and gases are expelled, giving the dam the impression of having just given birth;
and when the blindfold is removed, the first thing she sees is her foster calf. The
herdsman continues to cut her nose for 2 or 3 more days to prevent her from rejecting the calf on grounds of smell. For both she-camels and cows, an alternative is to
substitute a lamb or kid for the dead calf. All these operations may include shout-
ing at the dam, miming jackal attacks, and so forth, to try to trigger her protective
instincts toward the calf. To stimulate milk let-down in such dams, herders may
massage the teats or blow on the vulva. For sheep and goats, fostering is easy.
Herders merely stick their fingers into the dam's vagina, then rub their fingers over
her nose, and present her with the foster animal, on whom she thus smells her own
scent. Weaning practices consist of: tying a bark netting over a she-camel's teats
during the day; hobbling her so she cannot rise during the night; passing a cord
through the camel calf's upper lip and tying the cord to its teeth; muzzling cattle
calves; for both camel and cattle calves, making small gashes in the muzzle and/or
inserting a nail in the skin in such a way that the calf is pained whenever it tries to
nurse; or conversely, affixing a forked stick in the calf's nose so it pains the dam.
When it comes to breeding, camels are carefully selected for castration as pack or
riding animals according to a galaxy of criteria. For camels and, to a lesser extent,
cattle, pedigrees are tracked via individual camel names that reflect maternal ancestry and that do not change throughout an animal's life, even if it joins a different herd.
White camels and a special piebald strain with different-coloured eyes are particularly prized for salt caravaning. Twareg cattle are of a unique zebu race known as
Azawak that yields much milk by comparison, say, to Fulani Bororodji cattle. Cattle
are usually castrated using a bloodless method that, by crushing the testes with a
stick, diminishes chances of infection; and the operation is performed at the time of
year when animals are in best condition, i.e. the rainy season. Open surgery, in which
the testes are excised with a knife, is the norm for camels; and herders wait to
castrate camels until the end of the rains, so as to avoid the flies and humidity that
can promote infection. For sheep, only special individuals selected for fattening for
religious and other feasts are castrated; they are tethered next to the tent and fed milk
and porridge until they become 'enormous' (p. 176). Otherwise, in most Twareg
clans, the penises of both rams and bucks are simply tied to one side until the chosen
mating time arrives; after breeding, the penises are re-tied. In this way, does can be
limited to one birth per year instead of two; an alternative is to separate does into two

herds, to spread births into two seasons and thus ensure a constant supply of goat milk. But some Twareg clans exercise no control over goats, while others castrate them. Goats are generally kept at the home encampment, except for annual salt-seeking migrations. This volume goes on to present different Twareg groups' complex migratory cycles, herding strategies, animal exchanges, and so forth, along with chapters on virtually every other aspect of Twareg life.

Besche-Commenge, B. 1977. *Le Savoir des Bergers de Casabede* (2 volumes). Travaux de l'Institut d'Etudes Meridionales. Université de Toulouse-le-Mirail, Toulouse, France (2 volumes).

Unavailable for review.

Besche-Commenge, Bruno. 1986. Mythe, métis, ou rien, les 'savoirs naturalistes populaires' chassent d'abord les baleines. *Production Pastorale et Société* 18(Spring): 116–136.

Although primarily a philosophical discourse on the merits and extent of indigenous knowledge, this article also reports on the author's researches among agro-pastoralists in the Pyrénées Mountains of France, where farmers described many now-abandoned local animal healthcare and husbandry practices especially relating to breeding. Still, some traditions remain. For example, farmers will not take their animals to summer pastures on a Monday. We are not told why, however.

Bertrand-Rosseau, P. 1978. *Ile de Corse et Magie Blanche.* Publications de la Sorbonne, Paris, France. 173 pp.

Unavailable for review. However, according to Brisebarre 1985a, see especially Chapter 5, 'Magie Pastorale'.

Bhatnagar, Prafull. 1998. Farmer participatory research on ethnoveterinary practices: Approaches and experiences. In: E. Mathias, D.V. Rangnekar and C.M. McCorkle, with M. Martin (eds). *Ethnoveterinary Medicine: Alternatives for Livestock Development – Proceedings of an International Conference Held in Pune, India, 4–6 November 1997. Volume 2: Abstracts.* BAIF Development Research Foundation, Pune, India. Pp. 8–10.

Since 1984 the Indian organization Krishi Vigyan Kendram Badgaon (VBKVK) has been working on various aspects of goat husbandry and healthcare. Through its health umbrella, between 1991 and 1996 VBKVK has succeeded in reducing abortions from 18.6% to 4.8% and the mortality rate of kids from 21.3% to 5.8%. Although both VBKVK and goat-raisers alike recognize the importance of animal healthcare, modern veterinary services are not sustainable without outside intervention, especially from NGOs. As a cost-effective and practical solution to this problem, VBKVK decided to promote EVM. In 1996 it thus commissioned a study entitled 'Ethnoveterinary Practices for Goats in Mewar and Marwar Regions of Rajasthan'. The study addresses: documentation and verification; primary screening; qualification and material collection; validation trials; farmer participatory research; experience sharing and exchange; and a goat demonstration unit. Documentation was done in five districts selected with a view to the migration routes of the Rabaris, a tribe of traditional sheep- and goat-raisers famed for their

EVK. These districts were extensively toured to identify *guni*, i.e. local livestock healers. The study team informally interviewed about 100 *guni* and documented about 350 ethnoveterinary practices for 20 different goat health problems. Verification was done merely on the basis of internal and external consistency of the information. In some cases, the evolution of a given practice was traced in order to sort truly effective treatments from superstitions. At present, VBKVK experts screen the practices documented according to the following parameters: intensity and frequency of occurrence of the problem; conditions under which a certain remedy is preferred for a problem; effectiveness of the traditional remedy vis-à-vis modern medication; costs and availability of the ingredients; skills and expertise required to administer the remedy; and adverse and side-effects. Such screening is essential as the traditional knowledge is highly context-specific in nature and ingredients. However, one benefit of working across a large geographical area is that substitute ingredients, based on different areas' characteristic flora, are revealed. VBKVK plans to store certain, seasonally-available ingredients at its goat demonstration unit for future use. The author cautions that ethnomedical practices can be promoted as an alternative to modern healthcare only if they are effective under local husbandry conditions. A group of goat raisers will therefore test the selected practices under VBKVK guidance using participatory approaches from VBKVK in the cropping sector. The practices that pass FPR trials will then be shared with goat-raisers and local livestock development agencies generally.

Bhavsar, S.K., J.G. Sarvaiya, R.A. Patel, A.M. Thaker, M.P. Verma and J.K. Malik. 1998. Studies on wound healing activity of *Prosopis juliflora* leaf juice. In: E. Mathias, D.V. Rangnekar and C.M. McCorkle, with M. Martin (eds). *Ethnoveterinary Medicine: Alternatives for Livestock Development – Proceedings of an International Conference Held in Pune, India, 4–6 November 1997. Volume 2: Abstracts.* BAIF Development Research Foundation, Pune, India. Pp. 10.

Previous studies have shown that the leaf juice of *Prosopis juliflora* acts against some micro-organisms. This study evaluated the wound-healing activity of a 10% ointment of the leaf juice in calves with surgically-created wounds. The healing process was compared with that induced by a simple ointment of the carrier material only. The ointments were applied daily for 10 days and thereafter every second day until healing was complete. Treatment evaluation was based on clinical, histological and biomechanical studies. Wound tissue was collected at days 7, 14 and 28 after the start of treatment. In both groups, various clinical indices such as inflammatory reaction, granulation, and the contraction and epithelization of tissues at different time intervals were similar. There were no marked differences between groups in the localization of collagen or elastin fibres, mucopolysaccharide concentration, acid and alkaline phosphatase activities, or the tensile strength and extensibility of healing tissue at different stages of healing. In sum, results indicated no significant difference in the wound-healing effects of 10% ointment of leaf juice and the carrier-material ointment.

Bijwal, D.L. 1998. Effects of Nutrospel and oxytetracycline in hypogammaglobulinaemic calves. In: E. Mathias, D.V. Rangnekar and C.M. McCorkle, with M. Martin (eds). *Ethnoveterinary Medicine: Alternatives for Livestock Development – Proceedings of an International Conference Held in Pune,*

India, 4–6 November 1997. Volume 2: Abstracts. BAIF Development Research Foundation, Pune, India. Pp. 10.

The effects of Nutrospel, a commercial herbal immunostimulant, and the broad-spectrum antibiotic oxytetracycline were tested in 12 newborn hypogammaglobulinaemic cross-bred calves. The animals were divided into three groups of four each. The first group was fed with colostrum while the second and third groups received none. All calves of the second group were treated with oxytetracycline at a dosage of 5 mg/kg of body weight (bw) intramuscularly daily for 3 days at the age of 2 and 4 weeks. Calves of the third group were treated with 20 g Nutrospel daily orally in milk for 20 days and oxytetracycline at a dosage of 5 mg/kg bw intramuscularly daily for 3 days at the age of 2 and 5 weeks. All groups were examined for clinical and immunobiochemical changes at different intervals. Colostrum-fed calves were normal and healthy. Colostrum-deprived calves of the second group had a marked immunosuppression that was associated with clinical changes like diarrhoea and dehydration, and 75% mortality. Their levels of serum total proteins, globulins, gammaglobulins, glucose, calcium, iron, copper, zinc and manganese as well as their body weights were significantly lower than the first group's. In the third group, Nutrospel with antimicrobial therapy stimulated resistance and growth, as evidenced in the control of fever, diarrhoea, navel ill and mortality. In this group, the levels of serum total proteins, globulins, gammaglobulins, phosphorus, iron, copper, zinc and manganese, as well as their body weight were significantly higher than the second group's. Results indicated that the combined herbal/antibiotic therapy controlled infections and mortality of hypogammaglobulinaemic calves through antimicrobial, immunostimulatory and growth-promoting effects.

Bizimana, N. 1994a. Epidemiology, surveillance and control of the principal infectious animal diseases in Africa. *Revue Scientifique et Technique de l'Office International des Épizooties* 13(2): 397–416.

Spanning 21 ethnicities continent-wide, this article details traditional criteria and methods – the majority of which remain in use – for the recognition, prevention, and treatment of the principal infectious diseases of ruminants, equines, camels and chickens in Africa. Along with ethno-prognoses and post-mortem carcass handling for each disease discussed, ethnoaetiologies are noted. The latter include, contaminated standing water, muddy corrals, drought, infested pastures, inadequate nutrition, endoparasites, wild animals or their diseased carcasses, dust wallows and dung. Besides visual observation of symptoms, common diagnostic procedures include palpating, listening, smelling and testing the skin's elasticity. Medical responses vary by disease (e.g. tick removal, dew avoidance, ethnopharmaceuticals, flight) and by ethnicity. For instance, for rinderpest, Twareg and Somali pastoralists have homemade vaccinations; Fulani separate sick animals from the herd; and Turkana drench with infusions of *Euphorbia triaculeata*. Moors in Mali and Baggara in the Central African Republic have their own vaccines for CBPP, as do Kikuyu and Somali for CCPP. In Tanzania, cattle are given indigenous vaccinations against anthrax. In all these cases, vaccinations are performed using tissue or other materials from an infected animal which are applied to healthy animals in various ways, depending on disease and ethnic group: as an intranasal drench; by means of an incision; or, after some processing, an injection. Other ethnomedicines are prepared using plants, insects, earths and other materials such as milk, butter, honey, salt, manure, hot and cold water, heated stones and tarred and burnt linen. These may be administered as sprays, washes, baths, drenches, soups, poultices, smoke inhalations, etc. A partial, mechanical treatment for CCPP among Fulani is to close the mouth and one nostril of the affected goat and then blow into the other nostril while striking the rib cage on the side of the congested lung. Somali accompany CCPP treatments with faith healing by reading from the Koran. Also noted for various diseases are: Somali's use of charms; Twareg and Turkana scarification and bleeding techniques to allow the 'evil principle' of certain diseases to leave the body; Fulani's firing; slaughter as an occasional medical option; and the general extermination of rabid or potentially rabid dogs.

Bizimana, Nsekuye. 1994b. *Traditional Veterinary Practice in Africa.* GTZ, Robdorf, Germany. 917 pp.

This compendium of traditional veterinary practices in Africa includes chapters describing diseases and their treatments for cattle, horses, donkeys, mules, camels, goats, sheep, poultry, pigs and dogs. The chapters are divided by species. There are sub-chapters on the following: diseases of the skin, hair, feathers and horns; diseases of the circulatory system; alimentary system; respiratory system; urinary system; reproductive system; motor system; nervous system; sense organs; several organs; nutrition; and toxic substances. The appendices contain lists of the English and vernacular names of animal diseases, and botanical and vernacular names of medicinal and poisonous plants. In addition to plant-based treatments, blood-letting, washing, firing, cutting and other methods are described. As an example of the depth of this book, the contents of the chapter on 'Diseases of the skin, hair, feathers and horns' are given: non-infectious diseases (boils, perspiration, broken horns), infectious diseases (ringworm), and parasitic diseases (ectoparasites, fleas, flies, maggots, lice, mites and mange, ticks).

Bizimana, Nsekuye. 1998. Scientific evidence of efficacy of medicinal plants for animal treatment. In: E. Mathias, D.V. Rangnekar and C.M. McCorkle, with M. Martin (eds). *Ethnoveterinary Medicine: Alternatives for Livestock Development – Proceedings of an International Conference Held in Pune, India, 4–6 November 1997. Volume 2: Abstracts.* BAIF Development Research Foundation, Pune, India. Pp. 11–12.

With the development of modern medicine, especially after WWII, traditional medical practices have been increasingly replaced and overlooked at the international level, on the assumption that they are ineffective. By contrast, modern medicine was thought to be able to solve almost all human and animal health problems. But this overestimation of modern medicine changed in the course of the 'green wave' demand for natural drugs, foods and cosmetics that began in the 1970s, particularly in industrialized countries. The wave was triggered mainly by growing recognition of the adverse side-effects resulting from the increasing use of chemicals in various areas of life, including medicine. This movement has stimulated a reconsideration of traditional medical systems, since these are largely based on natural products. Coupled with the fact that modern medicine is too expensive for many developing countries, this reconsideration in the industrialized world led in the 1970s to WHO promotion of traditional medical systems, particularly by scientific research into the efficacy and active therapeutic principles of plants used in traditional medicine. Subsequently, thousands of such plants have been investigated; and in many cases, a correlation between traditional medical uses and pharmacological findings has been established and the active principles identified and isolated. Meanwhile some promising substances like the antimalarial artemisinin from *Artemisia annua* and the contraceptive gossypol from *Gossypium* spp. have been discovered; and taxol from *Taxus brevifolia* Nutt. has rapidly become a leading anticancer drug. Today herbal medicines are big business. The market for phytomedicines in the USA alone is currently estimated at over US $1 billion annually; and in the European Community, annual sales of herbal remedies recently exceeded US $6 billion. In contrast to traditional medicine for humans, however, traditional or 'ethno-' veterinary medicine has not yet won broad international R&D attention. Work in this field has been largely limited to cataloguing which plants are used for which purposes. But many plants used in human medicine are equally helpful for understanding and sustaining the use of veterinary medicinal plants. Thus, numerous researchers are now engaged in compiling data from the existing literature on the efficacy and the biological and pharmacological properties of African plants employed in both human and animal ethnomedicine. Huge amounts of data have come together and are valuable not only for Africa but also for other (especially tropical) areas, where many of the same species are found and used medically. This paper presents details on selected plants to show the correlation between traditional veterinary claims and chemical and pharmacological findings. A book with the complete results of this study of African pharmacopoeia is forthcoming.

Bizimana, N. and W. Schrecke. 1996. African traditional veterinary practices and their possible contribution to animal health and production. In: Karl-Hans Zessin (ed.). ***Livestock Production and Diseases in the Tropics: Livestock Production and Human Welfare. Proceedings of the VIII International Conference of Institutions of Tropical Veterinary Medicine held from the 25 to 29 September, 1995 in Berlin, Germany.*** Volume II. Deutsche Stiftung für Internationale Entwicklung, Zentralstelle für Ernährung und Landwirtschaft, Feldafing, Germany. Pp. 582–587.

This conference paper reports the results of a bibliographic study of the chemical and pharmacological properties of more than 30 plants used in African EVM. The plants are divided into four categories: antiparasitic, anthelmintic and molluscicidal, antibiotic and other. Findings are presented in tabular form by Latin plant name, traditional use(s), probable active principle(s) and pharmacological properties as reported in the literature. Illustrating for each category, the pungent oil of *Tagetes minuta* L. contains carvone, linaoöl, and other elements and is used as a fly repellent in southern and eastern Africa. In Nigeria and Madagascar, *Carica papaya* shoots and seed oil, which contain the vermicide papain, serve as anthelmintics. *Khaya senegalensis* stembark is used throughout West Africa to treat fevers, inflammations, diarrhoea and abdominal disorders in both humans and animals; it contains sterols and coumarins with antipyretic properties. And almost everywhere it is found in Africa, *Ricinus communis* L. seed oil is given to combat constipation; this oil's purgative effects have been known worldwide for centuries. Overall, findings reveal a clear correlation between the properties of such 'drug plants' and the veterinary purposes to which they are put in Africa. Yet in the face of pressures from veterinary faculties and the pharmaceutical industry, animal healthcare practitioners and veterinary authorities are indiscriminately promoting modern chemo-prophylactica and -therapeutica, not only for serious animal diseases but also for minor health problems. In consequence, 'Practical authentic know-how and skills acquired over centuries by the African population are about to be forgotten. It is all too likely that simple, efficient . . . and inexpensive methods, which the animals' keepers themselves can apply, will very soon vanish forever' (p. 582). To forestall such a sad state of affairs, the authors argue for promptly integrating traditional African veterinary medicine into formal animal healthcare systems so as to optimize the efficiency of both public and private veterinary services. To this end, they list several mechanisms for so doing, e.g. collecting and studying traditional practices, including them in university curricula, raising awareness, and facilitating information exchange between veterinarians and livestock keepers.

Black-Michaud, Jacob. 1986. *Sheep and Land: The Economics of Power in a Tribal Society.* Cambridge University Press and Editions de la Maison des Sciences de l'Homme, Cambridge, UK, and Paris, France. 231 pp.

This ethnography focuses on the political-economic organization of nomadic pastoralists in Luristan, Iran, and their relationships with sedentary agro-pastoralists. However, Chapter 3 briefly treats pastoral resources and production techniques, including production and processing of wool, meat and milk, flock composition, and general husbandry. The latter is described as apathetic and fatalistic due to the extremely low yields from Luri pastoralism. The author also finds Luri veterinary practices and knowledge very much lacking, in comparison with other Asian pastoralists. Despite chronic parasitism in their sheep and goats, the Lurs are unaware of parasitic life cycles and the hygienic measures these imply. They make only sporadic and ill-timed attempts at prophylaxes and treatments for parasitism, footrot and respiratory ailments using Western-world drugs which, because of their cost, are always administered too sparingly. The author likewise considers Luri breeding, feeding, predator control, trailing techniques (like throwing stones at the animals) and castration patterns irrational. Perhaps more interesting, however, he blames the imperfect extension of Western veterinary medicine for contributing to genetic deterioration of flocks by keeping alive sickly and deformed ewes that would otherwise have perished.

Blakeway, Stephen. 1993. Animal health: Community problem, community care. *Appropriate Technology* 19(4): 5–7.

Community animal healthcare (CAH) projects in Kenya use local knowledge of livestock healthcare and husbandry in training CAH workers. Community-chosen trainees learn about local ruminant diseases and both modern and traditional veterinary drugs and methods, and they are encouraged to use traditional treatments when appropriate. Some trainees are herbalists who keep their own medicinal herb gardens, although Kenyans tend to consider cultivated plants less powerful than wild ones. The text cites one example of an indigenous veterinary technique, in which Turkana pastoralists rub fat and blood into sores around lambs' mouths. The author offers the following insights on the role of EVM in CAH projects. 'If existing husbandry practices or treatments are coping with problems, there is no need to replace them. That does not mean that people should not have access to new information, but care should be taken not to give the blanket impression that modern drugs necessarily work better. . . . the loss of traditional knowledge not only deprives the local people of their most dependable treatments, it is also a loss to the wider world and can lead to the complete loss of plant species.' And 'The spiritual dimension of much traditional treatment is . . . often ridiculed, but it may well be that element which ensures that the environment is respected' (p. 6).

Blakeway, Stephen. 1997. EVK in Africa – An overview. Paper presented to the First International Conference on Ethnoveterinary Medicine: Alternatives for Livestock Development, Pune, India, 4–6 November 1997. Unpublished. 2 pp.

'Production systems that allow people to raise healthy animals in difficult circumstances are the bedrock of EVK . . . [Yet] it is only recently that outsiders have begun to appreciate the sophistication of most traditional husbandry systems . . . Sadly, this recognition has come at a time when extrinsic factors . . . are making many traditional practices more precarious, while not offering any real improvements or alternatives' (p. 1). In this context, the author outlines five major challenges facing ER&D in Africa today. First is the need to work with and develop EVK within local communities, so it can remain useful and relevant under changing circumstances. An example is HPI's work to establish nurseries of veterinary medicinal plants in Cameroonian communities. Second is to validate local remedies, again within communities insofar as possible, but also to the satisfaction of outsiders. The latter step is necessary in order to restore local confidence in useful aspects of EVK, which has often been sorely shaken by insensitive and unsubstantiated outsider criticisms. An example here is ITDG's confidence-ranking work on traditional veterinary treatments in Kenya. Third is the challenge of sensitizing the African veterinary profession and veterinary education system to the value of EVK and training them on how to approach EVK with an open-mind and a learning orientation. Teaching vets the principles of participatory R&D could be helpful in these regards. Fourth is protection of intellectual property rights such that ER&D does not end up being merely an extractive exercise. The recent award of a plant patent to an ethnic group in India may offer one solution to this challenge. Finally, and most difficult to define is the 'holistic challenge'. In its everyday use, EVK is inextricably linked with animal husbandry practices, animal welfare concepts, environmental management (including relations between livestock and wildlife), religious beliefs and parental education of children. But development projects in Africa typically focus on only one of these arenas. As a result, conflicts could arise between, for example, animal health and wildlife preservation initiatives; or disjunctures arise, as between animal healthcare and school curricula. The challenge is to view and tackle animal healthcare, including EVK, in a wider perspective that takes off from that of stockraisers themselves. The solution is more highly integrated studies that directly involve local communities.

Blakeway, Stephen, David Adolph, B.J. Linquist and Bryony Jones. 1999. The integration of ethnoveterinary knowledge into a community-based animal health project working with the Dinka and Nuer in Southern Sudan. In: E. Mathias, D.V. Rangnekar and C.M. McCorkle, with M. Martin (eds). *Ethnoveterinary Medicine: Alternatives for Livestock Development –*

Proceedings of an International Conference Held in Pune, India, 4–6 November 1997. Volume 1: Selected Papers. BAIF Development Research Foundation, Pune, India. Pp. 185–188.

Since 1993, a UNICEF livestock project in southern Sudan has been focusing mainly on vaccinations for rinderpest plus vaccination and treatment of a few other major diseases. To this end, it had established a system of community vaccinators. In 1996, the project commissioned a study of EVK among Dinka and Nuer stock-raisers there, to learn how EVK could be integrated into its community-based animal health work. Study findings were many and varied. Dinka and Nuer both have a rich vocabulary of animal health terms, although these terms vary within and between ethnicities. Both groups identify a wide range of health problems, and they boast a high level of EVK, although Dinka and Nuer healers known respectively as *atet* and *leert* naturally control more EVK than ordinary stockraisers. Healers' help is sought for setting broken bones, cutting lumps and performing dystocias (including foetotomies) and sometimes castrations. Healers are also more knowledgeable about plant medicines, which both groups use with confidence. But Dinka, who live in an area of greater plant diversity, employ more such medicines than Nuer; and Dinka herbalists called *ran wal* are particularly adept in their use. But healers generally receive little or no material reward for their assistance. Indeed, despite the existence of healer-specialists, EVK as a whole lies mostly within the public domain, where it is widely and readily shared. And some EVM tasks, like diagnosis, are often a group activity. Many women are knowledgeable about livestock disease, and they may collect, prepare and sometimes administer treatments. Partly as a result of the recent war, female-headed households are increasing in number, and thus more women are taking a larger role in animal healthcare than they did traditionally. On the basis of such findings as the foregoing, the study made a number of recommendations for integrating EVK into project work. First, it urged project personnel to discuss and gain support for building on EVK with local administrators and with donors, emphasizing to the latter: the long-term advantages of integrating EVK into healthcare initiatives; the need for more informal, unstructured, continuing-learning visits with stockraisers about their healthcare practices; and relatedly, the need for longer funding cycles. In terms of future R&D, recommendations were to: discuss with local healers how they might participate in EVK integration, e.g. in seminars to share their knowledge among themselves or as co-trainers in animal health courses; working with linguists and other disciplines, continue building a database of local knowledge of livestock diseases and generate dialect-sensitive dictionaries of EVK terms; translate the EVK resource manuals resulting from this study into local languages; identify confidently used veterinary botanicals, check them against existing databases and phytochemical studies, and canvass healers as to the efficacy of these and other traditional treatments; involve women more, e.g. as experts on smallstock or the early diagnosis of disease. At a larger level, it was recommended that the project investigate why, despite its otherwise sound development procedures, it had marginalized traditional healers and much local livestock knowledge. Since the conclusion of this initial EVK study, the project has moved forward on a number of these recommendations. For example, it has increased references to EVK in its training for community animal health workers; and it discovered that a number of the workers already recruited were in fact traditional healer-specialists.

Blakeway, Stephen, B.J. Linquist and David Adolph. 1996. *Nuer Ethno-Veterinary Knowledge – A Resource Manual: Findings of a Preliminary Study.* UNICEF Lifeline Sudan Southern Sector Livestock Programme, Nairobi, Kenya. 51 pp.

This manual is part of a larger study to investigate whether the work of the above-referenced UNICEF programme could be better integrated with local veterinary knowledge and practice. It records Nuer local knowledge and culture relating to livestock, including: men's and women's pastoral responsibilities; Nuer disease names and groupings plus animal health terms; and botanical and other treatments. 28 diseases or disorders for which there are plant remedies are cited. Only the local names of the plants are given.

Blancou, J. 1994a. Early methods for the surveillance and control of glanders in Europe. *Revue Scientifique et Technique de l'Office International des Épizooties* 13(2): 545–557.

Across centuries, much has been written about glanders [also known as farcy] because of the historical importance of equines as (especially military) transport and because of human susceptibility to the disease. By the beginning of the 20th century, however, glanders had been eradicated nearly everywhere except in some African and Asian countries. Even in an absence of a good understanding of the disease's aetiology and pathogenesis, astute controls were sometimes effected, e.g. by: segregation, quarantine or slaughter of infected animals; destruction of the *Actinobacillus'* reservoirs and vectors; safer handling of infected animals and virulent materials; and annulment of sales of diseased animals. Treatments for horses with glanders were multifarious and largely useless. In Europe, Egypt and Arabia they spanned, for example, praying, bloodletting, cauterizing lesions, fixing a sprig of hellebore under the skin, making the animal inhale origanum smoke, applying nettle leaves in an unspecified manner, and giving various vaccinations and injections.

Blancou, J. 1994b. Early methods for the surveillance and control of rabies in animals. *Revue Scientifique et Technique de l'Office International des Épizooties* 13(2): 361–372.

This article examines certain technical and scientific aspects of the pre-19th-century history of rabies in animals in light of current veterinary knowledge. The focus is on convergences and divergences in people's recognition of rabid animals and their risk avoidance and prevention/control strategies. Across 40 centuries, different people's surveillance and recognition of the clinical and post-mortem signs of rabies, pathogenesis, modes of transmission, susceptible species, and so forth varied greatly in substance and accuracy. General disease control measures instituted at one time or place included: muzzling dogs in 7th and 6th century Persia; as outlined in the Talmud and as legalized in much of post-Renaissance Europe, prohibition of straying; also in Europe, quarantine and observation; and almost everywhere, destruction of carrier animals. At least one, potentially effective, early vaccine, based on the saliva of a rabid dog, was developed by an 18th-century Italian. Medical prophylaxes for rabid animals were few and ineffective, ranging from administering plant-based medicines to amputation of various body parts.

Likewise for treatments. In practice, prior to the discovery of the rabies vaccine, the only way to combat rabies was with hygienic precautions, particularly the killing (including preventive killing) of rabid dogs.

Blomley, Tom. 1994. Indigenous agroforestry: *Melia volkensii in Kenya.* *Agroforestry Today* 6(4): 10–11.

In Kenya, Mbeere, Tharaka and Kamba farmers use an extract of the leaves of *Melia volkensii* as an ectoparasiticide for small ruminants. The extract is rubbed into goats' hides to control ticks and fleas.

Bocquené, Henri. 1986. *Moi, Un Mbororo: Autobiographie de Oumarou Ndoudi Peul Nomade du Cameroun.* Karthala, Paris, France.

In describing the nomadic pastoralist life of Fulani in Cameroon and Nigeria, this book briefly mentions *karfa*, a mixture of plants that is burned on the night fire in the middle of cattle camps, especially during migration (pp. 103, 144, 347). The smoke from the burning *karfa* is believed to strengthen cattle and to make them respectful of their masters and wary of strangers. Fulani also use green wood of any type to make their campfires smoky and thus drive away flies.

Bodding, P.O. 1925. Santal medicine. *Memoirs of the Asiatic Society of Bengal* 10(2): 394–426.

This article lists traditional veterinary prescriptions for cattle from the Santal Parganas district of India. Diseases cited include rinderpest, blackquarter, anthrax, dropsy, fractures, bloat and plant poisoning. Fractures, for example, can be plastered with a thick paste of *Helianthus annuus* W., *Marsilea quadrifolia* L. and *Vitis adnata* R. ground together; splints are then affixed. An alternative remedy is a mixture of *Artocarpus lakoocha* R. bark, *Euphorbia pilulifera* L. leaves, 5 long-legged spiders and 3 black peppercorns, all ground together. Bloat is alleviated by pouring a cup of human urine into the nostrils of the affected cattle. Alternatively, a switch of *Phyllanthus emblica* L. is passed three times over the animal in one breath and the abdomen is struck with the switch five times, after which the herdsman must go straight home without looking back. Antidotes for plant poisoning caused by ingestion of sorghum, castor leaves and linseed plants include preparations of the bark of *Gmelina arborea* Roxb. and *Bauhinia purpurea* L. (p. 403).

Bogdan, Ingeborg, A. Nechifor, I. Basea and Edith Hruban. 1990. Aus der rumänischen Volksmedizin: Unspezifische Reiztherapie durch transkutane Implantation der Nieswurz (*Helleborus purpurascens*, Fam. Ranunculaceae) bei landwirtschaftlichen Nutztieren. *Deutsche Tierärztliche Wochenschrift* 97: 525–529.

For more than 100 years, Rumanian farmers have used *Helleborus purpurascens* to stimulate the immunity of weak and sickly livestock. In spring – when animals are said to 'renew their blood' – farmers implanted a piece of the plant's root in the chest skin of cattle and horses and in the ear flaps of pigs and sheep for about 24 hours. This study examines the effect of this practice on the general condition and blood values of the four livestock species, in comparison with data from animals receiving placebo implants using the same site and methods as for the *Helleborus* root. In each species, three animals received the plant implant and three the placebo. Cattle showed weakness, fever and inappetence and a strong oedema around the implantation site. The latter was also found in horses. The general well-being of pigs and sheep did not seem to be affected and their local reactions were much weaker than those of cattle and horses. The number of red blood cells did not change except in cattle, where it increased. In all but cattle, leucocyte numbers increased significantly within the first 24 hours after implantation. In *all* species the percentage of neutrophils increased significantly and phagocytosis activity was six times higher than the values measured before beginning the experiment. For the placebo groups, the number of leucocytes in horses, sheep and pigs increased very slightly. There was no change in leucocyte composition in any species. In sum, findings suggest that *Helleborus* implants stimulate an immune response. Western medicine should consider this treatment for sheep and pigs but not for cattle and horses because of the latters' strong general and local reactions to it.

Bognounou, Ouétian. 1994. Réflexions sur les thérapeutiques traditionnelles en soins de santé animale et état des connaissances ethnobotaniques au Burkina-Faso. In: Kakule Kasonia and Michel Ansay (eds). ***Métissages en Santé Animale de Madagascar à Haïti: Actes du Séminaire d'Ethnopharmacopée Vétérinaire 'KAGALA', un Partage de Savoirs Burkina-Faso, Ouagadougou, 15–22 Avril 1993.*** Presses Universitaires de Namur, Namur, Belgium. Pp. 181–201.

This literature review notes aspects of traditional horse and cattle treatments and ethnobotanical knowledge among stockraisers in Burkina Faso. Difficulties in collecting EVK data are discussed, such as: identification of qualified informants, and especially over-reliance on educated Africans who in fact may know little about rural realities; language barriers, transcription problems and the lack of correspondence between ethnoscientific and scientific names and interpretations of disease; choice of methodology, such as large-scale surveys versus in-depth interviewing; the collection of voucher samples of plants at different seasons or stages of growth; shortcomings in botanical textbooks; time constraints on researchers' observing the preparation and administration of ethnoveterinary medicines; and finally, an overly 'Cartesian' stance toward the study of EVK. The chapter offers three extensive annexes on details of the plant species cited in the review, results of a survey of veterinary ethnopharmacopoeia, and a list of local healers' EVM secrets. An example of a traditional prescription for coughs in horses is *Cymbopogon schoenanthus* mixed with cattle manure, dog faeces, cotton seeds and chilli pepper; this mixture is placed in a pot with hot coals and administered as an inhalation. A healer treatment for fever in cattle consists of grilling a mixture of *Bombax costatum*, some cheetah skin, chilli pepper, sheanut butter, red millet and salt, and then applying the mixture in the form of a cross on the animal's tongue. Briefly mentioned in the text or the healer annex are hydrotherapies, surgical operations, foot/hoof toughening techniques, and controls on breeding.

Bollig, Michael. 1992. East Pokot camel husbandry. ***Nomadic Peoples*** 31: 34–50.

Pokot camel pastoralists of northwestern Kenya distinguish four types of diseases: pest-borne ills, transmitted by flies and ticks; 'diseases which are in the ground, in the dust, or in the grass'; ailments due to lack of salt; and supernatural ills such as the evil eye. Pokot believe the first two types result in 'bad' body fluids, which they purge by drenching with botanical laxatives. Lack of salt is said to cause ills such as unthriftiness and skin necrosis. For the former, camels are trailed to natural salt licks, or are given a sack of salty earth to lick. For skin necrosis, the entire plant of *Kleinia* sp. is ground, dissolved in water, and rubbed over the camel's body. Alternatively, the camel may be drenched with soda ash dissolved in water. Severe diarrhoea is treated either by burning a sheep's head, boiling it and feeding the soup or by drenching with an infusion of smashed unripe *Boscia coreacea* fruit. The latter three treatments have a purgative effect. A cure for pneumonia is feeding pounded *Cyperus alternifolius* bark, firing along the ribs, and washing the animal with a solution of soda ash. Altogether, the Pokot ethnopharmacopoeia includes 20 to 30 plants, as well as firing and minor operations, with blessings usually accompanying treatments. To ward against the evil eye, camel enclosures are built some distance away from the main homestead in order to keep calves out of envious visitors' sight. Mixed in with their traditional practices, Pokot frequently use modern medicines too.

Bollig, Michael. 1995. The veterinary system of the pastoral Pokot. *Nomadic Peoples* 36/37: 17–34.

Pokot pastoralists live in the semi-arid savanna of northwestern Kenya, where they keep cattle, camels, goats, sheep and donkeys. Pokot names for livestock diseases frequently represent the affected part of the body, refer to the cause of the disease, or are borrowed from other languages. Tables list causes of premature deaths among Pokot livestock, plus the vernacular and scientific names of some 40 livestock diseases. Herders understand the aetiology of most of these ills and seem to differentiate between vector-borne, contagious and deficiency diseases. The article details treatments for each disease and provides an overview of Pokot veterinary medicine that spans herbal and non-herbal treatments, manipulative techniques, and magico-religious practices. Pokot also use antibiotics and other commercial drugs, but often in the wrong dosages. Thus, projects to teach them more about when and how to use commercial drugs would be helpful.

Bolton, Ralph and Linda Calvin. 1985. El cuy en la cultura peruana contemporánea. In: Heather Lechtman and Ana Maria Soldi (eds). *La Tecnología en el Mundo Andino: Runakunap Kawsayninkupaq Rurasqankunaqa. Tomo I: Subsistencia y Mensuración.* Imprenta Universitaria de la Universidad Nacional Autónoma de México, México DF. Pp. 261–326.

An alternative title for this book chapter might have been 'Everything you ever wanted to know about guinea pig raising in the Andes'. Or at least, almost everything. Based on field research in the community of Santa Bárbara in Canchis Province, Department of Cuzco, Peru, the authors discuss in detail such topics as: sex, age, colour and pelt classifications for guinea pigs; their daily management, reproductive behaviour, and growth; ideal hutch composition by number, sex and age; and the animals' importance in human diet and ritual. With regard to management of guinea pig health, the authors note that the principal problems are louse and flea infestation and bites from poisonous spiders. Producers mainly combat these pests by keeping the animals in smoke-filled places, usually the family kitchen. In some instances, guinea pigs may also be treated with an unguent of llama fat. A mysterious disease known only as '*cuy* sickness' (possibly rabies), for which the people of Santa Bárbara have no cure, can wipe out entire hutches.

Additional aspects of *cuy* management include extra feeding for postpartum females and castration of aggressive males.

Bonfiglioli, Angelo Maliki. 1988. *Le Baton et la Houe: Introduction à l'Agro-pastoralisme du Sahel Tchadien.* Report prepared for the World Bank Project on the Social Dimensions of Adjustment, N'Djaména, Chad. 147 pp. [Working draft cited with permission of the author and of the World Bank.]

This report focuses on Chadian agropastoralists' social, economic, and political organization plus their cultivation and herding systems. One brief section deals with 'Herd Management and Animal Cures' (pp. 70–74). Principal among these are watering practices and mineral feedings, both of which are tailored to specific sex, age and reproductive classes. Feeding of salt and other minerals is accomplished by driving animals to pastures of mineral-rich or 'salty' forages and soil, watering them at wells known to have a high natron content (hydrated sodium carbonate), mounting long-distance caravans to collect natron, or purchasing natron. Many other aspects of herd management are also discussed, particularly herd composition and subdivisions, and grazing movements and strategies.

Bonfiglioli, Angelo Maliki, Yero Doro Diallo and Sonja Fagerberg-Diallo. 1988. *Kisal: Production et Survie au Ferlo (Sénégal).* Rapport préliminaire. Oxfam, Dakar, Senegal. 64 pp.

Kisal, or survival, has a central meaning in the life of the Fulani in Ferlo, a region of northeastern Senegal. This study describes the seasons of the nomadic year and seasonal work requirements for different family members. It also discusses Ferlo animal husbandry and agricultural activities. Pages 44–55 deal with nutrition and EVM. The herders differentiate between seasonal nutritional deficiencies and those which occur year-round. They believe that mineral deficiencies can cause weakness, leading to blindness, haemorrhages and internal parasitism. They have thus developed several strategies for supplementing their animals' diet with salt [see Bernus 1979]. According to the authors, Fulani concepts of disease can be grouped into the following categories: contagious diseases, diseases derived directly from the environment, nutritional deficiencies, diseases specific to certain animal species, and pathological conditions, which are the consequence of fate. Treatments include traditional medicines applied orally or topically, branding, cauterization, fumigation, surgery and massage. The pastoralists prevent diseases by quarantine, vaccination, nutritional improvements, magical antidotes and avoidance of infected areas.

Bonfiglioli, Angelo-Maliki, Yero D. Diallo and Sonja Fagerberg-Diallo. 1996. Veterinary science and savvy among the Ferlo Fulße. In: Constance M. McCorkle, Evelyn Mathias and Tjaart W. Schillhorn van Veen (eds). *Ethnoveterinary Research & Development.* Intermediate Technology Publications, London, UK. Pp. 246–255.

Taking an 'insider' point of view, this chapter overviews traditional knowledge and practice pertaining to cattle health among Fulße, a Fulani group of the Ferlo region of northern Senegal. Based on interviews, the second author – himself a member of a pastoral family – identified 35 emically recognized cattle 'diseases' and some 26 other conditions. Fulße concepts of animal health problems fall into four broad categories. First are contagious diseases: pleuropneumonias, FMD, blackleg, anthrax, rinderpest and a chronic botulism. Fulani say these can be spread by wild animals, the wind, odours in the air, sometimes the steam from cooking the meat of an animal dead of a contagious disease, and also by handling a healthy animal after touching a diseased carcass. Second are general sorts of diseases considered non-contagious, such as fevers, swellings, malnutrition and environmentally-linked ills. The latter refer to natural resources such as forages, water, soils and wildlife, reflecting Fulße's basic belief that a good environment promotes good livestock production while a bad one creates health problems. For example, poisoning, abortions and bloat can variously result from grazing sandy, toxic-plant-infested, littered (e.g. with plastic bags), and other kinds of 'bad' pastures. Other ills results from the heat, cold and poor forages of different seasons. Wildlife such as birds, ticks, flies and worms are known to contaminate pastures and cause certain diseases. The third category consists of health problems associated with particular sexes or ages of cattle, especially newborn calves and their dams. Last are accidents and sorcery, although the Pulaar language has no term for accidents as these are seen as 'fated' events. With the assistance of the third author, a linguist, all these conditions are presented here in the original Pulaar language. For each health problem, interviewees described its contagiousness, key symptoms, sea-sonal prevalence, causes or predisposing factors, and treatments. The authors divide treatments into preventive and curative ones, of which all Fulße know many. The keystone of preventive care, however, is the daily and seasonal movement of herds, so as to keep livestock camps and quarters clean and free of pathogen buildup, search out the lushest or especially nutritious grasses and clean water, keep stock away from ripening crops, and periodically lead the herd to sources of salt. A multipurpose prophylaxis is the feeding of special minerals, by animal health and age; e.g. salt may be mixed with water and bitter or salty leaves such as those of baobab, *Combretum* spp., and okra. A more specific prophylaxis is an indigenous vaccine for CBPP. Curative treatments include herbal medicines, bloodletting, piercing and incising the skin, bonesetting, branding, cauterizing, fumigation, massage and simple hydrotherapies. All kinds of treatment can also involve incantations and rituals. In addition, herders have access to local healers, known as *ñeeñduße* or *gannduße*, who specialize in treating certain unusual or complex diseases or, in the case of *bileejo* healers, ailments due to sorcery. To con-clude, the chapter describes how all of this carefully collected information was put to practical development purposes. Two booklets were produced in Pulaar on Fulße ethnoveterinary vocabulary, as readers for a national NGO's functional literacy program. Besides meeting the desperate need for training materials relevant to pastoralists' daily lives, the booklets implicitly acknowledged the value of Fulße culture and technology. This approach to literacy training provided students with a way individually to expand, and collectively to share and reaffirm, but also think critically about, their fund of local knowledge. The information in the booklets was also utilized in designing post-literacy classes in which participants learned to keep records on the livestock diseases in their area. This practical application greatly increased herders' interest in maintaining their literacy skills. It also empowered them to do more systematic epidemiological surveillance on their own, in turn enabling them to apply or coordinate their traditional (as well as modern) strate-gies of disease avoidance and control in more timely or effective ways. Herders' resulting skills and records could also facilitate the work of national epidemio-logical intelligence systems. Used by an international NGO (Oxfam) to train

Pulaar-speaking veterinary auxiliaries, the same booklets rapidly established a shared vocabulary and knowledge base between trainers and trainees. This significantly accelerated training and focused it on areas where all agreed that inputs of more 'outsider' veterinary information would be most useful.

Borthakur, S.K. and U.K. Sarma. 1996. Ethnoveterinary medicine with special reference to cattle prevalent among the Nepalis of Assam, India. In: S.K. Jain (ed.). ***Ethnobiology in Human Welfare.*** Deep Publications, New Delhi, India. Pp. 197–199.

Nepali immigrants into India's Assam State raise goats mainly for meat, and buffalo and cattle for dairy products. This article reports on 45 wild and cultivated plants plus associated ingredients (alum, common and rock salt) used in 32 Nepali prescriptions for treating these animals' urinary, gastrointestinal, respiratory, reproductive, endocrine, energetic and ectoparasitic problems, along with other ills such as burns, sprains and wounds. Precise details of prescription preparation and administration are given throughout. The study that generated these findings was based on a survey conducted iteratively between 1989 and 1994, spanning different seasons and geographic areas. The methodology is noteworthy for a number of features: data are based on firsthand reports from practitioners of veterinary medicine and on personal observations by the authors (both university botanists); the findings reported here were cross-checked with different informants; and only those remedies known to have been applied on at least five separate occasions were considered for further verification, which was done by the authors' follow-up observations of treatment efficacy.

Boutrais, Jean. 1988. ***Des Peul en Savanes Humides: Développement Pastoral dans l'Oest Centrafricain.*** Éditions de l'ORSTOM, Paris, France. 387 pp.

This volume deals with the lifeways and especially the stockraising activities of three major groups of Fulani in the humid savannas of western Central African Republic (CAR), as revealed in a 6-month field study in 1984. The three groups are Fulße, Mbororo and migrants from the general direction of Chad. Mbororo's main race of cattle is the red zebu, which has been carefully selected for hardiness and for a number of ethological traits such as attachment to its master, fear of strangers, 'disciplined' herding, and courage. However, the red zebu has little resistance to trypanosomosis and it requires large quantities of fresh forage; hence its masters' many pastoral movements. Mbororo also keep smaller numbers of white zebu of two strains (small and large) that hail from northern Nigeria and Chad. In CAR the big white zebu has nearly disappeared, but the smaller variety persists. Different clans and tribes of Fulani maintain different mixes of these and other cattle breeds. Mbororo in particular pay great attention to breeding and are able rapidly to change their animal 'materials'. One traditional way to obtain new genetic material is to exchange a large male animal for a heifer of another breed with passing cattle merchants on their way to urban meat markets. An Mbororo may also borrow a stud bull of a different race from a co-ethnic for 4, 5 or as much as 10 years, after which the bull is returned to its master along with a heifer in thanks for the loan. Sometimes members of related lineages make outright gifts of breedstock to each other, as well. A final mechanism is to graze one's herd near another herd with the desired traits, in hopes that the animals will mingle and mate naturally. Currently,

CAR Fulani are emphasizing interbreeding of red zebu with races that can survive on limited, dry forage, as people's access to pasturage and their migratory movements are increasingly constrained. Choices and mixes in breeds also vary according to a man's stage in life. Young men, who are able to go on long migrations, prefer fewer but bigger, albeit riskier, breeds in their 'stock portfolio'; but as they age and migrate less often or widely, they shift to more conservative investments in the form of greater numbers of smaller, more trypanotolerant animals. But for young and old alike, the subject of breeds and breedings is a passionate one they never tire of discussing; and Fulani experiment constantly with new crossings. Today, CAR Fulani maintain multiple races of cattle in the same herd. Along with castration, one method of controlling breeding is judicious selection of sale animals. Lately, however, some groups of Fulani have found themselves so pressed for cash with which to buy food that they are selling off healthy young breedstock (female as well as male), having already disposed of all their bulls, old cows and steers except for the steers trained as pack animals. However, Fulani still practice a 'social code' in which cows are lent to co-ethnics in need. And every herder disperses animals to other Fulani as a way to reduce losses to epidemics. Disease avoidance is also a consideration in migrations. But many CAR Fulani claim that their traditional migratory routes and areas are now all disease-ridden and overgrazed, and thus that herd movements today engender more ills than they avoid. This development is linked to increased privatization of land. Another change in traditional lifeways for CAR Fulani has been widescale abandonment of sheepraising due to predators (panthers, civets and dogs) and rustling. When it comes to healthcare for their cattle, Fulani happily pay for modern vaccines against epidemic diseases, although they also note that there have been problems with vaccine quality, corruption in the livestock service, and needless vaccinations of animals already immune to certain diseases. Many herders now give vaccinations themselves, although they confess they are often unsure of indications, proper dosages and injection techniques. For basic animal healthcare, CAR Fulani must rely on their own skills and resources, since the livestock service offers virtually no such care. They employ both traditional and, nowadays, mainly modern treatments. Among the former, the only examples of therapies given in this volume are: for diarrhoea, a decocted aqueous drench of *Stereospermum kunthianum* or sheanut-tree bark powdered together; and for wounds on the bottom of the feet, otitis and coccidiosis, firing with a hot iron. Preventive measures include regular feeding of salt or preferably natron, and manual de-ticking. The latter is a major activity of men, women and children throughout the wet season. Today, traditional medicine is being abandoned or forgotten by a majority of CAR Fulani. In part, this may be because Fulani no longer have access to some of the medicinal plant species they knew in their northern homelands. But Fulani have also come to consider various local treatments unreliable – whether because Fulani have been swayed by modern medicine or because local remedies cannot combat the diseases of Fulani's new humid-savanna environment is not clear. Despite their adoption of modern medicines, CAR Fulani have an imperfect understanding of their use, as evidenced by their: injecting terramycin for gastrointestinal parasites; giving *all* injections intravenously; administering injectible drugs via intra-nasal drenching, as done for many traditional medicines; using trypanocides as a panacea; halving the dosage of vermicidal pills, regardless of animal age or weight; giving water-soluble drugs in dirty water or even in beer. Also noted is a trend to creative techno-blending of the two medical traditions. For example, in lieu of their traditional bark-based medicines, Fulani will mix modern antidiarrhoeals in with animals' natronized drinking water. In fairness, the author observes that herders desire not only greater access to modern drugs they can themselves administer, but also training in the drugs' proper use. Thus he strongly recommends mass training for pastoralists in this regard.

Boutrolle, M.J.G. 1797. *Le Parfait Bouvier.* Geffier Jeune, Paris.

This antique volume is organized into three parts by cattle, sheep and horses. It mentions 30 plant species used in French livestock remedies of the period.

Bowen, Robert. 1997. Something from Somaliland . . . . *Vetaid Newsletter* 16 (winter): 3.

In planning for a livestock development programme among one group of Somali agropastoralists, Vetaid interviewed local people about their priority stockraising problems. Interviewees underscored their difficulty in purchasing veterinary drugs from petty traders. To illustrate, elders led Vetaid personnel to one man who told how a trader sold him what was supposedly an anthelmintic drench. When the man drenched his 25 sheep with the drug, however, seven of them promptly died. Because he had no previous experience with the drug and was unable to read the instructions on the container, the unfortunate stockraiser had no way of knowing that – whether out of ignorance or unscrupulousness – the trader had instead sold him a poisonous tick-dipping compound!

Brag, S. and H.J. Hansen. 1994. Treatment of ruminal indigestion according to popular belief in Sweden. *Revue Scientifique et Technique de l'Office International des Épizooties* 13(2): 529–535.

Remedies for ruminal indigestion of cattle have been recorded in Sweden for several centuries. In folkloric texts, some 44 treatments are reported by 75 contributors. The prescriptions make use of animal, vegetable and mineral *materia medica* such as frogs, camomile tea and hydrochloric acid. One remedy was for the farmer to chew a cow's fodder for it, and then give it to the animal. Another was to feed cud from a healthy animal. Such cud was considered to be a living organism, whereas in animals that ceased ruminating, the cud was presumed to have 'died'. The logical solution therefore was to replace it. These explanations make good sense in that fresh cud from a healthy animal can in fact renew the sick animal's ruminal flora and fauna. But this scientific understanding of rumen ecology has only recently come to light, after centuries of effective folk practice. The pharmaceutical industry has now developed drugs for ruminal indigestion that contain dried rumen content (*Extractum ruminis siccum*) along with other elements such as vitamins, glucose and yeast.

Bretting, P.K. 1984. Folk names and uses for Martyniaceous plants. *Economic Botany* 38(4): 452–463.

This article surveys anthropological and botanical literature from fieldwork in the Americas on the Martyniaceae. Of ethnoveterinary interest is Guatemalans' use of the sticky foliage of *Martynia annua* L. to remove lice from fowl. This practice helps explain common names for *M. annua* in Mexico, where it is known as 'flea hunter', 'flea killer', 'flea leaf' and 'fisherman of fleas'.

Brisebarre, Anne-Marie. 1978a. ***Bergers de Cévennes: Histoire et Ethnographie du Monde Pastorale et de la Transhumance en Cévennes.*** Editions Berger-Levrault, Paris, France.

Unavailable for review.

Brisebarre, Anne-Marie. 1978b. La médecine vétérinaire traditionelle du berger de transhumance en Cévennes. *Le Courier de la Nature* 75: 4–12.

The centuries-old transhumant routes of modern-day Cevenol shepherds of southern France mimic those of wild animals in the annual move to summertime mountain pastures. During transhumance, shepherds must depend entirely upon their own resources for protecting and curing their sheep. They know medicinal plants and other remedies against scabies, mastitis, colds, fever, intestinal parasites, fungal infections, colic, footrot and snakebite. For example, mastitis may be treated by rubbing a camphorated pomade on the udder and/or fumigating the animal with burning *Sambucus nigra* L. Medicinal teas are particularly popular. One example is a tea of *Arundo phragmites* L., to help an aborted ewe expel the foetus and placenta and avoid infection. Also figuring in certain treatments are non-plant ingredients like human urine, ammonia, gunpowder, honey, cuttle-bones, lizard droppings and snake meat. Shepherds also use mechanical treatments and simple surgical methods such as: lancing abscesses; for certain infections, slitting the skin of the tail or the ear in order to insert medicinal plants in the incision; piercing the rumen to relieve meteorism while tying a stem of *Helleborus foetidus* L. in the mouth to cause salivation and oral explusion of stomach gases; and for dogs as well as sheep, surgically removing cataracts, and setting and splinting fractures. When coenurosis is detected, the affected sheep are slaughtered and all the herd dogs are dosed with *Cucurbita maxima* Duch seeds to purge them of the parasite by which they help transmit the disease to sheep. Some shepherds have the ability to heal snakebites by laying hands on the stricken sheep and by incantations. To build immunity against snakebite, shepherds make sure their sheep graze *Capsella bursa-pastoris* L. and *Sarothamnus scoparius* L. Antivenin properties in the flowers of the latter have been scientifically confirmed. Other practices, such as hanging bells or talismans around sheeps' necks or suspending bouquets of flowers in the folds, are believed to ward off injuries and various diseases. However, some commercial treatments are beginning to replace traditional ones – e.g. penicillin instead of teas or chemical baths for footrot instead of homemade pastes; and Cevenol shepherds' ethnomedical know-how is in danger of disappearing.

Brisebarre, Anne-Marie. 1979a. La Caussenarde des Gerrigues. Paper presented to the 26 April Colloque sur les Zones Marginales et les Races Rustiques. Société d'Ethnozootechnie, Maison Nationale des Éleveurs, Paris.

Unavailable for review. But according to Brisebarre 1978b and 1979b, the Caussenarde is an endangered breed of rustic sheep in France that is known for its ability to browse.

Brisebarre, Anne-Marie. 1979b. La médecine vétérinaire traditionnelle des bergers des Cévennes. ***L'Action Vétérinaire*** 1: 17–20.

Cevenol shepherds of France employ three types of ethnoveterinary treatments singly or in combination: plant-based, mechanical and magical. Examples of the first type are: purging taenia infestions in dogs with pumpkin seeds (*Cucurbita maxima* D.); drenching any diarrhoeal animal with a preparation of *Tanacetum annuum* L.; for thrush, drenching the fasted sheep with human urine or giving it *Adiantum capillus veneris* L. or *Ceterach officinarum* Willd. Colic is treated with *Tanacetum annuum* L. and *Mercurialis annua* L. is used as a purgative. Colds and chills are treated with *Sambucus nigra* L. and *Agrimonia eupatoria* L., respectively. Sheep mange is cured on moonless nights with a topical application of juniper oil, sulphur and petrol. A multipurpose mechanical treatment entails placing a tourniquet on the ailing sheep's tail and inserting a piece of *Helleborus foetidus* L. or *Euphorbia characias* L. into an incision in the tail until an abscess forms. Shepherds believe the plant material will draw infection away from other parts of the body and, upon removal, will also remove the disease. Viper bites are generally treated by incantations and/or laying on of hands by shepherds reputed to have this gift. Talismans may be placed on some of the flock as a prophylaxy against lightning, falling rocks and hail. Along with still other treatments, the use of medicinal bouquets is also discussed.

Brisebarre, Anne-Marie. 1984a. À propos de l'usage thérapeutique des bouquets suspendus dans les bergeries cévenoles. ***Bulletin d'Ethnomédecine*** 32(4): 129–163.

French shepherds of the Cevennes use bouquets of two different plant species to treat lambs with a certain fungal infection of the mouth. One of the species, *marcioure*, can be collected and hung in the sheepfold by the shepherd himself. For the other species, *san cap*, this must be done by a healer. Both plants have a strong odour. Stockowners also go on pilgrimages to obtain bouquets at chapels dedicated to saints linked with the protection of livestock. These bouquets are believed to forestall or cure diseases, and to enhance flock fertility. Different plants are used to treat and prevent different diseases. Other non-plant objects – such as saint-blessed ribbons and stones, toads, vipers and salamanders – are also suspended within the folds or barns. Depending on the purpose, practices vary by where and how the bouquets are placed, who positions them, which plants or objects are used, and whether magic or religious formulae are recited to reinforce the healing process.

Brisebarre, Anne-Marie. 1984b. Le recours à Saint Fleuret, guérisseur des bestiaux, à Estaing (Aveyron). ***Ethnozootechnie*** 34: 59–76.

St Fleuret, a local saint in Southern France, plays an important role in the life of stockowners in this area. They believe he protects their herds from disease and injury and enhances flock fertility. Once a year, farmers go on a pilgrimage to St Fleuret's chapel and have him bless bread and salt to feed to their animals. Stockowners also use home remedies, mainly derived from plants, against common illnesses such as indigestion, swelling and warts. For more complicated cases, they call upon skilled neighbours, blacksmiths, or healers. Veterinarians are consulted only for epizootics, caesarean sections and diseases that are associated with modern, intensive methods of stock raising. The author also discusses changes in traditional animal husbandry in the Cevennes.

Brisebarre, Anne-Marie. 1985a. La médecine vétérinaire populaire en France: Aperçu bibliographique. *Production Pastorale et Société* 16: 101–108.

Ethnoveterinary descriptions can be found in publications about local animal husbandry, ethnomedicine, folk religion and holy healers, medicinal plants, magic and sorcery, and the history of veterinary medicine. The author distinguishes two user groups of EVM. In one group, the knowledge is transmitted from generation to generation. The other group is comprised of modern stockowners who make use of traditional veterinary practices. This bibliography lists publications from the past 20 years on EVM in France. It contains five entries on practices and beliefs in folk medicine in the whole of France, 23 about specific regions, six on veterinary medical plants, eight on veterinary medicine and religion, and 17 on veterinary medicine and magic.

Brisebarre, Anne-Marie. 1985b. Les bouquets thérapeutic en médecine vétérinaire et humaine – essai de synthèse. *Bulletin d'Ethnomédecine* 35(3): 3–38.

Herders in different parts of France treat and prevent certain human and livestock diseases with hanging bouquets of plants, flowers or sometimes other objects. The author has compiled a list of 15 plants and 3 animals (toads, vipers and salamanders) used in this fashion to treat livestock diseases that affect skin and other external body parts. Fourteen of these plants are also employed as topical remedies for skin diseases. Plants used as bouquets have one or more of the following characteristics: thorns, a strong odour, natural toxins, and some similarity to the symptoms of the disease being treated. The logic behind the practice of hanging bouquets is the 'law of signatures' based on the principles 'like evokes like' and 'like cures like', i.e. sympathetic magic.

Brisebarre, Anne-Marie. 1985c. Élevage et médecine vétérinaire dans les pays d'Afrique et à Madagascar. *Production Pastorale et Société* 16(Spring): 109–112.

A large majority of theses on veterinary medicine produced in France between 1970 and 1984 that pertain to Africa are listed in this bibliography. Though not all based on firsthand field research, many are authored by natives of the country they treat. Here, 63 theses are listed by nation within the following geographic categories: the Maghreb, the Sahel, East Africa, other African states and Madagascar. The species dealt with include camels, donkeys, goats, horses and sheep. Topics span almost every possible subject, e.g.: stockraising in general, nomadism, rangelands, cultivated pasturage, browses, nutrition, reproduction, watering, species-specific diseases, zoonoses, animal traction, Islamic slaughter rites and food preparation, fattening operations, marketing, other economic or social considerations, veterinary health legislation, and the roles of veterinarians in national development.

Brisebarre, A.-M. 1987. Pratique et insertion sociale d'un berger-guérisseur cévenol. *Bulletin d'Ethnomédecine* 39(2): 135–151.

Cevenol sheep raisers customarily hang bouquets of plants in their folds to ward off or cure livestock diseases. One of these plants, known as *san cap*, is hung to combat mouth sores (French *bouchise* or *muguet*) among newborn lambs. This plant is exclusively controlled by specialized shepherd-curers. Based on interviews with one such curer, the author describes the ritual inspection of ailing lambs by the curer, his mode of collection and preparation of the bouquet, secret incantations, and more. As the bouquet dries up, presumably so does the disease. The author also explores the curer's social role vis-à-vis his fellow shepherds.

Brisebarre, Anne-Marie. 1989a. Déprise, maîtrise, reprise, une pratique vétérinaire 'traditionnelle' dans la modernité. *Anthropologie Sociale et Ethnologie de la France* BCILL(44): 395–404.

This article presents two modern-day case studies of the preservation and extension of the French ethnoveterinary practice of hanging bouquets of plants in sheep-folds to cure or prevent certain sheep diseases [see also Brisebarre 1984a, 1985b, 1987]. In the first case, a young shepherd – formally trained in ovine husbandry yet traditionally charged with directing the annual transhumance of his community's flocks – modified and adopted a demystified and profane version of such bouquets' use, with the result that many other shepherds followed his lead. In the second case, a veterinary field agent did likewise with another species of plant, but now also rubbing the sores of afflicted animals with the plant before hanging it up in the folds. He actively extended this practice among his client group as an alternative to an unsatisfactory Western vaccine. The author analyses these events first in terms of the technological and cognitive syncretisms they represent; and second in anthropological terms of cultural brokering and the roles and attributes of leaders that spearhead adoption and diffusion. She concludes with the observations that many young veterinarians in France are gaining interest in EVM and that, in merging with scientific praxis, the latter shows a tenacious vitality.

Brisebarre, Anne-Marie. 1989b. La célébration de l'ayd el-kébir en France: Les enjeux du sacrifice. *Archives de Sciences Sociales des Religions* 68(1): 9–25.

This is a discussion of the ritual slaughter of sheep for the feast of ayd el-kebir, which is held throughout the Islamic world and in France's North African community. In response to the emergence of a new market that demands special types of animals for sacrifice, French shepherds have modified some of their traditional husbandry and practices. For instance, they leave off castrating and docking ram lambs in order to meet Islamic requirements for intact animals.

Brisebarre, Anne-Marie. 1989c. Le quotidien et l'accidentel: Les éleveurs et la santé de leurs bestiaux au XIXème siècle. In: *Homme, Animal, Société III: Histoire et Animal.* Presses de l'Institut d'Études Politiques de Toulouse. Pp. 257–277.

This is a historical treatise on veterinarians, empirical healers and farmers' own animal healthcare innovations in rural France in the 19th century. The latter are illustrated by one shepherd's discovery that feeding his flock willow bark cured their fasciolosis. He later learned from his local doctor that the bark contains salicylic acid – a well-known tonic in 1859, and the origin of today's aspirin. For meteorism, health professionals and farmers employed separate but similar methods. The former drenched with bleach, alcohol or ammonia while the latter preferred cheaper liquids such as solutions of saline, soap or ash in water, or pungent plant-based drenches of aniseed, camomile, juniper, leeks, onions and peppermint. Meteorism could also be treated mechanically by placing a twig in the ailing animal's mouth to stimulate jaw movement or by throwing water on its head and left flank. When all else failed, the left side of the ruminant's abdomen was pierced with a knife; then a canula made from the hollow stem of elder or reed was inserted to release the trapped gases. In 1857, the system of troca and cannula passed from local into modern knowledge via a process of instrumentation; i.e. the tools were produced commercially and sold in a box. The author notes how, by the end of the 19th century, veterinarians had won a monopoly over all diseases legally denoted as contagious; but stockraiser-healers and other local specialists remained as people's 'first recourse' for their everyday animal healthcare needs. This 'division of labour', as it were, persists in parts of France today.

Brisebarre, Anne-Marie. 1996. Tradition and modernity: French shepherds' use of medicinal bouquets. In: Constance M. McCorkle, Evelyn Mathias and Tjaart W. Schillhorn van Veen (eds). ***Ethnoveterinary Research & Development.*** Intermediate Technology Publications, London, UK. Pp. 76–90.

Since the 14th century, French shepherds have hung preventive and curative 'bouquets' of medicinal flora, fauna and other items from the rafters of their barns, folds and homes. French ethnomedicine has long held that air can carry agents of disease and thus, by logical analogy, can also transmit corresponding treatments, e.g. via diffusion of substances believed to be associated with a bouquet's 'smell', even if humans may be unable to detect the smell. This chapter overviews the application of such bouquets to livestock (and also human) ailments, based both on bibliographic research and on field interviews with shepherds of western and central France and the Cevennes. Findings demonstrate the widescale distribution, diversity of forms (wreaths, faggots and crosses, as well as bouquets), and variety of plants and other *materia medica* employed in these treatments. Analysis reveals that bouquet ingredients generally manifest one or more of four emically-assigned characteristics: a strong odour; toxicity or venomousness; aggressiveness, e.g. prickly or thorny plants; or some perceived similarity to the disease they are designed to treat, e.g. pustules, white scales, brown spots, etc. Plants of 26 species, animals of three types (vipers, toads and salamanders), and various religious items (medals, consecrated ribbons and other objects blessed by a priest or obtained on a pilgrimage) are identified as common bouquet components. Vegetal bouquets must always be hung up fresh, preferably when the plants are in flower and hence at peak biological activity; in like vein, faunal bouquets must employ freshly-killed creatures; and religious objects must be suspended as soon as they are brought home. The bouquets are primarily used to combat dermatological conditions, especially in seasonal situations of sharp temperature changes, crowded winter quarters, or spring lambing. If analysed in terms of the old ethnomedical law of signatures, bouquets can be interpreted as operating on any of four principles: like cures like, e.g. malodorous ailments are treated with foul-smelling plants such as stinking hellebore; like follows like, e.g. as organic bouquets slowly dry up, disintegrate, and flake away, so do the patient's scabs or squamae; like repels like, e.g. the carcasses of repulsive animals drive off other repulsive creatures like lice, fleas, mites, etc.; and opposites mediate, e.g. bringing wild, natural materials from 'outside' into the domesticated, human-made 'inside' of a crowded fold can beneficially mediate the boundary of the skin, which separates the patient's external and internal environments, as it were. Until the 1970s, the use of bouquets was confined to the traditional livestock sector, where their collection, creation and handling was the semi-sacred domain of specialists. However, certain medicinal bouquets have now gained some popularity in modern ovine production systems, especially for combatting ecthyma among lambs. Developed and diffused both by veterinary technicians and by professional groups of shepherds, in some areas the practice has successfully replaced a modern vaccine of unreliable availability and questionable efficacy. Moreover, stockmen's groups have begun to agitate for scientific research on the mechanisms and validity of medicinal bouquets.

Brown, Jean. 1990. Horn-shaping ground-stone axe-hammers. *Azania* 25: 57–67.

Pokot pastoralists shape the horns of selected adult 'name' oxen and goats into at least 25 styles (for cattle). This article details the steps involved in the operation. It is performed only by men recognized as especially skilled at it, who use stone axe-hammers that have been handed down in their families through generations. The procedure begins by throwing and tying the animal, and smearing several layers of dung on the axe-hammer. The latter act is said to soften the coming blow and thus avoid brain damage, reduce pain, prevent sorcery and speed recovery. Illustrating for the horn-style known as *nukurion*, the operator then smashes the skull at the base of the horns to loosen them. The blows are delivered along the lines of wet dung he has first traced as guides around each horn. Next he applies a smouldering stick to each horn tip in order to soften the tip before notching it with a knife. The horns are then manœuvred into the desired position and tied firmly with a bark rope wound between the notched horns in a repeated figure-eight. After this, the whole assemblage is thickly plastered with dung. The dung eases the immediate pain and keeps off insects and birds while the skull bones knit. Finally, the animal is untied, assisted to stand, and bled of 3 to 4 l of blood by shooting a stopped arrow into the jugular vein. Such horn operations date back to at least 3500 B.C. Egypt. But they are still widely practised today among Nilotic pastoral groups throughout southern Sudan and East Africa, where the animals thus cosmetically modified have immense cultural and personal significance. When performed by experts, reportedly the operation has no long-term adverse sequelae.

Brown, Stu. 1989a. Pest control using natural insecticides. Unpublished manuscript. Mennonite Central Committee, Kawimbe, Zambia. 3 pp.

In Zambia, a number of plants are used as natural pest controls. Tobacco is burnt as a fumigant for livestock ectoparasites and stored crops. *Gnidia kraussiana* is most widely known as a fish poison, but it is also effective against ticks when the pounded root is added to water and sprayed on livestock. The seeds of *Sesbania aegyptica* are also used as an acaricide.

Brown, Stu. 1989b. Use of utupa (*Tephrosia vogelii*) for control of ticks on cattle. Unpublished manuscript. Mennonite Central Committee, Kawimbe, Zambia. 12 pp.

Tephrosia vogelii leaves contain rotenone, a selective acaricide that kills ticks. Rotenone can be leached from the leaves by pounding them so as to break the cuticle and then soaking them in water. Rotenone is also preserved in dried leaves of *T. vogelii*; when acaricide is needed, water is simply added to the pounded leaves and the mixture sprayed on cattle with a hand sprayer or spray race. Moreover, the plant can be intercropped with maize, Zambia's staple foodgrain. The use of the roots of *Gnidia kraussiana* is also mentioned as an acaricide.

Buldgen, A., M. Piraux, A. Dieng, G. Schmit and R. Compère. 1994. Les élevages de porcs traditionnels du bassin arachidier sénégalais. *World Animal Review* 80/81(3–4): 63–70.

To establish the demographic and zootechnical parameters of local pig production units, a survey was conducted on 115 farms in villages and towns of Senegal's groundnut basin. Local husbandry practices include castrating boars at 4 months using a razor and then disinfecting the wound with salt, ash and petrol. Piglets are weaned at 2 and 3 months in villages and towns, respectively, simply by removing them from the sow and selling them. Although pigs were kept extensively in all cases, their foraging was also universally supplemented by feeding such items as kitchen scraps, baobab and cabbage leaves, millet, rice, sweet potatoes, tomatoes and yams.

Burridge, M.J. and C.W. Schwabe. 1977. Hydatid disease in New Zealand: An epidemiological study of transmission among Maoris. *The American Journal of Tropical Medicine and Hygiene* 26(2): 258–265.

Although this article deals with comparative social epidemiology rather than ethnoveterinary medicine, it is referenced here in order to illustrate the cultural, social, biological and economic implications of livestock diseases and their control – and what can happen when local veterinary knowledge is deficient. The article reports on an epidemiological study conducted in New Zealand to determine why the risk of hydatid disease was six times greater among Maori sheepraisers than among their European counterparts in New Zealand. It was found that Maori treat their work and pet dogs equally whereas European farmers do not allow workdogs into their homes. Also, Maori landholdings are so fragmented that ranges have become increasingly unproductive and thus there is no incentive for Maori to build adequate slaughterhouses. As a result, dogs readily gain access to raw offal. (For another example of ethnic differences in the incidence of hydatid disease among shepherds, see Araujo et al. 1975 on Basques in California.)

Bustamante, José. 1982. La gallina de los huevos verdes. *Minka* 8(Aug): 9.

This brief article enumerates the many advantages of raising the naturalized *chusca* or *criolla* chicken of the Andes rather than importing 'improved' breeds from outside the region. In addition to the *criolla*'s resistance to rain and cold, its ability to forage for most of its feed, and its relatively high productivity under such harsh conditions, the author (a veterinarian) notes its resistance to all manner of disease, including respiratory and stomach ailments, diarrhoea and parasites. He opines that the breed's only serious health problem is lice, and offers a home remedy based on a vinegar and lemon-juice wash.

Bustinza Choque, Victor and Clemente Sánchez Viveros. 1985. Formas de tratamiento tradicional de la sarna de alpacas. In: Victor Bustinza Ch. et al. (eds). *Proyecto Piel de Alpaca: Informe Final.* Universidad Nacional del Altiplano, Instituto de Investigaciones para el Desarrollo Social del Altiplano, Convenio UNA-NUFFIC, Puno, Perú. Pp. 80–84.

With the Spanish conquest of Peru, well-controlled Inca systems to manage the health and productivity of both domestic camelids (llama and alpaca) and wildlife were destroyed, leading to epidemic disease. Particularly devastating was the spread of mange resulting from biting or burrowing ectoparasites that ruin the fibre and may even kill the camelid. Yet some Inca veterinary therapies remained; and rural producers invented new ones to confront this growing problem. This chapter overviews six mange treatments used by Andean smallholders. The treatments involve varying combinations of pig fat, rancid camelid grease, boiling-hot lard, fermented urine, sulphur, stove ash, soot from earthen cookpots, masticated coca leaf, and old motor oil, sometimes along with powdered commercial products like DDT. These therapies are evaluated for their probable effectiveness and relative advantages in relieving pain and itching, healing the lesions, and destroying the parasites. Three additional 'semi-scientific' preparations used on large alpaca-producing estates in the early and mid-1900s are likewise described and evaluated. These involve ingredients such as sulfur, potassium carbonate, fresh lard, barbasco, baking soda and diesel oil. The authors conclude that, in general, all these treatments are beneficial but serve primarily in the early stages of the disease or in mild cases. They recommend further research into the properties of some of these ethno-therapies, along with other items in the folk pharmacopoeia like *tarwi* and *muña*. However, the authors suggest that genetic control may be the most important research need.

Butcher, Catherine. 1994. Extension and pastoral development: Past, present and future. *Pastoral Development Network Paper* No. 37d. Agricultural Administration Unit, ODI, London, UK. 17 pp.

In this overview of extension and pastoralism in relation to paravet programmes, the author recommends that paravet treatments combine introduced technology with pastoralists' own veterinary remedies, as well as their ethnodiagnostic skills. This is recommended because, in most pastoral societies today, Western drugs have become a *de facto* part of local veterinary systems, based on pastoralists' independent experimentation with such drugs' usefulness and effectiveness.

Buxton, Jean. 1973. *Religion and Healing in Mandari.* Oxford University Press, Oxford, UK.

Mandari nomadic pastoralists of the Horn of Africa consider most cattle diseases to have natural causes, and herders demonstrate considerable empirical knowledge of such diseases (cf. pp. 4–11, 317–323). So when Mandari diagnose infectious diarrhoea, for example, they isolate the infected herd and modify their grazing patterns. However, cattle's health is also thought to be affected by the actions and dispositions of their human owners and of supernatural beings. Thus, non-empirical diagnoses include envy, sorcery, breaches of female prohibitions, and the doings of ghosts. The evil eye explains cattle infertility, poor milk yield and calf mortality. In terms of husbandry practices, Mandari never shelter their cattle because they move daily from pasture to pasture. Stud bulls are said to lead herds and their herdsmen to grass and water. Most male stock are castrated, but some are especially chosen for neutering to become display oxen. These oxen have distinctive markings; and their owners perform elaborate cosmetic horn surgery on them to produce specific horn conformations. Such oxen are intimately identified with the young men who look after them, and ox and man are inseparable for many years. Special cattle rites are held whenever a valuable animal or a whole herd is threatened by disease or other dangers. The rites involve rubbing ashes on the animals' back while offering prayers. Chickens, goats, or a young ox may occasionally be sacrificed on behalf of herd health. Only cattle receive medico-religious attention; diviners are not called upon to treat small stock. Because of their great spiritual as well as economic value, cattle are incorporated into the realm of human socio-religious experience.

Byler, Emma. 1991. *Plain and Happy Living: Amish Recipes and Remedies.* Goosefoot Acres Press, USA.

The Amish are North American farmers who make extensive use of traditional human and veterinary medicine. In the section on 'Animal Ailments and Their Care' (pp. 130–133), this book lists several Amish remedies for cattle, poultry, horses, dogs and cats. Diarrhoeal cattle are drenched twice a day with blackberry root tea. Pennyroyal leaves are used as an insecticide. For poultry, the leaves are placed in the cracks of the chicken coop; alternatively, tobacco juice made from chewing tobacco and water can be poured into the cracks. Horses, dogs and cats can be washed in pennyroyal tea to keep off flies and fleas. For dogs and cats, dusting their coats with and/or feeding them brewer's yeast works as an acaricide. An anthelmintic made of epsom salts, sulphur, saltpetre, cream of tartar and sifted wood ash is administered in horses' feed. To tame and calm horses, cumin seed may be added to their nosebag. A traditional prescription for scours in calves is a drench of soda, ginger, cloves, nutmeg, cinnamon and water, administered in a bottle. Alternatively, raw eggs may be added to a calf's milk at the first sign of scours. Finally, horses can be prevented from chewing wood by putting wood ash or vinegar in their feed.

Caballero Osorio, Abel A. 1984a. Efecto del aceite esencial de muña en el control del *Haematopinus suis*. In: Abel A. Caballero Osorio and Marco A. Ugarte (eds). *Muña: Investigación y Proyección Social.* Instituto de Investigaciones UNSAAC-NUFFIC, Cuzco, Perú. Pp. 17–19.

Pediculosis produced by the ectoparasite *Haematopinus suis* is a major problem in family-level swine raising in highland Peru. This chapter reports the results of an experimental study to test the relative effectiveness of three different home treatments for pediculosis: essence of *muña* (*Minthostachys andina*) oil in a detergent solution; *muña* oil alone; and kerosene. Results revealed that all three were effective. However, the first was slow-acting; and the third, while having the advantage of killing the parasite's eggs, predictably produced considerable skin irritation. The authors therefore recommend the use of *muña* oil alone, a plant that has no toxic effects for either animals or people and that forms part of the human diet in the Andes. [See also Caballero Osorio 1984b.]

Caballero Osorio, Abel A. 1984b. Uso del aceite esencial de muña en el control de la sarna de alpacas (géneros *Sarcoptes, Psoroptes*). In: Abel A. Caballero Osorio and Marco A. Ugarte (eds). *Muña: Investigación y Proyección Social.* Instituto de Investigaciones UNSAAC-NUFFIC, Cuzco, Perú. Pp. 20–25.

Veterinary scientists and alpaca raisers alike agree that ectoparasitic mange (Spanish *sarna*) is economically one of the most damaging diseases in Peru's alpaca fibre industry. But the smallholders who produce the bulk of the nation's fibre crop rarely have access to dipping structures; and in any case, they cannot afford the requisite commercial pharmaceuticals. Hence the rationale for this study of the ectoparasiticidal properties of oil of *muña*, a native plant widely used throughout the Andes to combat a multitude of ailments in both humans and animals. Three topical treatments were tested on three groups of alpaca, with a fourth group as controls. The first treatment consisted of 100% *muña* oil, the second of *muña* oil along with the water in which it was extracted, and the third of diesel oil. Results revealed an effectiveness of 100%, 20% and 40%, respectively. The author concludes that topical applications of *muña* oil represent a highly effective, non-toxic, broad-spectrum therapy for mange in alpaca. Moreover, such treatments are well-suited to smallholders' economic situation and animal management system.

Cabaret, J. 1986. *Phytotherapie Vétérinaire: 167 Plantes pour Soigner les Animaux.* Editions du Point Vétérinaire, Maisons-Alfort, France. 192 pp.

Unavailable for review.

Cabrol, A. 1984. Lexique pastoral du Languedoc oriental. *Folklore* 38(2–3): 30–72.

Unavailable for review.

Cáceres Vega, Edgar. 1989. *Fasciola Hepatica: 'Enfermedad y Pobreza Campesina'.* Imprenta Metodista, La Paz, Bolivia. 201 Pp.

In biological, epidemiological, socioeconomic, nutritional, clinical, etc. terms, this book presents a thorough-going scientific study of hepatic distomatosis and its accompanying diarrhoeal syndrome in rural people of Bolivia. Page 66 notes the publication of various studies in the early 1900s on the effectiveness of an extract of the plant *Aspidium Filix-mas* (Spanish *helecho macho*) in combating adult forms of fasciola in both humans and animals. Reportedly 30 000 sheep were successfully treated with this extract. Additional studies cited are page 44 in C. La Page, 1975, *Parasitología Veterinaria*, Editorial Continental, México, and V. Turner, 1961, 'Fasciola Konja', *Veterinaria Glasvik* 15: 399, Belgrade, Yugoslavia.

Campos, Jesús, Victoria Jayme and Nicandro D. Yslas. 1989. Estudio del género *Brickellia* o hierba del becerro y su aplicación en la cunicultura. In: Gerardo López Buendía (ed.). *Memorias: Segunda Jornada sobre Herbolaria Medicinal*

en Medicina Veterinaria. Universidad Nacional Autónoma de México, Facultad de Medicina Veterinaria y Zootecnia, Coordinación de Educación Continua, México DF, México. Pp. 92–95.

Brickellia spp. or 'calf's herb' is a uniquely American genus that grows as far north as Canada and as far south as Bolivia and Brazil. It has long been used in Mexico to make infusions to treat diarrhoea in both humans and animals. Although its chemical composition has been exhaustively researched, pharmacological studies have been lacking. This published conference paper helps fill that gap by evaluating *Brickellia* for its action against gastrointestinal problems in rabbits, which are potentially a cheap source of much-needed protein for Latin America's poor. *In vitro* trials on *B. pendula*, *B. veronicaefolia* and *B. secundiflora* plus *in vivo* trials on the latter indicate that extracts of the leaves are active against bacterial diarrhoeas and that they positively affect the contractive activity of the small intestine.

Carlier, Ana B. de. 1981. *Así Nos Curamos en el Canipaco: Medicina Tradicional del Valle del Canipaco, Huancayo, Perú.* Producción Gráfica Color Jesús Ruiz Durand, Huancayo, Perú. 180 pp.

This book opens with an 81-page description of home remedies for human ills in the Canipaco region of Peru's Huancayo Department. It then lists 121 plants plus a number of animal species and minerals figuring in these remedies. Each item's Latin name is given, along with a brief description of its physical appearance, mode of employment, and a colour plate of the item. There is little mention of ethnoveterinary applications aside from the use of *jaya-shipita* to treat liver fluke in herd animals. [See also Córdova 1981.] However, plants that are poisonous to animals are noted, along with the use of *tantal* as a living fence to keep animals out of cultivated fields. The primary value of this book for ethnoveterinary research lies in the excellent colour plates, which are potentially of great assistance in identifying plants used in animal medicine in other parts of the Andes.

Carter, William E. and Mauricio Mamani P. 1982. *Irpa Chico: Individuo y Comunidad en la Cultura Aymara.* Empresa Editora Urquizo S.A., La Paz, Bolivia. 459 pp.

This wide-ranging ethnography deals with almost every aspect of life in an Aymara community of highland Bolivia. However, only a few pages (111–120) discuss stockraising – the tremendous economic and social importance of the community's sheep, llama, alpaca and cattle; their pasturing patterns; milk production and utilization; description of a failed poultry project; and so forth. With regard to livestock diseases, the authors note only that those of supernatural origin are the most greatly feared. Comets that fall on Tuesday or Friday and evil spirits are believed to cause *p'uju usu* (an undefined ailment). Stockowners are also very fearful of *k'iwcha kururu*, a liver fluke.

Casaverde, Juvenal. 1985. Calendario alpaquero. *Minka* 16(Mar): 18.

This article briefly outlines the annual cycle of alpaca management tasks among Andean herders: the herd fertility ceremony in August, shearing in November–December, birthing and breeding in January–March, dipping in April, and culling and castrating in June–July. The author mentions that during shearing the herd is also treated for mange (Spanish *sarna*, Quechua *qarachi*) with topical applications of alpaca fat or old motor oil, as well as commercial veterinary products.

Casaverde, Juvenal. 1988. *Comunidades Alpaqueras del Sur Andino: Una Introducción a su Estudio.* Informe Técnico No. 3. Proyecto Alpacas, COTESU/IC, Puno, Perú. 57 pp.

This technical report is composed of nine chapters covering the distribution of alpaca in Peru, community life and economy among Puneño alpaca raisers, herding and husbandry tasks, natural pastures, livestock, trade and markets and complementary activities in the region. Pages 45–48 deal with animal health. Seven major ailments afflicting alpaca in the area are outlined: *q'echa* (diarrhoea), *qarachi* (different types of mange), *ishu kuru* (strongylosis), *fiebre* ('fever'), *aftosa* (foot-and-mouth disease), *k'utu* (cysticercosis) and *qocha* (hydatidosis). Stockowners' eclectic use of both Western and Andean treatments for these diseases are described. The author notes the main reasons cited by Puneño alpaca raisers for their animals' many ills: the poor nutrition of the dry season weakens the herds; commercial drugs are too costly for regular use, and few people know how to administer them properly; and stockowners' diagnostic skills are limited.

Casimir, Michael Jan. 1982. The biological phenomenon of imprinting – its handling and manipulation by traditional pastoralists. *Production Pastorale et Société* 11: 23–27.

Pastoralists are aware of the importance of odour for the bonding between mother and offspring. They have developed several methods to continue to obtain milk from animals whose young have died. These methods can be grouped in three categories: dummies, blocking of the olfactory system, and use of force. Casimir illustrates each category with examples from the literature.

Castillo, L. and M. Ansay. 1998. Approache de la problématique: La santé traditionnelle. Unpublished summary report of Work-session I of the 'Atelier Ressources Animales' of Projet CIUF/CUD meetings on 'Gestion Intégrée par les Acteurs Locaux des Ressources Physiques, Végétales et Animales pour une Qualité de Vie et un Développement Durable'. University of Liege, Faculty of Veterinary Medicine, Liège, Belgium. 16 pp.

This work-session report highlights the creation of a PRELUDE databank on traditional medicine comprised of approximately 5000 prescriptions, mostly from the Great Lakes region of Zaire. [See also Baerts et al. 1996.] The databank is designed to serve as a source of 'raw materials' to be 'put to the test' in pharmacology, phytochemistry and biology by comparing its entries of plant species across six measures of 'coherence': botanical, veterinary, human-medical, phytochemical, pharmacological and toxicological. To date, analysis of the databank has generated a list of 'remarkable plants' according to their frequency of citation by informants, the specificity of uses for which they were cited, and similarity of use in veterinary and human medicine. Also discussed are different possible uses of the databank and its findings in animal-health-related interventions between and across scientists and stockraisers such as in: establishing nurseries of medicinal plants; diffusing high-coherence prescriptions among local practitioners; encouraging production and trade of prepared ethnomedicines; building electronic EVK networks internationally; promoting EVK seminars and exchanges among all interested groups; suggesting new EVK research thrusts; and more. In the process, the report establishes a new terminological distinction between *sachants* (local people wise in traditional medicine) versus *savants* (academicians who study EVK). The report also offers an illustrative question-guide for ER&D, matrices for cross-site comparison of responses, and advice on participatory approaches to the subject and subsequent research themes. Some of these elements are illustrated in a mini-case-study of VSF work in Bolivia. There, research revealed that people considered FMD a serious and contagious disease. They said it was especially prevalent during the rainy season and was due either to standing water on grazing grounds or to a 'virus'. As FMD therapy and prophylaxis, they respectively applied kerosene to the lesions and sometimes gave commercial vaccinations. This information allowed the VSF project to include FMD in its surveys – identifying it by its local name and locally recognized symptoms – and then to evaluate corresponding training needs.

Catchero, Daisy L. and Jim L. Orprecio. n.d. *A Case Study Report of the Community Animal Health Volunteer Training Program in the Philippines.* In-house report. HPI, Laguna, Philippines. 8 pp.

This report on an HPI paravet project in the Philippines notes the project's commitment to, and successful implementation of, the collection, production and dissemination of information on indigenous herbal medicines [see HPI/Philippines n.d.], other local treatments, and basic animal healthcare throughout the project life. This information has especially been shared with paravet trainees, to use in their practice, but also with ordinary stockraisers. Such ethnoveterinary options are particularly important given the lack of local outlets for modern veterinary inputs in the project area, and the project's own inability to ensure sustainable supply of same to its paravet trainees.

Catley, A.P. 1997. Adapting participatory appraisal (PA) for the veterinary epidemiologist: PA tools for use in livestock disease data collection. In: E.A. Goodall and M.V. Thrusfield (eds). *Society for Veterinary Epidemiology and Preventive Medicine: Proceedings of a Meeting Held at University College, Chester on the 9th, 10th and 11th of April 1997.* Pp. 246–257.

In the early 1970s, the recognition that formal systems of inquiry such as questionnaires were of limited value when working with rural communities in developing countries gave rise to a variety of RRA and PRA techniques. This paper explores the application of participatory appraisal (PA) techniques to the collection of both qualitative and quantitative epidemiological information in such communities, illustrating from two PA tools used in community-based animal health projects in Somalia. One is a scoring/ranking procedure to determine the relative importance stockraisers assigned different animal diseases there; the same technique was also used to determine the relative use values and other characteristics stockraisers attributed to their five species of herd animals (camels, sheep, goats, cattle, donkeys), based on 42 indicators that interviewees themselves defined. Health-related indicators included susceptibility to disease, animal hygiene, water and forage requirements, and more; emic economic indicators also appeared, such as 'easy to sell', 'good' for earning additional income, and 'sale value'. The second technique is a seasonal calendar, in this case constructed with stockraisers to outline their knowledge of seasonal variations in livestock infestation by seven different kinds and classes of ticks. Also outlined here are the basic components of a PA training course, which workers should learn before endeavouring to use PA in the field, plus a table of different types of PA tools that can be applied to gathering different types of veterinary epidemiological and economic data.

Catley, Andy and Robert Walker. 1999. Somali ethnoveterinary medicine and private animal health services: Can old and new systems work together? In: E. Mathias, D.V. Rangnekar and C.M. McCorkle, with M. Martin (eds). *Ethnoveterinary Medicine: Alternatives for Livestock Development – Proceedings of an International Conference Held in Pune, India, 4–6 November 1997. Volume 1: Selected Papers.* BAIF Development Research Foundation, Pune, India. Pp. 189–201.

Livestock figure in every aspect of Somali economy and culture. Somali pastoralists' EVK has been documented since at least the 1950s, although rarely has this information affected the design of livestock-related aid programmes. This paper summarizes the literature on Somali ethnoveterinary language and practices. It then relates traditional healthcare and management systems to veterinary privatization and paravet projects in the 1990s. Studies of newly emerging private veterinary services in Somaliland have underscored local concern about the loss of traditional skills and over-reliance on imported veterinary pharmaceuticals. Despite a governmental vacuum, both veterinary service delivery and livestock production in Somalia are changing. The paper argues that although aid agencies will continue to promote Western-style veterinary services in Somali-occupied areas, the resilience of the Somali livestock economy at both household and national levels is based on traditional veterinary, herding and husbandry skills that should therefore be acknowledged and supported.

Catley, Andrew, Patricia Delaney and Hunt McCauley. 1998. *Community-based Animal Health Services in the Greater Horn of Africa: An Assessment.* USAID Office of Foreign Disaster Assistance in cooperation with the USDA Famine Mitigation Activity, Washington DC, US. 68 pp.

In discussing CAHW programmes in the Horn of Africa, this assessment notes that 'While traditional veterinary practitioners are not completely integrated, . . . their involvement is sometimes sought' (p. 19). It informs that the PARC-VAC (Participatory Community-based Vaccination and Animal Health) Project actively solicits information about EVK during its initial assessment and subsequent dialogue with participating communities. This information, which includes local disease terms and treatments, is then utilized to tailor other community dialogue presentations and CAHW training curricula. The UNICEF Operation Lifeline Sudan (OLS) programme also pays attention to local veterinary knowledge and practice. EVM-related lessons learned and recommendations from these assessments include the following. As shown by research in Ethiopia and as corroborated in other parts of the Horn, the importation of Western biomedicine can overshadow traditional practices. Thus, such programmes 'should take special care to validate and support EVK and traditional veterinary practice, even while training in western bio-medical practice' and also 'consider issues of indigenous copyrights and the return of proprietary information in usable format for the affected populations' (p. 64). The authors add that more should be done to incorporate the full range of ethnoveterinary knowledge and practice into data collection and training in order to enhance treatment options and strengthen local capacity. Finally, 'Linkages between CAHWs and human health should be pursued diligently' (p. 67), giving due recognition to the complexity of such linkages, their unique sociocultural circumstances, and the timing and phased levels of incorporation of a human-health component. Usually the latter takes place after animal health services are firmly established. To this end, CBAH programmes such as PARC-VAC and OLS should collaborate with NGOs and other partners already experienced in the human health sector, continuing the characteristically participatory and on-the-ground approach of CBAH initiatives.

Catley, Andy and Ahmed Aden Mohammed. 1995. Ethnoveterinary knowledge in Sanaag region, Somaliland (Part I): Notes on local descriptions of livestock diseases and parasites. *Nomadic Peoples* 36/37: 3–16.

A pastoralist dictionary of livestock ailments was compiled based on a survey in Sanaag region, Somaliland. Some 150 diseases are described and categorized under the following headings of disorders: oral, enteric, systemic, musculoskeletal, respiratory, reproductive, parasitic, nervous, udder, skin, eye, foot, poor body condition, sudden death and abscesses. A tick life-cycle is diagrammed in this article, detailing Somali names for different tick species and their life-cycle stages. The goal of the study was to correct previous, over-simplistic translations of Somali words into English or scientific names. Investigation of the literal meaning and use of Somali disease terms helped highlight pastoralists' extensive EVK, including sophisticated understandings of disease transmission that helped them elaborate rules to limit the spread of disease on rangelands. This research also brought to light detailed local knowledge of certain diseases' epidemiology and pathology that was of considerable diagnostic value. Finally, it provided useful inputs for designing veterinary training exercises and extension materials.

Catley, Andy and Ahmed Aden Mohammed. 1996a. Ethnoveterinary knowledge in Sanaag region, Somaliland (Part II): Notes on local descriptions of livestock diseases and parasites. *Nomadic Peoples* 39: 135–146.

As part of an animal health programme in Sanaag region, Somaliland, details of over 70 livestock treatments were collected and categorized into groups as discussed in Catley and Mohammed 1995. Treatments made use of some 30 plant remedies as well as branding, firing and cauterization. To ward against or treat mineral deficiencies, people lead their animals to salty wells or feed them salty soups, broths, other liquids and browse. Interviewees also reported that grazing camels on *Salsola foetida* and *Salsola crasse* for 10 days provides these animals with sufficient salt for 8 months. In general, Somalis choose and use grazing and drinking areas carefully, with disease prevention in mind. For example, at wells, healthy and sick animals are separated; and often each family brings its own drinking pan to water the animals at the well. Kraals are regularly mucked out, as

Somalis say the dung attracts ticks. Medico-religious practices also figure in live-stock healthcare. For example, some respiratory ailments are treated by reciting Koranic verses while spitting into a bowl and then pouring the sputum over the patient. A general measure to protect animals from disease and ill-fate is to adorn them with amulets bearing Koranic texts.

Catley, A.P. and A.A. Mohammed. 1996b. The use of livestock-disease scoring by a primary animal-health project in Somaliland. *Preventive Veterinary Medicine* 28: 175–186.

Participatory rural appraisal (PRA) can be used as an informal livestock disease scoring tool. PRA is useful for understanding local animal health priorities and is an appropriate technique for information gathering in pastoral societies. [See related publications by Catley and co-authors.]

Catley, A.P. and Ahmed Aden [sic]. 1996c. Use of participatory rural appraisal (PRA) tools for investigating tick ecology and tick-borne diseases in Somaliland. *Tropical Animal Health and Production* 28: 91–98.

This article describes the application of PRA methods to the collection of local-knowledge and scientific data on tick ecology and tick-associated livestock health problems in Somaliland. PRA can also be used to elicit information from herders and brokers at local livestock markets on how tick-borne diseases affect the sale price of livestock and animal products. Linking all such information to the cost, frequency and seasonality of acaricide treatments can help in the formulation of workable tick control strategies.

CEDECUM/PRATEC-CEPIA. 1988. *Tecnología Aymara: Revaloración del Saber Campesino.* Serie Eventos Campesinos. Servicios Editoriales Adolfo Arteta, Lima, Perú. 85 pp.

One in a series of publications aimed at shoring up the eroding base of indigenous Andean knowledge [see also PPEA-PRATEC 1989, PRATEC 1988a&b, PRATEC 1989 and PRATEC-CEPIA 1988], this book focuses on the Aymara peoples of Peru's Puno Department. In addition to discussing major themes and methodol-ogies for 'technology rescue', the volume presents three technologies in detail, all of which concern ethnoveterinary practices. No. 68 describes the long-standing use of a decoction of the *ajana ajana* plant to combat pulmonary and intestinal para-sites in ruminants and humans. No. 69 details a cure for bloat in cattle involving a decoction of various herbs with barley and cooking oil. Technology No. 70 pre-scribes a hot plaster of seven plants ground together with lime and water, used to treat fractured bones in both animals and humans.

Celestino-Husson, Olinda. 1985. Éleveurs Aymaras des punas de Puno. *Production Pastorale et Société* 16(Spring): 85–94.

This article consists of a French-language summary of several works by Félix Palacios Ríos, including Palacios Ríos 1985 and 1988.

Centro de Capacitación de la Mujer Campesina and World Concern Latin America. 1995. *Indigenous Women, Andean Knowledge, and Livestock*

Production. In-house report. CCMC and World Concern, Santa Cruz, Bolivia. 49 pp.

In a survey of highland Bolivian women's EVK conducted by World Concern and the CCMC training centre for rural women, interviewees discussed their treatments and rituals for llama, sheep, cattle and hogs. They also discussed castration, marking and docking procedures. Some examples of treatments included: drenching with an infusion of ground papaya seeds to expel tapeworms; bathing tick-infested animals with *yarita* tea; and for bottle-jaw, rubbing a mixture of urine, salt and ashes into the affected area, and then cutting out the swelling and filling the wound with ashes. Sheep are docked in the belief that this will fatten them by directing more nutrition to the rest of the body, rather than to the tail. Docking is performed by tying a band around the tail at the third vertebra and then amputating at this point. One year old llamas are weaned by placing a stick in the nasal septum to prevent nursing. A treatment for bloat is to drench with tea made from the oil of human hair. Animist rituals pervade many aspects of animal healthcare in the Bolivian highlands. To take one example, when people station a herd of male llama to graze alone on a hillside, they chew a small amount of coca leaves, bury the leaves in the ground near the herd, and pray to the local animist spirits to care for the unattended llama and protect them from foxes and condors until the owner returns.

Cerrate de Ferreyra, Emma. 1980. Plantas que curan las heridas del hombre y los animales. *Boletín de Lima* 3–4: 1–12.

This article identifies and describes 15 plants commonly used in Peru's Ancash Department to treat injuries and ailments of both humans and animals. Descriptions include names, plant architecture, habitat and application details. The plants are use to treat fractures, wounds, sore throats, gastric ulcers, saddle and pack sores, cracked hooves, and kidney, bladder, liver and other problems.

Chahar, L.S. and L. Singh. 1997. Local wisdom in veterinary medicine. In: Anil Gupta (ed.). *International Conference on Creativity and Innovation at Grassroots for Sustainable Natural Resource Management, January 11–14, 1997: Abstracts.* Indian Institute of Management, Ahmedabad, India. P. 79.

The authors of this paper are two farmers from India's Uttar Pradesh State. They offer a selection of their villages' animal healthcare practices, as verified by a local veterinarian and as commented on by scientists (in parentheses). For retained placenta in buffalo, the cure is feeding: 1 to 2 litres of the animal's own colostrum (this calcium- and energy-rich milk may help restore the exhausted cow); about 2 kg of *Ficus religiosa* or sugarcane or bamboo leaves (they might provide some oestrogenic activity); 0.5 to 1 kg of linseed or *Carum copticum* seeds boiled in 2 kg of water (possibly some uterotonic value). For stomach pain accompanied by inappetence and constipation, cattle are fed *Cleome icosandra* L. seeds crushed in jaggery (perhaps with some analgesic effects). For footrot and FMD hoof lesions in cattle, villagers clean the hooves and apply several drops of petrol thrice daily for 3 days (petrol repels flies and forms an oily barrier against infection). For myiasis, people feed *Lantana camara* or *Calotropis gigantea* L. leaves. The latter are given between bread slices to make them palatable, or they can be tied on the infested body part (no clear response).

Chakrabarti, Amalendu and Rahul Amin. 1998. Prevention of ketosis in cows with polyherbal preparation. In: E. Mathias, D.V. Rangnekar and C.M. McCorkle, with M. Martin (eds). ***Ethnoveterinary Medicine: Alternatives for Livestock Development – Proceedings of an International Conference Held in Pune, India, 4–6 November 1997. Volume 2: Abstracts.*** BAIF Development Research Foundation, Pune, India. P. 13.

Ketosis is a production disease of dairy cows that can substantially reduce milk yields. This study tested two traditional but commercially formulated polyherbal preparations for ketosis on 28 cows that were at least 8 months pregnant and had ketone bodies in the urine along with mild levels of hepatic lipidosis (borderline ketosis). The cows were divided into four groups of seven each (treatment groups A1, B1, C1 and a control group). Clinical signs and biochemical profiles of all four groups were monitored before and after treatment and 2 weeks after calving. Group A1 was treated with 30 ml of Livol PFS daily for 14 days. Group B1 was treated with 30 ml Livol PFS Plus daily for 14 days and 10 g of Hb Strong twice a day for a week. (Both are polyherbal drugs marketed by M/s. Indian Herbs, Saharanpur.) Group C1 received propanediol, a conventional drug, at a dosage of 100 ml twice daily for 7 days. Controls received no treatment. In group B1, ketotic features disappeared and remained absent even 2 weeks after calving. In contrast, A1, C1 and control animals showed ketotic features following calving. Results indicate that the combination of Livol PFS Plus and Hb Strong is more effective than the other treatments. The paper discusses details and advantages of preventive aspects of such herbal preparations versus conventional drugs for post-parturient production diseases.

Chander, Mahesh and Reena Mukherjee. 1994. Traditional agricultural and animal husbandry practices for sustainable agriculture in [the] Kumoun Hills of Uttar Pradesh. ***Journal of Rural Development*** 13(3): 443–449.

In the hill region of India's Uttar Pradesh State, the plant *Urtica dioica* is fed to lactating buffalo to enhance their milk production. Fermented wheat flour or fermented bananas are given to restore weak and/or anaemic animals. Draught oxen and horses are drenched with human urine in order to improve their strength and vigour. Saline or smoke tar is applied topically to animals with ticks. Pigeon excrement – said to contain oestrogen – is fed to cows and buffalo to bring them into heat. For indigestion or tympani, stock are fed ground coriander seeds. FMD is controlled by isolating the infected animals and fumigating them by burning scrapings from horses' hooves. A prophylaxy for FMD is to feed spider eggs.

Chauhan, Vijay and Astad R. Pastakai. 1996. Stemming erosion of knowledge: A case of horse husbandry. ***Honey Bee*** 7(1): 14.

With the end of colonialism and the breakdown of the feudal system in India's Gujarat State, horses began to disappear from farms. With them went a vast fund of indigenous knowledge of horse husbandry. This article recuperates three healthful plant recipes for horses. To enhance equine agility and energy, a daily bolus of the following mixture can be given in jaggery in a ratio of 1:1 750 g each of sugar, *Vetiveria zizanoides* and *Trachyspermum* spp. seeds, and 150 g of almonds. To increase blood supply, a daily bolus of the following compound is recommended: 5 kg *Trigonella foenum* seeds, 1.5 kg of *Trachyspermum* seeds, 1.5 kg *Vernonia anthelmintica*, 0.75 kg *kalu* (?), 0.5 kg turmeric powder, 0.25 kg black salt, and 0.25 kg ginger powder mixed 2:1 with jaggery. A daily feeding of 50 g of jaggery, 1 egg, 15 g of ghee, and 25 g of ginger powder mixed together in jowar flour strengthens horses' legs.

Chavunduka, D.M. 1976. Plants regarded by Africans as being of medical value to animals. *Rhodesian Veterinary Journal* 7(1): 6–12.

This paper describes the preparation and administration of ethnoveterinary medicinal plants and gives examples of their traditional curative and preventive uses. The appendices list the scientific, English, Shona and Ndebele names for 53 plants and indicate the plant parts used, the reasons for administering the medicine, the animal species involved, and the method of administration.

Chavunduka, D.M. 1984. Delivery of animal health and production services – general aspects. In: D.L. Hawksworth (ed.). *Advancing Agricultural Production in Africa.* Proceedings of CAB's First Scientific Conference, Arusha, Tanzania, February, 1984. Pp. 262–266.

This paper describes problems of overgrazing and overstocking, land tenure, and animal breeding in African countries. Organizing producers into cooperatives and collectives, instituting patterns of short-duration grazing, and improving pastures might help alleviate these problems. Veterinary services should emphasize production methods and disease prevention in addition to clinical care. More training facilities for research and extension workers are needed; and communication among researchers, extensionists and producers must be improved. Page 262 mentions that stockowners still use a wide range of traditional remedies. A limitation within traditional medicine, however, is the poor understanding of disease causation. Therefore, extension services should work to improve dissemination of aetiological information.

Chiang, Tse-sheng. 1979. Control and treatment of animal diseases by traditional Chinese drugs. *Dairy Science Handbook* 12: 18–24.

Details of traditional Chinese mono- and poly-prescriptions are here presented for eleven types of disorders in horses, mules, donkeys, cattle, buffalo and sheep. Impaction of the colon and caecum in horses is cured by a combination of beating, palpating the rectum, and feeding a compound of rhubarb, sour orange, betel, magnolia and sodium sulphate. This last ingredient promotes intestinal motility. Wounds are dressed with plants that have haemostatic properties. An injectable haemostatic can be produced from *Panax pseudoginseng* and *Nelumbo nucifera*. In Tibet, sheep with the lungworm *Dictyocaulus filaria* are given a tracheal injection of *Usnea longissima* in solution.

Chino Vargas, Soledad, Patricia Jácquez Ríos and Abigail Aguilar Contreras. 1989. Experiencias en el estudio etnobotánico y la herbolaria medicinal en veterinaria de la región de Quimixtlan, Puebla. In: Gerardo López Buendía (ed.). *Memorias: Segunda Jornada sobre Herbolaria Medicinal en Medicina Veterinaria.* Universidad Nacional Autónoma de México, Facultad de Medicina Veterinaria y Zootecnia, Coordinación de Educación Continua, México DF, México. Pp. 40–48.

The study of traditional medicine is important for recuperating local knowledge about the medicinal use of natural resources, which can in turn contribute to solving some of a nation's current health problems and to better managing its flora and fauna. Based on 18 months' research on a variety of ethnobotanical and ethno-zoological issues among mestizo residents and traditional healers in the Quimixtlan region of Mexico's Puebla State, this conference paper presents five plants used in drenches, baths or topical applications to treat rabies in dogs, unstip-ulated diseases in turkeys and chickens, and wounds and intestinal disorders in unspecified animal species. To combat evil eye in livestock, people tie a protective red ribbon about the necks of animals considered to be at risk. Also noted are numerous wild and domesticated animals and animal products used in local treat-ments for human diseases. A few examples are: armadillos, buzzards, coyotes, foxes, rats and rattlesnakes; and eggs, cheese, pork and chicken fat. The authors comment that the people of this zone have no access to modern veterinary medicine.

Chinthu, T.U., B.K. Narainswami and Sheeba Revi. 1998. Ethnoveterinary medi-cine for dairy cows. In: E. Mathias, D.V. Rangnekar and C.M. McCorkle, with M. Martin (eds). *Ethnoveterinary Medicine: Alternatives for Livestock Development – Proceedings of an International Conference Held in Pune, India, 4–6 November 1997. Volume 2: Abstracts.* BAIF Development Research Foundation, Pune, India. Pp. 13–14.

This paper reports on a 1997 study of ethnoveterinary treatments among local healers of south Kerala, India. For cows with FMD, healers smear *Azadirachta indica* (neem) oil boiled with *Brassica juncea* (mustard) seeds on the affected parts, and they feed the animals a gruel of cooked rice and *Cuminum cyminum* (cumin) seeds. Rinderpest is treated with a 'cocktail' of drenches: *Oxalis cornicu-lata* juice in salted buttermilk; *Murraya koenigii* leaves roasted in a mud pot and mixed with a little water; and a porridge of rice and *Aegle marmelos* extract. To control dysentery, *Tragia involucrata* leaves cooked in fermented bran and mixed with *Curcuma longa* L. (turmeric) are fed, along with the water from boiled *Murraya koenigii* leaves. Cows with stomach pains are fed young *Piper betle* L. (areca nut) shoots, *Capsicum frutescens* L. (green chillies), and *Terminalia chebula* in human urine. A decocted drench of dried ginger controls coughs. External parasites are controlled by topically applying a mixture of *Datura stramonium* and *Tinospora cordifolia*. Feeding *Elephantopus scaber* leaves in buttermilk counter-acts tapioca-leaf poisoning, after which the afflicted cows are run, massaged with hot water bags, and drenched with hot sugar-water. Flatulent cows are fed a mixture of milk, onions and *Annona squamosa* leaves. While ethnoveterinary medicines are eco-friendly and cheap, they are tedious to prepare. Also, prescrip-tions and dosages await standardization.

Chittawar, D.R. and K.N.P. Rao. 1981. Some observations on the treatment of canine mycotic dermatitis with indigenous drugs. *Indian Veterinary Journal* 58: 990–991.

Himax^{TM}, Teeburb^{TM}, and Vegecort^{TM} are Ayurvedic medicaments that have been commercialized in India. This article discusses clinical trials on the three drugs' efficacy in treating fungal dermatitis in domestic animals. Combinations of the drugs were found to be efficaceous against *Trichophyton* spp. and *Microsporum* spp.

Choquehuanca Rodríguez, Senón. 1987. Principales enfermedades en ovinos y alpacas y tratamientos en uso en la comunidad de Quishuara. In: *Anales del V Congreso Internacional de Sistemas Agropecuarios Andinos.* Editoriales A. Arteta for CIID, ACDI, and PISA, Lima, Perú. Pp. 414–415.

This abstract of a paper by an SR-CRSP veterinarian reports on a preliminary study of the incidence of and local therapies for sheep and alpaca diseases in a peasant community of Puno, Peru [see also Bazalar and McCorkle 1989]. For both species, parasitism accounted for more than 50% of livestock losses. Indigenous treatments included: application of llama fat and stove ash after washing with a decoction of the *accana* plant for different types of mange; drenching with *huamanlipa* tea for verminous gastroenteritis; for pyosepticaemia, painting the navel with live lime; for conjunctivitis, eye drops of human milk or of blood from the afflicted animal, plus washes with water collected from three different sources; a plaster of salt, sugar and native plants for fractures; and for locoweed poisoning, drenching with a solution of salt and ash made from the same loco.

Choquehuanca, Zenon, Genaro Yarupaitan and Constance M. McCorkle. 1989. Uso de plantas nativas en la sanidad animal en una comunidad campesina de Puno. In: Hernando Bazalar and Constance M. McCorkle (eds). *Estudios Etnoveterinarios en Comunidades Altoandinas del Perú.* Lluvia Editores, Lima, Perú. Pp. 71–82.

Authored by an SR-CRSP zootechnician, botanist and anthropologist, the first half of this chapter overviews the ethnopharmacopoeia of a community of sheep and camelid herders of Peru's Puno Department. The focus is on the most important sylvan plants these herders employ in a variety of infusions, decoctions, plasters, washes and smoke cures to treat their animals' many ills – reportedly with considerable success. The second half of the chapter describes the results of experimental studies scientifically to evaluate the efficacy of three local pharmacotherapies used to treat gastrointestinal parasites in sheep: drenching with decoctions of *akhana, huamanlipa* (both *Senecio* spp.) or the two combined. All three therapies significantly reduced faecal egg counts in comparison to controls. As of day 17 post-treatment, reductions were 55%, 63% and for the combination, 70%, respectively; for controls, this figure was 18%. Between days 17 and 31, counts began to rise again, but much more slowly for treated versus non-treated animals.

Choudary, C. 1990. Use of indigenous medicine in poultry. *Pashudhan* 5: 24,28.

This brief article promotes six commercial preparations of traditional herbal prescriptions for poultry in India. The preparations cure liver disorders, helminthosis, gout, loose droppings and ectoparasites (lice). The article also notes another indigenous, but not yet commercialized, poultry medicine. To wit, wet and dry fowl pox lesions can be topically treated with a decoction of neem tree bark that has been pounded and soaked overnight and then mixed with jaggery (crystallized sugar).

Cihyoka Mowali, Augustin. 1994. Expérience en pharmacopée vétérinaire traditionnelle au Bushi (Kivu/Zare). In: Kakule Kasonia and Michel Ansay (eds). *Métissages en Santé Animale de Madagascar à Haïti: Actes du Séminaire* *d'Ethnopharmacopée Vétérinaire 'KAGALA', un Partage de Savoirs Burkina-Faso, Ouagadougou, 15–22 Avril 1993.* Presses Universitaires de Namur, Namur, Belgium. Pp. 265–274.

The Bushi region of Zaire is one of agropastoralism, where a consortium of NGOs is investigating EVM as a supplement to commercial veterinary inputs, which are rarely available. This article opens with a list of common animal health problems recognized by agropastoralists of the area. A brief overview of local medicaments for livestock is then offered. The author reports that about 30 of the plants cited by Bushi residents as being employed in livestock remedies appear to have some efficacy. The plant parts used are mainly roots, leaves or bark. The main modes of preparation are maceration, decoction and infusion. Non-plant ingredients include various salts, clays and limestone. Rituals may accompany treatment; and people recognize certain contra-indications. The article concludes with two tables. The first lists the Latin and local names of 44 species of plants used in animal health-care in the region. The second outlines treatments for 14 common livestock ailments. Interestingly, nearly all treatments consist of complex polyprescriptions. For example, one remedy for diarrhoea involves nine different plant species, and another for constipation coupled with loose teeth calls for seven.

Cihyoka, Augustin M. 1996. Actes des journées Kagala. *Lettre du Sous-réseau PRELUDE 'Santé, Productions Animales et Environnement'* 9(Jan): 2–3.

This article reports on an EVM workshop held in Zaire in 1994/1995 and attended by stockraisers, farmers and healers for the purpose of exchanging their knowledge of veterinary medicinal plants. In the course of their discussions, participants agreed on treatments they consider helpful for four livestock disease clusters: FMD; ECF; piroplasmosis, babesiosis and anaplasmosis; colibacillosis and salmonellosis. For each, the article describes modes of transmission, clinical signs, species affected and medicinal plants utilized. Workshop participants also agreed that people usually turn to their traditional veterinary medicines first, not only because they are cheaper than modern ones but because people have confidence in them; but sometimes both types are employed simultaneously. Also discussed were the plant proportions in polyprescriptions, the standardization of measures, and dosing regimes. It was agreed that rule-of-thumb proportions for polyprescriptions are: 60% of the principal plant(s); 30% of reinforcing plants; and 10% of other plants or ingredients for ancillary conditions such as fever, weakness, etc. Standardized measures were set as per the sizes of familiar local drinking-glasses and bottles. Likewise for dosage size and frequency for small ruminants and young calves versus adult cattle. Finally, the group also made plans for traditional healers and 'farmer researchers' to: offer and also track, validate and record herbal livestock treatments and patient outcomes; exchange their findings with one another and with development and documentation centres; and in the longer term, establish gardens of veterinary plants and open dispensaries for these plants as well as for basic modern drugs.

Cisse, F. 1992. Rapports techniciens et eleveurs ruraux. In: G. Tacher and L. Letenneur (eds). *Proceedings of the Seventh International Conference of Institutions of Tropical Veterinary Medicine, Yamoussoukro, Ivory Coast: Volume I.* Pp. 81–84.

Among the problems encountered in setting up paravet services in Kita, Mali was stockraisers' mistrust of veterinarians, paravets and their wares. Partly as a result of having been repeatedly duped by vendors who sold them fraudulent veterinary products, stockraisers had 'totally lost confidence in the efficacy of these products' (p. 83).

Clater, Francis. 1811. *Every Man His Own Farrier: Or, the Whole Art of Farriery Laid Open.* W. Lewis, London, UK. 360 pp.

This old-time book on English blacksmithing contains over 200 prescriptions for ailments of horses. A few examples are the following. An astringent for sprains and strains was comprised of camphor, nitre, wine vinegar, turpentine, white lead powder and aquafortis. A 'green ointment' for cooling and softening tumours, wounds or swellings of wounds was compounded of wormwood and elder and plantain leaves bruised together in a mortar and then boiled in hog lard over a slow fire. Once crisped, the leaves were strained out of the mixture. Also described are methods of bloodletting, firing and rowelling.

Claus, Gilbert J.M. n.d. Camel diseases and the traditional methods of treatment in use among the Ghrib camel breeders of the northwestern Tunisian Sahara. Unpublished manuscript. Department of Languages and Cultures of the Near East and North Africa, Section Arabic and Islamic Studies, University of Gent, Gent, Belgium. 12 pp.

Ghrib Bedouin of the Tunisian Sahara are nomadic camel herders. This document describes nine categories of camel disorders, their diagnoses and treatments as recognized and applied by Ghrib. The categories span: lameness; ailments of the skin and eyes; nervous, respiratory, digestive, circulatory and urinary problems; and injuries, mainly due to packs. Seven different types of lameness alone are noted. These are treated by various combinations of cauterization, bleeding and incisions into which salt is inserted. For skin diseases, like mange and scabies, the affected areas may also be cauterized and/or daubed with DDT, plant tars (especially broom, *Retama duraeginista barbara*), used motor oil, unspecified oils mixed with sulphur, butter melted with date syrup, butter or olive oil mixed with *Thuya tetraclinislariks* leaves, and still other preparations. A cataract-like condition is treated by surgical removal; inflamed eyes are dusted with powdered pepper or tobacco. For respiratory ailments, camels may be fed a porridge or crushed wheat and butter, and covered against the cold. For digestive-tract disorders like a swollen palate or buccal abscesses, the affected area is pricked or incised and dressed with salt. An example of circulatory problems is hypertension, which is diagnosed by a camel's lowered head, flushed body parts, and desire to graze only at night; the remedy is to drench with olive oil and melted butter. A male camel that grazes on *Genista saharae* may suffer from urine retention. In such cases, the herdsman inserts a thin reed [a sort of indigenous catheter] into the camel's penis and then sucks on the reed to induce urination. For injuries or wounds on the front of the hump, the herder presses out the pus and then dusts the area with pounded tea leaves or the ashes of burnt date pits. Strains, cricks or sprains are cured by cauterization with a red-hot iron. The author also reports that, to date, he has collected some 1100 Ghrib terms pertaining to camels, including scores that deal with camel anatomy and physiology as appreciated by herders' experience in slaughtering.

Claxton, John and Philippe Leperre. 1991. Parasite burdens and host suscepti-bility of zebu and N'Dama cattle in village herds in Gambia. *Veterinary Parasitology* 40: 293–304.

Helminth and tick burdens among Gambian villagers' herds of N'Dama cattle were compared with parasite burdens in zebu cattle introduced into the same herds. The authors concluded that observed differences in susceptiblity to endemic endo- and ectoparasites between the two breeds could not be wholly attributed to zebu's naturally lesser adaptation to such environmental disease challenges. Rather, data pointed to [anthropogenically?] enhanced innate resistance factors in the N'Dama cattle.

Cockrill, W. Ross. 1974. Management, conservation and use. In: W. Ross Cockrill (ed.). *The Husbandry and Health of the Domestic Buffalo.* FAO, Rome, Italy. Pp. 283–312.

Several traditional types of buffalo castration around the world are described in this chapter. Reportedly, the most common method is to pound the testicles with a heavy stone or a flat metal bar. Sometimes the neck of the scrotum is tightly clamped between two flat bamboo strips and the clamp is pounded instead. A tra-ditional Javanese instrument, the *pasurnam*, consists of three iron bars in which the scrotum is enclosed and to which pressure is then applied. In the Amazon delta, castration may be effected by a tight elastic band around the testes or by knife and emasculator. Besides castration, the author also comments on the difficulty of drenching buffalo; and he mentions people's use of a bamboo tube to administer human urine as a general tonic.

Cole, D.P. 1975. *Nomads of the Nomads: The Al Murrah Bedouin of the Empty Quarter.* AHM Publishing Corporation, Arlington Heights, Illinois, USA.

Unavailable for review. According to Hjort and Dahl 1984, however, this work con-tains considerable information on health-related aspects of camel management.

Coly, Raphael. 1994. Enquête ethnomédicale vétérinaire au Sénégal. In: Kakule Kasonia and Michel Ansay (eds). *Métissages en Santé Animale de Madagascar à Haïti: Actes du Séminaire d'Ethnopharmacopée Vétérinaire 'KAGALA', un Partage de Savoirs Burkina-Faso, Ouagadougou, 15–22 Avril 1993.* Presses Universitaires de Namur, Namur, Belgium. Pp. 153–156.

Findings from an ethnoveterinary survey in Senegal are presented in tabular form in this chapter. Fulani (Pulaar) names for 16 livestock diseases are given, along with their French glosses and the clinical signs and causes as recognized by stock-raisers. For each disease, a traditional plant remedy is listed, including its method of preparation, side effects and the geographical locales where the plant(s) can be found. A total of 14 medicinal plant species are mentioned. For example, *Cissus quadrangularis* is cited for three horse ailments: colic, mange and strangles (dis-temper). For colic, the plant is pulverized, filtered and administered *per os.*

Mangey horses are bathed with an aqueous maceration of the plant. For strangles, the plant is administered as a fumigant. Interestingly, all but one of the plant remedies is a monoprescription.

Combe, G.A. 1926. *A Tibetan on Tibet.* T. Fischer Unwin, London, UK.

Page 129 mentions that Tibetan pastoralists tapped certain blood vessels in the necks of yaks, to obtain blood for human consumption and to make the animals stronger.

Comisión Organizadora de Criadores de Alpaca de la Provincia de Caylloma. 1985. *Alpaqueros de Caylloma: Problemas y Alternativas.* DESCO – Centro de Estudios y Promoción del Desarrollo, Lima, Perú. 68 pp.

Focusing on alpaca raising in Caylloma Province, Department of Arequipa, this booklet discusses constraints, husbandry practices, fibre marketing and processing, the role of technical assistance, and opportunities for further development of alpaca production in the region. Pages 23–30 deal with local management techniques and animal health. Birthing practices consist of disinfecting the navel with iodine, tying it off with a piece of homespun, and drenching newborns with herbal decoctions against diarrhoea and with infusions of coca against the cold. Weaning techniques include tying a flap of plastic over the young alpaca's forehead or inserting a stick in its nose. With regard to alpaca diseases, the greater resistance of the *huacaya* breed to pneumonias is noted, in contrast to the *suri* breed. Eleven major categories of ills afflicting alpaca in the area are outlined, along with the Quechua names of these diseases and stockowners' therapies of choice (both indigenous and Western commercial). The booklet makes two important observations. First, alpaca raisers of Caylloma report that climatological changes in recent decades have promoted more and sometimes heretofore unknown alpaca diseases in the region. Second, knowledge and use of traditional treatments with herbs and other native substances are rapidly disappearing.

Cook, A.J.C. 1991. Communal farmers and tick control: A field study in Zimbabwe. *Tropical Animal Health and Production* 23: 161–166.

Intensive dipping of cattle to control tick-borne diseases precludes development of endemic stability to such diseases. Alternative control strategies have been recommended that reduce dip frequency and permit the expression of natural tick resistance. However, such strategies imply cattle-owner acceptance of higher tick burdens. In this study, 107 Zimbabwean communal farmers were queried as to their views on tick dipping. On balance, they preferred to continue automatically prescribed dipping rather than to adopt strategic or threshold dipping [as Sahelian pastoralists do in their own ectoparasite strategies], modern vaccinations or [as in other parts of Africa] tick-resistant cattle breeds.

Córdova, Pedro. 1981. Así curamos el ganado en el Canipaco. *Minka* 5(Jan): 11.

In this brief article, a producer from Peru's Huancayo Department offers two home remedies used in his village to cure liver fluke and septicaemia in herd animals. The fluke cure is based on an extract of the herb *jaya-shipita* [see also Carlier

1981]. The septicaemia treatment consists of bathing the afflicted animal for five days with a herbal decoction and drenching with another made from salt, burnt brown sugar and three different herbs.

Córdova, Pedro. 1982a. Enseñanzas de Don Pedro. *Minka* 8(Aug): 6.

Pedro Córdova is a respected local livestock curer who lives in a community in highland Peru, where he treats animals for free – although grateful villagers thereafter never fail to send him small gifts of potatoes and other foodstuffs. This kind of tangible community recognition is 'worth more than all the money that Bayer and other pharmaceutical companies earn', he says. Don Pedro used to prescribe such companies' products, but often they failed to work because, he confesses, much of the time he didn't really understand the directions. So Don Pedro turned to traditional medicinal herbs instead, along with other simple ingredients like lard, soap and urine. These seemed to work better, and people preferred them because they were much cheaper than commercial drugs. Don Pedro comments that, although there is a great deal of research going on in order to help farmers like himself, most of it 'is pure story-telling' that makes no use of traditional knowledge and has little relevance to farmers' problems.

Córdova, Pedro. 1982b. Nuestra vaquita en el campo. *Minka* 8(Aug): 7.

In this article, a respected local healer gives advice to farmers of highland Peru on the breeding and peri-natal care of cows and calves, as performed with 'affection and love'. Among other, more conventional advice, he recommends drenching newborn calves with a mixture of fresh urine, black soap and *Cestrum hediondinum* juice if they show signs of agitation. To treat retained placenta, he has the cow lick a preparation of toasted *zuela de zapato* [?] mixed with salt. For people wishing to upgrade their herd's milk production, he recommends crossing local cows with Brown Swiss studs, as this breed is better adapted to the Andes' altitude and climate.

Cornuau, C. 1989. Les bouquets suspendus . . . Magie? Sorcellerie? N'y a-t-il rien d'autre . . . ? *Bulletin de l'Alliance Pastorale* Mar: 23.

In the Cevennes region of France, bouquets of holly are hung from the rafters of sheepfolds to ward against fungal infections of the flock. The bouquets should be hung during the first six days of the new moon; thereafter, infections supposedly regress as the moon wanes. Other practices, such as hanging up of box leaves blessed on the Christian feastday of Palm Sunday, are also thought to protect man and beast.

Crane, Eva. 1990. *Bees and Beekeeping: Science, Practice and World Resources*. Comstock, Ithaca, New York, USA. 603 pp.

Humans have been keeping bees for over 4500 years. The most universal of traditional hives has been in use since 2500 B.C. and is still found the world over. It is a horizontal fixed-comb structure, in contrast to Northern Europe's upright structures. In ancient Greece of 400 B.C. to 600 A.D., hives were made of tapered cylindrical pots. In today's East Africa, hives consist of horizontal hollow logs suspended from a tree branch, out of reach of bee predators. A similar sort of hive is used in Java. In Thailand, to prevent swarming, beekeepers tether the queen bee to a new hive with a fine thread; her workers will then follow her, after which she is untied. Similar procedures are found in Burma and Vietnam, where the tether consists of a human hair. The type and construction of hives is largely determined by local materials and conditions. All beekeeping cultures control considerable ethnoentomological and ethnometeorological knowledge. In hot climates, for example, horizontal hives prevent overheating by allowing the bees to spread out to the ends of the structure. Traditional fixed-comb hives are less likely to spread pathogens between colonies than modern, moveable-frame ones (although the latter were already known in Greece in 1682). This is because the moveable frames are easier to transport around a country than entire hives. However, moveable designs have become increasingly popular because they facilitate swarm control, honey harvesting, and inspection and manipulation of colonies while the bees are out foraging. The modified African long hive is an example of techno-blending, introduced as a transition from a fixed to a tiered-frame design. Long hives have many advantages: they are cheaper to build; they can be readily modified to suit local conditions (as the author describes for England, Ecuador, Mexico and Uganda); and every frame is accessible without disturbing the others. Extra materials needed include: bamboo or other sticks to support the combs, and wire mesh or nylon netting. Water feeders can be made from the perforated cap of a plastic bottle, or a clean wet sponge.

Crees, Jim. 1995. Southern Sudan: Will Vetaid help in the homecoming to Bor? *Vetaid Newsletter* 12(Summer): 2.

A Vetaid representative visiting Dinka refugees who had returned to their long-contested 'no-man's-land' grazing grounds in warring southern Sudan commented that their cattle looked to be the fattest and healthiest in the country. Displaying their indigenous ecological, nutritional, parasitological and epidemiological savvy, Dinka replied that this was because the pastures had been abandoned for some time. Thus they were lush with grass; infective parasites had long since died out; and no other livestock had been around to reinfect the pastures or spread any kind of disease.

Crees, Jim. 1996. More tales from Kenya. In: Peter Fry (ed.). *Vetaid Book of Veterinary Anecdotes.* Vetaid, Edinburgh, UK. Pp. 96–100.

Detailing his experiences as a veterinarian in Kenya, the author recounts what he terms 'the curse of the phantom flukes' – a case in which he was called in to treat a herd of exotic cattle that had suddenly begun to lose weight dramatically. The veterinarian was dubious about the owner's diagnosis of liver fluke, given that the farm had no marshy land; but he administered the usual flukicide nevertheless, although the owner glumly predicted that all the animals would waste away and die no matter what. Dung samples at the time of the vet's initial visit indicated massive fluke infestation, while samples from a return visit showed no trace of fluke eggs, as a result of treatment. Yet all the herd expired. When the last two animals died, the vet performed a necropsy. Findings revealed all the classic signs of liver fluke, except that there were no flukes in the swollen tubes of the shrivelled livers. The only explanation was that proferred by neighbours, who avowed the deaths resulted from another's jealousy of the owner's stockraising success. The author termed the event 'the most clear-cut case of a malicious curse affecting livestock that I have come across in 25 years in East Africa' (p. 97). In recounting another experience, the author notes that a Western commercial drug (Stilboestrol), which was very popular in East Africa for bringing cows into heat, had long been banned in Europe because European men suffered [in unspecified ways] from eating the meat of cattle so treated.

Croxton, S., V. Lewis, P. Mulvany, L. Pridmore, B. O'Riordan and H. Wedgwood with J. Bell. 1996. *Livestock Keepers Safeguarding Domestic Animal Diversity through their Animal Husbandry.* ITDG Food Security Programme. ITDG, Rugby, UK. 16 pp.

The combination of rural peoples' environmental knowledge and livestock management techniques helps maintain domestic animal diversity, via stockraisers' recognition and evaluation of genetic characteristics, types and breeds of livestock; their understanding of how plant and animal genetic resources interact, and their design of husbandry systems accordingly; and their ethnoveterinary know-how. With regard to breeding and genetics, people have evolved a number of livestock races that are exceptionally well-adapted to their environment. Examples include: Scottish North Ronaldsay sheep, which thrive on seaweed during the winter and thus are one of the few breeds to fatten during the winter in such northern climes; China's Taihu pig, which survives on its own foraging and averages litters of 16; Yakut horses of Siberia that can survive at −70°C; and Africa's Ankole cattle, which have been bred to resist ECF. To this list can be added the various trypanotolerant cattle, sheep, and goats of West Africa [see ILRAD 1985]. Indeed, virtually every pastoral group has developed a distinct animal breed to suit its specific needs.

Cueva-Abena, Nita. 1996. *Paraveterinary Medicine: An Information Kit on Low-cost Health Care Practices.* IIRR, Silang, Cavite, Philippines. 4 booklets of 53, 60, 60, and 18 pp.

Written by a practising rural veterinarian 'in the simplest language possible for the convenience of the intended user – the animal health practitioners or "para-vets" working in isolated rural communities' (Vol. 1, p. i), as the first of the four booklets in this information kit pragmatically points out, 'It is neither practical nor necessary to call a veterinarian for every little thing that goes wrong with your animals' (p. 47). The four booklets are entitled *Restraining Animals and Simple Treatments, Basic Husbandry Practices and Veterinary Care, Disease Control and Treatment,* and *Herbal Medicine for Animals.* Based on fieldwork across a year in the Philippines Cavite Province, the third and the fourth volumes offer some botanical and other alternatives to Western medicine (the author's term) for health problems of cattle, buffalo, small ruminants, swine and chickens. Booklet 4 lists 15 medicinal plants and their uses in combatting ecto- and endo-parasites, plant poisoning, warts, anaemia, wounds, bloat, coughs, colds, fevers and diarrhoeas. Booklet 3 often indicates whether these herbal treatments are curative or merely palliative, along with diseases for which Western medicine is the only effective option. Booklet 2 notes the following 'indigenous practices in castrating animals' (p. 49). A traditional way for farmers to castrate bulls is the *pukpok* method, in which the testicles are crushed using a large stone or a hard piece of wood. To stop the bleeding from castration and also to reduce the risk of infection, farmers apply wood ash or hot, cooked rice to the wound. People believe that castrating during a full moon will make the wound heal faster. They may also throw the testicles onto a hot tin roof in the belief that, as the tissue quickly dries up, so the castration wound will quickly heal. Also noted in Booklet 2 is the advisability of clipping piglets' milk teeth to avoid harm to the nursing sow. This booklet describes a home-made insecticide of *Gliricidia* leaves, vinegar and laundry detergent in water for combatting the mites, ticks and lice that plague livestock.

Cunningham, A.B. and A.S. Zondi. 1991. *Cattle Owners and Traditional Medicines Used for Livestock.* Investigational Report No. 69. Institute of Natural Resources, University of Natal, Pietermaritzburg, South Africa. 35 pp.

A survey of ethnoveterinary practices in KwaZulu, South Africa revealed extensive use of some 50 plant and 10 animal species plus other items (disinfectants, potassium permanganate, salt, vaseline) as *materia medica* among Zulu pastoralists. Both mono- and poly-prescriptions are prepared and administered to cattle by herders, herbalists (*izinyanga*) and diviners (*izangoma*). The percentage of interviewees employing each treatment cited is given. Retained placenta in cows can be remedied in three ways. The most popular method (62% of interviewees) is to beat the hindquarters gently with a spear, presumably to induce uterine contractions. Alternatively, the cow may be drenched with diced, boiled and sieved *Gunnera perpense* root. Or *Crinum* sp. and *Rhoicissus digitata* bulb and tuber can be diced, boiled and applied to the abdomen while still hot. For eye problems, the favourite treatment (48%) is to blow powdered cuttlefish shell through a pipe into the eye. Snail shell, salt and *Aloe cooperi* may be added to this prescription. Damaged teats are rubbed with monitor-lizard, white-rhinoceros or whale fat, vaseline or freshly ground *Senecio serratuloides* leaves. The author notes the difference between symbolic and physiological uses of the various ingredients in Zulu's ethnoveterinary pharmacopoeia. Although the Zulu word for cuttlefish translates literally as 'faeces of the moon', this interpretation should in no way mask the real physiological value of cuttlefish treatments for human as well as livestock eye disorders in southern and western Africa. Monitor lizards (*Varanus* spp.) represent strength and are thought to steal milk directly from cows; but their fat does help heal damaged teats.

Cunningham, James G. 1969. Traditional veterinary medicine at the edge of the Sahara. *Veterinary Scope* 25(1): 22–24.

Traditional veterinary practices of Hausa and Fulani in northern Nigeria include phytotherapy, bloodletting, medico-religious techniques, surgery and indigenous vaccination. Of particular note in this article is a Twareg technique of camel contraception, in which a stone is placed in the uterus.

Cunnison, Ian. 1966. *Baggara Arabs: Power and the Lineage in a Sudanese Nomad Tribe.* Clarendon Press, Oxford, UK.

Appendix 4 of this ethnography on the Baggara [also spelled Baqqara] Arabs deals with cattle brands. Branding is the most common veterinary treatment for cattle. Medicinal brands are quite distinct from those used for animal identification. Both types have their own design and locations. Moreover, the medicinal brands are usually more coarse (p. 208).

Curasson, G. 1947. *Le Chameau et ses Maladies.* Vigot Freres, Paris, France. 462 pp.

Pages 38–41 of this book on camel diseases and their treatments deal with EVM. Traditional treatments are based on empirical knowledge passed on from generation to generation. Camel herders diagnose diseases by inspection, touch and odour. They are aware of the contagiousness of certain diseases and they know that insects can transmit diseases. Traditional surgical methods consist of cauterization, bleeding and bonesetting. Arabs as well as Hindus inoculate their camels against camel pox (pp. 56–57). Other diseases are prevented by amulets or verses from the Koran. Cures for internal diseases follow the principle of 'like evokes like'. For example, treatments of pepper, milk and butter for respiratory diseases are given intranasally. The author views most such treatments as ineffective, but acknowledges the herders' observational acumen. It has led to their use of tar for scabies and their discovery of the transmission of trypanosomosis by flies. Other chapters of this book deal with Western-style veterinary medicine, but they occasionally refer to traditional methods, e.g. salt feeding (p. 167) and herders' belief that *Enartocarpus clavatus* is toxic to camels (p. 179). Pages 426–427 discuss cauterization and bleeding.

Curry, J.J., B.D. Perry, J.M. Delehanty and S. Mining. 1992. Improving animal health care delivery through the use of ethnoveterinary knowledge in coastal and highland Kenya. In: P.W. Daniels, S. Holden, E. Lewin and S. Dadi (eds). *Livestock Services for Smallholders: A Critical Evaluation of the Delivery of Animal Health and Production Services to the Small-scale Farmer in the Developing World – Proceedings of an International Seminar, Yogyakarta, Indonesia, 15–21, November 1992.* INIANSREDEF, Bogor, Indonesia. Pp. 220–223.

This conference contribution in essence constitutes a revised and compressed version of Delehanty 1990.

CUSO. 1987. Untitled. Unpublished list of ethnoveterinary plants collected in Nong Pho, Thailand. Nong Pho Dairy Cooperative, Ratchaburi, Thailand. 14 pp.

This list of 30 plants was collected in the dairy-cattle region of Nong Pho, Thailand by a CUSO volunteer. Some of the plants used in livestock treatments in the region are: *Allium sativum* L., *Anamirta cocculus* W., *Annona squamosa* L., *Heliotropium indicum* L., *Ocimum sanctum* L., *Zingiber cassumunar* R. The local, botanical and English names are given for each plant; and pharmaceutical uses and active ingredients are cited, where known. The uses of each plant part (seed, flower, vine, fruit, leaves, bark, root, etc.) are discussed as well. General comments are given on mode of preparation, along with detailed prescriptions for nine livestock ailments: haemorrhagic septicaemia, mastitis, colds, stiff legs, bloat, FMD, sore throat, bloody stools and 'parasites'. For each of these conditions, more than one prescription is given, with a listing of the plants and other ingredients to be included. Examples of non-plant ingredients are sugar, salt, rice-whiskey and coconut milk.

Dahl, Gudrun and Anders Hjort. 1976. *Having Herds: Pastoral Herd Growth and Household Economy.* Stockholm Studies in Social Anthropology No. 2. Department of Social Anthropology, University of Stockholm, Stockholm, Sweden. 335 pp.

This study illustrates economic aspects of herd management among pastoral households in the Middle East and Africa. It describes the composition and growth of herds of cattle, camels, sheep and goats; their food production capacity; and their relative advantages and disadvantages. An extensive review of the literature presents information on the selection of breedstock (p. 29), bleeding (pp. 171, 193, 218), and calf rearing (p. 186), to mention only those passages relating directly to EVM.

Dakshinkar, N.P. and D.B. Sarode. 1998. Therapeutic evaluation of crude extracts of indigenous plants against mange of dogs. In: E. Mathias, D.V. Rangnekar and C.M. McCorkle, with M. Martin (eds). *Ethnoveterinary Medicine: Alternatives for Livestock Development – Proceedings of an International Conference Held in Pune, India, 4–6 November 1997. Volume 2: Abstracts.* BAIF Development Research Foundation, Pune, India. P. 14.

Local application of crude extracts of garlic, neem and *sitaphalas* 1:10 volume/weight were effective against sarcoptic mange in dogs. Recovery rates for the three plants were 54%, 67% and 44% respectively; and the average numbers of days required for complete cure were 22 ± 0.6, 27 ± 1.7 and 28 ± 1.9 days. All treatments were refractory in treating *Demodex* spp. infection.

Dakshinkar, N.P., D.B. Sarode and A.S. Rao. 1998. Comparative evaluation of herbal anthelmintics in calves. In: E. Mathias, D.V. Rangnekar and C.M. McCorkle, with M. Martin (eds). *Ethnoveterinary Medicine: Alternatives for Livestock Development – Proceedings of an International Conference Held in Pune, India, 4–6 November 1997. Volume 2: Abstracts.* BAIF Development Research Foundation, Pune, India. P. 14.

Thirty-six 12-to 16-month-old Sahiwal × Jersey heifers naturally infected with *Haemonchus contortus* were randomly divided into five groups and treated as follows: no treatment (T); powdered neem leaves (T1); powdered *Moringa oleifera* seeds (T2); M/s. Indian Herbs Broad Spectrum Anthelmintic (IHBS) powder (T3); and the chemical Morantel Citrate (T4). The mean numbers of eggs per gram of faeces (epg) as well as haemoglobin and serum iron and copper were recorded on days 0, 7, 14, 21 and 28 after treatment. As of day 28, only in group T4 were epg counts significantly lower than on day 0. The haematobiochemical parameters did not differ significantly in any of the groups.

Damiel, James. 1969. *A Study of Buffalo Husbandry Practices Prevalent among Farmers of Hissar Block.* MS thesis, Haryana Agricultural University, Hissar, India.

Unavailable for review.

Dar, R.N., L.C. Garg and R.D. Pathak. 1965. Anthelmintic activity of *Carica papaya* seeds. *The Indian Journal of Pharmacy* 27(12): 335–337.

In India and elsewhere, papaya seeds have traditionally been claimed, and now scientifically demonstrated, to have anthelmintic activity. Papaya seed powder has previously been shown to have half the anthelmintic activity of piperazine when used in suspension, and nearly equal potency as an aqueous seed extract. Earlier authors identified carpasemine (benzyl thiourea) as the main chemical component responsible; but later studies suggested it might be an artifact of benzyl isothiocyanate. This article reviews further chemical research and describes a series of experiments using *Ascaris lumbricoides* to isolate the main component responsible for this activity: benzyl isothiocyanate. Carpasemine turns out to have much less activity. Other findings of interest are that: the yield of carpasemine is much lower if extracts are not made from freshly powdered seeds; and both skin and internal tests of benzyl isothiocyanate in rabbits showed no signs of toxicity.

Das, S.N., K.P. Janardhanan and S.C. Roy. 1983. Some observations on the ethnobotany of the tribes of Totopara and adjoining areas in Jalpaiguri District, West Bengal. *Journal of Economic and Taxonomic Botany* 4(2): 453–474.

This article cites 84 species of angiosperms used by tribes in West Bengal, India for food, fish poisoning, cattle fodder and human and livestock ethnomedicine. In the latter regard, *Arisaema tortuosum* seeds are given with salt for colic pain in goats, while the roots serve as a cattle anthelmintic. *Duchesnea indica* is also cited as a cattle medicine, but no further details are given.

Dash, M. n.d. -a. About the Mongolian traditional veterinary science. Unpublished manuscript. No agency or place of publication given. 7 pp.

This paper presents a historical review of Mongolian ethnoveterinary practices for cattle, horses and sheep, along with indications of the continuing use of EVM in Mongolia today. The practice of veterinary medicine in Mongolia has been documented from at least the 10th century A.D. Ancient magical and medical veterinary methods are recorded not only in early medical/veterinary texts but also were, and are still, encoded in sutras. Mongolian EVM is based on the principle of opposites, akin to Chinese medicine's yin and yang. Key diagnostic and treatment dichotomies include internal versus external signs, depression versus excitement, and cold versus hot syndromes. Taken together, they indicate which organ system may be malfunctioning. The veterinary pharmacopoeia incorporates animal, vegetable and mineral *materia medica*, as well as surgical, physical and magical treatments. The first three categories include milk, meat, bone, bile, horns and bones of wild animals; various plants; and soot, ashes, sulphur, copper and silver. Surgical treatments span bonesetting, bloodletting, castration, cauterization and suturing, as in sewing up wounds in camels' soles. Physical techniques include enemas for camel-calf and foal constipation and the use of cold and hot compresses for unspecified conditions. Magical treatments are divided into charms, fortune telling, incense, shamanism and exorcism. For acute mastitis, an exorcist creeps up to the animal at night, scratches its udder three times with a bear paw, and thrice repeats an incantation. Sheep bloat is exorcised by a man's sitting on the sheep facing its tail while waving a wolf or fox skin around the sheep's head and chanting an incantation. Traditional Mongolian, Chinese and Indo-Tibetan veterinary medicine all operate on the yin/yang theory of disease. However, Mongol traditions do not include acupuncture.

Dash, M. n.d. -b. Mongolian traditional veterinary science. Published abstract. No agency or place of publication given. 2 pp.

This is a shorter, published version of the above-referenced unpublished manuscript.

Davies, Jeremy. 1992. A life in the day of Seetha. ***Vetaid News*** 7(summer): 2.

In describing the care that an Indian woman, Seetha, gives her one precious dairy buffalo, this article notes that she takes the animal every day to a wallow, where she gives it a good rub-down with a handful of rice straw.

Davis, Diana K. 1995. Gender-based differences in the ethnoveterinary knowledge of Afghan nomadic pastoralists. ***Indigenous Knowledge and Development Monitor*** 3(1): 3–4.

A survey of gender-based differences in EVK among Afghan Pashtun nomadic pastoralists found that women have at least as much such information as men, but women's and men's knowledge lie in different spheres. Women tend to know more about healthcare for newborns and for animals too ill to transhume with the rest of the herd, who are therefore left with the women at the tent site. Women are also responsible for preparing slaughtered animals and as a result they can cite twice as many types of internal parasites as men. In addition, women help with dystocias and the manual removal of ectoparasites.

Davis, Diana K., Karimullah Quraishi, David Sherman, Albert Sollod and Chip Stem. 1995. Ethnoveterinary medicine in Afghanistan: An overview of indigenous animal health care among Pashtun Koochi nomads. ***Journal of Arid Environments*** 31: 483–500.

Animal diseases, plants and minerals of veterinary importance to nomadic Pashtun Koochi of Afghanistan are discussed in this article. Examples of plants used in livestock medicine are *Mallotus philippensis* and *Berberis vulgaris*. *Mallotus philippensis* fruit is used as a treatment for tapeworms in goats. *Berberis vulgaris* roots and stems are administered for coughing, pneumonia, sunstroke and trauma. Minerals include alum and especially copper sulphate. The latter, which occurs naturally in the desert regions of Afghanistan, is administered for health problems as diverse as endoparasitism, diarrhoea, enterotoxaemia, pneumonia, frostbite and sunstroke. The standard procedure is to dose each sheep or goat with approximately 1 g of copper sulphate. Koochi also make use of traditional vaccination and surgical techniques, along with amulets and prayers. In an effort to prevent the spread of anthrax, when an animal dies suddenly, a gun is fired over the remainder of the flock – as though they might die suddenly as from being shot. This act may relate to the law of signatures, which postulates that like, cures or prevents like.

Day, Christopher and J.G.G. Saxton. 1998. Veterinary homeopathy: Principles and practice. In: Allen M. Schoen and Susan G. Wynn (eds). *Complementary and Alternative Veterinary Medicine: Principles and Practice.* Mosby, Inc., St Louis, Missouri, USA. Pp. 485–513.

Introduced in the early 1800s, veterinary homeopathy takes a holistic approach and employs extreme dilutions of medicaments, in contrast to conventional medicine's mechanistic and reductionistic approach using highly invasive techniques and drugs. Today, veterinary homeopathy is particularly popular in Europe. While demand for it among the public is burgeoning, it has not yet won scientific acceptance, however. In large part this is because of the paucity of scientifically acceptable clinical trials, due to lack of funding plus the difficulty of designing such trials for a system of medicine that relies on individualistic prescriptions rather than on blanket treatments. Thus, a highlight of this book chapter is its report of a number of clinical trials, conducted by the senior author, that demonstrate good response to homeopathic medication. These trials span prophylactic or therapeutic treatments for dystocia and mastitis in cattle, canine tracheobronchitis, and porcine stillbirths. Also detailed here is the careful case-study approach that veterinary homeopathy takes to each patient and its problem. The author further lists disease-types × patient-species that he feels homeopathy is well able to treat. Along with herbal medicine and acupuncture, he notes that homeopathy is perhaps particularly relevant to farm animals in light of current concerns about dangerous drug residues in foodstuffs. A six-page table presents a brief guide for selecting helpful homeopathic remedies in common veterinary situations. These include not only physical ills but also a wide range of behavioural and 'mental' problems in animals. The chapter concludes with an overview of recent research on the effects and effectiveness of veterinary homeopathic treatments plus a list of eight US and UK associations or teaching groups active in this variety of EVM.

Dayrit, Ricardo El. S. 1990. Plant-based medicine for livestock (water buffalo/carabao). In: Lyn N. Capistrano, Janet Durno and Ilya Moeliono (eds). *Resource Book on Sustainable Agriculture for the Uplands.* IIRR, Silang, Cavite, Philippines. Pp. 132–136.

Filipino stockraisers are returning to their traditional veterinary phytotherapies, drawing upon local herbalists' knowledge. This chapter cites some 40 plant species used in mono- and poly-prescriptions to treat approximately 25 common ailments of water buffalo – e.g. wounds; gastrointestinal, respiratory, urinary and eye disorders; fevers and sprains; and more. Seven botanical ectoparasiticides are listed, including topical application of cashew-nut oil. To take a different example, tobacco is applied with saliva as a poultice to staunch bleeding wounds. Besides plant materials, sugar and kerosene figure in a few prescriptions. Overall, decoctions and drenches appear to be the most common mode of preparation and route of administration, respectively.

Delehanty, James. 1990. *Local Knowledge of Cattle Diseases in Kaloleni Division, Kilifi District, Kenya: A Report to KARI and ILCA.* ILRAD, Nairobi, Kenya. 79 pp.

This report details the findings from the author's intensive study of local knowledge of disease aetiology, conditions, prevention and cure among 158 Mijikenda cattle-keepers of coastal Kenya's Kaloleni Division. In total, interviewees volunteered 144 discrete syndromes of cattle. However, many of the terms elicited were mere sign descriptors, rather than true disease names referring to culturally codified complexes of clinical signs. This is because, as recent adopters of cattle, Mijikenda lack a cultural and practical tradition of cattle lore and expertise. For example, they have very inadequate understandings of the vectors and causes of many cattle diseases. Naturally, there was little correspondence between Mijikenda and Western disease names. Moreover, Mijikenda terminology varied considerably across interviewees. However, using a novel methodology that combined epidemiology and linguistics, the author analytically identified ten major 'syndrome clusters'. [For methodological details and an in-depth discussion of one syndrome, see Delehanty 1996.] These roughly referenced helminth infection, calf and adult theileriosis, trypanosomosis, diarrhoea, fever, boils and skin lesions, and weight loss. Overall, Mijikenda label diseases using native words plus colonial and modern veterinary terms they learned from extensionists and veterinarians. Consequently, Mijikenda sometimes distinguish a Western disease name and its seeming local-language equivalent by applying them to acute versus chronic forms, to manifestations in certain ages of cattle, to different stages of progression, or even to entirely different diseases. Epidemiological investigations revealed that, sometimes also, native terms – and certainly their frequency of citation – reflected the extent or endemicity of a disease. Often, this correlated with whether cattle-keepers lived in drier or wetter parts of the Division. In conclusion, the report offers a 'cautious . . . inter-linguistic lexicon of disease terms in Kaloleni, useful, potentially, in a variety of veterinary extension contexts' (p. iv). Otherwise, extensionists risk fruitlessly recommending interventions for Western-named disease X (the term extensionists know) that goes by local name Y or, in local parlance, may even refer to an entirely different disease, Z. The author therefore recommends conducting a lexical survey early in regional veterinary campaigns, so that farmers do not misinterpret the aims of and need for the campaign simply because extensionists do not know the right words to use. Such surveys need not be time-consuming, and they are readily amenable to computerized organization and analysis as per the methods described in this report. Further, they can reveal previously unsuspected or underestimated animal health problems, especially in regions where veterinary research is lacking.

Delehanty, James M. 1996. Methods and results from a study of local knowledge of cattle diseases in coastal Kenya. In: Constance M. McCorkle, Evelyn Mathias and Tjaart W. Schillhorn van Veen (eds). *Ethnoveterinary Research & Development.* Intermediate Technology Publications, London, UK. Pp. 229–245.

This chapter presents the methodology and illustrative results of a 1989 study of the technical and contextual knowledge of bovine diseases among cattle-owning farmers of Kaloleni Division, Kilifi District, Kenya. Research centred on three broad questions: can information on livestock diseases be gathered from stock-raisers quickly and systematically, and be analysed in such a way as to provide rigorous scientific support, rather than mere anecdote, to veterinary epidemiologists and others concerned with regional animal health? Can such information be used in lieu of expensive laboratory diagnostic surveys and other measures to determine variable disease risk? And, how can EVK findings best be presented in order to be useful for extensionists? The 158 subjects of the study were mostly Mijikenda farmers, a majority of whom had only recently taken up cattle raising. They were systematically interviewed as to: how well they recognized the clinical signs of a range of livestock maladies, how they encoded these signs as 'diseases', and what patterns of disease occurrence they identified; their ethno-aetiologies and knowledge and use of traditional preventive and curative treatments. As interviews were conducted in KiSwahili and six dialects of KiMijikenda, both of which have borrowed disease terms from English, translating local aetiologies and disease names into Western disease categories required devising a three-tiered analysis of its own. The author assigned a convenient English gloss as an overarching ethno-scientific category of disease – for example, 'tick disease' – under which he identified terminological classes of synonyms by language, with further dialectal variations grouped under each language. Ultimately, with computerized assistance, it was possible to locate the total of 144 discrete disease names elicited in three broad disease clusters: theileriosis, helminthosis and diarrhoea. The further analysis of the theileriosis cluster is presented here by the three major ethnoscientific categories identified: *ngai*, considered a disease of calves; 'tick disease', which was said to attack adult as well as young cattle; and 'East Coast Fever' (ECF), a term that embraced tick-borne disease in all cattle ages plus other maladies and that was used by farmers with greater extension contacts and membership in a formal dairy association. It was possible to link these terms to various agroclimatic and other factors. Multiple lessons were learned from this research. One is that a more quantitative approach, beginning with computerized data entry, can ease the organization and analysis of inherently untidy ethnoveterinary information, while ensuring accurate replication of local descriptive nuances in the database, facilitating production of a lexicon that correctly reflects local classificatory knowledge, and speeding the more refined analysis of related terms. Another lesson is that the first step in any disease control campaign should be to bridge the various cognates in a disease cluster by pointing out to farmers their aetiological, and thus treatment, inter-relatedness. Another is that it is more practical for veterinary workers to adjust to stockraisers' own disease vocabulary than to superpose common or scientific English names because the latter only add to terminological confusion when it comes to communication between the two groups. Further, the author tentatively concludes that, with further testing, the methodology described here might be used in lieu of laboratory diagnostic surveys, assuming some modifications and refinements to the methodology, such as: truly random and larger sampling; careful collection of baseline as well as lexical and ethnodiagnostic/clinical data from informants; and targeted clinical observations or laboratory diagnostics to confirm presumed associations between ethnoscientific and scientific disease categories. The chapter concludes with four general principles for veterinary epidemiologists and especially extensionists. First, any campaign to control a given disease should be identified to the general public as aimed at the entire range of locally named ailments likely to correspond to that disease. Second, labels in every relevant language should be used. Third, where there is doubt whether a local term X corresponds, or sometimes corresponds, to the scientifically defined disease, explain to the public that the latter could be X. Fourth, a campaign should elucidate the clinical signs of the disease in question, since some stockraisers lack precise ethnoscientific definitions beyond the most obvious clinical signs.

Delgado Ortega, Crescencio. 1989. Plantas medicinales utilizadas en el estado de Nayarit por ejidatarios compesinos [sic] para curar sus animales. In: Gerardo López Buendía (ed.). *Memorias: Segunda Jornada sobre Herbolaria Medicinal en Medicina Veterinaria.* Universidad Nacional Autónoma de México, Facultad de Medicina Veterinaria y Zootecnia, Coordinación de Educación Continua, México DF, México. Pp. 49–65.

Whether on the coast or in the sierras of Mexico's Nayarit State, few formal veterinary services are available to smallholder stockraisers. In any case – asks the author – why turn to drugs offered by commercial pharmaceutical houses, which only sell back at 'stratospheric prices' the botanical and other resources that they took from ancient native peoples and Nature in the first place. Moreover, such products often have noxious side effects. Although many advances of modern medicine must be applauded, chemical-pharmaceutical labs have turned much of medicine into the patented exploitation of poor and middle-class people. Particularly where such labs are foreign ones, an alternative is '. . . ourselves to become the producers of our own medicaments, adequate to our health needs, our own resources and technology . . . and not necessarily following the shopworn procedures that rich societies impose upon the rest [of us]' (p. 50). To this end, the author reports on 16 plants used by Nayarit stockraisers to treat their sheep, goats, pigs, cattle, burros, horses, household and hunting dogs and fighting cocks: *Argemone mexicana, Aristolochia odoratissima, Barkleyanthus salicifolius, Bocconia arbórea, Brosimum alicastrum, Commelina pallida, Coutarea latiflora, Crescentia alata, Euphorbia prostrata, Guázama tomentosa, Lophophora williamsii, Matricaria chamomilla, Ruta graveolens*, and [no Latin names given] 'avilla', 'corteza de Nanchi', 'cuate', 'hierba del alacran', garlic, lemons/limes and coconuts. Detailed for each plant are: its geographic distribution both within and outside Mexico; its active principles; the parts utilized; and its mode of preparation and administration for which ills in which species. Sometimes combined with other ingredients like honey or alcohol, the plant materials are prepared as drenches, rubs, plasters, washes, and in one case, an injection (given around the edges of warts to remove them). These medicaments serve as, e.g., sedatives, vermifuges, purgatives, emmenagogues, antispasmodics, tonics, analgesics, styptics, disinfectants, abortifacients, galactagogues and much more. A sampling of the livestock ills treated includes colics, anaemia, respiratory ailments, bites and stings, eye disorders, tendon and muscular problems, burns and bullet and other wounds.

deMaar, Thomas W. n.d. The animal doctor – the other ones. Unpublished paper.

'For thousands of years, a multitude of societies have pondered, experimented and succeeded with an impressive array of medicinal plants, therapeutic techniques and special practices designed to protect their animals' (p. 1). Beginning with his observation of EVM as a youth in Switzerland, the author reflects on the fact that, even though veterinarians like himself have personally witnessed the success of seemingly strange-looking brown medicines in old wine bottles wielded by traditional stockraisers, vets have relegated such experiences 'to the old trunk of fun stories to tell in the evenings' (ibid.). Seduced by commercial marketing and advertisements, vets ignore what their own eyes tell them, and continue to reach for a handy pill or syringe. This paper argues for greater attention to early and alternative veterinary medicine and briefly reviews and illustrates the following options: acupuncture, herbalism, homeopathy, holistic medicine/naturopathy, traditional vaccinations and rituals. [For greater detail, see deMaar 1992.] In a discussion of science versus tradition, the author notes that allopathic medicine is very effective and that doubtless many traditional livestock remedies are not. That said, however, for developing countries allopathic veterinary medicine poses many problems. It requires adequate foreign currency, whether to purchase the machinery and raw materials to manufacture 'high-tech' drugs in-country or to import them; and if they are imported, political stability, open borders, honest custom agents are necessary. Likewise for the physical and human infrastructure to distribute and administer the drugs, including expensive professional training programmes for veterinarians. After all that, if for any reason the supply of imported drugs is interrupted, stockraisers can suffer a disaster. These problems argue for a closer look at the relative efficacy and economics of alternative medicine. For example, researchers at Gujarat Agricultural University in India have proven a herbal antiseptic and an antifungal ointment dubbed Melicon-V to be of equal efficacy to nitrofurazone but at only 50% to 70% of the cost. This is the challenge: to determine which of the multitude of traditional medicaments and practices are actually beneficial. To do so, steps must be taken to preserve not only the *materia medica* but also the knowledge of beneficial treatments. Otherwise, as happened with Sioux Indian herbals in the American Dakotas, even though the plants continue to grow along the roadside, the knowledge of their uses has been forever lost. One method of gathering and preserving EVK might be to train traditional healers to keep their own records. In sum, whether in Switzerland or Somalia, for more self-sufficient and sustainable animal production, 'The need is for any veterinary or animal husbandry project to include a component to account for and study traditional practices and treatments' (p. 6).

deMaar, Thomas W. n.d. The healing herbs. Unpublished paper.

Many cultures revere their herbal medicines as gifts from the gods. Somali tribal healers show their reverence by never allowing their shadows to fall upon the medicinal plants they tend and harvest. Because of botanicals' great and semi-sacred value, many societies impose restrictions and taboos on their harvesting and use in order to ensure a continued supply. The potentials hidden in traditional knowledge of plant and other medicines is immense. To take one proven example, in 1991 researchers in Malaysia announced that a certain herbal preparation known as *prajana* successfully induces oestrus in cattle in 73% of cases. Herbal remedies given to pregnant animals in Cameroon have been found to be exceptionally high in calories, thus furnishing the extra energy vital for healthy pregnancies and births. Somali camel herders feed their animals a mixture of certain plants and crumbled rocks to provide their camels with key minerals. The author urges increased research attention to such EVM along two fronts: technology and local knowledge, the latter with careful attention to every detail of local collection, preparation and use of medicinal plants. In fact, interest in botanicals is already growing, via, e.g.: communication centres like NAPRALERT, a computer databank at the University of Illinois-Chicago that is affiliated with WHO; international pharmaceutical houses like Boehringer and Sanofi, both of which recently acquired companies specializing in herbal remedies; and increasing numbers of conferences on herbal treatments. The benefits of greater attention to traditional pharmacotherapies may take various forms: the development of new drugs for humankind (and their livestock) as a whole; and cost-savings on expensive imported veterinary medicines for cash-strapped farmers. Indeed, the author foresees a day when 'importation of essential medicines could become as simple as providing packets of seeds and instructions in their use' (p. 2).

deMaar, Thomas W. 1992. Ask what's in those bottles. *Ceres: The FAO Review* 24(4): 40–45.

'There are hundreds of documented accounts of animals cured by traditional practitioners in many . . . corners of the world' (p. 136). This article in the official magazine of FAO presents a lively selection of the extensive veterinary pharmacopoeia and techniques of such practitioners worldwide. Allopathic medicines can be replaced or complemented with acupuncture, homeopathy, naturopathy and holistic medicine. For example, holistic approaches to animal healthcare [which are the norm in most non-Western societies] look beyond the moment of biomedical treatment to also ensuring that, afterwards, the patient is encouraged to drink plenty of water, is tempted with tasty feeds, sheltered from the elements, and provided with companionship and other stimuli to make it 'want to thrive again' (p. 42). Physical therapy such as massage, exercise and bone manipulation furnish further alternatives or complements to Western pharmacotherapy. For instance, for abdominal inflation in animals, *Dhami* healers of Nepal prescribe massage and forced exercise while old British farmers give their affected cattle 'a ruddy good gallop round the paddock' (ibid.). Nor should traditional vaccinations be forgotten. European farmers of not long ago invented an effective wart vaccine consisting of inoculating young animals with homogenized warts from older animals [which practice provided the basis for modern wart vaccines]. Many stockraising peoples know that mixing young animals in with sick ones can sometimes immunize the young, although people acknowledge that such exposure is a 'hit or miss' proposition. Traditional management practices can also be important in preventing or controlling animal disease. For instance, Maasai of Kenya know to keep their cattle away from wildebeest, which are carriers of malignant catarrhal fever. Of course, every society of the world has employed plants in animal healthcare. To take a few examples, Ugandans tie bouquets of amaranthus, comfrey and other plants in their poultry houses for chickens to peck at; these greens are rich in vitamin A, which is lacking in the birds' other feeds and which produces eggs with bright yellow yolks. To repel flies, wise old Ugandan farmers burn marigold around livestock pens. For cattle bloat, Mexicans tie a branch of bitter *Polakowskia tacacco* in the animal's mouth to induce salivation; saliva buffers the stomach, while the oral insert encourages chewing, which promotes the release of stomach gas. Finally, rituals, chants, prayers, dances, symbols painted on the patient's body, and so forth, are a common feature of traditional treatments. Some rituals form part of a complex diagnostic procedure as is the case in traditional Chinese medicine. Others help practitioners to remember volumes of complex remedies, as in India's Ayurvedic medicine. And given that animals, as well as humans, can suffer psychosomatic ills (examples are mysterious diarrhoeas in horses and excessive thirst in dogs), it is conceivable that certain ritual acts may help assuage such conditions. Beyond these functions, rituals may serve other useful purposes such as revealing practical animal healthcare and husbandry acumen, facilitating diplomatic interchange between practitioners, and acting as a basis for the introduction or explanation of new, scientific medical techniques to people. Whether for such seemingly extra-medical interventions or for more biomedically-oriented traditional practices, 'the mere fact of [their] survival over hundreds of years should be a strong indication that these methods were tested enough times to be significant' and that it is thus unwise 'to simply ignore every treatment that has not been developed in the laboratory' (p. 40). At the same time, however, the author cautions that 'Many so-called folk cures may be no better than "quack" methods, while others, for example acupuncture applied by the unskilled, may even be dangerous' (ibid.). He recommends keeping an open mind and judiciously mixing or choosing between EVM and modern veterinary medicine. In China, for instance, people first treat lack of cycling in sows with acupuncture combined with management changes that provide more exercise and increased social contact with the boar and other anoestrous sows. These traditional methods cure as much as 80% of the sows. High-priced Western hormonal therapies are then used only on the remaining 20%. Even where traditional cures are not 100% effective, they may be more appropriate than costly commercial drugs. In illustration, analysis of antiparasitic herbs used in Nigeria indicates they may achieve a kill rate of anywhere from 58% to 92%; but the benefits of using a purchased drug with 90% to 100% effectiveness must be balanced against the drug's additional cost, given that low-grade parasitic burdens are usually not a serious problem in developing country livestock systems and thus may not warrant the extra expense.

deMaar, Thomas W. 1993. Zoopharmacognosy: A science emerges from Navajo legends. *CERES: The FAO Review* 143(Sep/Oct): 5–8.

As part of their ethnomedical knowledge for both humans and livestock, native peoples like the Navajo may take note of the self-medicating behaviours of wild and/or domesticated animals. Scientists have embarked only fairly recently on systematic zoopharmacognosy research. But peoples who depend on animals for their livelihoods noticed animal self-medication early on. For example, European gypsies have long maintained that it is important to allow their domestic animals to roam free so that the creatures can choose their own plants for medicinal, as well as nutritional, properties.

DENR/IIRR/FF. 1990. *Agroforestry Technology Information Kit.* International Institute of Rural Reconstruction, Silang, Cavite, Philippines.

This information kit is a predecessor of IIRR/DENR/FF 1992. Its section on livestock production includes information on plant-based livestock medication, documenting a survey of 43 plants used by Filipino farmers in their livestock healthcare. Coconut has many applications: the water of unripe coconuts serves as an oral rehydration therapy for feverish or anorexic animals. A drench of coconut oil or milk is used as a dewormer or to alleviate bloat or constipation. The husk and shell are carbonized, pulverized, and administered orally to halt diarrhoea. Finally, coconut oil cooked with ginger is spread on open wounds. [See related paper by Dayrit 1990.]

Deore, P.A. 1998. Use of herbal preparations in clinical and sub-clinical mastitis. In: E. Mathias, D.V. Rangnekar and C.M. McCorkle, with M. Martin (eds). *Ethnoveterinary Medicine: Alternatives for Livestock Development – Proceedings of an International Conference Held in Pune, India, 4–6 November 1997. Volume 2: Abstracts.* BAIF Development Research Foundation, Pune, India. P. 15.

Mastitis is an udder inflammation that, in its subclinical form, causes greater milk production losses than clinical cases. Routinely, clinical and subclinical mastitis is treated with antimicrobials both intramammarily and parenterally. However, the use of antimicrobials over long periods has triggered chemoresistance accompanied by even greater doses of antimicrobials and thus increased drug residues in milk and increased biohazards to consumer health. Four veterinarians tested the oral herbal preparation Titali-M (Mycon Pharma, Pune) in subclinical and clinical cases of mastitis in 56 dairy cattle and buffalo under field conditions. After Titali-M treatment, both the quantity and quality of milk improved; and swelling of the udder was reduced considerably within three days. Titali-M has anti-inflammatory and microbicidal properties.

Deore, P.A. 1999. Different approaches for alternate systems of animal healthcare. Paper presented to the International Seminar on Integrated Approach for Animal Health Care, 4th–6th February 1999, Calicut, Kerala, India.

This paper gives details of 26 different types of alternative treatments for animals. They include homeopathy, acupuncture, acupressure, iridology, osteopathy, Shiatsu massage and reflexology among others.

Desai, P.U. 1998. Effect of *Annona squamosa* seed preparations on house flies. In: E. Mathias, D.V. Rangnekar and C.M. McCorkle, with M. Martin (eds). *Ethnoveterinary Medicine: Alternatives for Livestock Development – Proceedings of an International Conference Held in Pune, India, 4–6 November 1997. Volume 2: Abstracts.* BAIF Development Research Foundation, Pune, India. P. 15.

House flies and other ectoparasites can transmit diseases. *Annona squamosa* or 'custard apple' is a tropical tree that reportedly helps heal wounds and keep off lice. This study tested the effects of various *A. squamosa* seed preparations on housefly eggs, larvae and adults, using Zurich, Chinese and WHO strains of flies according to standard breeding and maintenance methods. The seeds were applied in powdered concentrations of 10%, 15% and 20%; aqueous or acetone solutions, and in boiled and unboiled preparations in edible oil. The powdered form had a marked effect on larvae and eggs. In particular, it remarkably reduced egg-hatching percentages; and this effect increased with increasing concentration of the powder. Concentrations of the powder above 10% showed variable larvicidal activity, which is pertinent to the treatment of myiasis. The aqueous solutions had some effect on egg hatching, but the acetone preparations were superior. Adult flies also seemed susceptible to the acetone preparations. The contact treatment on adult flies showed variable effects on all three strains of flies. In sum, custard-apple powder is reasonably useful in fly control and thus on the diseases these insects can transmit.

Devi, Gayatri and C.S. Sisodia. 1969. Effect of ether extract of *Juniper communis* [sic] on sarcoptic mange in sheep. *Indian Journal of Animal Sciences* 39(4): 345–348.

In India, a clinical trial on *Juniperus communis'* efficacy against sarcoptic mange applied an ether extract of the plant and linseed oil daily to lesions in a treatment group of 20 sheep. A control group was treated daily with a commercial antiscabies drug. At the end of a month, all traces of mange had disappeared in both groups. The trial's write-up doesn't differentiate between the active ingredients in the juniper and the linseed.

DeVries, James. 1990. Passing on the gift of know-how in Cameroon. *Sharing Life* Summer: 1,8.

The author briefly describes his visit with an elderly Fulani livestock healer who is participating in an HPI livestock development project in Cameroon. There, HPI has organized an Ethnoveterinary Council of 14 such knowledgeable men. They meet to share their professional secrets with each other, with younger Fulani herders, and even with farmers of other ethnicities. Moreover, in a revolutionary step, these healers have agreed to have their medicines and treatments recorded, most for the first time, so as to preserve their knowledge for the future.

Dewasi, Dewa Ram. 1992. Prevailing animal health care services to Raika camelherders [sic] in Pali District, Rajasthan (India). In: John Young (ed.). *A Report on a Village Animal Health Care Workshop – Volume II: The Case Studies.* ITDG, Rugby, UK. Pp. 55–57.

This brief workshop contribution notes a Raika method for diagnosing camel trypanosomosis. Herders make a ball from sand on which the suspect animal has just urinated; if the sample gives off a sweet and pungent odour 2 to 4 hours later, the diagnosis is positive. However, Raika have no traditional methods for treating this disease. This is not the case for the other major camel disease, mange. This they cure with a variety of home remedies, usually containing petroleum products. Specialized healers also administer firing for mange.

Dietvorst, D.C.E. 1996. Farmers' attitudes towards the control and prevention of anthrax in Western Province, Zambia. In: Karl-Hans Zessin (ed.). *Livestock Production and Diseases in the Tropics: Livestock Production and Human Welfare. Proceedings of the VIII International Conference of Institutions of Tropical Veterinary Medicine held from the 25 to 29 September, 1995 in Berlin, Germany.* Volume I. Deutsche Stiftung für Internationale Entwicklung, Zentralstelle für Ernährung und Landwirtschaft, Feldafing, Germany. Pp. 330–335.

Since 1990, anthrax has broken out in Zambia's Western Province every year, despite annual vaccination campaigns. Interviews to learn about farmers' attitudes toward this disease were conducted in 25 veterinary camps with over 200 farmers, 80 of whom were women, and with veterinary and agricultural field staff. Findings revealed that farmers' EVK (or lack thereof), their husbandry and herding strategies, and household consumption practices are all implicated in this continuing problem. Farmers encountering anthrax for the first time naturally had little knowledge of it. Moreover, they blamed vaccination campaigns for carrying the disease from corral to corral. Not unreasonably, they thought this was the mode of transmission because already-infected cattle that were sometimes vaccinated in the middle of an outbreak died practically upon being vaccinated. However, these farmers said they soon realized such animals would have died anyway, and later came to accept vaccination of their animals. Other farmers agreed to vaccinations for all but their work oxen, which they had been told to let rest for 2 weeks after treatment; but because rest was not an option during the ploughing season, people refused vaccination for oxen if it came at this time of year. In performing their ploughing or transport duties, however, oxen move frequently from camp to camp, sometimes transmitting anthrax. An even more widespread transmission mechanism is the requirement that hired herders present the skin and also sometimes the head of any animal that has died under their care to its owner in proof of herder honesty. This means that cattle dead from anthrax are dragged back to the village for skinning and butchering, or at the very least, their meat and hides are carried to the owner's homestead. Thus, the soil is contaminated across long distances and the anthrax spores are distributed in or near human settlements. Moreover, virtually everyone eats the meat of such animals, including people who know they should not. Since cattle deaths from anthrax are so swift, animals often die in good condition; thus people risk eating them because they simply cannot afford to forego such a valuable amount of food. But farmers' knowledge of anthrax overall and of its transmission to humans, as well as between animals, was generally very limited. They normally recognized only the swollen spleen as being infective for humans, and could identify few other post-mortem signs.

Diiriye, Mohamed Farah. 1984. Camel trypanosomiasis in Somalia. In: Mohamed Ali Hussein (ed.). ***Camel Pastoralism in Somalia: Proceedings from a Workshop Held in Baydhabo, April 8–13, 1984.*** Camel Forum Working Paper No. 7. Somali Camel Research Project, Mogadishu, Somalia, and Stockholm, Sweden. Pp. 83–90.

This paper lists various local names for camel trypanosomosis in Africa and Arabia and notes that some peoples make a conceptual and semantic distinction between chronic and acute forms of this disease. Stockowners link the former with tsetse flies and the latter with diptera species other than tsetse. Among Somali camel owners, trypanosomosis is known as *surra*. They recognize several specific signs and symptoms, including a distinctive unpleasant smell and affected animals' habit of facing into the sun in the afternoon. Camel owners' use of various Western drugs to combat trypanosomosis is noted. Sometimes overdosing leads to night blindness. The drugs also have undesirable side effects and, according to the herders, can cause an animal's neck to break.

Dinçer, F. 1988. Some notes on the treatment of human and animal diseases in the folklore of Turkey and the Balkan countries. ***Deutsche Tierärztliche Wochenschrift*** 95: 419–420.

This brief historical review of Turkish and Balkan human and animal ethnomedicine discusses the recurring plagues of rinderpest from at least the 16th century to 1932, when the disease was finally eradicated from the area. As there were no effective tangible treatments, stockraisers turned to religion for help. In the Christian era, holy water was poured over the affected animals. This technique was also adopted by Moslems, who read Koranic verses over water to purify it before sprinkling it over the animals. During the Middle Ages, as a general healthcare measure, people and herd animals drank oil from church lamps. Turkish healers (*ocak*) of both humans and animals cured digestive disorders by striking the patient's abdomen with prayer sticks; they treated blackleg by poking hot sticks at the patient. *Ocak* also specialized in giving vaccinations by smearing patients' skin with infective material. Still today, Yörüks who migrated from central Asia make a vaccine against sheep pox from the vesicle fluids of diseased animals. Similarly, they vaccinate goats against enterotoxaemia, piroplasmosis and pneumonia by smearing the skin of healthy animals with a suspension of diseased animals' blood and internal organs.

Djarwaningsih, Tutie and Tahan Uji. 1992. Pemanfaatan jamu untuk penyakit ternak di tiga desa propinsi Jawa Timur. *Prosiding Seminar dan Lokakarya Nasional Etnobotani, Bogor, Indonesia, 19–20 February 1992.* Departemen Pendidikan dan Kebudayaan, Departemen Pertanian dan LIPI, Bogor, Indonesia. Pp. 90–96.

This paper reports the results of an unspecified number of interviews on the use of traditional medicines in three villages of East Java. Farmers there keep cattle, horses and goats but hardly any buffalo because the villages lie at 700 m or more above sea level. Farmers use at least 44 plant species to treat and prevent diseases in their livestock. The paper discusses similarities and differences among the three villages. The appendices list the Latin and Indonesian names of all these plants and describe 34 local remedies for cattle, 17 for horses, and four for goats. For cattle, the prescriptions cover bloat, diarrhoea, worms, constipation, poisoning, eye diseases and reduced appetite. Remedies are presented for worms, constipation, diarrhoea, fever, poisoning, skin diseases, eye problems and flu in horses. For goats, prescriptions are given for diarrhoea, poisoning, skin diseases and reduced appetite. The paper also details several mixtures for keeping cattle and horses healthy and in good body condition.

Dobie, J. Frank. 1950. Indian horses and horsemanship. *Southwest Review* 35(Fall): 265–275.

This article describes the relationship between American Indians and their horses. In the process, it occasionally mentions ethnoveterinary practices. For example, to make a horse long-winded, its nostrils are slit (p. 268). Tender-footed horses are treated by applying the smoke and heat of burning wild rosemary so as to harden their feet (p. 269). Smudge fires are set to protect the animals from insects (p. 271).

Doepmann, Felix R. 1996. Zur Quellenproblematik der traditionellen Tierheilkunde bei den Peul-Nomaden (Westafrika). In: Johann Schäffer (ed.). *Aktuelle fachhistorische Forschung Beruf und Geschichte: Bericht der Tagung am 27. und 28. Oktober 1995 in Hannover.* Deutsche Veterinärmedizinische Gesellschaft e.v., Fachgruppe 'Geschichte der Veterinärmedizin', Giessen, Germany. Pp. 22–33.

This chapter critically analyses written sources on the history and development of traditional animal healthcare among Peul nomads of West Africa. Botanical, geographical and anthropological rather than veterinary documents comprise the majority of such sources, although the earliest ones consist mainly of travel reports and writings by colonial officers. Especially after World War II, field-based ethnographies and botanical studies proliferated. During the 1970s and 1980s, several synthesizing compilations on traditional African medicine were published. More recent are interdisciplinary studies about local beliefs concerning disease, diagnosis and healing with regard to blending Western and traditional veterinary medicine. The author points out that nearly all sources are by Europeans, and thus the documents reflect their writers' background and the prevailing views or Zeitgeist of their era. He warns that the content of all such documents must therefore be judged critically. This is particularly true for the earliest, 'primary' sources, which are so frequently cited and re-cited.

Doepmann, Felix R. 1997. *Traditionelle Tierheilkunde in der Sudanzone: Studien zur Aporetik mündlich tradierter Medizinsysteme.* Doctoral dissertation. Fachgebiet Geschichte der Veterinärmedizin und der Haustiere, Tierzärztliche Hochschule Hannover, Germany. 132 pp.

In a critical review of the literature, this dissertation discusses the historical development, medical systems, disease causes and classification, healers, technology (including pharmacology, toxicology, vaccination, surgery and reproduction), husbandry methods and magico-religious practices in traditional veterinary medicine in Africa's Sudanian zone. It also notes that Western concepts of animal welfare cannot be applied to other cultures, because the human–animal relationship varies greatly across cultures. The author concludes that future scientific approaches to African veterinary medicine must be closely interrelated with the respective cultural system and must take account of historical, anthropological and linguistic, as well as biomedical and husbandry, elements.

Doepmann, Felix R. 1998. Tales from the outposts? The 'ontology' of written sources on traditional veterinary medicine in Africa. In: E. Mathias, D.V. Rangnekar and C.M. McCorkle, with M. Martin (eds). *Ethnoveterinary Medicine: Alternatives for Livestock Development – Proceedings of an International Conference Held in Pune, India, 4–6 November 1997. Volume 2: Abstracts.* BAIF Development Research Foundation, Pune, India. P. 16.

Literature on traditional veterinary medicine in Africa was reviewed critically, mostly for therapies. Studying written texts gives insight into how authors interpret these sources. Examples from the works of anthropologists, linguists and veterinarians show that they may differentially interpret the ethnoveterinary treatments described. This review reveals that there is no one traditional veterinary medicine; rather, every culture has its own specific healing system. Thus, techniques for diagnosis, prevention, therapy and rating of medical outcomes differ across systems. This point is illustrated for time reckoning, disease classification and livestock values among different cultures. Examples from WoDaaße, Twareg and Nuer traditional veterinary medicine include rectal examination, haematoscopy and macroscopic examination of faeces and urine. For instance, some stockraising peoples aptly note that the blood of animals with anthrax does not clot.

Domingo, Ines Vivian. 1998. Medicinal plants for animal healthcare. *Footsteps* 34: 6–9.

This short article briefly describes simple, on-farm techniques and measures for preparing homemade poultices, decoctions, powders, etc. and for drenching ruminants, pigs and chickens. It then presents 17 plant-based prescriptions commonly used in EVM throughout the tropics. Ailments span anaemia, bloat, diarrhoea, ecto- and endoparasitoses, wounds and myiasis, poisoning, dehydration, and cough, colds and fevers. The 17 plants include many food (e.g. banana, bitter gourd, coconut, garlic, guava, tamarind, turmeric) and other product species (e.g. betel nut, camphor) as well as wild plants.

Donald, A.D. 1994. Parasites, animal production, and sustainable development. *Veterinary Parasitology* 54: 27–47.

Ecologically sustainable development aims at reducing environmental degradation while enabling economic development. This article suggests several approaches for achieving this goal in livestock production. Cattle can be bred for trypanotolerance, as in the N'Dama and the Shorthorn breeds of West and Central Africa. Biological control of parasites can replace chemical insecticides. For example, dung beetles have been imported to Australia, where they destroy faecal deposits and, with them, the larvae of nematodes that parasitize cattle. It should also be possible to exploit the nematophageous fungi that occur naturally in faeces in order to reduce the maturation of nematode eggs into infective larvae on pasturelands. Aspects of traditional animal health and husbandry systems have long operated on similar such principles [abstractor's note].

Dorantes, José Antonio and Carlos Peraza. 1988. El valor de uso de las plantas medicinales en el ganado caprino. In: Luz Lozano Nathal and Gerardo López Buendía (coordinators). *Memorias: Primera Jornada sobre Herbolaria Medicinal en Veterinaria.* Universidad Nacional Autónoma de México, Facultad de Medicina Veterinaria y Zootecnia, Coordinación de Educación Continua, México DF. Pp. 130–133.

This article appears to be mistitled, since no mention is made of goats. Instead, the authors briefly discuss three themes: colonial and capitalist impacts that have led to a deprecation of non-Western medical traditions; the cultural and regional specificity of the use of veterinary medicinal plants; and methodological and social-philosophical directions for the study and use of folk pharmacopoeia.

Downs, James F. 1964. *Animal Husbandry in Navajo Society and Culture.* Vol. I. University of California Publications in Anthropology. University of California Press, Berkeley, California, USA.

Navajo Indians pay little or no medical attention to their dogs (p. 29). But they do try to prevent their sheep from breeding before mid-October, so that lambs are born in late spring when forage is abundant and temperatures are mild. To control mating, Navajo shepherds tie aprons over their rams' genitals (p. 35). Horses with sprains and bruises on the feet and legs and other disabling disorders are rested. Most Navajo men know how to treat a dislocated shoulder and how to remove lampers in the roof of a horse's mouth. Both these operations were reported by

Franciscans in 1910. More severe injuries in horses are treated with methods similar to those used for humans by curers with supernaturally sanctioned powers. These curers belong to the horse medicine cult (pp. 55–56).

Drury, Susan. 1985. Herbal remedies for livestock in seventeenth and eighteenth century England: Some examples. *Folklore* 96(2): 243–247.

This article is a rich source of information on traditional veterinary practices in rural England of the 1600s and 1700s for horses, cattle, sheep, pigs and poultry. The remedies blend phytotherapy (over 30 plant species are cited), other *materia medica*, and magic with complicated conditions stipulated by local wisemen or 'cow doctors'. For eye infections in cattle and horses, powdered ivy (*Nepeta glechoma*) mixed with ale and honey and then strained was recommended. Farcy (cutaneous glanders) in horses was cured by first drenching the patient with ale and rue (*Ruta graveolens*) and then placing a little aquavitae and rue juice into the horse's ears, secured with wool. Several treatments were based on the common notion worldwide of transferring disease from a patient to an inanimate object. For foot problems, for instance, turf cut from where the ailing animal had trod was hung out to dry in the belief that once the turf was completely desiccated, the foot would be cured. To take another example, shrews were thought to cause limb paralysis in cattle by running over their backs; burying a live shrew in a hole in an ash tree and then touching the paralysed limb with a branch from the tree supposedly transferred the disease to the tree. Cattle plagues were warded off with amulets, fumigation with juniper, and bouquets of onions.

Dubois, D. 1984. Quelques saints vétérinaires de Picardie-Nord. *Ethno-zootechnie* 34: 77–85.

This article details the history of cults to a number of 'veterinary saints' [see also Brisebarre 1984b, Millour 1984 and Villemin 1984] in northern Picardie, France. The saints were, and in some cases still are, believed to protect and cure livestock. Today, for example, pilgrimages are made by pickup truck, and picture postcards of the saints are displayed in stables throughout parts of France, Belgium, Holland and Germany. The author describes the symbolic importance of such practices, and notes that prudent stockowners have recourse *both* to saints and to veterinarians.

Duerr, Cynthia. 1998. Survey of pack animal health care in Petén, Guatemala. In: Magdalena Escamilla Guerrero, Rosa María Parra Hernández and Angélica María Vargas (eds). *3er. Coloquio Internactional sobre Équidos de Trabajo.* División de Educación Contínua, Facultad de Medicina Veterinaria y Zootecnia, Universidad Nacional Autónoma de México, México DF, Mexico. Pp. 102–111.

In the jungles of Guatemala's Petén region, pack animals are essential to peasant survival. Based on a 1998 survey of 50 pack animal owners in the environs of one Petén town, this article reports on peasants' husbandry practices, animal healthcare problems, and access to veterinary services for their horses and mules. Findings revealed that people supplement these animals with maize when it is in season and with certain high-protein tree leaves. All but 36% of the sample bathe their equines with some regularity. Only 43% said they routinely clean and remove stones from the hooves; the remainder did so only for visibly lame animals. Respondents as a whole cited their most common pack-animal ills as follows, as per the author's interpretation of disease descriptions: strangles (22 respondents), colic (19), black-widow spider bites – possibly confused with laminitis (8), clostridial infections (8), other infections and sores (6), fistulous withers (6), foot abscesses (5), and often as a result of anthrax, accident or sudden death (5). Rarer problems included snake, tick and bat bites. There was no match whatsoever between this list and that given by local veterinarians, however. Many home remedies were described to the author, but only one is mentioned in this paper: facial neurectomy to treat fistulous withers [an operation of doubtful benefit for this problem]. Ninety percent of respondents said they had treated sick pack animals with commercial medicaments purchased from agro-supply stores, and 72% said they consulted a vet at least once in a while. In fact, however, there are exceedingly few vets in the area. Apparently, people categorized conversations with supply-store staff as consultations with veterinary personnel.

Dupire, Marguerite. 1957. Pharmacopée Peule du Niger et du Cameroun. ***Bulletin de l'I.F.A.N.*** 19(3–4): 382–417.

This article describes medico-religious charms and talismans plus botanicals and other ethnomedical practices employed by Fulani in Niger and Cameroon to protect, treat and promote fertility among themselves and their herds. Ordinary stockraisers as well as paid healer-specialists (*bokao*), holy men and certain castes (*griots*) and cults (*bori*) make and use these items and treatments, as inherited from relatives, revealed by friends, or purchased from itinerant traders and holy men. A majority of botanical prescriptions involve plant materials brought from afar, especially from parts of northern Nigeria that have been inhabited by Fulani for over 500 years. The author groups ethnomedical practices into eight categories. First are charms for human and herd prosperity, based on complex rituals utilizing sympathetic magic and performed on especially propitious days. However, many such charms and rituals also involve acts such as feeding foodstuffs and minerals. For livestock, these include items like groundnuts, fruits, certain wild leaves presumed to have special nutritional or lactogenic properties, and salt or natron. Second are cures. In livestock, scarification is used to cure congestion and heat stroke in all animals. But scarification of camels must be performed by Twareg or Bouzou specialists. Cauterization with a hot iron is a universal remedy. Natron and certain salts are given as purgatives. Examples of plant remedies for livestock are: a decoction of *Bauhinia* spp. leaves for diarrhoea; for intestinal worms, dried *agugu* fern soaked in milk (also reportedly used as an effective human vermifuge by Europeans); and bean juice to help extract maggots from wounds. The third category consists of treatments to promote fertility, labour and lactation. For example, cows that fail to lactate after parturition are fed powdered *Loranthus* or *Calotropis procera* with natron to trigger milk flow. For a cow whose calf has died, women massage the udder and smear it with a preparation of *Acacia tortilis* roots so it will not harden. Remedies against sorcery or diseases due to genies constitute the fourth category. One lengthy such prescription is described for warding off spells cast on calves' tethers in order to kill the calves. Powdered gypsum is applied to lightning burns, which are also attributed to sorcery. Sorcerers and genies are also believed to be implicated in epidemics of pasteurellosis. To combat this disease, a healer specializing in it may be called in to dance three times around the herd while uttering incantations. Alternatively, the animals may be made to sniff perfume or to ingest a decoction of *Entada sudanica* bark pounded with droppings from a wild boar and a black donkey. In addition, the campsite is permanently abandoned, along with all tack and other livestock paraphernalia like troughs. Indeed, Fulani assign supernatural causes to most diseases with central nervous system signs, such as pasteurellosis, blackquarter and coenurosis. For the latter ill in calves, a decocted drench of pepper, the odiferous *Cymbopogon giganteus* plant, and boar, elephant and civet dung is given. Additionally, the patients are fumigated in order to drive out the offending genies. In general, along with fumigation, Fulani use especially caustic, toxic, bitter, peppery, strong-smelling or allergenic plants in remedies for supernaturally-linked ills. The fifth and sixth categories consist of love potions, aphrodisiacs and puberty rites. The author does not indicate any applications of such treatments to livestock, however. Seventh is snakebite prophylaxes and cures, the latter typically involving incisions near the bite. Eighth and last are 'diverse charms' to ward against blows, wounds and livestock predators. In summary, the author makes the following observations. The Fulani pharmacopoeia is seldom divorced from magic, astral and lunar influences, days of the week, and verbal acts. Although Fulani may assign a supernatural origin to certain diseases, they also recognize other or accompanying natural causes linked to foods, feeds, water, and insects. And 'Many magical recipes are associated with empirical precautions' while 'rare are . . . empirical and natural techniques that are not surrounded by magical prescriptions' (p. 414). Further, Fulani are quick to adopt medical practices and preparations from outside sources; they are equally quick to reject prescriptions that prove ineffective or healers that prove incompetent. On the other hand, there are Fulani 'bush veterinarians' who can make expert diagnoses of, e.g., respiratory ills merely by tapping an animal's ribs or smelling its breath. The article concludes with a discussion of the interplay between medical magic and science in terms of Fulani shifts from nomadism to sedentarization and from animism to Islam.

Dupire, Marguerite. 1962a. Des nomades et leur bétail. *L'Homme* 2(1): 22–39.

Based on the author's field research in 1951–1952 among Bororo (WoDaaße) Fulani pastoralists in Niger, this article focuses on the centrality of these people's red, long-horned and semi-savage zebu cattle as 'the bone around which the meat' of Fulani life is organized. EVK observations of interest include the following. Stud bulls are selected at 3 to 4 years of age according to whether they have long lyre-shaped horns, a large and strong body, a dark coat, and above all a dam of exceptional milk-producing prowess. Bulls of the *bororoji* breed are generally preferred. To avoid fighting and accidents within the herd, Bororo keep few bulls – sometimes only one per fraternal herd. People without a suitable stud can borrow one *gratis* from a relative for several months. For a fee in millet or milk, they can also rent the services of a desirable bull from another pastoralist who specializes in breeding. In this way, the dangers of herd inbreeding can be diminished. *Azawak* cows are preferred to *bororoji* as they are longer-lived and higher-producing. Thus the ideal mating is between a *bororoji* bull and an *azawak* heifer. A Bororo family may also keep one *azawak* steer as a pack animal, due to this breed's greater strength. These steers are usually purchased from another ethnic group, the Bouzou, who raise and train them. Every animal in the herd has its own name, usually based on phenotypic characteristics but often reflecting its ancestry. Consequently, sometimes a white animal may be named 'red' if its forebears were red. When an animal is sold, the new owner never changes its name. Thus any 10-year-old child can easily identify all the animals in his/her own and nearby families' herds, along with much of their pedigree. The names act in part as a sort of universal stock record. Rightly or wrongly, Bororo assign various genetic (e.g. fecundity) and magical (e.g. good or bad luck) qualities to different phenotypic features of their cattle. The author discusses these at length and provides a summary table. The remainder of the article is largely devoted to a discussion of the complex matrix of often competing cattle use and inheritance rights, obligations, and sentiments within and across household members such as husbands, senior and junior wives, sons and daughters. Among other things, these considerations sometimes make it difficult to decide upon what animal to sell when the need arises.

Dupire, Marguerite. 1962b. *Peuls Nomades: Étude Descriptive des WoDaaße du Sahel Nigérien.* Institut d'Ethnologie, Musée de l'Homme, Paris, France. 336 pp.

An entire section (pp. 99–108) of this ethnography is devoted to disease classifications, ethnoaetiologies and veterinary practices, both empirical and magical, among the Bororo WoDaaße of Niger. These pastoralists accurately diagnose rinderpest, which they name by its principal symptom (diarrhoea) and endeavour to halt through quarantine measures. The aetiology of pasteurellosis, the most devastating disease at the time of writing, was generally unknown to the WoDaaße. Often ascribing it to genies, stockowners sought to combat it with a powerful oath, as well as quarantine, branding and recourse to shamans. Anthrax, believed to be produced by ingesting dangerous plants, is named *ladde*, 'bush'. In effect, the bush is contaminated wherever a carcass with the disease has lain. While they avoid such places, the Bororo have no effective cure for anthrax. Three-day sickness (ephemeral fever) in cattle is ascribed to bad pasturage or contaminated water rather than to tsetse vectors. It is treated by bleeding the ears, as is also CBPP. Butter, milk and urine are injected into the nostrils to cure piroplasmosis. For acute anaemia, the muzzle and mouth are bled. Other conditions recognized and treated with magic, herbal preparations, cauterization, bleeding or other remedies are coenurosis, dysentery and other intestinal troubles, wounds, fractures, loose horns, albinism and snake bite. The Bororo sometimes call upon Twareg specialists to treat their camels. The author offers several important generalizations. Bleeding is an almost universal cure. Supernatural (including both black and white magic) and natural techniques are usually combined in therapeutic and prophylactic practice. In both humans and animals, neurological and paralytic conditions are generally ascribed to magical causes. Fetishes play a major role in the promotion of herd growth and, along with word magic, in protecting livestock from predators. Most important, the author notes that the veterinary arts among these Nigerien WoDaaße are currently 'in crisis'. Many useful traditional techniques like indigenous vaccination have been lost while Western veterinary medicine has been only imperfectly extended and assimilated.

Dutton, Roderic. 1998. Jordan's Badia: Local knowledge has little relevance to livestock development. Paper presented to the Tropical Agricultural Association Seminar on Local Knowledge in Tropical Agricultural Research and Development, 26 September 1998. Durham University, Durham, UK. 2 pp.

This paper argues that local knowledge is irrelevant to R&D on sheep-raising in the Jordanian panhandle, given that traditional Bedouin pastoral systems and lifeways are being wiped out by vast political-economic changes. Indeed, the author wonders if sheep-raising in this area will be able to survive at all as a profit-making enterprise in the face of tough Israeli and Australian competition. If it does, he says, it will be thanks only to adoption of 'external' productivity-increasing veterinary, breeding and feeding techniques with which local people 'have no traditional familiarity' (p. 2). [See also Abu-Rabia 1994.]

Dwivedi, S.K. (ed.). 1998. *Techniques for Scientific Validation and Evaluation of Ethnoveterinary Practices. ICAR Summer Short Course (August 3–12, 1998).* Division of Medicine, Indian Veterinary Research Institute, Izatnagar 234122, Uttar Pradesh, India. 119 pp.

The 26 lectures presented at the above-referenced course are compiled in this volume. The lectures can be roughly grouped as follows. Seven discuss general aspects of EVM, review its history and status in India, or give examples of EVM found in ancient Indian texts. Three focus on ethnobotany and the documentation or selection of ethnoveterinary practices. Six present laboratory and clinical methods for validating the efficacy, side effects and other characteristics of medicinal plant preparations. Finally, four lectures address the place and importance of NGOs, farmers' and women's participation in ER&D and in the field application of findings.

Dwivedi, S.K. 1999. Evaluation of indigenous herbs as antitrypanosomal agents. In: E. Mathias, D.V. Rangnekar and C.M. McCorkle, with M. Martin (eds). *Ethnoveterinary Medicine: Alternatives for Livestock Development – Proceedings of an International Conference Held in Pune, India, 4–6 November 1997. Volume 1: Selected Papers.* BAIF Development Research Foundation, Pune, India. Pp. 108–114.

A scan of the Indian ethnomedical literature reveals a number of herbs claimed to be effective for managing recurrent, intermittent and malarial fevers plus spleno- and hepatomegaly. Along with anaemia and jaundice, most of the foregoing symptoms are characteristic of trypanosomosis (surra). However, neither ancient Ayurvedic literature nor publications on folk or tribal medicine in India mention this disease, even though it is economically important in camels and horses there. Nevertheless, if scientifically validated, some of the herbs that traditional healers use to treat these symptoms could prove helpful against *Trypanosoma evansi*. To this end, the following such indigenous plants were screened *in vitro* and *in vivo* against *T. evansi*: *Achyranthes aspera, Aristolochia indica, Azadirachta indica, Caesalpinia bondeculla, Calotropis procera, Cannabis indica, Cassia occidentalis, Cissampelos pareira, Cyperus rotundus, Datura alba, Eclipta prostrata, Embelia ribes, Holarrhena antidysenterica, Hydrocotyle asiatica, Moringa pterygosperma, Nyctanthes arbor-tristis, Ocimum sanctum, Parthenium hysterophorus, Pongamia glabra, Smilax china, Streblus asper, Tinospora cordifolia* and

Xanthium strumarium. The plants were prepared as fresh juices and aqueous and alcoholic extracts. At a 1:20 dilution, the fresh juices of *A. indica* stem, *P. hysterophorus* flowers, and *X. strumarium* leaves possessed 100% trypanocidal activities *in vitro*; the alcoholic and aqueous extracts of these same plant parts were also 100% effective in concentrations of 500 and 1000 mg/ml. Extracts prepared from the different parts (i.e. flower, leaf, bark, stem or root) of all other plants showed no significant antitrypanosomal activities. For the *in vivo* trials, mice were inoculated with 10^4 trypanosomes intraperitoneally and treated with preparations made from individual parts of plants. The tests showed that no plant material could clear the mice of trypanosomes. All experimental animals died within 6 to 10 days of infection. Treatments with alcoholic extracts of the seeds of *C. indica* (250 mg/kg), *N. arbor-tristis* (300 mg/kg) and *X. strumarium* (100 mg/kg) significantly prolonged the infected mice's mean survival time. *Calotropis procera* and *P. hysterophorus* were found to be highly toxic to the experimental animals. Based on these preliminary investigations, it is difficult to pinpoint a single plant that could alleviate surra in animals. Therefore, polyprescriptions of herbs possessing antipyretic, anti-inflammatory, hepatoprotective and antianaemic properties *in vivo* and antitrypanosomal activity *in vitro* should be tested in cattle, horses, camels and dogs experimentally infected with trypanosomes. In sum, the author argues that in countries where surra is rare, expensive commercial drugs that destroy 100% of the parasites may be feasible. But in poor countries where surra is enzootic, inexpensive plant-based remedies that control parasite proliferation and alleviate surra symptoms may be a more realistic option.

Dwivedi, S.K. and M.C. Sharma. 1985. Therapeutic evaluation of an indigenous drug formulation against scabies in pigs. *Indian Journal of Veterinary Medicine* 5(2): 97–100.

A clinical trial of an Ayurvedic miticidal drug was carried out in India to test this traditional prescription. This consisted of *Abrus precatorius*, *Allium cepa* (onion), *Allium sativum* (garlic), *Citrus lemonum* (lemon), *Curcuma longa* (turmeric) and camphor, all mixed into a sesame-oil base and topically applied to pigs with sarcoptic mange. Daily application of the drug for 5 consecutive days completely eliminated the infestation; moreover, after 30 days no reinfestation was evident. The onion and garlic exhibited miticidal and antiseptic effects due to their sulphur content; the lemon and camphor were effective against the pruritis associated with mange; and the turmeric reduced itching. The trial was undertaken on 11 piglets, four of which were the control group.

Dwivedi, S.K. and M.C. Sharma. 1986. Studies on a herbal preparation against scabies in indigenous pigs. *Indian Journal of Veterinary Medicine* 6(1): 51–53.

This is a revised and updated version of Dwivedi and Sharma 1985, with substantial data tables added.

Dy, Baldwin L. 1989. List of herbal prescriptions from the Philippines. Unpublished manuscript. HPI/Philippines, Manila, Philippines. 5 pp.

This paper names treatments for 14 disorders of large and small ruminants involving over 40 plants. Many of the plants are familiar ones like bamboo, coconut, guava, jackfruit, papaya and tobacco. A few examples of treatments are the following. For wounds and swellings caused by thorns, the stem juice and pounded leaves of *Tabernaemontana pandacaqui* are mixed with coconut oil and applied topically. For carabao and cattle rope burns, *Macaranga tanarius* juice from a 10 cm stem is infiltrated into the wound. For forehead wounds, a tobacco leaf or a decoction of *Solanum nigrum* is applied.

Dy, Baldwin L. 1998. Ethnoveterinary medicine and therapeutics: Defining their context and potentials. In: E. Mathias, D.V. Rangnekar and C.M. McCorkle, with M. Martin (eds). ***Ethnoveterinary Medicine: Alternatives for Livestock Development – Proceedings of an International Conference Held in Pune, India, 4–6 November 1997. Volume 2: Abstracts.*** BAIF Development Research Foundation, Pune, India. P. 17.

This paper draws veterinary scientists' attention to the importance of natural, traditional medicines in the development of new prototype drugs. It stresses the overall adequacy of the veterinary medical approach as a research strategy, illustrating with recent research findings on EVM. Indeed, the basic postulates of modern organic chemistry and other sciences can help interpret and extrapolate the ethnomedical theories that underpin the effective use of EVM. This is because, in both substance and form, the basic medical rationale behind EVM resembles most such postulates. Of course, in laboratory testing care must be taken to duplicate the precise methods and application of traditional medicines. For example, some traditional herbal remedies in Chinese and Filipino medicine that have antimicrobial properties *in vitro* may not exert this effect *in vivo* unless they are prepared in very specific ways and/or mixed with certain other ingredients. An illustration of all the foregoing statements is the common use of finely ground coconut-shell charcoal in coconut oil for deworming young animals. As per standard organic chemistry processes, the charcoal acts as an absorbent and the oil as a demulcent. When this mixture is rubbed on the dam's tongue and teats and then ingested with her milk, newly-hatched nematode larvae in the young animal are absorbed by the charcoal and held in place by the oil until evacuated in the faeces; the oil also serves as a purgative in this regard. Clinical trials bear out the traditional use of this treatment is appropriate mainly for neonates that have not received colostrum. Thus, understanding traditional medicines as they are handled and applied by practitioners can help illuminate disparate laboratory findings. In conclusion, the author notes the further need to formulate and institutionalize R&D policies and programmes for animal healthcare based on their relevance, appropriateness and cultural compatibility for stockraisers.

Dyson-Hudson, V.R. 1960. East coast fever in Karamoja. *Uganda Journal* 24: 253–259.

Karimojong agropastoralists in Uganda naturally avoid grazing their cattle where East Coast Fever is rife. But conditions favouring grass growth also favour the tick that is ECF's vector; thus herds may be tempted into areas where the grass is lush but heavily tick-infested. If one animal contracts the fever in such an area, Karamajong promptly move the whole herd to alternative pastures.

Gittens, Clarke. 1990b. Let them run wild. *Farmer's Weekly* 4 May: unpaginated. 3 pp.

This article continues from Gittens, 1990a. Farmers breeding Nguni cattle in Swaziland advocate the multi-sire herd approach. They argue that under extensive conditions this approach is the most natural and effective one. The herd is run on a survival-of-the-fittest basis; the animals are undisturbed, unvaccinated, and dipped only when required by law.

Glatzle, Albrecht. 1990. Futterresourcen im Sahel. In: Horst S.H. Seifert, Paul L.G. Vlek and H.-J. Weidelt (eds). *Tierhaltung im Sahel. Symposium 26–27. Oktober 1989.* Göttinger Beiträge zur Land-und Forstwirtschaft in den Tropen und Subtropen, Heft 51. Forschungs- und Studienzentrum der Agrar- und Forstwissenschaften der Tropen und Subtropen, Georg-August-Universität Göttingen, Germany. Pp. 153–170.

This paper reviews fodder resources of the Sahel and discusses how the fodder base is influenced by different animal production systems, and vice versa. For example, pastoralists keep mixed herds in order to optimize the use of available fodder, given that different species prefer different plants. The author concludes that measures are needed to preserve Sahelian forage and water resources and to reduce risk for pastoralists. But to achieve sustainable improvements in the resource base, external inputs would be required. These would intensify herds' exploitation of suitable areas, thereby relieving grazing pressure on marginal lands. However, adoption of external inputs would mean abandonment of a purely subsistence economy. The paper concludes with a list of possible solutions to selected problems and the corresponding constraints.

Glazier, Dana. 1982. *Herding Dynamics Study: Profile of a Wodaaße Herding Unit of the North Dakaro Region, Niger.* In-house report. Niger Range and Livestock Project, Tahoua, Niger. 138 pp.

The health of animals in one WoDaaße pastoralist herd was assessed. One finding of ethnoveterinary interest was WoDaaße give a protein supplement of millet chaff every 2 or 3 days to cows weakened by lactation. Some calves also received this supplement but mixed with goat milk to form a gruel. Weak ewes are supplemented with a mix of cotton seed and millet chaff.

Gokhale, S.B. 1998. Traditional beliefs effecting [sic] cattle breeding: An analysis of field records of cattle breeding centres. In: E. Mathias, D.V. Rangnekar and C.M. McCorkle, with M. Martin (eds). *Ethnoveterinary Medicine: Alternatives for Livestock Development – Proceedings of an International Conference Held in Pune, India, 4–6 November 1997. Volume 2: Abstracts.* BAIF Development Research Foundation, Pune, India. P. 20.

As in many parts of the world, Indian farmers strongly believe that the position of stars and the phases of the moon influence climate, crop and livestock performance. They therefore organize much of their agricultural work according to their traditional, *panchang* calendar, which is based on such astronomical phenomena. Indian farmers further believe that factors like the direction in which an animal is facing at the time of insemination can influence conception. To verify these beliefs, field data were collected for 6175 cattle at breeding centres in one district of India between 1981 and 1991. Analysis revealed an overall village-level conception rate of 47.4 ± 2.3%. Cows facing east and north showed significantly higher conception rates than those facing west and south. The effect of direction was more pronounced in local cows than in crossbreds. Conception rates were highest during full moons, and lowest during new moons. Also, cows inseminated on Wednesdays and Thursdays showed significantly higher conception rates than those inseminated on Fridays. Significantly higher and lower differences in conception rates were also found according to key *panchang* dates or periods of insemination. Further data and analysis are needed to interpret local notions of astronomical influences on livestock breeding so as to determine how or if traditional beliefs may help inform, and thus increase the effectiveness of, field programmes.

Goldschmidt, Walter. 1986. *The Sebei: A Study in Adaptation.* Holt, Reinhart and Winston, New York, New York, USA. 162 pp.

A member of the Kalenjin language group that includes such groups as the Pokot, Kipsigi and Nandi of Kenya, Sebei are today sedentarized agropastoralists who inhabit the north slope of Uganda's volcanic Mount Elgon and the plains at the mountain's foot. They raise cattle, sheep, goats and chickens. Sebei bleed their cattle for blood for human consumption and, rightly or wrongly, as a prenatal therapy for cows. People collect salt for their livestock from the caves of Mount Elgon, or drive their herd to salt licks. Sebei keep mental stock records, as it were, in the form of 'cattle lineages' that mirror those of Sebei families' lineages; and every Sebei knows the name of every head of cattle in the household herd along with each animal's unique habits, virtues and faults. Stud bulls are selected according to their dams' calving and milking prowess. Sebei households exchange heifers and sometimes goats in an age-old and sometimes three-generations-long contract known as *namanya*. The recipient household in this relationship cares for the heifer and all her progeny until the contract is terminated, in return for the heifers first-born female calf and harvest rights to all the milk produced by the original heifer and her progeny. Of their explanations for this practice, one is social and the other is that *namanya* spreads the burden of pastoral labour plus the risks of disease, rustling, and raiding so that a given household is unlikely ever to lose all its cattle. However, *namanya* has the added benefits of damping inbreeding and allowing villagers living on the slope to exploit the plains forage by handing animals over to Sebei there.

Gomero, Luís. 1989. Unpublished field notes. Faculty of Veterinary Medicine, Universidad Nacional Mayor de San Marcos, Lima, Peru. 2 pp.

This brief communication lists various ethnoveterinary practices noted by the author – a student of veterinary medicine – during discussions with National Agricultural Institute scientists, producers, veterinary professors and others in Peru. In Peru's Cajamarca Department, farmers treat their cattle and sheep against ectoparasites like mites and fleas using the bitter water left from steeping *Lupinus mutabilis*. Some rabbit ranchers cure diarrhoea by feeding *Salix alba* leaves and stalks, administered to fasting animals for 3 days or until the diarrhoea ceases. In Arequipa Department, cattle with meteorism are fed, or drenched with an infusion of, leaves and the slim stalks of *Schinus molle*; reportedly within minutes, the patient begins to belch, thus expelling the offending gases. Various treatments for retained placenta are reported from both coast and sierra, as described by nuns and producers. They centre on drenching with infusions of parsley or orange leaves or stinging nettle (*Urtica* spp.).

Gómez Rodríguez, Juan de la Cruz. 1985. *Tecnología del Pastoreo en las Comunidades del Cañon del Colca.* Central de Crédito Cooperativo del Perú, Arequipa, Perú. 77 pp.

In this study of camelid herders of the highland Colca Canyon of Peru's Arequipa Department, the anthropologist-author encapsulates the history of camelid husbandry from pre-domestication through Incaic and colonial times to today. Focusing mainly on alpaca, he describes various aspects of natives' traditional camelid care. They keep three races of alpaca: Huacaya, Suri and Macusani. The animals are systematically rotated up and down the mountains according to seasonal climatic and pasture conditions, but without herd subdivisions other than by colour. Some pastures are irrigated. When it comes to birthing, people assist alpaca only if there is a problem. Annual ear-marking takes place once a year and consists of notching the ear and threading brightly coloured yarn through it. People reportedly do not keep track of alpaca pedigrees and, when studs are selected, pay little attention to animal age or weight. As a result, birth defects are not uncommon. At shearing time, tools vary by economic means: smallholders still use ancient obsidian or quartz knives; slightly wealthier ones wield glass, tin or metal tools; only the richest people can afford steel scissors. Since people have little access to formal veterinary services, they rely mainly on fetishes like necklaces of quinces hung around the animals' necks (to ward against diarrhoeas), prayers and offerings to the gods, and of course traditional plant medicines. They have several such medicines for diarrhoeas and FMD [no Latin names given]. FMD lesions are also treated with methylene blue, urine or lard, and the animals are drenched with mallow/hollyhock water. Mange is cured with alpaca, llama or pig fat, cooking oil or burnt engine oil. Eye conditions are treated with sugar. Ethnoaetiologies of endoparasitism centre on climatic conditions like drought and damp, and on contact with the manure of introduced species (cattle, sheep, horses).

Gonda, Sam. 1992. Proposed community livestock development project in Dodoth County, Kotido District, Karamoja, Uganda. In: John Young (ed.). *A Report on a Village Animal Health Care Workshop – Volume II: The Case Studies.* ITDG, Rugby, UK. Pp. 39–49.

This proposal notes its intent to include reliable ethnoveterinary medicines plus appropriate traditional healers of animals and their EVK in paravet curricula and training.

González Vite, Juan, Lilian Morfin Loyden, José Ma. Ramírez Linares and Demetrio García Rojas. 1989. Determinación de anabólicos para el incremento de producción de carne. In: Gerardo López Buendía (ed.). *Memorias: Segunda Jornada sobre Herbolaria Medicinal en Medicina Veterinaria.* Universidad Nacional Autónoma de México, Facultad de Medicina Veterinaria y Zootecnia, Coordinación de Educación Continua, México DF, México. P. 108.

Medicinal plants may offer alternatives to the current use of animal-fattening hormones and antibiotics, which are causing consumer concern over harmful residues in meat products. To this end, two concentrations of anabolics from *Cinchona pubescens* were subjected to a controlled comparative study in piglets. Findings revealed that a 10–60 concentration of *C. pubescens* significantly increased weight gains.

Gounder, P. 1998. How long will the wisdom of Pulla Gounder survive? *Honey Bee* 9(1): 9–10.

Pulla Gounder is a 65-year-old Tamil farmer and herbal healer of livestock who is descended from a family of four generations of such healers. Some of his practices are detailed here. For better let-down in milking, he recommends covering the teats and udder for two days with a handful each of *Alternanthera sessilis*, *Kedrostis foetidissima* and *Sida acuta* leaves ground together and mixed in cow butter. He feeds fevered animals one whole, ground *Tephrosia purpurea* plant (including the root) mixed with gingelly oil. Feeding five to ten macerated, crushed *Abrus precatorius* seeds expels placentas. A plaster for fractured legs is made from boiling together two partially burnt *Aegle marmelos* fruits ground up with *Agave americana* leaves and bandaged around the broken limb. Inappetence is cured by a paste of equal portions of *Cissus quadrangularis* and salt pounded together, spread over the patient's tongue, and also fed as a small bolus. Several other farmers' ethnoveterinary remedies are also listed here. For indigestion in cattle, one is to place a betel leaf smeared with castor oil on the tongue and then press a hot iron spatula over the leaf; reportedly, this removes small red-coloured growths inside the mouth. Remedies for persistent diarrhoea include feeding: *Bassia longifolia* leaf extract; 3 kg of steamed *Paspalum scrobiculatum* grains; or burnt *Datura metel* pods. If the latter treatment fails, the animal is diagnosed as having rectal cancer. Finally, for eye injuries, drops of the diluted liquid from pounding together a handful of *Cleome pentaphylla* leaves with 10 pepper seeds are squeezed through a muslin cloth into the eye.

Gourlet, Sylvie. 1979. *Les Plantes en Médecine Vétérinaire Populaire.* Doctoral thesis, Veterinary Science, Université Paul-Sabatier, Toulouse, France. 117 pp.

Based on library research and field surveys, this thesis reviews both past and present folk veterinary remedies among shepherds of the French Pyrenees. Literally hundreds of such remedies are presented, organized into 13 heuristic categories: general condition; fevers; skin; eyes; accidents and trauma; locomotive apparatus; infectious diseases; and reproductive, digestive, respiratory, urinary, cardiovascular and nervous systems. An annex alphabetically lists 150 of the indigenous plants utilized in these remedies, along with the conditions they are popularly used to treat and their known pharmacological action, if any. The author opines that some are effective, particularly for relatively benign ailments, but that some are not. She also notes the usual problems with folk botanical nomenclature [see, e.g. Esparza B. 1988] and the fact that most disease names are symptomatic rather than aetiological. While the thesis recognizes the existence of supernatural aspects of EVM in France, it chooses not to treat them. Two important observations are: this veterinary tradition is in large part one of poor people who cannot afford expensive drugs; and 'this survey came 40 years too late' (p. 4) in that, even in the most remote corners of the mountains, a great deal of ethnoveterinary knowledge has been completely erased.

Gowda, S.K. 1998. Biological effects of neem (*Azadirachta indica*) derivatives in animals. In: E. Mathias, D.V. Rangnekar and C.M. McCorkle, with M. Martin (eds). ***Ethnoveterinary Medicine: Alternatives for Livestock Development – Proceedings of an International Conference Held in Pune, India, 4–6 November 1997. Volume 2: Abstracts.*** BAIF Development Research Foundation, Pune, India. P. 21.

Neem (*Azadirachta indica*) is a hardy and highly esteemed evergreen plant native to the Indian subcontinent. The parts of the neem plant that are used in livestock nutrition and medicine include the leaves, bark, seed kernel and oil. Numerous chemical compounds and their derivatives (like azadirachtin and nimbicidin) have been isolated from neem; and their biological and other properties (like bitterness) have been identified. Because bitter compounds generally exhibit repellent, sterilizing and antifertility effects on insects, they often figure in manufactured pesticides. Neem products have been screened in experimental animals, where they have shown varied effects. Hypoglycaemic, anti-inflammatory, anti-infective and antinematodal effects of neem derivatives are well documented. Aqueous extracts of neem seeds, bark or leaves exhibit potent immunostimulant activity through both humoral and cell-mediated response. The spermicidal action of neem oil in the vaginal tract of rats and monkeys is well understood. Processed neem seed cake is known to be a good protein supplement in livestock feed. When fed to rats, rabbits and chicken for sufficiently long periods, however, the raw seed cake has caused tissue damage as well as physiological changes including antitesticular action. Limited seed-cake feedings to layers did not affect egg production, but levels above 15% of the diet reduced egg production and affected erythropoiesis. Azadirachtin has shown dose- and tissue-specific inhibition of glutathione S-transferase and reduced glutathione and UDP-glucuronyl transferase activity in liver, lung, kidney and brain of rats. In view of its many beneficial effects, neem has a promising role in animal health and production.

Grandin, Barbara E. 1985. Towards a Maasai ethno-veterinary. Unpublished paper. ILCA, Kenya. 5 pp.

ILCA studies have shown that Maasai often misuse Western drugs. This will probably continue for the foreseeable future, because providing adequate Western-style veterinary services to pastoralists is difficult. To solve this problem, pastoralists themselves could be given some veterinary training – either a few individuals in depth as para-veterinarians, or many herders less intensively. Also, understanding of local concepts could greatly improve communication between pastoralists and their trainers. The author outlines how enumerators and veterinarians together can collect information on Maasai knowledge of diseases and traditional treatments.

Grandin, B.E., P.N. de Leeuw and M. de Souza. 1991. Labour and livestock management. In: Solomon Bekure, P.N. de Leeuw, B.E. and P.J.H. Neate (eds). ***Maasai Herding: An Analysis of the Livestock Production System of Maasai Pastoralists in Eastern Kajiado District, Kenya.*** ILCA Systems Study No. 4, Addis Ababa, Ethiopia. Pp. 71–82.

One morsel of animal healthcare among Kenya's Maasai is briefly noted in this text. To wit, ticks are removed by hand from cattle in order to reduce tick burdens, rather than specifically to prevent tick-borne diseases.

Grandin, Barbara, Ramesh Thampy and John Young. 1991. *Village Animal Healthcare: A Community-based Approach to Livestock Development in Kenya.* Intermediate Technology Publications, London, UK. 52 pp.

This booklet overviews the development and outcomes to date of ITDG's Kenya Livestock Programme in its 'barefoot vets' or *wasaidizi* training efforts. These provided basic information on the diagnosis, prevention and treatment – including some traditional herbal remedies – of simple diseases. Four out of more than 12 such ITDG-sponsored projects are discussed in this booklet. Preliminary surveys of farmers in Meru District noted a decline in recourse to traditional livestock healers (*mugaa*) and, among ordinary stockraisers, a generally low level of EVK. Traditional treatments incorporated into *wasaidizi* training there were thus limited to herbal medicines for worms, wounds, mange and ticks. In contrast, there were no such healers among Pokot pastoralists of Baringo District, where stockraisers themselves controlled considerable traditional as well as modern knowledge of livestock diseases and treatments; and as a point of pride, they preferred to diagnose and treat their animals themselves. Training programmes there had to be retooled accordingly. Yet a different situation was found among WaKamaba mixed farmers of Machakos District. They had many, and more highly valued, traditional healers. Thus, these individuals were closely consulted on training design, and were encouraged to take part in courses. For a fourth project, in Samburu District, preliminary data suggested that emphasis should perhaps be placed on the establishment of small drugstores, where trainees could help diagnose diseases, give veterinary advice and sell medicines.

Grandin, Barbara and John Young. 1994. Ethnoveterinary question list. In: Kate Kirsopp-Reed and Fiona Hinchliffe (eds). *RRA Notes Number 20: Special Issue on Livestock.* IIED, London, UK. Pp. 39–46.

This article focuses on the collection and use of ethnoveterinary data in the context of community-based animal health (CBAH) training programmes in Kenya. The authors drew up an ethnoveterinary question list to elicit information on local people's disease nomenclature, symptoms, causes, and traditional and modern treatments for livestock ills. Stage I of the data collection was done to gain background information on the local production system and help design the question list itself. Informants were asked which livestock species they kept, the breeds and ages, and then the names, seasonality, severity and incidence of diseases that attacked their herds. Stage II consisted of administering the question list itself, which elicited more information on particular diseases by asking about the species, age and sex of affected animals, as well as about each disease's aetiology, prevention and cure. In Stage III, findings were then analysed to decide whom to train in the CBAH programme, and what training content to include. For example, whether for traditional or modern medicine, basic healthcare information and techniques shown by the question list to be already familiar to a particular group of stockraisers would be excluded from the curriculum in order to focus on subjects new to trainees. In this way, training could be made more relevant to local people's needs and could proceed more rapidly.

Grandin, Barbara E. and John Young. 1996. Collection and use of ethnoveterinary data in community-based animal health programmes. In: Constance M. McCorkle, Evelyn Mathias and Tjaart W. Schillhorn van Veen (eds). *Ethnoveterinary Research & Development.* Intermediate Technology Publications, London, UK. Pp. 207–228.

This chapter describes the design and step-by-step application of a flexible interview guide that can be posed to farmers, pastoralists, butchers, vets and other livestock workers to collect ethnoveterinary information. Originally developed by ITDG/Kenya, data collected by the guide were then used as part of a package of techniques to arrive at a 'minimum dataset' for the design of community-based animal healthcare (CBAH) training and extension programmes. The other techniques include literature reviews, participant observation, wealth ranking and progeny histories. The Ethnoveterinary Interview Guide (EIG) consists of two parts. The first section collects gender-sensitive background information on livestock, husbandry practices and local-language names for diseases of the area. This information is necessary for framing EIG questions in culturally comprehensible ways, for selecting appropriate EIG informants and groups, and ultimately for analysing the EIG data. For example, a basic understanding of local livestock categorizations is necessary in order to pose sensible questions about what types of animals are affected by which diseases. Maasai distinguish three animal-age and two physiological categories, for instance. Also necessary is information on seasonal changes, which directly affect livestock nutrition and health. In selecting EIG informants among Maasai pastoralists and WaMeru farmers, background information revealed the need to include some Maasai women in interviews in order to capture their specialized knowledge of ailments in young stock; WaMeru interviews were divided equally between men and women in stockraising households, as the sexes shared more nearly equal ethnoveterinary responsibilities. Background information also indicates whether men and women are best interviewed in mixed- or same-sex groups. Disease names require particularly careful investigation due to differences among informants in their livestock knowledge and experience, languages and dialects, contact with other ethnicities, semantic overlaps, and conflation of names for body parts with names for diseases. For example, KiKamba *metho* can mean 'eye', 'conjuctivitis' or 'inflammation from a cobra's spitting into the eye'. Maasai *oltikana* can refer collectively to ECF, heartwater and redwater, which are all tick-borne diseases with similar signs; however, Maasai can add adjectives to distinguish which type of *oltikana* they mean. Conversely, they have two different words for ECF, depending upon the age category of the afflicted animals. It may also be necessary to do some disease rankings to avoid biases in stockraiser reporting of the most frequent, dramatic, acute, or current diseases. Once all pertinent background information has been collected and specific diseases decided upon for further investigation, depending upon producer needs and CBAH programme goals, the second part of the EIG consists of ten questions. (1) What species, breeds, ages and sexes of animals are affected by this disease? (2) Is there seasonality to the appearance of the disease? (3) Does it affect one animal, group of animals at the same time? Is it contagious or infectious? (4) What causes the disease? (5) Are there ways of preventing/avoiding it, and if so what? (6) Describe the main symptoms, their order of progression, and timing. (7) Are traditional treatments available? What are they, where/how are they obtained, and what is their effect? (8) Same questions again as in (7) but for modern treatments. (9) What happens if the animal is not treated? (10) When did you last have/hear of an animal with this disease? What did you do and what happened to the animal? For each question, the authors describe how to administer it, what kinds of responses and problems to anticipate, and how to interpret the answers. A real-life example of the ten questions as administered to one disease (trypanosomosis) among one pastoral tribe (Pokot) is also given. Also discussed are criteria for selecting good local-language interviewers and different ways to organize, analyse and apply the ethnoveterinary data collected. Applications span informed selection of: CBAH trainees by gender, age, healer/stockraiser status, etc.; training approach, depending upon the depth of trainees' and their prospective clients' existing veterinary knowledge – modern as well as traditional – and the match between the two in techniques and terminologies; course content, based above all on stockraisers' expressed needs but also on effective local treatments and ineffective use of modern treatments. ITDG/Kenya is also exploring application of EIG findings to help government veterinary departments improve their epidemiological and drought-early-warning monitoring by collecting information in herders' indigenous disease vocabulary. The EIG has proven particularly helpful, however, in bringing to light stockraisers' difficulties with modern drugs. For example, it was found that Samburu often calculate the dosages and dipping concentrations of potent modern drugs by trial-and-error; and because they consider aqueous Western drugs less powerful than viscous ones, Samburu may overdose with the former, risking toxicoses, and underdose with the latter, encouraging chemoresistance. Both Pokot and Maasai were prone to give stock potentially dangerous 'cocktails' of modern drugs in hopes that one or another or the combination would be sure to work. Moreover, Pokot were found to administer a trypanocidal tablet under the skin, rather than dissolving and injecting it as the drug was designed to be used. Moreover, Kenyan pastoralists do not always know to give different kinds of injections at different sites (subcutaneous, intramuscular, intravenous).

Green, Edward. 1972. Preventive medicine in dogs and man: Matawais of Suriname. Field notes shared in a personal communication to McCorkle. 1 p.

This communication details two preventive herbal medicines for dogs in Surinam. The first neutralizes snake poisoning in dogs and people. Certain plants are cooked together and 'made more powerful' by adding the head and tail of a snake to the mixture. The resulting medicine is applied to the skin or is eaten. 'Jaguar medicine' can also be administered to protect dogs from having their viscera eaten by jaguars; supposedly a jaguar that approaches a protected dog becomes weak or dies.

Green, Edward C. 1998. Etiology in human and animal ethnomedicine. *Agriculture and Human Values* 15(2): 127–131.

Considerable common ground exists between modern medical and traditional African aetiologies of disease. Moreover, in any given culture, human and animal medicine share theories about the range and nature of causal categories of illness, and the same indigenous healers treat people and livestock with essentially the same medicines, materials and methods. These overlaps are not generally recognized, however, because of the low regard in which Western-trained doctors and veterinarians hold traditional African medicine. African ethnomedicine classes diseases as either natural or supernatural, transmissible or contagious, chronic or curable. Africans typically attribute sudden inexplicable disease and death to supernatural causes. Diseases that are biomedically classed as contagious and that Africans perceive as chronic, curable, or preventable, however, are generally dealt with in naturalistic – and often biomedically successful – terms by Africans. Along with a keen understanding of disease transmission in both people and livestock, Africans also demonstrate some knowledge of zooprophylaxis. For example, in some cultures certain animals are believed to act as a sort of lightning rod, deflecting illnesses from their human owners and/or soul-mates. Such beliefs may be linked to Africans' empirical observation that contact with an animal disease that is nonpathogenic for humans may confer immunity to people challenged by a closely related disease. The classic example is the cowpox-smallpox relationship. Thus, it is wrong simply to dismiss all African ethnomedical concepts as witchcraft and superstition. Rather, a biomedically more sophisticated appreciation of such concepts can put them to work in designing healthcare delivery systems and, especially, preventive health education campaigns.

Greslou, Francois. 1989. Visión y crianza campesinas de los animales andinos. PRATEC, Lima, Perú. 32 pp.

This paper offers a general overview of earlier work on camelid pastoralism in the Andes, divided into four themes: characteristics of pre-Colombian pastoralism, consequences of the Spanish invasion and capitalist expansion, contemporary Andean pastoralism and culture, and their re-invigoration. The author mentions the role of sacred figurines of camelids in the annual reproductive and protective rites for herds and the preponderant use of home remedies for camelid ailments among Andean (agro)pastoralists. More importantly, however, he makes the sensitive point that, given camelids' profound and pervasive role in Andean culture and ideology, illness and death among these species are seen not just as economic or natural phenomena (as in the case of alien animals like sheep and cattle), but rather as an expression of the anger of deities or of cosmological turmoil. Many indigenous veterinary and herd management strategies are dictated by this perception, as opposed to a notion of stock raising as a purely profit-oriented enterprise.

Grigore, E. and I. Mihale. 1981. Fitoterapia – Unele rezultate obtinute si perspectiveie a pentru medican veterinaria. *Revista de Creõterea Animalelor* 31: 58–61.

Entitled 'Phytotherapy – Results and Prospects in Veterinary Medicine', this article mentions *Mentha piperita* (mint), *Urtica dioica*, *Achillea millifolium* and *Matricaria chamomilla* for treating livestock digestive problems in Romania. *Tilia cordata*, *Sambucus nigra* and *Zea mays* are discussed for respiratory ills, and *Hyoscyamus niger*, *Atropa belladonna* for nervous-system disorders. *Adonis vernalis* and *Capsella bursa-pastoris* are used for cardiac problems. General information concerning the plants' preparation is also given, along with the results of some experiments carried out on them at the Institute Pasteur. The authors find that various of the herbal treatments discussed are useful as antibacterials, endo- and ecto-parasiticides, cutaneous fungicides and galactagogues.

Groulade, M. 1978. Review of 'Médecine vétérinaire traditionnelle dans le Centre-Ouest' by M. Fournier. ***Revue 'Aguiaine'*** Special Number (Sep): no page numbers available.

A study conducted in France by a Ms Fournier reportedly covers both past and present ethnoveterinary practices there, including: the appearance of farriers; healing saints for livestock and other protections against sorcery and black magic; folk superstitions; home remedies; and the role of veterinarians. The study's conclusion highlights the 'mysterious complicity, a tacit understanding' that occurs between smallholder stockraisers and their animals in central-west France.

GTZ. 1994. ***Marsabit Development Programme Project Activity Report (July 1993–August 1994).*** Ministry of Agriculture, Livestock Development and Marketing, in cooperation with GTZ, Marsabit, Kenya. 107 pp.

For the livestock health component of the above-referenced project, staff designed a number of health, nutrition, breeding and other production interventions for local sheep, goats and poultry. But aside from some pharmacological disease controls, they were unable to identify any production or husbandry strategies for camels that would improve upon herders' own. Just the opposite was the case for beekeeping, for which local people had a tradition of 'honey hunting' but not husbandry.

GTZ. 1995. ***Marsabit Development Programme Project Activity Report.*** Ministry of Agriculture, Livestock Development and Marketing, in cooperation with GTZ, Marsabit, Kenya. *Ca.* 111 pp.

In this integrated rural development project with Boran, Burji and Rendille peoples of northern Kenya, some of the livestock activities centred on improved breeding and paravet training. With respect to the former, the project endeavoured to introduce Galla bucks and Black Head Persian rams to Rendille. However, both breeds suffered high mortality rates, such that all the participating stockraisers asked the project to introduce more of the local Gabbra breed of goats and sheep instead. The introduction of Rhode Island Red cocks and pullets fared somewhat better, however. With regard to the paravet program, after some initial experimentation and disappointments with trainee selection, 'a new selection criteria [sic] was . . . set to cover those pastoralists who have knowledge of traditional veterinary practices' (p. 22).

GTZ. 1996. ***GTZ Internal Project Report: Marsabit Development Programme.*** Ministry of Agriculture, Livestock Development and Marketing, in cooperation with GTZ, Marsabit, Kenya. No. of pages unknown.

This internal report notes that an EVK survey was conducted in the Marsabit and Moyale Districts of northern Kenya, where the Marsabit Development Programme operates. Starting from EVK information thus gathered, the longer-term aim of the project is to include useful EVK in training curricula for herder paravets.

Guèye, El Hadji Fallou. 1997. Diseases in village chickens: Control through ethno-vetinary [sic] medicine. ***ILEIA Newsletter*** 13(2): 20–21.

In this article, the Afro-Asian Network for Rural Poultry Development based in Senegal and the University of Ibadan, Nigeria reports on members' experiences with ethnoveterinary medicines in several African countries. In Senegal, farmers combat endoparasites in chickens by putting *Capsicum* sp. extracts and the leaves or bark of *Azadirachta indica* A. Juss. in the birds' drinking water. In Cameroon, *Kalanchoe crenata* and leaves of *Carica papaya* have proved successful in treating coccidiosis and other diarrhoeas, respectively. Togolese farmers use various infusions of *Peltophorum ferrugineum*, ground pepper, and the bark of *Adansonia digitata* to cure diarrhoea. Pepper (*Piper guineense*) is widely prescribed for coughs. A study in Cameroon found the bark of a creeping species of *Combretum* to have nematocidal properties in naturally infested village chickens. Reports from southern and eastern Africa claim that aqueous extracts of *Nicotiana glauca* can help chick embryos survive influenza infections. Applications of sheanut (*Butyrospermum parkii*) oil control ticks, lice and red ants by suffocating them. Infusions of *Borreria verticillata* leaves are used to treat diseases affecting locomotion in poultry. Also noted are: in Zimbabwe, sprinkling a cold infusion of *Annona senegalensis* roots in hen runs to repel snakes; in Nigeria, placing *Cucumis pustulatus* fruits in chicks' drinking water to ward off hawk attacks; and more.

Guillaumet, J.L. 1972. Note sur la connaissance du milieu végétal par les nomades de la basse vallée du Wabi Shebelle (Ethiopie). *Journal d'Agriculture et de Botanique Appliquée* 19(4–5): 73–84.

This article notes three ethnoveterinary phytotherapies known to nomadic pastoralists in Ethiopia. One is the use of *Cadaba glandulosa* leaves to treat wounds, particularly hyena bites. Another is an unidentified root to increase milk production. Finally, the same root may be inserted into a cow's vulva to stimulate milk let-down.

Gultom, D.S. Prawirodigdo, W. Dirdjopratono, Muryanto and Subiharta. 1991. The use of traditional medicine for small ruminants in Central Java. In: E. Mathias-Mundy and Tri Budhi Murdiati (eds). *Traditional Veterinary Medicine for Small Ruminants in Java.* Indonesian Small Ruminant Network, SR-CRSP, Central Research Institute for Animal Science, Agency for Agricultural Research and Development, Bogor, Indonesia. Pp. 13–27.

Some 50 farmers in the highlands and lowlands of Central Java were interviewed about their traditional veterinary practices. Approximately 130 prescriptions for 19 different disorders of small ruminants were collected. The prescriptions were prepared from locally available plant materials such as banana, basil, guava, jackfruit, mango, papaya and tea. The diseases treated were diarrhoea, bloat, scabies, conjunctivitis, worms, hoof infections, orf, milk fever, poisoning, dystocia, low milk production, post-partum haemorrhaging, anorexia, myiasis, influenza, sprains, fever, anoestrus and reduced fertility. Some traditional medicines are now also produced commercially. One is a tonic to promote livestock health, strength and disease resistance, which is made up of *Alstonia, Centella, Curcuma, Eucalyptus, Phyllanthus, Retrofraca* and *Zingiber*.

Gupta, Anil. 1997. Roots of creativity and innovation in developing societies. In: Anil Gupta (ed.). *International Conference on Creativity and Innovation at Grassroots for Sustainable Natural Resource Management, January 11–14, 1997: Abstracts.* Indian Institute of Management, Ahmedabad, India. Pp. i–xxxviii.

Section E in this introduction to the collected abstracts of the above-referenced conference gives an apt example of how everyone stands to benefit from collecting and disseminating EVK via cross-cultural and regional linkages such as the India-based local-knowledge network, 'Honey Bee'. Mongolian pastoralists are known to make their own, highly nutritious mineral blocks out of onion leaves, wheat germ, sodium bicarbonate and dried milk. A Scottish scientist discovered that the block is also rich in selenium. A mineral that is vital for many aspects of livestock health and especially for calf survival, selenium is notably deficient in Mongol forages. All these facts were noted in the Honey Bee newsletter. Meanwhile, it was learned that the livestock of Canada's Akwasasne Indians suffer from lack of selenium. Here, says the author, is a case where a technique elaborated by people of one world region, studied by someone from an entirely different one, and disseminated by a group from yet another can help stockraisers on yet a different, distant continent to solve their local veterinary problems.

Gupta, Anil, Jyoti Capoor and Rekha Shah. 1990. *Inventory of Peasant Innovations for Sustainable Development: An Annotated Bibliography.* Centre for Management in Agriculture, Indian Institute of Management, Ahmedabad, India. Pp. 55–71.

Gupta, Capoor and Shah's bibliography contains nine chapters on farmers' knowledge relating to: plant protection, water and land management, livestock, cropping, horticulture, climate, farm implements and general agronomy. A number of abstracts in the livestock chapter relate to ethnoveterinary medicine. Some of these are reproduced in the present bibliography under their author(s) name(s).

Gupta, Anil K. and Kirit K. Patel. 1994a. Survey of innovations in Gujarat Part VIII. *Honey Bee* 5(2): 14–18.

In India's Gujarat State, a Muslim healer who is much revered even by his Hindu neighbours cures yoke galls with an extract of *Triumfetta rotundifolia*, sometimes mixed with the bullock's saliva: this is massaged into the sore area for 15 minutes twice daily until a cure is effected. For urinary blockages in livestock, another local healer drenches with the ashes of 20 to 25 peacock quills in 500 ml of water, followed by the milk of 1 to 2 green coconuts; if urination does not occur within 40 minutes, he drenches again with tea. To bring animals into heat, Gujarat farmers feed them freshly chopped *Euphorbia* sp. roots every day for 8 to 10 days, as these roots are classed as 'hot' in hot/cold ethnomedical theory. Minor wounds on udders are dressed with castor oil and coconut-husk ash. A drench of *Ziziphus mauritiana* ash in water induces expulsion of the placenta; alternatives are a filtrate of *jinjara* (?) leaves or the boiled tassles of 20 to 25 maize cobs. An age-old galactagogue is 10 kg of fresh *doddi* (?) vines. For diarrhoea, crushed *Syzygium cumini* seeds are fed. To repel lice from poultry, *Vitex negundo* leaves are scattered about the farmyard.

Gupta, Anil K. and Kirit K. Patel. 1994b. Survey of innovations in Gujarat Part IX. *Honey Bee* 5(3): 14–15.

To promote conception in buffalo cows, Gujarat farmers drench them in the fifth and ninth months after calving with 1 kg of sugar, 500 g of *majith* (?), and the juice extracted from 2 kg of *Cordia* sp. leaves, all in 3 l of water. The same recipe halved and using only 2 l of water is given to cattle at 5 and 9 months postpartum. To 'clean the uterus' of small ruminants that have just aborted, farmers drench with crushed young *sipda* (?) twigs boiled in buttermilk. For prolapsed uterii, people say a drench of 250 to 300 g of crushed cactus tips in 700 g of buttermilk is effective in 60% to 70% of cases. To prevent milk fever, farmers feed chalk dust (lime) and limit the withdrawal of colostrum. To prevent occlusions in milk flow, they drench with an aqueous filtrate of a certain latex-ful creeper. Remedies for internal parasites in very young calves consist of week-long regular drenches of 50 g of salt in 500 ml of buttermilk, and/or feedings of *rati bhindi* (?) leaves or sesame. Bullocks with intestinal worms receive the latter two items along with 250 g of white onion for a week. Bloat is treated with pellets of 200 g of crushed *Madhuca indica* flowers in 100 g of jaggery. Rotted horns are cut away, and the stubs are dressed with 100 g of castor oil, followed by an application of 50 g of urea fertilizer mixed with either [unspecified] hair or 50 g of *Vernonia anthelmintica*. The stubs are then bandaged with a cotton or leather wrapping. Several such dressings are required for complete healing. An expert bonesetter, who works *gratis*, manually sets fractures, massages the area with sesame oil or iodex, splints it with bamboo or wood, and then repeats the sesame massage for 5 days.

Gupta, Anil K., Kirit K. Patel and Jitendra H. Suthar. 1995a. Survey of innovations in Gujarat Part XIII. *Honey Bee* 6(3): 11–14.

Gujarat farmers of India feed the entire plant or sometimes just the boiled root juice of *lajamani* (?) to break up gallstones in bullocks. Five to 10 g of pigeon or chicken droppings fed daily for several days reportedly induces heat in buffalo heifers; likewise for 2 to 3 kg of papaya fruit or, alternatively, *chapati* bread with several grasshoppers. Dislocated joints are massaged twice a day for a week with four pellets of camphor dissolved in 500 g of hot sesame oil. A well-known Muslim veterinary healer skilled at difficult livestock deliveries renders these services cost-free 'round the clock'.

Gupta, Anil K., Kirit K. Patel, Jitendra H. Suthar, Vijay Chauhan et al. 1995b. Survey of innovations in Gujarat Part XIV. *Honey Bee* 6(4): 11–13.

Valo (?) is a common cattle disease of the monsoon season in India. It is characterized by inappetence and continual salivation. A traditional treatment, said to be effective within 2 days, is to rub the animal's back with 500 to 700 g of salt for half an hour and then force it to inhale the smoke of a burning gunny/grain sack and sawdust from *Dalbergia sissoo*, wood over a charcoal fire. The fire is built in a container and the animal's muzzle is simply held above it.

Gupta, Anil K., Kirit K. Patel, Jitendra H. Suthar, Vijay Chauhan et al. 1996a. Survey of grassroots innovations part XVI. *Honey Bee* 7(2): 13–15.

During the monsoon, a farmer in south Gujarat, India drenches his animals that have diarrhoea with a filtrate prepared from approximately 500 g of pounded *Ficus racemosa* bark mixed with with 500 ml of banana juice, followed an hour later by a drench of 250 ml of peanut oil. According to the scientific literature, all of these ingredients are in fact beneficial in treating diarrhoea. Two other men's remedies for yoke gall consist of an extract of crushed *Aerva tomentosa* (a wild pasture plant) or of *Mucuna prurita* leaves, applied thrice daily for 5 to 6 days.

Gupta, Anil K., Kirit K. Patel, Jitendra H. Suthar, Vijay Chauhan et al. 1996b. Survey of innovations in Gujarat Part XVI. *Honey Bee* 7(3): 15–16.

A farmer from North Gujarat reports his treatment for myiasis. Applying sugar crystal to the wound brings out the maggots, which can then be removed by hand. Then wash the wound with a cooled decoction of *Acacia nilotica* bark and dress it with cotton wool dipped in castor seed oil. Repeating the whole treatment for up to a week will completely heal the wound.

Gupta, Anil K., Kirit K. Patel, Jitendra H. Suthar, Vijay Chauhan et al. 1996c. Survey of grassroots innovations part XVII. *Honey Bee* 7(4): 15–17.

To treat urinary blockages in animals, a healer in India uses 500 g of crushed *Bryophyllum* leaves in 500 ml of water. About 250 ml of the filtrate is given twice daily for 8 to 10 days.

Gupta, Anil K., Kirit K. Patel, Jitendra H. Suthar, Dilip Koradia et al. 1997. Survey of innovations in Gujarat Part XVII. *Honey Bee* 8(1): 9–11.

Indian farmers give 500 g of *Citrullus colocynthis* fruits to animals with urinary blockages from kidney stones. In north Gujarat, horses suffering from inappetence, stomach aches, or other gastric troubles are fed 100 g of mango flowers in water or 50 g of powdered teak seeds in water. In south Gujarat, farmers heal FMD wounds in a week by applying a thick black fluid made from burning dried cowdung cakes around a partially buried pot filled with *Dalbergia sissoo* tree bark and water. A traditional Indian practice to ensure placental expulsion within an hour is to feed 10 to 15 live *Ficus benghalensis* primordia with 100 g of *bajra* flour. A teaspoon of dried and powdered earthworms in 200 ml of milk helps cure calves of intestinal worms. For eczema in camels, donkeys and horses, the leaf juice or a decoction of *Calotropis gigantea* is applied to the skin.

Gupta, J.C. nd. Livestock Treatment by Indigenous Medicines. Unpublished paper. 5 pp.

This paper lists some 20 polyprescriptions from India that employ locally available plants and minerals for an assortment of livestock diseases. For example, to induce heat, stock are given 1 g of copper sulphate added to jaggery, wheat flour or rice; an alternative is 1 kg of carrots, barley or lentils. These preparations are fed daily for 40 days. Mange is treated with a topical lotion of sulphur, quick lime and water.

Gupta, Jagdish C. 1998. Experiences of practising ethnoveterinary medication in villages in Uttar Pradesh. In: E. Mathias, D.V. Rangnekar and C.M. McCorkle, with M. Martin (eds). *Ethnoveterinary Medicine: Alternatives for Livestock Development – Proceedings of an International Conference Held in Pune, India, 4–6 November 1997. Volume 2: Abstracts.* BAIF Development Research Foundation, Pune, India. Pp. 21–22.

In India the veterinary arts have a long tradition. Several early Indian kings and leaders – like King Nal, Shalihotra and Nakul – were regarded as excellent veterinary physicians. Before the discovery of antibiotics in the 1950s, Indian veterinary hospitals routinely treated their patients with local herbs, spices and chemicals. And whenever veterinarians are not available in rural areas, animals are often treated with ingredients available in village shops or the kitchen. Based on the author's 40 years of veterinary practice using herbal as well as other treatments, he recommends such ingredients as the following for at-home use by Indian stockraisers who cannot access any other veterinary assistance: astringents – *Acacia catechu*, chalk, *Aegle marmelos*, rice; appetisers – black salt, *Swertia chirata*; expectorants – liquorice (*Glycyrrhiza glabra*), ammonium chloride; wounds and injuries – alum, marigold; urinary diseases – potassium nitrate; parasitic diseases – areca nut, copper sulphate; deficiency diseases – proteins, minerals, vitamins; retention of placenta – bamboo leaves; tympanitis – linseed, turpentine, sodium biocarbonate. With regard to infectious diseases, prophylactic indigenous vaccinations are advised for all animals according to season and locality. The author notes that all the foregoing ingredients are normally readily available to India's farmers. In the full text, the local as well as Latin plant names are given; also, many more ingredients identified only by local names are listed.

Gupta, S.P. and A. Gupta 1989. *Local Innovations and Farmers' Practices in Rainfed Eastern Uttar Pradesh (District: Faizabad), India: An Annotated List of Farmers' Knowledge.* Pp. 1–31.

Traditional veterinary practices from Uttar Pradesh, India reported here include: giving a mixture of ghee and pepper to animals with sore throats; curing septic toes by washing them with water in which the bark of a certain tree has been boiled; firing pustulent gums with a hot iron rod and then dressing the gums with turmeric and mustard oil. [Abstract based on Gupta et al.'s 1990 annotated bibliography.]

Grupo Talpuy. 1992. Conversando entre todos aprendemos. *Minka* 30&31: 26–28.

Drawing upon Andean farmer testimonies gathered in the course of fieldwork by the NGO Grupo Talpuy, this article describes how development communication is most effective when as many family and community members as possible take part in information exchange and play a hands-on role in learning, alongside scientists and developers. This lesson is illustrated by experiences while re-introducing a traditional pumpkin-seed anthelmintic for cattle. In one demonstration *cum* experiment, everybody got involved. With household and neighbourhood children looking on, first the seeds were ground in a mortar. The children then fetched the water for making an infusion of the pulverized seeds. An elderly lady strained the solution. A male passerby on his way to visit a relative also stopped to help, saying 'I want to see too. Will it really work?' The passerby then helped the owner of the experimental bull hold the animal while a young man administered the pumpkin-seed drench. Another farmer present detailed his own successes with the treatment, describing how he now feeds pumpkin seeds to his pigs as well. Meanwhile, a medicinewoman supervised, giving instructions on how to tilt the bull's head back and to turn the drenching bottle just so – all the while reminiscing on how she became a curer. The article makes the larger points that not all learning takes place in universities, and that scientists have much to learn from farmers as well as vice versa. Or as one farmer puts it, 'We learn best when we all learn together' (p. 27).

Hadani, A. and A. Shimshony. 1994. Traditional veterinary medicine in the Near East: Jews, Arab Bedouins and Fellahs. *Revue Scientifique et Technique de l'Office International des Épizooties* 13(2): 581–597.

Among the Semitic peoples of the Near East, traditional healers of both humans and animals are numerous. They include: Jewish *kohanim* (priests) or *chachamim* (bearers of knowledge); Arab *derwish*, *chatib* (makers of amulets and tokens), *medjabar* (orthopaedists) and *attar* (herbalists); and last but not least, shepherds themselves. This article describes both ancient and traditional texts, measures and treatments concerning parasitic and infectious diseases of livestock, including medical, surgical, hygienic and kosher procedures, plus early legislation to prevent cruelty to animals. Following are examples of traditional treatments still in use today. To treat mange and other skin conditions in camels, Bedouin have many alternatives: topically applying any of the following – powdered *Plantago psyllium* leaves, a concoction of *Calotropis procera* leaves, sulphurous water, or automotive lubricant; covering the patient's body in calcareous soil; or washing the animal in the water in which olives have been soaked. To repel flies and mosquitoes, green wood is burnt or the animals are covered with mud. A unique treatment for flea infestation is to tie a ball of wool to an animal's nose or forehead and then slowly push the animal into a bath of water; the fleas congregate in the wool, which is then destroyed. Bedouin keep poultry with the explicit aim of the birds' eating ticks and other insects that transmit both livestock and human diseases. To remove bot larvae, Israeli shepherds administer tar in the drinking water; and using a cloth soaked in a salt-and-lemon solution, they manually detach leeches clinging to the pharynx. Shepherds in hilly areas of Israel have an astute system of grazing certain slopes only every third year, in order to avoid the most infective stage in the life cycle of the *Ixodes ricinus gibbosus* tick, which transmits a paralysing caprine disease. Knowing, too, that the ticks prefer the head and neck area, for added protection shepherds tie a rag soaked in kerosene around their goats' necks [much like the flea collars worn by pets in the developed world]. Bedouin have an astute, centuries-old ecological understanding of seasonal gastroenteritis, which they ward against using modern anthelmintics and/or a twice-annual drench consisting of water in which a fish steeped in sheep manure has been boiled. Also noted is Arab shepherds' appreciation of anthrax's soil longevity and of its human health hazards. Bedouin and Fellah recognize many other bacterial diseases, including glanders, for which they have a two-pronged treatment. For FMD, Arab cattle raisers have various responses: keeping affected animals on muddy soil, separated from healthy ones; conversely, vaccinating the whole herd by letting first infected and then healthy, cattle drink from the same large pot or by wiping the latters' mouths with a rag soaked in the water; and/or keeping the local Baladi breed of cattle, which is believed to be more resistant to FMD. Sheep pox is prevented by a vaccination that entails soaking a string in water with a few, crushed papules from an infected animal and then passing the string through the auricle using a needle. Some Bedouin and Fellah also used to vaccinate children against chicken pox by exposing them to camel pox. Examples of Arab surgical and other methods include: bleeding, performed by bruising the skin or by passing a homemade needle through the jugular vein; for metritis-induced infertility in horses, flushing the uterus with hot water and soap; and for a veritable galaxy of ills (mastitis, wounds, fractures, snakebite, pneumonia, bottle-jaw, lungworms, bots, coenurosis and more) branding with a red-hot nail. This last procedure is typically performed by women. Also included in this article are lists of plant-based remedies and toxic plants known to Bedouin and Near Eastern stockraisers, respectively.

Hadgu, Kassaye. 1992. Decentralized village animal health care in Dalocha District, southern Shoa region, Ethiopia. In: John Young (ed.). *A Report on a Village Animal Health Care Workshop – Volume II: The Case Studies.* ITDG, Rugby, UK. Pp. 50–54.

Future plans are noted here for this ActionAid and Ministry of Agriculture programme to ask its trained Community Veterinary Agents to collect herbs used in traditional livestock medicines for expert evaluation and [presumably] incorporation into future training curricula.

Hadrill, David. 1989. Vets in Nepal and India – The provision of barefoot animal health services. In: *The Barefoot Book: Economically Appropriate Services for the Rural Poor.* Marilyn Carr (ed.). Intermediate Technology Publications, London, UK. Pp. 13–19.

In Kutch, western India, *deshis* are the traditional human and animal doctors. A local rural development organization is training them to use primary animal health-care kits (PACKs) containing basic veterinary equipment and ten drugs that are readily available from local chemists. This training adds to *deshis*' traditional knowledge and professional status by increasing the range of livestock conditions they can treat.

Hadrill, David and Haroon Yusuf. 1994. Seasonal disease incidence in the Sanaag region of Somaliland. In: Kate Kirsopp-Reed and Fiona Hinchliffe (eds). *RRA Notes Number 20: Special Issue on Livestock.* IIED, London, UK. Pp. 52–53.

In a joint ActionAid/Vetaid project, a participatory seasonal disease calendar was drawn up with herder and elder focus groups in the Sanaag region of Somaliland in order to identify: the different diseases prevalent in their herds of sheep, goats and camels; the seasonal incidence of these diseases; and those that herders considered most important, as ranked by their placement of 0 to 3 stones in the appropriate cell of the calendar. The calendar was organized according to the four emically-recognized seasons of the year across the horizontal axis and the local names of important diseases down the vertical axis. From the information thus collected, the project was able to develop a Primary Veterinary Assistant training plan organized around only the most common and/or important diseases, as defined by herders themselves. In general, people scored infrequent but often-terminal infectious diseases as more important than common ailments, such as helminthosis, that

cause production losses. When coupled with knowledge of herders' grazing movements as elicited during participatory mapping exercises, the calendrical disease
data also made for more effective project planning of a drug distribution program
for Sanaag.

Haile-Mariam, Mekonnen, Birgitta Malmfors and Jan Philipsson. 1998. Boran –
Indigenous African cattle with potential. *Currents* 17/18: 38–43.

Borana pastoralists of Ethiopia's Boran Plateau depend for their survival upon the
breed of Boran cattle they have husbanded across hundreds of years. Indeed, 'in
the evolution and development of Boran cattle the role of their owners, the Borana
people, can not be overestimated' (p. 40). The Boran is one of the most productive
indigenous breeds of East African cattle and one of the few African breeds to have
been introduced to other parts of the world (notably Australia and the USA). It is
an extremely hardy animal, able to withstand regular shortages of water and feed,
to walk long distances in search of sustenance and to digest exceptionally low-
quality forage. Boran cows have a long reproductive life and good maternal
instincts; their calves are able to thrive and grow under conditions that exotic or
even cross-bred Borans cannot; and the steers have a higher level of lipoprotein
lipase activity in the subcutaneous fat depot than animals sired by other breeds. In
addition, Boran are tolerant to heat stress, some ticks and tick-borne diseases and
other tropical diseases. As the frequency and severity of droughts in Ethiopia
increase, however, the breed faces genetic dilution. Under drought conditions, the
most productive, lactating and twinner cows and their calves perish first. Also,
recent droughts have forced pastoralists to sell larger numbers of animals than in
past in order to purchase needed supplies of foodgrain at ever higher prices. Worse,
in a desperate attempt to minimize the numbers of animals sold while maximizing
their cash earnings, Boran stockraisers may have begun to sell off some of their
best animals, thus removing the most desirable genes from the breeding pool. And
under post-drought pressures to re-stock, pastoralists have broken with breeding
tradition and begun to exchange Boran bulls and steers for non-Boran heifers from
the highlands. If such practices continue, the indigenous purebred could disappear.

Hajare, S., S. Chandra, S.K. Tandan and J. Lal. 1998. Anti-inflammatory activity
of *Dalbergia sissoo* leaves. In: E. Mathias, D.V. Rangnekar and C.M. McCorkle,
with M. Martin (eds). ***Ethnoveterinary Medicine: Alternatives for Livestock
Development – Proceedings of an International Conference Held in Pune,
India, 4–6 November 1997. Volume 2: Abstracts.*** BAIF Development Research
Foundation, Pune, India. P. 22.

This study tested the anti-inflammatory activity of an alcoholic extract of
Dalbergia sissoo leaves in different models of inflammation in rats. The extract
was orally administered at dosages of 100, 300 and 1000 mg/kg. In the carrageenin-induced, hind-paw oedema models, the extract significantly inhibited
acute inflammation at the 300 to 1000 dosage levels. Furthermore, these two
dosages significantly inhibited dye leakage in acetic-acid-induced vascular perme-
ability. The extract also significantly reduced the weight of granulamous tissue
from chronic inflammation induced by cotton-pellet granuloma. No ulcerogenic
effects on the gastric mucosa of the rats were recorded during acute and chronic
gastric irritation tests. The study concluded that the alcoholic extract of *D. sissoo*

leaves produces significant anti-inflammatory effects in different models of inflam-mation, with no adverse side effects on the gastric mucosa.

Haldar, Avijit. 1998. External parasites: Protecting your livestock. *Footsteps* 34: 12–13.

The use of commercial pesticides from the last century to the present is briefly reviewed here. Previously, pesticides were based on such materials as sulphur, tobacco and arsenic [which were also common in ethnoveterinary treatments]. In the 1940s, chemicals such as DDT and chlorinated hydrocarbons replaced these earlier materials. Now known to be very dangerous both to livestock and humans, these chemicals have been banned in most countries. Organophosphates were the next to be developed, but their handling still requires close attention to safety. Today, the safest known pesticides are synthetic pyrethroids. Even more recently, injectible systemic pesticides have been developed for livestock. But along with the pyrethroids, they are very expensive. In advising on how to protect livestock from ectoparasites, the author suggests first trying a common ethnoveterinary treat-ment: a paste of water and dried neem-leaf ashes, smeared on animals every 2 weeks. If this is not effective or practical, animals can instead be dipped or sprayed with an appropriate commercial pesticide. People lacking a spray pump can apply the product with a paint brush or with a cloth or sponge on the end of a stick. Also noted are 12 'do's and don'ts' for the safe and environmentally healthy handling of pesticides.

Halpin, Brendan. 1981. Vets – Barefoot and otherwise. *Pastoral Network Paper* No. 11c. Agricultural Administration Unit, ODI, London, UK. 7 pp.

When great lethal epidemics in livestock are mostly under control, other diseases that are more difficult to diagnose gain greater economic importance. Preventing such diseases is usually cheaper than curing them, but measures should be based on sound epidemiological studies. This requires investigative teams consisting of a veterinarian and a laboratory technician, plus basic laboratory equipment. Such a team should cooperate with agronomists and soil scientists and should become familiar with the pastoralists' language and customs. Because existing animal health services are rarely appropriate to the needs of pastoralists, pastoralists them-selves should be recruited as veterinary health workers or 'barefoot animal health assistants'. The 'BAHAs' could improve the dialogue between pastoralists and the government. Also, unlike most government functionaries in developing countries, BAHAs would be less reluctant to live in the bush. Where available, local healers should be selected for this task. Their training should be of a practical rather than of a 'classroom' type and it should be conducted in the local language. At the first stage, only simple procedures would be taught, such as wound care, elementary suturing and medication. Later, annual meetings could introduce topics such as tick control and calf care. BAHAs would not replace the government service, but they would link its local veterinary workers more closely with the pastoral community.

Hamed, Khan Shaheen. 1998. Traditional veterinary wisdom: Practices from rural Medak, A.P. *Honey Bee* 9(2): 17–18.

This article is the first in a new series on local veterinary practices observed in the Medak region of India's Andhra Pradesh State, where a regional development organization has set out to document all such practices and scientifically validate them. The present article deals with three important livestock diseases: FMD, tympany and diarrhoea, for which seven local treatments each are presented in a corresponding set of three tables. For each treatment, the tables specify: the plant; where known, its Latin name; other ingredients; the quantities of all ingredients; method of preparation, dosage; and the source farmer who reported the treatment. In addition, citations as to plant activity from pharmacological and pharmacognostic publications and databases are given.

Hamed, Khan Shaheen. 1999. Traditional veterinary practises in rural Medak, India. In: E. Mathias, D.V. Rangnekar and C.M. McCorkle, with M. Martin (eds). *Ethnoveterinary Medicine: Alternatives for Livestock Development – Proceedings of an International Conference Held in Pune, India, 4–6 November 1997. Volume 1: Selected Papers.* BAIF Development Research Foundation, Pune, India. Pp. 57–59.

Cost, inaccessibility and other problems associated with conventional animal healthcare systems have led to the rediscovery of traditional rural wisdom on this subject. Ethnoveterinary practices are often cheap, safe and based on local resources and know-how. Unfortunately, these often-useful alternatives are disappearing because they are passed on from generation to generation through oral rather than written communication. With the aim of preparing a manual of simplified, effective traditional veterinary treatments from one part of India's Andhra Pradesh State, the author collected and documented information on EVM by disease and treatment there. Since several treatments exist for each disease, an effort was been made to validate treatments on an empirical basis by keeping quantitative and qualitative records of cases and their treatments. To date, details of 160 indigenous veterinary treatments have been collected for 24 animal diseases. In illustration of this initiative, this paper presents six such remedies for diarrhoea in livestock, along with the corresponding case records and farmers' own estimations of the treatments' efficacy.

Hammel, Roland. 1995. *SECADEV: Working with Agro-pastoralists in Chad.* Arid Lands Information Network (ALIN), Dakar, Senegal. 40 pp.

In 1991, the Chadian NGO SECADEV began working with pastoralists in the Oum-Hadjer region, in a follow-on to the earlier Oxfam-funded Ishtirak development programme there. The latter led the way in paravet training, which SECADEV is continuing. This booklet notes that SECADEV encourages communities to select paravet trainees who already have a solid hands-on knowledge of common diseases. In the Oum-Hadjer region, these are usually older men. SECADEV also underscores the importance of listening to community definitions of the livestock health problems that need solving [i.e. those that traditional EVK cannot adequately deal with] and of finding out what trainees and stockraisers already know about animal healthcare before designing curricula. Otherwise, as SECADEV found in its first training effort, trainees 'already knew about 60% of the course before they came to be trained' (p. 12). This NGO recommends starting training by making a list of the diseases and symptoms that trainees already recognize and getting participants to agree on a common name for each disease. Also noted here is pastoralists' extensive knowledge of forage resources. They know which plants are good for milk production, which are most palatable to different livestock species and the season of the year when a given wild forage is at its most nutritious. However, their knowledge was less acute when it came to the nutritional value of dry-season food supplements like millet stalks and groundnut leaves and stems. Interestingly, among these Chadian agropastoralists, often local plant names duplicate scientific ones semantically. For instance, the local Arabic name for *Dactyloctenium* spp. means 'fingers' just as the Latin genus name does.

Hammond, J.A., D. Fielding and S.C. Bishop. 1997. Prospects for plant anthelmintics in tropical veterinary medicine. *Veterinary Research Communications* 21(3): 213–228.

This article reviews anthelmintic plants currently in use in tropical veterinary medicine and notes the frequent lack of scientific evidence for their effectiveness. The case for such plants as a means of overcoming some of the serious limitations of manufactured anthelmintics is outlined [see other annotations by Fielding and Hammond]. Reasons why anthelmintic plants are not generally used in veterinary medicine, in contrast to their greater acceptance in human medicine, are considered. One is the fact that such treatments are generally less toxic than commercial drugs and thus often less lethal to helminths. The authors also caution against over-enthusiastic and -simplistic acceptance of botanical anthelmintics. In the absence of scientific research, worms observed to be expelled in the faeces after dosing with such remedies can not be confidently attributed to the action of the botanical administered. Expulsion could be due to other factors, such as animals' self-medication via consumption of anthelmintic pasture plants, or to the natural excretion of old, dead worms. The authors thus discuss various strategies for developing reliable plant anthelmintics, particularly the need for *in vivo* trials to identify which plants are truly effective and suitable for general use. Eleven such species are suggested as good candidates for further evaluation: *Artemisia maritima, Caesalpinia crista, Melia azedarach, Mallotus philippensis, Chrysanthemum* sp., *Matteuccia orientalis, Carica papaya, Heracleum* sp., *Hedysarum coronarium, Aloe barteri, Terminalia avicennioides* and *Diospyros mollis*.

Hammond-Tooke, W.D. 1962. *Bhaca Society: A People of the Transkeian Uplands, South Africa.* Oxford University Press.

Pages 266 to 271 of this anthropological study make brief reference to how Bhaca protect their livestock from sickness and accident. Removing and cooking the foetus of a freshly killed jackal, grinding and mixing it with medicines and then burning the mixture in the fold is believed to protect sheep from this predator. Cattle are protected from lightning by burying a tortoise shell at the entrance to their kraal; the rest of the tortoise is burnt and the smoke allowed to waft over the cattle.

Harouna, Souley. 1996. La médecine vétérinaire traditionnelle Africaine: Réalite et modernisme. *Lettre du Sous-réseau PRELUDE: Santé, Productions Animales et Environnement* 9: 4.

This short article presents a sampling of ideas and information based on a 1933 volume [title not given] about traditional Fulani practitioners of veterinary medicine in Macina, Mali, written by a Mr Falley Koumaré. Indigenous vaccinations and other prophylactic measures are highlighted. In what Fulani termed 'sale of the disease', material from an infected animal (the seller) was employed to immunize a healthy one (the buyer). The most common such technique was for CBPP. Reportedly borrowed by Fulani specialists from Twareg and Mawre herders, it entailed inserting a bit of the seller's lung, previously macerated in milk for 2 to 3 days, into the buyer's forehead using a sterilized penknife. In indigenous FMD vaccinations, rock salt was rubbed over the lingual lesions of the seller and then over the tongue of the buyer. Indirect vaccination was also practised. Stockraisers purposely exposed their calves to animals with CBPP or rinderpest in order to stimulate a natural immunity in the calves. In addition, Fulani elaborated strict rules of quarantine for herds with contagious diseases and for newly purchased stock. The author notes that the Pulaar language employs the categorical term *hindous* 'spirit' for all such contagious and infectious diseases with invisible agents but patent signs. Despite this 'spirit' notion, from such operations and rules as the foregoing, it is clear that Fulani enjoyed considerable empirical understanding of many of the same principles and procedures for contagious bacterial and viral disease as those underpinning modern veterinary medicine.

Hatch, John K. 1983. *Our Knowledge: Traditional Farming Practices in Rural Bolivia. Volume I: Altiplano Region.* Rural Development Services under contract to USAID, New York, USA.

Pages 144 to 169 of this volume provide local livestock knowledge on Bolivia's Altiplano region. Cattle, sheep, llama, donkeys, pigs and guinea pigs are discussed in terms of uses, breeding, nutrition, castration, marking, diseases and special rites. Llama diseases described here include external parasites, cracked hooves and trichinosis. The first is cured by dipping, the second by applying lard or engine grease to the hooves and the third has no known local cure. Llama are castrated at about 2 years of age when the moon is full. Water is withheld from the animal for a day after castration, in the belief that the risk of infection is reduced thereby.

Hatch, John K. 1986. *Our Knowledge: Traditional Farming Practices in Rural Bolivia. Volume III: Tropical Lowlands Region.* Rural Development Services, Bethesda, Maryland, USA.

In Bolivia's tropical lowlands, rural families all keep cattle, small ruminants, pigs, poultry and dogs. This volume notes several local practices to help cows expel the placenta (cf. pp. 134–140). One technique is to tie the cow's legs and drench her with a purgative of cactus juice and salt water. Another is to reach into the vagina and simply yank the placenta free. Alternatively, a thin rope with a flat rock attached to one end can be tied to the placenta and left to dangle until gravity pulls out the placenta.

Heffernan, Claire. 1990. *The Dynamics of Livestock Healthcare among the Samburu Pastoralists of Northern Kenya.* MSc thesis, School of Veterinary Medicine, Tufts University, North Grafton, Massachusetts, USA. 23 pp.

Phytotherapies, branding and venipuncture (bloodletting) are common veterinary practices among Samburu pastoralists in Kenya. Local specialists, usually elders, are called in for obstetrics, to perform foetotomies and, more rarely, caesarean sections – although most births entail little more than aiding the cow by pulling on the calf's nose as soon as it is visible. Clans are known for their specific knowledge of e.g. eye diseases, finding lost animals, or making a cow accept her calf. Samburu have great skills of disease diagnosis, e.g. they can differentiate between CBPP and other respiratory diseases. The author also notes that neighbouring Rendille place hot stones on the abdomens of animals suspected of worm infestations.

Heffernan, Claire. 1994. Livestock healthcare for Tibetan agro-pastoralists: Application of rapid rural appraisal techniques. In: Kate Kirsopp-Reed and Fiona Hinchliffe (eds). ***RRA Notes Number 20: Special Issue on Livestock.*** IIED, London, UK. Pp. 54–57.

PRA and RRA were conducted in a village of Tibetan agropastoralists of Nepal in order to understand their primary animal healthcare delivery system, cultural beliefs about livestock disease and healing, seasonal migrations, husbandry techniques and community demand for veterinary inputs. Open-ended interviews were held with key informants who were identified by villagers as being especially knowledgeable in animal healthcare and with individual stockraisers. Key informants included the son of the village animal doctor, the mayor and an animal shaman from a neighbouring village. All three easily detailed the clinical signs and seasonal occurrence of the diseases they deemed most common; but only the shaman was able to indicate disease processes in internal organs. Post-mortem signs are generally unknown due to religious restrictions on the slaughter of sick animals. Moreover, the carcasses of sick animals are never butchered and consumed; they are simply buried. Stockraiser interviewees were voluble about husbandry practises but reluctant to discuss diseases. Apparently this was partly because they felt themselves unqualified to advance an opinion, given that illness is closely linked with spiritual matters, for which certain Buddhist cleric-healers should be consulted instead. Similarly, ethnoveterinary treatments are considered the purview of these and other specialized healers. Unlike stockraisers in other parts of the world, these Tibetan interviewees claimed not to treat sick animals themselves. However, they did provide rankings, symptoms and ethnoaetiologies for what they considered their most serious animal health problems. They particularly pointed to plant poisoning from a certain lowland grass. This despite the fact that many people naming this as their main disease problem did not own the type of stock that would be exposed to it (i.e. pack yak); and those who did own pack yak all knew to avoid the poisonous grass. Key informants' rankings were quite different from ordinary stockraisers'. The former tagged diarrhoea as the number-one disease and linked it to poor nutrition. The author concludes that, for cultural-ideological reasons, stockraisers were unwilling or unable to discuss certain ills and disease details clearly. She therefore cautions that disease ranking exercises can be complex and that the resulting data should not be taken at face value divorced from their socio-cultural context.

Heffernan, Claire. 1997. Tibetan veterinary medicine. ***Nomadic Peoples*** NS 1(2): 37–54.

Written records of Tibetan veterinary medicine date from the 7th century A.D. but there are few recent descriptions. This article examines present-day animal healthcare among agropastoralists of Tibetan ancestry in two communities of northeastern Nepal. They keep bovines (yak, cattle), small ruminants, equines and in one community, camels. Both groups practise varieties of Buddhism and animal healing is strongly grounded in religion – so much so that laymen will rarely practise or even discuss it. Religion also influences animal welfare practices and special roles assigned to animals, as well as ethnoveterinary modalities. Tibetan veterinary medicine developed in tandem with its human counterpart and the two share many of the same concepts and treatments. Diseases of all species are classified according to several interlocking taxonomies, one of which groups ailments into four basic categories according to whether they are triggered by actions in a previous life, actions in this life, spirits, or diet and behaviour. In Buddhist thought, most animal ills fall under the spirit category. Negative supernatural forces are believed to cause illness by entering the body through any of the nine orifices (ears, eyes, nose, mouth, genito-urinary). To cure such ills, the highest order of animal healthcare provider is called upon, a *sngag*. This is a Buddhist lama with years of study and the power to contact spirits and divine disease aetiologies. Once he has divined the cause, the lama looks up the disease's treatment in medico-religious texts and then he proceeds accordingly. *Sngag* veterinary (and human) treatments range from exorcisms, through amulets and fetishes to be worn on the animal's neck or ears, to herbal remedies. All *sngag* treatments are accompanied by powerful *mantras*. Another type of livestock healer is the *lha-rje*, a layman who has acquired limited curative powers for specific diseases via a dream or vision and who is also familiar with Ayurvedic medicine. A *lha-rje* may also have learned a few *mantras* from a *sngag*. Any treatments involving *mantras* and herbal cures on the part of these two types of healers are accompanied by a certain sort of ceremony. Beyond their ritual components, such ceremonies often entail acts with possible biomedical benefits – such as having the patient inhale the smoke from burning paper on which *mantras* have been written, or feeding the paper to the animal along with salt and crushed barley in water. Third are Tibetan animal doctors. They are mostly former nomads and sons of nomads who are now refugees in Nepal and who acquired their ethnoveterinary knowledge from owning vast herds in Tibet before the Chinese invasion. These men have no special spiritual standing. They deal primarily in herbalism, obstetrics and minor surgery such as bloodletting. For instance, stock are usually bled before they are moved to a significantly different altitude. Also noted is the veterinary use of moxibustion, especially for lameness, fractures and abscesses. Although there are differences in the two communities' EVM customs according to their historical backgrounds, stock-raisers in both usually call in a Tibetan animal doctor first. If none is available, their next choice is a local animal healer [presumably an *lha-rje*, but the article is unclear on this point]. Only if a patient worsens or if a spiritual causation is strongly suspected do people turn to a *sngag*, as *sngag* services are very expensive. However, access to traditional animal healers today is limited because a number of such men have died and younger men are not interested in the profession. Yet even among wealthy stock-raisers, there has not been a corresponding growth in interest in Western veterinary treatments. The author hypothesizes that this is so because, while Western medicines can treat the symptoms of disease, people feel they do not address the root causes, which are spiritual. The article discusses a number of common livestock ailments, along with their ethnoaetiologies, -diagnoses and treatments, plus correlates in human ethnomedicine. To take just one example, the ailment most frequently mentioned by healers and herders alike is diarrhoea, for which they cited ethnoaetiologies ranging from witches, through poor-quality food and water, to the ingestion of plastic bags. Depending upon animal age, variety of diarrhoea diagnosed and presumably healer type, treatments may span, e.g.: placing ashes of burned juniper flowers on the muzzle for the patient to inhale the smoke; giving ground *Prunus armeniaca* seed in the feed; and to reduce accompanying fever, administering a concotion of musk-deer scent glands and a lowland camphor-based remedy in water. The article also briefly overviews: yak breeding and yak × cattle hybridization practices and preferences in the two communities; animal welfare beliefs and behaviours; and the role of 'scapegoat' animals in diverting harmful supernatural forces away from people and communities.

Heffernan, Claire, Ellen Heffernan and Chip Stem. 1996. Aspects of animal healthcare among Samburu pastoralists. In: Constance M. McCorkle, Evelyn Mathias and Tjaart W. Schillhorn van Veen (eds). ***Ethnoveterinary Research & Development.*** Intermediate Technology Publications, London, UK. Pp. 121–128.

Based on field research in 1987–88, this chapter reviews concepts of livestock disease and healing among Samburu pastoralists of northern Kenya. Four major topics were studied: (1) traditional and current management practices and productivity problems; (2) pastoralists' views on the aetiology, symptomology, prevalence, zoonotic properties and economic importance of different diseases; (3) herders' recourse to traditional versus modern veterinary medicine; and (4) Samburu knowledge of and access to the latter. Attention was also given to historical and socioeconomic aspects of livestock healthcare in the region. With regard to (2), research revealed that, relying upon clinical signs and/or post-mortem lesions, Samburu can definitively diagnose a number of livestock ills. These include, e.g.: Nairobi sheep disease and rinderpest; diseases that share very similar symptoms, like ECF versus trypanosomosis or CBPP versus other respiratory ailments; and afflictions that take acute and peracute forms, like anthrax. Elders and specialists are also expert at obstetrics and bonesetting. Samburu stockraisers are well-aware of the role of insects like ticks and flies in disease transmission and they take specific measures to avoid or combat them such as carefully selecting herding sites or burning infested rangelands. Samburu generally do not attribute livestock disease to punishment by supernatural beings. And while they do believe some animals (and people) are 'fated' from birth to fall ill or die from disease, this belief often logically attaches to animals that are weak and sickly from an early age. However, one management outcome of this belief is that Samburu rarely separate sick animals from the rest of the herd. Also, Samburu knowledge of zoonoses appears to be sketchy. Ethnotherapies span venipuncture, branding, a mastitis treatment in which sheep fat boiled in water is rubbed warm on the udder and of course herbal medicines. Examples of the latter are: *Albizia anthelmintica* or a decoction of *Kyllinga flava* for intestinal parasites; a bath of milk, water and *Psiadia punctulata* leaves to prevent lice in newborn calves; a decoction of crushed tea leaves, sugar and water as an eyewash for conjunctivitis. Concerning (3), Samburu employ both traditional and modern medicines. The latter are particularly sought-after for any newly introduced disease for which no ethnoveterinary treatments exist. Most Samburu also participate in livestock vaccination campaigns. In general, Samburu seem to be adopting more of modern medicine, but this makes for some problems. One is that, perversely, the need to earn cash in order to purchase commercial pharmaceuticals threatens livestock production by draining off key young-adult male labour for herding. Relatedly, as young men take over elders' traditional roles of knowing about and providing veterinary inputs and treatments, elders' status and authority are severely eroded, further fraying the fabric of Samburu social organization. Another problem is that the young men's knowledge of the specificity, posology and administration of commercial pharmacotherapies is at best imperfect. For example, they sometimes kill animals by overdosing or overdipping; and they often give injections at the wrong site, using the same needle and syringe for all medications on all animals, without sterilization. Moreover, pastoralists' main source of commercial pharmaceuticals is the black market, which of course offers no assurance of drug quality. Samburu difficulties with commercial drugs are exacerbated by the paucity and the technical and social-informational inadequacies of formal veterinary treatment and extension services in the region. The authors conclude that part of the solution lies in training selected herders (including elders) as paraveterinarians who could provide treatment services and drug education to their peers. Moreover, paravets could relay much-needed epidemiological intelligence to the national veterinary department. Differential training is recommended for men and women, according to their traditional pastoral roles. For example, women are in an ideal position to detect early signs of diseases specific to milk animals and to monitor and ward against certain kinds of zoonoses because women are the milkers and processors of animal products.

Herbert, W.J. 1974. ***Veterinary Immunology.*** Blackwell Scientific, Oxford, UK.

Page 4 of the chapter on 'The early history of immunology' describes *dashe*, a traditional and effective Fulani method of vaccinating cattle against CBPP. The author notes the failure of similar attempts to vaccinate cattle against rinderpest in 18th century Europe.

Hermanns, Matthias. 1948. ***Die A Mdo Pa-Grosstibeter: Die sozialwirtschaftlichen Grundlagen der Hirtenkulturen Innerasiens.*** Philosophische Fakultät der Universität Freiburg, Freiburg, Switzerland.

If a yak calf dies, the A Mdo Pa, a Tibetan people, keep its stuffed skin near the mother so that she will continue to produce milk (p. 128). Horses are usually castrated before they are a year old, either by tying the spermatic cord with a tendon or singeing it off with a hot needle; skin is never incised. The author also describes castration methods used by neighbouring peoples for horses and reindeer (pp. 231–232).

Hernández y López, Jorge A. and Abigail Aguilar Contreras. 1989. Experiencias en el estudio etnobotánico y la herbolaria medicinal en veterinaria de la región de Misantla, Veracruz. In: Gerardo López Buendía (ed.). ***Memorias: Segunda Jornada sobre Herbolaria Medicinal en Medicina Veterinaria.*** Universidad Nacional Autónoma de México, Facultad de Medicina Veterinaria y Zootecnia, Coordinación de Educación Continua, México DF, México. Pp. 20–26.

Based on a literature review followed by field research with traditional healers and local stockraisers, three aspects of ethnoveterinary practice and belief were studied among the Totonac and mestizo population of the Misantla region in Mexico's Veracruz State: (1) ailments of domestic animals, (2) animals that can cause illness in humans and (3) animal-derived *materia medica* for treating livestock and/or human diseases. With regard to (1), 16 conditions (spanning rabies, poxes, fevers, intestinal disorders, obstetric problems, ecto- and endoparasites, burns and wounds) afflicting one or more domestic species (cattle, horses, pigs, chickens, dogs) are enumerated, along with their local treatments and medicaments. The latter employ not only wild plants but also food plants, minerals (salt, sulphur, lime), lards, colostrum and in one instance, a commercial drug (terramycin). These materials may be administered as feeds, drenches, powdered topical applications, pomades, plasters, baths, washes, necklaces and in one case, an injection (of cow's milk into chickens with pox). For (2), informants listed: flies that transmit malaria; rabies and scabies from dogs; fleas; intestinal parasites; snakebite; and a unique disorder experienced by children who inhale the reek of livestock giving birth. Items in (3) included rattlesnakes and various wild avian and canine species. The authors note in passing that formal veterinary services are available only in the county seat, not in the countryside.

Herrera, Fortunato L. 1941. *Sinopsis de la Flora del Cuzco: Tomo Ia y Tomo Ib, Parte Sistemática.* Supremo Gobierno del Perú, no place of publication given. 264 and 528 pp. (two volumes).

A botanical study of the flora of Peru's Cuzco Department, these two volumes briefly mention several plants of ethnoveterinary interest, including: species that are toxic to guinea pigs (Vol. Ia, p. 239), cattle and sheep (Vol. Ib, p. 273), or camelids (*Coriaria thimifolia* HBK, known in Quechua as *miyo-miyo* or *llama-miyo*, Vol. Ib, p. 292); and an infusion of *Apurimacia incarum* Harms (Quechua *chacanhuai*), to treat liver fluke (Vol. 1b, pp. 275–276).

Hess, Carmen G. 1992. *La Racionalidad de una Economía Agropecuaria: Una Contribución hacia el Desarrollo en los Páramos Ecuatorianos – Proyecto de Fomento Ganadero-PROFOGAN.* Serie Técnica No. 2. Sistemas de Producción. Ministerio de Agricultura y Ganadería (MAG) and GTZ, Quito, Ecuador. 178 pp.

Section 3.6 of this report on the PROFOGAN livestock development project outlines the animal production system of Quechua Indians of highland Ecuador. It deals mainly with sheep and llama, although Quechua keep up to ten livestock species, including pigs, chickens, guinea pigs, cattle, donkeys, horses, mules and goats. Findings are based on 27 interviews conducted in the principal study community in 1990. The system is one of rangestock operation in which women and children see to daily grazing. Animals are given no mineral supplements. Stock are corralled nightly, sometimes in draughty wooden corrals, where they are guarded by dogs and occasionally family members. There is some attention to controlled breeding for llama, but little for sheep. Only 33% of stockraisers castrate their sheep (ideally during the new moon) and then only to tame or fatten them; 78% castrate their llama, however. For sheep, this operation is performed by an experienced family member. But for llama as well as for horses and cattle, a 'native veterinarian' called a *huihua yachac* healer (lit. 'one who is wise about animals') is hired. Sixty-seven percent dock their sheep, for reasons that include eliminating 'bad blood' from a sick or thin animal as well as for the breeding, hygiene and identification benefits of docking. In general, though, people consider sheep less able than llama to survive all such operations. Human assistance in parturition is minimal; but sometimes newborns are taken into the home during heavy storms. Overall, llama experience far fewer health problems and lower neonate mortalities than sheep. Interviewees cited conjunctivitis, pneumoenteritis, whitlow (*panadizo*) and ectoparasites as their major ovine health problems. Quechua ascribe most of these conditions to natural causes like heavy rain, cold winds, blows and introduced epidemics. But diarrhoeal and wasting diseases – due largely to endoparasitoses – are generally attributed to an animal's being near an angry human, having an unlucky owner, or drinking water touched by a rainbow. Besides salt and herbal drenches, endoparasite treatments include beating the sick animal with branches and other items in order to drive out the invading human anger, bad luck, or rainbow spirit. According to the project veterinarian, many local treatments are in fact helpful. Examples are: for conjunctivitis, salt and water; for pneumoenteritis, salt, lemon, or a drench of camomile, mint and eucalyptus leaves; for mastitis, lard applications; and for whitlow, drenching with sugarcane liquor or lemon. But this vet feels that many remedies for parasites are not effective. Yet a majority of interviewees rejected commercial endoparasiticides, believing that such drugs kill, rather than cure. However, Quechua do use some other modern veterinary pharmaceuticals. The report also mentions a few local health and husbandry practices for swine, horses, donkeys and guinea pigs. For example, *huhia yachac* successfully treat horses for wounds and glandular problems; donkeys receive special feedings of stovers; and people castrate their guinea pigs with a razor blade and then sew up the incision with needle and thread.

Hess, Carmen Gisela. 1994. *Development and Communication: Reflections on Cross-Cultural Encounters in Highland Ecuador.* Doctoral dissertation, Department of Anthropology, Harvard University, Cambridge, Massachusetts, USA. 365 pp.

Research among agropastoral Quechua Indians of Ecuador revealed how developers' ecological and veterinary appraisals of cropping and sheepraising 'clash head-on with central themes of the farmers' assessment' (p. iii). Illustrating mainly from EVM, these cross-cultural encounters are analysed for ways to promote more effective communication and cooperation between developers and farmer-stockraisers that overcome 'epistemological incompatibilities between different cultures and world views' (p. iv). The study shows that livestock development is not merely a technical matter that can be addressed in ignorance of stockraisers' overall cultural system. Even when people are keen to receive technical assistance for their stockraising, they often reject Western-scientific advice because it simply does not make sense, is impractical, or seems outright foolish in terms of ethnomedical theories. This point is illustrated by comparing Western and Quechuan beliefs and practices about genetic selection, nutrition, husbandry and healthcare of livestock plus meat and manure production (see Hess 1997). The author concludes that most local husbandry and healthcare practices (or the lack thereof) can ultimately be explained in terms of an overarching cultural notion of health as a balance of inner and outer forces. These forces are linked to disease agents that may be naturalistic (hot/cold), social (e.g. adultery, neglect of civic duties), or supernatural (mountain spirits, rainbows, sinister persons, bad luck). Thus, while some Quechuan ethnoveterinary responses may be effective from a technical point of view, others are not. All too often, agricultural and social scientists gloss over the latter because they want to demonstrate the 'rationality' of local agro-techno-ecological behaviours in Western scientific terms and/or because they do not trouble to investigate how seemingly 'irrational' practices in fact fit rationally into a people's overall worldview. The result is development failure, at the root of which lies an egregious communicative failure – not in the sense of developers' talking and listening to their clients but in an ultimate hermeneutic sense. Drawing upon the work of Paulo Freire and Jürgen Habermas, the author suggests that the only way to achieve true dialogue is to shift from instrumental to communicative rationality. First, developers must exclude all economic, political and social power differentials from their cross-cultural encounters; second, all interlocutors' worldviews must be mutually investigated, understood and accepted as equally valid by all. In the process, jointly intelligible and culturally non-offensive linguistic expressions must be identified and used; and all parties to the dialogue must be truthful and sincere. Only then, through uncoerced communication, can a democratic consensus on instrumental action – such as changes in veterinary practices – be reached.

Hess, Carmen G. 1997a. Becoming a development anthropologist. *Entwicklungsethnologie* 6(2): 77–92.

Based on the author's R&D experiences in the Ecuadorian Andes, this article illustrates the kinds of mis-communications that can occur when developers attempt, even 'successfully', to introduce new healthcare or husbandry techniques into traditional systems. Throughout the Andes, guinea pigs are usually raised in the family kitchen, where they are allowed to roam freely. A zootechnician on a project in highland Ecuador sought to introduce simple wooden dividers into guinea pig quarters in order to separate females from males and thus control their reproduction. The structure was also designed to improve hygiene. But people rejected the idea because the dividers took up too much space in the kitchen, which is where visitors are almost invariably received and entertained on cold days and nights. At last, the president of one community agreed to try the dividers in another part of his homestead. The zootechnician was gratified by the president's willingness to adopt this 'scientifically rational' approach to animal husbandry. The technician was even more elated when the president later acknowledged that his innovation in fact dramatically reduced the incidence of disease and death in his guinea pigs. However, the technician never took the trouble to investigate why the president decided to adopt the new technique in the first place, nor how the president explained the improved health of his animals. In fact, both were predicated upon Andeans' belief that the presence of upset, angry or aggressive people in the proximity of livestock can unwittingly trigger animal disease. Yet one of the main jobs of a community president in the Andes is to receive such individuals, hear them out and try to resolve their complaints. When queried by the author, the president explained that the zootechnician's suggestion seemed like a good idea because it would remove the guinea pigs to another location than the kitchen, where they were so often exposed to angry visitors. This was quite a different perception from the technician's, who had simply assumed that the president must have understood and recognized the superior scientific knowledge behind the introduced technology, along with its breeding and hygiene benefits.

Hess, Carmen G. 1997b. *Hungry for Hope: On the Cultural and Communicative Dimensions of Development in Highland Ecuador.* Intermediate Technology Publications, London, UK. 113 pp.

Revised for publication in the Intermediate Technology Publications series on Indigenous Knowledge and Development, this book covers much the same ground as the 1994 doctoral dissertation on which it is based. In illustration of the point that definitions of 'rational' animal health and production behaviours are culture-bound, the author recounts how – against their better judgment – some Quechua Indian agropastoralists of the Ecuadorian Andes allowed a development NGO to vaccinate their sheep against endoparasitoses, after which quite a number of the animals died 'from cold', said their owners. Most of the sheep would have probably died anyway. But local people took the deaths as proof of their hot/cold ethnomedical theories: injections are considered 'cooling' medicines that should be administered only for 'hot' diseases, which endoparasitism is not. The NGO's goal had been to demonstrate to people the efficacy of such injections and it went to great pains to explain everything about parasitism and its management in the local, Quechua language, to perform all procedures correctly and use high-quality vaccines. But because the NGO did not take local belief systems seriously – instead assuming that 'rational' people would see for themselves the treatment benefits – in the end it simply reinforced Quechua distrust of the technology. Beyond discussing such profound conceptual and communicative disjunctions across cultures, the book also details many health-related aspects of Quechua sheepraising. Although pastures are acutely deficient in minerals, Quechua give sheep no supplements whatsoever. Breeding is largely uncontrolled, with the result that ewes mate too young. Rams are rarely castrated and then only very late (age 14 to 18 months), often using a dirty knife and without washing the hands or applying any disinfectant; the wound is merely dressed with vegetable or pork fat to ward off 'cold'. Docking is also done late if at all and often at the wrong site to reap its hygienic and tupping benefits. Humans render ewes and lambs no pre- or post-partum assistance. However, sheep milk is prized and people do take care to milk only the best ewes and to leave enough milk for their lambs. Corrals are not kept very clean. Overall, sheep suffer from very poor health – as Quechua themselves agree. A random sample of 20% of all sheepraising households in the study village identified five major health problems of sheep, ranked by occurrence. Four of these are described. First was conjunctivitis, which if left untreated often leads to death from falls in the mountainous terrain. All respondents in the sample treated for this problem, using a variety of eyewashes they deem effective: the juice squeezed from *Alchemilla orbiculata* plants; human breast milk or llama urine; lukewarm water with salt or an antacid like Alka-seltzer or Sal Andrews; any medicine containing penicillin dissolved in the urine of a llama or a human infant; or commercial antibiotics like Terramycin or sulpha drugs. Second was ectoparasitism in the form of keds. Only a third of stockraisers said they treated for keds, whether with generic (usually DDT-based) insecticides, creosote or kerosene. They added that the results are limited. Project veterinarians observed that treatment timing is haphazard, instead of being done just after shearing. Third was diarrhoea, mainly due to enteritis or endoparasitism, which people diagnosed, respectively, by the presence of mucus or blood in the faeces. Forty-six percent reported treating this problem. A few did so successfully with veterinary antibiotics. But most did so unsuccessfully with homemade drenches of: lemon juice in water; sodium bicarbonate; infusions of eucalyptus leaves, camomile or fresh corncobs; or sulphur in a local rum. One woman's cure was to bed infected sheep for several nights on medicinal plants. Lastly, 83% of respondents said they cured footrot effectively by washing with commercial veterinary disinfectants or hydrogen peroxide, lemon juice or sugar-cane alcohol, plus massaging the foot with lard, to relieve the pain. While Quechua Indians link many of their animals' ills to climatic and other natural phenomena, ultimately they see illness in terms of a complex medical model that involves various supernatural agents, hot/cold imbalances in the body and the inborn spiritual strength of different classes and ages of animal (and humans). This model lies behind many other healthcare behaviours. For example, newborn lambs' navels are dressed with lard to stop 'cold' agents of disease (like moonlight) and other disease-causing forces from entering the body through the umbilical wound. The model provides the underlying emic rationale for all healthcare practices, whether naturalistic-seeming or not. For example, 'smelly substances' like garlic, coriander, urine, kerosene, etc. figure in many Quechuan treatments because they are believed to drive off evil spirits that can sicken animals and people. Stockraisers explain that this is why, for example, kerosene works against keds, because the keds are sent by a certain rainbow spirit. But the same model accounts for other, seemingly bizarre ethnoveterinary treatments such as beating a sick animal, bedding it on nettles or putting stinging hot pepper in its anus, for which the therapeutic goal is to make invading spirits so uncomfortable that they will depart the patients' bodies. Unless developers fully understand the internal logic of local ethnomedical theories, it will be difficult to transfer many useful Western healthcare techniques to peoples who hold non-Western models of disease causation.

Higgins, A.J. 1983. Observations on the diseases of the Arabian camel (*Camelus dromedarius*) and their control: A review. ***Veterinary Bulletin*** 53(12): 1089–1100.

Combining information from the literature and clinical experience, this review describes the aetiology, clinical findings, diagnosis, treatment, control and prevention of six classes of camel disease: protozoan, ectoparasitic, endoparasitic, viral, bacterial and fungal. Herders generally are astute at recognizing at least the acute forms of all their camels' ills; before animals reach the acute stage, however, owners often sell or slaughter them. Camel raisers also know to avoid known areas where trypanosomosis lurks, i.e. mostly wet or marshy regions where *Tabanus* spp. and other biting flies breed. If such areas are unavoidable, herders at least try to visit them only during minimal fly activity. Ethnoveterinary practices mentioned include: manually removing ectoparasites such as ticks and maggots; dressing maggot-infested wounds with a mud plaster sometimes containing various local herbs; removing bladderworms with a special tool; feeding or grazing animals on salty sand and salt-bush; vaccinating for camel-pox with a crude vaccine from scabs of infected animals, which is rubbed into the scarified lips of calves. A particularly effective milk-plus-scab emulsion is reported from India. For feared diseases such as trypanosomosis and sarcoptic mange, however, people prefer modern drugs. But they do not always understand the use of such drugs. For example, they have been known to apply undiluted acaricides directly to a camel's skin and even to drench camels with these drugs!

Hirsch kind, Lynn. 1998. Cross-cultural cows: A comparison of conceptions of cattle across time and space. In: E. Mathias, D.V. Rangnekar and C.M. McCorkle, with M. Martin (eds). ***Ethnoveterinary Medicine: Alternatives for Livestock Development – Proceedings of an International Conference Held in Pune, India, 4–6 November 1997. Volume 2: Abstracts.*** BAIF Development Research Foundation, Pune, India. Pp. 23–24.

The basic goal of ethnoveterinary R&D is to improve human well-being by improving livestock health and productivity via holistic analysis of, and consequently reasoned interventions in, animal management systems. Ideally, such analyses entail defining and understanding health and illness in terms of the biophysical, sociocultural, religious, economic, educational, political and even legislative systems in which humans and animals are embedded. In practice, however, such holism has proven elusive. Particularly seductive is the assumption that Western concepts of what a given animal species is, does and means are universal. This paper points out that these concepts vary significantly across cultures, particularly in relation to socioeconomic conditions. Ethnoveterinary researchers must fathom how animals are culturally cognized as a prerequisite to understanding how animals are positioned, interacted with and deployed in various agricultural or other livelihood systems. In illustration of this point, the author describes and compares 'the concept of cattle' in five sociocultural systems: peasant farmers of highland Ecuador, Hindu farmers of India, Nuer pastoralists, North American ranchers and Hebrew pastoralists of Biblical times. In each, the conceptual construct of cattle is traced to its agroecological/biogeographic, social, economic, cultural and historical underpinnings; and the observed (etic) system of cattle management is explained in (emic) terms of local knowledge and meanings, showing how the management system is an outcome of these multiplex underpinnings. Cattle are 'positioned' in terms of their locus in farming, herding or ranching systems, which are in turn placed in the framework of local, regional and national ecology, society, economics, culture, etc. Following Mary Douglas' work on human/animal relationships, cattle are categorized as an extension of human socio-organizational categories. Since human social organization is a variable product of multiple causation, logically the same holds true for cultural perceptions of animals. The goal of the present study is to trace out how conceptual categories of animals become concretized in livestock management and healthcare systems. The larger lesson is that the notion of a cow (or any animal domesticate) as a machine to convert kilo-calories into other, univalent or universal biological objects like meat, milk and fibre, or into monetary forms is specific to commercial ranching in urban-industrialized societies. It is not a cross-culturally valid or useful notion. Thus it can be actively misleading when applied in other settings.

Hittalagida. 1996a. Coconut, calving and conserving seeds: *Hittala Gida*. **Honey Bee** 7(1): 7.

Taken from the Kannada-language version of the *Honey Bee* newsletter, this article reports on seven ethnoveterinary measures from Kannada-speaking parts of India. To bring cows into early heat, feed them a kilogram of *munduga* (?) sprouts daily; to avoid abortion, make sure cows do not eat *banifoo* (?) leaves; to facilitate calving, feed the dams 1 kg of sugarcane trash (i.e. bagasse); for prolapsed uterus, simply push the organ back inside after first smearing your hands with the juice from several handfuls of *Mimosa pudica*; and to increase milk yields, feed dams 1 kg of cooked *byne* (?) tubers every day for a month after calving. To prevent intestinal worms in calves, give them 100 g of powdered papaya seeds in 1 l of water. To drive off cattle ticks, spread the leaves, flowers and stems of *Lantana camara* on the floor of the cattle shed.

Hittalagida. 1996b. Sour buttermilk, soothing shells and cleaning souls! *Honey Bee* 7(2): 11.

Traditional Indian treatments for two cattle disorders are described here, as reported in this Kannada-language version of the *Honey Bee* newsletter. Calves often suffer from lower jaw swellings that prevent them from eating. A traditional remedy is to burn the rim of a dry coconut shell and tie it around the calf's neck for two weeks. For bullocks with sprained necks, a paste of flakes of bath soap mixed with eggwhite is spread on the neck, where it hardens uncomfortably, causing the animal to kick out and twist about; after two or three applications, these movements set the sprain right.

Hittalagida. 1997. Mimosa restores uterus and cashew increases bio-gas. *Honey Bee* 8(3): 8.

Besides a mimosa treatment for prolapsed uterus (see Hittalagida 1996a), this article notes: a drench for bacterial infections of livestock (and humans), composed of the juices extracted from pepper, garlic and *Tylophora asthmatica* and *Capparis brevispina* leaves, given in buttermilk or goat milk; a drench to cure asthma, prepared by fermenting chopped *Withania somnifera* storage tissues, *Gynandropsis pentaphylla* leaves, *Cissus quadrangularis* stems, white onions, pepper and ginger – all placed in an earthen pot buried for several days in a manure pit and then mixed 1:1 with buttermilk to make up 1 l; and a topical wound paste made of crushed-together neem and *Acorus calamus* leaves, a few garlic cloves, several naphthalene balls and the carbon powder from used batteries.

Hittalagida. 1998. Bell the rat: Do away with the cat! *Honey Bee* 9(2): 8.

From this Kannada-language version of *Honey Bee* come the following ethnoveterinary treatments: wound dressings of mud or, alternatively, ash of burnt dried dung mixed with kerosene; for dysentery, feeding a handful of salt in cattle feed or in 4 l of water; and for expelling worms, feeding 20 crushed garlic bulbs with a pinch of salt.

Hjort, Anders. 1984. Notes from subsequent discussions with elders, Bonka Baydhabo. In: Mohamed A. Hussein (ed.). ***Camel Pastoralism in Somalia: Proceedings from a Workshop held in Baydhabo, April 8–13, 1984.*** Camel Forum Working Paper No. 7. Somali Camel Research Project, Mogadishu, Somalia and Stockholm, Sweden. Pp. 137–145.

Hjort reproduces statements of elders from camel-herding communities made during discussions at a workshop on camel pastoralism in Baydhabo, Somalia. The discussions covered various aspects of animal husbandry, breeding, marketing (also compared with other livestock species), meat and milk production and diseases. The local names of 23 diseases are presented, along with the clinical symptoms of most and the treatments for a few.

Hjort, Anders and Gudrun Dahl. 1984. Significance and prospects of camel pastoralism. In: Mohamed Ali Hussein (ed.). *Camel Pastoralism in Somalia: Proceedings from a Workshop held in Baydhabo, April 8–13, 1984.* Camel Forum Working Paper No. 7. Somali Camel Research Project, Mogadishu, Somalia and Stockholm, Sweden. Pp. 11–36.

The section on 'Management and Labour' in this workshop paper notes several health-related aspects of 'camel complex' in Africa and Arabia. In comparison with cattle, camels demand more frequent and correctly spaced 'salt cures'. Camel calves are very vulnerable to the poor nutritional quality of their dams' milk that results if herds are kept stationary. Likewise, if corrals are not moved constantly, calves easily fall prey to diseases transmitted by ticks that breed in the dung of the corrals. As preventive health measures, camel camps are moved every week to 10 days and camels are kept separate from cattle. Fodder intake of post-partum camels is carefully monitored to ensure good milk supply for calves. Birthing itself requires the attention of an experienced herder. Normally only one stallion per herd is used for breeding. Herd subdivisions and specialized care and grazing are provided for camels of different sexes and ages as well as for different species. For example, post-partum camels and their young and weak or sick animals are kept in the camp. The authors make the important point that 'The camel and camel husbandry are obviously fields which are under-researched, both from social, economic and veterinarian perspectives' (p. 31).

Hockings, Paul. 1980. *Sex and Disease in a Mountain Community.* Vikas Publishing House, New Delhi, India.

This book on human ethnomedicine and reproduction in India contains an appendix on 'Veterinary Practice' in which the author reports on suckling and health problems of buffalo and cattle and the corresponding folk therapies. For example, buffalo calves that have difficulty digesting their dam's milk are given opium or a preparation of barberry root juice, bean leaf, salt and butter; also, the calf is kept immobile after eating. To cure cattle calves of this problem, the tips of their ears are cut off. *Hotte bigiyalu* 'swollen stomach' is treated with barberry root juice and ground chili peppers. A related condition, *kundu*, is treated by an elderly man who strokes the animal with a special rod and prays, accompanied by ritual bathing and spitting. A complex cure for two contagious diseases, *be:koko* (mouth disease) and *pitcalu* (watery dung), involves entire villages' ceasing work for three days to pray while a priest or elder ritually manipulates a number of plants and oversees burnt offerings. Each day, all village cattle are made to walk through a line of bonfires. An eye ailment, *kan:belle*, is treated with tobacco juice mixed with salt and water. Finally, epidemics are attributed to sorcery by other tribes.

Hodnebo, K. 1981. *Cattle and Flies, a Study of Cattle Keeping in Equatorial Province, South Sudan, 1850–1950.* Bergen University Papers, Bergen, Norway.

Unavailable for review.

Hoffman, Matthew (ed.). 1998. *The Doctors Book of Home Remedies for Dogs and Cats.* Rodale Press, Emmaus, Pennsylvania, USA. 403 pp.

This book contains 1005 safe and useful home remedies for dogs and cats, including pet-training and grooming techniques as well as practical emergency treatments. Endorsed by a vice president of the Humane Society of the United States as 'strictly under good veterinary advice', the treatments are collected from the 'private' or 'secret' knowledge and 'own at-home pet cures' of more than 200 top veterinarians, animal trainers and breeders in the USA. The preparations and techniques employ locally available materials and are either based on longstanding tradition or are recent innovations. Examples of remedies include the use of: garlic and brewer's yeast to repel fleas; baby oil to smother ear mites; cranberry juice to relieve urinary tract infections; carrots to clean dogs' teeth; garlic to correct digestive disorders or invigorate pets; cottage cheese to assuage vomiting; vegetable oil to remove burrs; oatmeal to moisturize dry, itchy skin; petroleum jelly feedings for cats with hairballs; old clothing to keep wounds clean; a frozen rag to soothe teething pain; and a tennis ball to cure flatulence. Also noted is the selective use of over-the-counter analgesics, vitamins and other drugs for humans that can be given to pets as well. Further, the book gives home diagnostic tips, such as pinching the skin to gauge dehydration, examining the gums for signs of internal bleeding and for a variety of ills, smelling the animal's breath. For instance, a sweet, fruity scent could signal diabetes; a urine-like smell might mean kidney disease; and accompanied by vomiting, inappetence, abdominal swelling, or jaundice, a generally foul odour could indicate a liver disorder.

Holden, Sarah, Steve Ashley and Peter Bazeley. 1996. *Improving the Delivery of Animal Health Services in Developing Countries: A Literature Review.* Livestock in Development, Somerset, UK. 96 pp.

This volume tackles the debate over how best and most sustainably to deliver a variety of public- and private-good animal health services in developing countries. Based on empirical data, it explores various scenarios of the relative roles of government agencies, private enterprise and 'third-sector' entities. The latter are comprised of NGOs plus membership organizations such as cooperatives, customary institutions and other grassroots associations (e.g. associations of traditional healers). The authors note that the oldest form of animal health services consisted of locally provided prophylactic, therapeutic and curative treatments to individual stockraisers. These early clinical services were traditionally provided on a fee basis, in keeping with their private-good nature. Today they remain an important – indeed, often the only – source of veterinary advice and treatment for many people in the developing world. In some cases, these 'indigenous' clinical services have absorbed new knowledge from Western veterinary medicine and have evolved into more modern practices. In most cases, however, divided by differences in education, traditional and modern veterinary medicine have remained separate, resulting in two parallel services: one based on traditional medicine and found in rural areas; the other, the urban veterinary graduate operating in urban areas.

Holt-Wilson, Nell. 1996. *The Potential of Beekeeping as a Means for Facilitating Rural Development in the Wenchi District, Ghana.* MSc thesis, IERM, University of Edinburgh, Edinburgh, UK. 56 pp.

Bees can live in cavities that are dark, cool, stable and large enough for expansion – in other words, in environs that mimic hollows in tree boles. Therefore clay pots, gourds, barrels, hollowed logs and jerrycans can all be adapted to house bees. Bee shelters are as varied as the environments in which bees are kept. In Ghana, calabashes are hollowed out and several small holes are drilled in the shell for bees to enter and leave. The neck of the calabash is baited with wax, cow dung, lavender and the froth of millet or maize beer. The calabash is then hung in a shady place (e.g. in a tree or under the eaves of a house), where a swarm will usually colonize it within weeks.

Honey Bee. 1991. Animal husbandry practices. *Honey Bee* 2(1): 20–22.

Traditional Indian veterinary and husbandry practices are described in this article along with prescriptions for FMD, ulcers, rabies, urinary disorders, retention of placenta, ectoparasites and fractures. Methods to prevent, control and cure FMD are particularly diverse. As an FMD prophylaxis, people may drench the cattle with wine in the belief that the wine will keep the disease at bay, just as good Brahmins avoid alcohol. FMD therapies include: rubbing the hooves and mouth with a boiled salt solution, with jaggery, with a paste of *Clerodendrum multiflorum* leaves, or with tobacco seeds and camphor pellets; pouring fresh milk over the hooves; doing likewise with lime water and also standing the animals in lime water; feeding *bajra* (?) with edible oil for 3 to 4 days, or the macerated, crushed bark of the *Commiphora mukul* and *Butea monosperma* trees, or 50 g of *Trachyspermum ammi* L. with 100 g of jaggery and 25 g of tea powder all suspended in 0.5 l of water; tying fresh *Capparis decidua* tree tips boiled in oil between the cleft of the hoof; walking the animals through, or tethering them in, hot sand; and placing fish scales in the manger. Animals with rabies-like symptoms are fed *Calotropis procera* leaves. Stock having difficulty urinating are drenched with a filtered decoction of barley or lemon water and once urination begins, with plain tea. Retained placenta is prevented by immediate post-partum feeding of several *Abrus precatorius* seeds with boiled *bajra* or a decoction of *Syzygium cumini* bark. Ectoparasites like ticks and lice are a problem during winter and in arid areas, when stock are not shorn and where water for bathing the animals is scarce. Treatments consist of topical application over the entire body of 5 g of tobacco powder in 50 g of edible oil, or of kerosene in edible oil. Neck ulcers on newly trained bullocks are dressed with powdered *C. decidua* wood charcoal or with boiled and cooled edible oil. Fractures are dressed with honey, ghee and a few goat hairs and then tightly bandaged; alternative dressings are a mixture of salt, jaggery and turmeric powder or a paste of macerated *Sisymbrium* sp. seeds. Also noted are various drought-resistant fodders used by Indian stockraisers, including: *Acacia arabica* pods; leaves of *Azadirachta indica, Leucaena leucocephala, Madhuca latifolia, Mangifera indica, Sesbania sesban* and *Soymida febrifuga*; *Tamarindus indica* twigs and leaves; and *moth* (?) tubers.

Honey Bee. 1992a. Animal husbandry practices. *Honey Bee* 3(1): 17–18.

Various local Indian treatments are reported here, along with observations on them by Indian livestock specialists. In the early stages of a disease known as *galsundha*, characterized by a swelling of the throat, the patient is fed dried *Madhuca indica* flowers and crushed *Phoenix sylvestris* bark along with green fodder in an amount of 150 to 250 g per day, with the bulk of this being the bark. The animal swallows this feed very slowly due to the bark's offensive smell and the patient's painful throat. Traditional animal doctors (*deshi*) treat more advanced cases of *galsundha* by feeding 150 to 200 g of the foregoing flowers and bark pounded together with *karval* (?) spines, *Holarrhena antidysenterica* bark and either the bark or fruit of *Dendrophthoe* spp. Alternatively, *deshi* may paste pounded *karval* spines externally on the swollen parts of the throat. These treatments are continued every 1 or 2 days until recovery, reportedly usually in about a week. Flatulence is a particular problem for livestock during the monsoon season in India. Remedies include oral administration of: onions and *Annona squamosa* leaves in whey; equal quantities of onions and turmeric powder mixed in twice the volume of whey; 200 g of onion, 100 g of *ajma* (?) and an unstipulated quantity of the aerial roots of the banyan tree, *Ficus benghalensis*; 100 g each of pounded onions and *Scilla* spp. bulbs, after first smearing the patient's tongue with salt; and 100 g of edible oil, 200 g of water and 10 g of kerosene. Scientists note that most of these ingredients have one or more actions, as surfactants, carminatives, stimulants or antibacterials; and reportedly scientists wholeheartedly endorse the onion and turmeric remedy. A soothing and carminative remedy for gastric disorders is to feed 10 g of *asafoetida* in 500 g of edible oil. Constipation can be cured in a day by feeding a paste of *Gardenia resinifera* leaves and *Dendrophthoe falcata* seeds; the latter are known to have a laxative effect and to store well. An alternative treatment for constipation is to feed a mixture of *Salvadora* spp. leaves, boiled wheat and *Acacia* spp. pods.

Honey Bee. 1992b. Animal husbandary [sic]. *Honey Bee* 3(2): 20–22.

Numerous Indian treatments for livestock are listed here, with commentary on many of them by Indian animal scientists and veterinarians. For bovine FMD, remedies consist of: washing the hooves with warm salt solution and then applying ash from burning old leather shoes that has been sieved through cotton cloth and mixed with sesame or groundnut oil; likewise applying 50 ml of juice from the fresh tips of *Pongamia pinnata* branches, a plant that scientists note has antiseptic, maggoticide and insect-repellent properties; pasting the hooves for several days with *Diospyros cordifolia* fruits that have been warmed in hot ashes and then crushed and cooled; and applying 50 to 100 ml of oil from boiled *Schleichera oleos* fruits to the hooves and inside the mouth, and then withholding food and water for a couple of hours. As an FMD prophylaxis, cattle are fumigated with smoke from burning fish; alternatively, they can be fed dried fish with wheat bread. Skin diseases are treated by: spraying spent, boiled engine oil on the skin – which scientists say is effective for mange; and for dry skin, bathing the animal with warm water and then applying fresh *Clerodendrum phlomidis* leaf juice. Nose drops of *Solanum surattense* fruit juice are given for colds; and for fevers, an aqueous drench of powdered *Soymida febrifuga* bark. Diarrhoea treatments span: feeding 10 kg of boiled *Paspalum scrobiculatum* millet; amputating a portion of the tail and boiling it in oil; branding and acupuncture; and for especially malodorous diarrhoea, drenching for 3 to 5 days with a filtered decoction of the thorny weed,

Echinops echinatus. Scientists are dubious about the benefits of all these diarrhoea remedies, however. Likewise for a drench of donkey faeces in water as a remedy for food-poisoning, which usually stems from excessive ingestion of castor leaves or immature sorghum. Treatments for urinary and respiratory problems, respectively, are: drenching with 500 g of sodium bicarbonate in 1 l of water; and 3-to 4-day feedings of ruptured *Corchorus* spp. leaves to work oxen with laboured breathing. Using the same schedule, cattle and buffalo cows that fail to come into heat or to conceive are fed several *Semecarpus anacardium* seeds or fruits; available from consumer stores, these feeds are said by farmers to cure the problem in less than 2 weeks.

Honey Bee. 1993a. Animal husbandry. *Honey Bee* 4(1): 13–16.

This article lists treatments for ten disorders of livestock in India, along with scientists' commentary on whether elements of the treatments are valuable or not. Here, their commentary is summarized in a parenthetic 'yes', 'no', or 'maybe'. Two FMD remedies are described and evaluated as follows: walking the animals on hot riverbed sand (no) and then washing the hooves with a neem decoction (yes); and applying a paste of equal proportions of fresh *Aristolochia bracteolata* and *Annona squamosa* leaves to the hooves (maybe, due to the hydrocyanide content of the latter). Treatments for prolapsed uterus in late pregnancy are: washing the organ with fresh onion juice (no, the juice is an antiseptic but also an irritant), replacing the organ (yes), forcing the cow to stand (yes, this relieves abdominal pressure) and then feeding 2 to 3 kg of boiled *Amorphophallus campanulatus* tuber (yes, because the tubers have stomachic, carminative, tonic, emmenagogue, nutritional and other properties). In addition, a rope net may be tied around the body to keep the organ in place (yes, this is also a standard scientific practice); and the cow may be kept in her shed in such a way that her rear end is elevated (yes). To stimulate first heat, across 8 to 10 days heifers are fed 10 kg each of pearl millet and *Vigna aconitifolia* boiled in water (no comments). For retained placenta, cows are fed: fresh *Madhuca indica* flowers, crushed and heated over a slow flame or dried and then soaked in water, in combination with 500 g of *Garcinia indica* fruit extract and 2 to 3 kg of cooked rice. An alternative is a dry fodder with 1 kg of pearl millet or wheat and some ghee, all in hot water. Farmers swear by the first of these two treatments and note that cows who graze pastures where *M. indica* grows rarely suffer from retained placenta; they add that larger quantities of *G. indica* can be toxic. Scientists point out that such 'compare and contrast' observations on farmers' part is one way that local technical knowledge is developed and evaluated. Skin diseases of cattle are treated with a paste of scrapings from the inner bark of *Acacia nilotica*, applied for 7 to 10 days. Datura leaves pounded with jaggery (cooked crystallized sugarcane extract) are plastered over tumours; with several successive applications, reportedly the tumour bursts (no comments). Broken horns are mended by bandaging them with long strands of human hair and pasting a preparation of *Bombax ceiba* and *Eleusine coracana* over the broken edges (no comments). Diarrhoea is treated with drenches of crushed *Ventilago denticulata* root and *Syzygium cumini* bark in water, or fresh *Soymida febrifuga* leaves that have been soaked in water for an hour (no comments). Open wounds are dressed with: 100 to 150 g of curd mixed with 25 g of natural indigo (yes, *Indigofera articulata* has antihelminth properties), but indigo is becoming difficult to find; a paste of the ash from burning together small pieces of old shoe leather, coconut meat and tar (maybe, thanks to tannin in the leather); or a paste of the leaves of *A. squamosa* (yes, see above) and *Momordica charantia* (yes, due to alkaloids). Ulcerated hooves are dressed thrice daily for several days with a hot paste of fresh jaggery (no comments). Special feeds and fodders are given for a variety of purposes: *Prosopis cineraria* and *Acacia nilotica* pods, to heighten milk production (maybe); fresh primordia and immature cotton bolls, to increase the fat content of milk (yes, due to the high fat content of the bolls and the laxative and lactogenic effects of cotton seed); cactus and other xerophytic plants that have been cleaned of thorns, pounded, soaked in water and mixed with molasses and salt, to diminish stress during periods of scarce forage (maybe); likewise for 2 kg of dried *M. indica* flowers boiled with cotton bolls (yes, the flowers are rich in sugar and the Indian Veterinary Research Institute at Izantnagar recommends feeding buffalo madhuca seed cake); and dried datepalm nuts, to enhance the performance of work oxen (no comment).

Honey Bee. 1993b. Animal husbandry and livestock. *Honey Bee* 4(2&3): 22–24.

A variety of Indian ethnoveterinary practices are reported here. People give constipated cattle 250 g of dried *Terminalia chebula* fruits in 1 l of water. Diarrhoea is combatted by drenching with 100 to 200 g of *Ficus hispida* root filtrate for 2 to 3 days. Calves with worms receive a drench of pounded *Asparagus* sp. roots early in the morning or feedings of pounded *Enicostema hyssoplifolium*; also, infested calves' milk intake may be restricted. A widely known appetite stimulant for all stock, but especially after parturition or illness, is a daily, 8-to-10-day-long drench of 100 g of white alum dissolved in water. To enhance milk yield and butterfat content, cows are regularly fed leaves and twigs of the *Taverniera cuneifolia* tree (also said to reduce the time between calvings), *Tinospora* sp. and other forest vines, or pounded fennel seeds soaked in water. A filtered decoction of 400 g each of empty cotton bolls and roots boiled in 2 to 3 l of water and given several times at half-hour intervals reportedly triggers prompt expulsion of the placenta. To prevent prolapse of the uterus, farmers feed cows castor oil, jaggery and a certain clay in varying combinations and doses, according to the stage of pregnancy and the severity of parturition problems. The latex of *Argemone mexicana* applied twice daily for several days cures septic wounds; alternatives are a paste of mercuric oxide in sesame oil or crushed *Aristolochia bracteata* leaves. Different sides of a *sundarsol* (?) leaf heal clean wounds and boils. A 1:1 mix of sesame oil and sugar is rubbed on arthritic parts of camels twice daily for several days. In the very early stages of rabies, feeding the afflicted dog 10 leaves of *Calotropis* sp. and jaggery several times hourly may be helpful. General poultry remedies are made of each of the following items, pounded and given in the birds' drinking water: a certain bark known as *beda*; onion; rice smeared with kerosene; *Curcuma* sp. tuber; and *Cuscuta reflexa*.

Honey Bee. 1993c. Honey bee hums. *Honey Bee* 4(2&3): 16.

Both farmer and scientist readers of this Indian journal of local knowledge recommend the following as cattle feeds to relieve stress, promote weight gain and/or increase milk yields or butterfat content: the lower fronds of coconut palm leaves; the boiled tubers and stem-bark of tapioca; mango peels and kernels; and 600 g of powdered *Prosopis juliflora* seeds mixed 1:10 with rice bran, fed twice weekly.

Honey Bee. 1993d. Livestock and animal husbandry. *Honey Bee* 4(4): 17.

Readers of this journal wrote in with the following local livestock treatments in India. To prevent yoke galls on a new bullock, first apply a paste of burnt *Cordia* sp. ash in water to the parts of the body where the yoke will rest. Fumigation of the mouth area by burning sloughed-off material from horses' hooves is said to relieve the buccal lesions of FMD. To prevent abortion, at the first signs of pregnancy daily give the animal 500 g of crushed *Limonium acidissima* leaves with 200 g of sugar in 1 l of water, for 21 days. A swollen udder can be relieved in 24 hours by 200 g of termite soil in boiled water (whether administered as a drench or a wash is unclear). An effective poultice for fractures in humans as well as livestock is two spoonfuls of turmeric powder mixed with one egg, applied to the fracture site and covered with *Cordia gharaf* leaves and a bandage. An alternative is to dress the site with soft, partially baked bread of *Eleusine coracana* and bandage it with *akota*-tree bark.

Honey Bee. 1996. Indigenous knowledge about a plant parasite: Vakumba (Makar) a parasitic plant of tobacco. *Honey Bee* 7(4): 6.

In India, a parasitic plant known locally as *vakumba* or *makar* (?) attacks the root of tobacco plants. Small quantities of this plant's shoots are fed to cattle to improve milk quality. However, this practice promotes the parasite's spread to other fields, as its spores pass undigested into cattle dung.

Hooft, Katarina van't. 1988. *Investigación Preliminar de la Producción Avícola a Nivel Casera.* Project Report MIDINRA (Ministry of Agriculture and Land Reform), Esteli, Nicaragua. 10 pp.

Based on 2 months' field interviews in 1988 with 18 men and women poultry raisers in 14 rural communities of Nicaragua's Estelí zone plus clinical observation and lab sampling among their flocks, this manuscript describes local systems of poultry management: flock composition, breeds, reproduction rates, feeds, infrastructure, production and earnings, diseases, treatments used and poultry-raising customs and beliefs in general. Findings of ethnoveterinary interest include the following. Only people producing eggs for sale use any commercial feed supplements; but at times, even they cannot afford such supplements. The birds are not cooped at any time. Hens are generally culled after 1.5 to 2 years of production. Inbreeding is a problem, but is not locally recognized as such. Fleas, mites and endoparasites are universal in Estelí flocks. Every 6 to 8 years, all the birds in a community may be wiped out by an outbreak of infectious disease such as Newcastle, coryza, or cholera. Other common but less devastating diseases are fowl pox, 'white diarrhoea' (possibly salmonellosis) and a respiratory condition called *moquillo* 'distemper'. Chicks in particular suffer from the depredations of coyotes, foxes and hawks; and a number die from being accidentally stepped on by pigs and people. Vampire bats injure chickens of all ages; and theft is a big problem. In general, people appeared to know little about preventing or controlling disease in their flocks, whether by traditional or modern means. However, they reported several popular treatments for *moquillo*: placing drops of lemon juice, cooking oil, castor or other oils on the birds' beaks; and putting *achiote*, salt, or Sulfathiazol in their drinking water. Research also revealed that when poultry raisers do decide to take treatment measures, women usually have recourse to home remedies. Men are more likely to use commercial drugs, especially antibiotics.

Hooft, Katrien van't. 1995. *Interface between Local Knowledge and Western Scientific Knowledge in Family Level & Extensive Livestock Keeping: Research Based on 2 Casestudies in Nicaragua and Bolivia.* MSc thesis in Management of Agricultural Knowledge Systems, Wageningen Agricultural University, Utrecht, The Netherlands. 168 pp.

Based on several years' research with a variety of groups practising extensive stockraising in Nicaragua and Bolivia, this thesis explores how local and Western knowledge of animal husbandry and healthcare interact from both farmers' and extensionists' viewpoints. Findings revealed that in responding to variable macro- and micro-influences in their social, economic and political environments, both these actor groups combine both types of knowledge, although farmers are the more dynamic in this regard. Certainly, stockraisers are not interested only in re-evaluating their local knowledge. They themselves recognize that it is not always adequate to cope with changing circumstances. Thus they are eager to learn about new options, which they can selectively blend into their existing production systems. The author warns that development projects that draw upon solely one or the other kind of knowledge are bound to fail. After a critical review of existing sociology-of-knowledge theory, development attitudes toward variant knowledge bases and related topics, this thesis discusses its multi-pronged methodological approach. It then presents two country case studies. A sampling of findings is as follows. In general, all Nicaraguan farmers except absentee landowners maintain and use traditional knowledge of veterinary treatments (e.g. for mastitis and intestinal disorders) and range ecology (e.g. poisonous plants, field management for livestock nutrition). However, wealthier farmers are more open to Western technologies that involve purchased inputs like urea and molasses or crossbred dairy cattle. Poorer farmers with smaller herds use more labour-intensive strategies. For example, they store maize stover and bean threshings for dry-season fodder, whereas richer farmers simply graze their stock on these crop byproducts in the fields. Poorer farmers are more open to adopting new but low- or no-cost strategies on analogy to their existing ones, such as improved conservation measures for storing feed sorghum or cultivation of dryland sugarcane for forage. Women raise backyard pigs and poultry, with wealthier households receiving and responding to more extension attention. Examples of EVM mentioned for Nicaragua are: applying lemon and salt on the skin between hooves infected by a spider bite; using other plants to treat retained placenta and calf diarrhoea; to control ticks, burning cattle dung in the corrals where stock are quartered overnight; giving lemon juice and unspecified herbs for various chicken diseases; plastering and splinting fractures with the leaves and bark, respectively, of a certain tree; castrating bulls only during the waning moon so as to reduce bleeding and packing the wound with salt so that the added pain will limit the steer's movement for several days; and surgically correcting undescended testicles in horses. This last operation is performed by local castration specialists. These individuals also employ herbal medicines and they have learned to handle some modern veterinary techniques such as injections. Moreover, all said they are interested to acquire more Western veterinary skills. In Bolivia, three different ethnic groups were studied in the same Amazon lowlands: one forest Indian tribe, the Yuracaré; and two immigrant groups, consisting of Trinitarios from the Beni plateau and Colonos from the Andean highlands. Yuracaré only recently adopted pigs and chickens, although they have long raised dogs and tamed wild animals such as turkeys and a certain 'wild chicken'. The latter are kept for killing snakes and sounding the alarm when predators approach, while dogs provide general protection for livestock and people. Yuracaré attribute diseases to evil spirits and curses, which their ethnoveterinary treatments of purging, bloodletting and fumigating are designed to remove. So far, Yuracaré have had virtually no access to Western veterinary medicine. Trinitarios had a long tradition of stockraising in their Beni homeland, which they continued in the lowlands. However, all their cattle and horses were lost in a flood. At the time of research, women were raising pigs and poultry, as well as gardens of medicinal herbs with which to treat them. As a group, Trinitarios have little recourse to modern medicine for livestock. Colonos came to the area with extensive EVK, but because of the sharply different Amazonian agroecology they could not put much of it into practice. Indeed, they could not maintain their ruminants or guinea pigs in the new environment, where they were reduced to only pigs and poultry. Even with these species, they encountered entirely new health problems, such as vampire bats that bite sows' teats so severely that they cannot nurse. In their new circumstances, Colonos are understandably more open to Western techniques, such as new types of chicken coops and breeds and occasional veterinarian visits for pigs. In the latter case, however, Colonos endeavour to learn the vet's techniques so they can apply them themselves thereafter. When queried at an extension event about their home remedies for livestock, Colonos told the author [a veterinarian] 'We have not come all this way to talk about what we already know. We want to hear what you know' (p. 134). They agreed to exchange knowledge on this basis. An example of Colonos' EVM is a variety of treatments for canine demodicosis that consist of rubbing the skin with various combinations of kerosene, creolene, a crop insecticide and black machine oil. After the author responded to a demand for a Western treatment for this problem, Colonos tried it and declared they preferred it. They found it had fewer side effects than their home remedies and yet was cost-effective for their much-esteemed dogs, who protected their chickens. Also described in this thesis is the author's work with paravet programmes in the two countries.

Hooft, Katrien van't. 1996. Farmers, extensionists and the relation between indigenous knowledge and scientific knowledge in extensive livestock production: Experiences from Latin America. *Indigenous Knowledge and Development Monitor* 4(1): 17.

In studying six different groups in Bolivia and Nicaragua, the author found that all combined indigenous and modern/scientific stockraising knowledge and inputs in one way or another. Thus, separating the two kinds of knowledge is a sterile exercise. Rather, development efforts should focus on assisting stockraisers to find the right balance between the two. Outsiders like technicians and extensionists can help people analyse and experiment with all available options, but the final decision as to what mix of technologies and practices to adopt should (and does) rest with the stockraiser. Especially for extensive stockraising in the South, 'modern' technologies – which were elaborated mainly for intensive production in the North – may not all be appropriate for smallholders' situation. For example, modern veterinary medicine may have few practical and economic responses to parasitic diseases of livestock raised under a low-input rangestock regime. On the other hand, indigenous knowledge may be stymied in the face of epidemics like Newcastle disease.

Hooft, Katrien van't. 1999. Relation between ethnoveterinary and western knowledge in family-level livestock keeping (examples from Bolivia). In: E. Mathias, D.V. Rangnekar and C.M. McCorkle, with M. Martin (eds). *Ethnoveterinary Medicine: Alternatives for Livestock Development – Proceedings of an International Conference Held in Pune, India, 4–6 November 1997. Volume 1: Selected Papers.* BAIF Development Research Foundation, Pune, India. Pp. 25–29.

Animals are vital to the survival of the vast majority of rural Bolivian families, who rely upon a wide range of food and work animals (cattle, sheep, goats, pigs, guinea pigs, donkeys, horses, chickens) in close conjunction with other agricultural and non-agricultural products and activities. Their stockraising, cropping and off-farm strategies combine both traditional and modern methods in a mix that is almost as varied as the number of families themselves. The growing need for cash, which touches even the most remote rural village, has forced this mix. The influence of a cash economy is also reflected in local human and veterinary medical practice. To understand the relation between traditional and modern veterinary medicine in such contexts, one must look at stockraising under different, family-level circumstances taking into account the following variables at a minimum: market versus non-market objectives in stockraising; different uses of different species; industrialized-style intensification in one species while still raising others under traditional management regimes; family members' differential livestock management and decisioning responsibilities; family-wide socioeconomic circumstances, stockraising objectives and changes in both these factors; ecological conditions and shifts; cultural and religious considerations; the influence of development projects; basic characteristics of the health problems confronting each livestock species; and availability of Western versus traditional veterinary medicines and experts. In Bolivia, the rapid loss of EVK is a sad reality that argues for urgent interventions to counteract this process; but EVK research in Bolivia has been limited by researchers' general ignorance of ethnoveterinary alternatives due to the hegemony of Western-style education and, for the few researchers working in ethnoveterinary R&D, their isolation from the scientific mainstream. Moreover, once embarked on ER&D, researchers and developers must also beware of falling into a merely academic exercise that ignores family survival strategies, which combine traditional and Western elements to fit their specific livelihood circumstances.

Horowitz, Michael M. 1982. On listening to herders: An essay on pastoral demystification. In: *Third International Symposium on Veterinary Epidemiology and Economics – Arlington, Virginia, USA, 6–10 September 1982.* Veterinary Medicine Publishing Company, Edwardsville, Kansas, USA. Pp. 416–425.

In discussing livestock development among nomads in the dry tropics, this paper debunks popular myths about herders' behaviours and production outcomes, such as irrational herd-size expansion, low herd productivity, rapacious exploitation of rangelands and backward-bending supply curves. The author notes that strictly veterinary interventions enjoy a much higher level of development attention and nomad acceptance than most other kinds of Western livestock interventions, e.g. in range management or in off-range marketing infrastructure and strategies like feedlots, abattoirs, herder co-ops, etc. In a nutshell, nomads often reject such Western-centric management notions because they provide no increased (and frequently only decreased) benefits for herd health, nutrition, production and/or income over and above traditional practices. A case in point is herders' gentle burning of rangelands, which discourages scrub and therefore keeps down pests and associated pest-borne diseases while at the same time encouraging the growth of grasses. The benefits to livestock of burning, as described in several in-depth technical studies, include: a regrowth of more biomass of higher quality; maintenance of grass tussocks, which burning leaves untouched due to their green foliage and isolation; and an increase in available protein from under 5% to about 20%. Failure to 'listen to herders' on the ecological rationale and the many benefits of such traditional practices 'leads to inevitable and unnecessary conflict between project officials and . . . producers' (p. 420). The author encourages veterinarians to pay more attention to herders' opinions on such topics, and gives as an example the complex relationships between particular animal health, nutritional and disease statuses and seasonal cycles of climate, water quantity, fodder quality and thus herder movements and behaviours. In particular, based on his extensive field experience in the dry tropics of West Africa, the author reports that herders perceive veterinarians as being disinterested in nutrition-related diseases. For example, pastoralists have long recognized a certain nutritional syndrome linked to the young grass of the early rainy season. But this problem (a cobalt deficiency) was not 'discovered' by national researchers until the 1980s and then only thanks to discussions with herders. For dealing with such to-them-familiar conditions, nomads typically have practical experience that can be helpful in designing more universal solutions. Thus herders trained as veterinary assistants or auxiliaries can help provide a cost-effective animal health delivery system. The paper concludes that the already-good record of veterinary medicine in livestock development can be further improved by firmly grounding veterinary science in the ecology and sociology of pastoral production.

Horst, K. ter. 1986. Poultry improvement in rural areas of developing countries: Matching technical demands with social facts. Unpublished manuscript. The Netherlands Assisted Poultry Improvement Project, Department of Livestock Services (Poultry), Ministry of Livestock and Fisheries, Dhaka, Bangladesh. 50 pp.

In Bangladesh, chickens are marketed for a variety of reasons, beyond an immediate need for cash. These include disease, poor productivity, unmanageably large flocks, or imbalances in flock composition. Excess male birds, pullets, old layers, non-productive hens and large birds are all candidates for sale. In other words, poultry sales are part of an overall husbandry strategy for controlling health and other problems by culling undesirable birds from the flock.

Horwood, David. 1998. A gene for fluke resistance? *Partners in Research for Development* 11(May): 10–11.

Drawing upon research initiated in 1990 by a team of Indonesian and Australian scientists, another such team working in Java later confirmed that the Indonesian Thin Tail sheep breed is resistant to the tropical liver fluke *Fasciola gigantica*. Moreover, once exposed to this parasite, Thin Tails acquire immunity. In other words, they do not merely have some physiological defence system but rather are innately immune. Further research revealed that this resistance is controlled by a major gene. This means that eventually the gene could be introduced into other livestock species that lack such immunity. Similar breeds of sheep in Malaysia and Thailand might be likewise immune.

HPI. 1989. Vaccine against rinderpest. *Heifer Project Exchange: Appropriate Livestock Technology for a Developing World* 51(Nov/Dec): 2.

This brief note describes a new rinderpest vaccine developed in the US for on-farm use. Once one animal has been immunized with the vaccine, more vaccine can be obtained simply by scratching this animal's abdomen to form a scab. The scab is then removed, soaked in saline solution and inserted into an incision made for this purpose on another animal.

HPI. 1990. Stable fly control. *Heifer Project Exchange: Appropriate Livestock Technology for a Developing World* 52(Jan/Feb): unpaginated.

A biological pest control for flies and some ticks can be prepared from herbal ingredients that leave no chemical residues in milk. It is made by grinding into a paste 4 kg each of old neem leaves, sliced *Languas Galanga* roots and the stems and leaves of citronella grass, adding 40 l of water as grinding progresses. This mixture is then stored overnight and then filtered. The resulting solution is mixed with water in a ratio of 1: 40–60 and sprayed on buildings, grounds, or directly onto animals.

HPI. 1992. Strip cup. *Heifer International Exchange: Appropriate Livestock Technology for a Developing World* 67(Jul/Aug): 3.

A study from an unidentified country showed that chickens are valuable for parasite control, in that they eat large numbers of ticks from the ground, where more are to be found than on herd animals; but chickens also peck ticks directly off of recumbent cattle.

HPI. 1993a. Strip cup. *Heifer International Exchange: Appropriate Livestock Technology for a Developing World* 70(Jan/Mar): unpaginated.

Rabbits raised in cages are particularly prone to parasitism. To keep away ants and disease-bearing pests, free-standing raised cages can be built on stilts steeped in used motor oil. Also noted is an effective dewormer for goats made from diluting a paste of *Leucaena leucocephala* seeds in water.

HPI. 1993b. Strip cup. *The Heifer Project Exchange: Appropriate Livestock Technology for a Developing World* 72(Jul/Sep): 3.

Scientists in the US have discovered that chickens can control weeds in Michigan orchards as effectively as herbicides. Not only do the chickens cut farmers' costs thereby; they also provide another marketable product. Similar research on geese as a means of controlling weeds and diversifying income are underway in Alaska.

HPI. 1994. Strip cup. *The Heifer Project Exchange: Appropriate Livestock Technology for a Developing World* 74(Jan/Mar): 3.

A project at the Asian Rural Institute recommends mixing 1% charcoal, by weight, in with animal feeds as an effective digestive. A by-product of charcoal production, wood vinegar, is also given to chickens as a coccidiosis prophylactic.

HPI/India. 1995. *Booklet on Indigenous Medicines for the Treatment of Simple Diseases of Ruminants.* HPI/India, New Delhi, India. 34 pp.

This booklet divides the Indian veterinary pharmacopoeia into six categories of materials: alkaline (e.g. sodium carbonate), acidic (e.g. hydrochloric acid), metallic (e.g. copper sulphate), vegetable (including kitchen spices such as pepper, coriander, clove), animal (e.g. horse hair) and oils/fats (including vaseline). An example of a metallic treatment is the removal of warts by using a matchstick to drip 2 or 3 crystals of copper sulphate in water on the wart. An alternative treatment using animal materials is to cut off blood supply to the wart by tightly tying a thread of three strands of horse hair around it, after which the wart will eventually dry up and fall off. With regard to vegetable materials, some 50 plants used to treat nine classes of ruminant disease are listed.

HPI/Philippines. n.d. Common (Philippine) and scientific names of medicinal plants, plant parts used, ailments, methods of preparation and administration and approximate dosages. Photocopied handout. HPI, Manila, Philippines. 9 pp.

As per its title, this photocopied handout presents useful Filipino prescriptions for treating livestock ills. The prescriptions employ a total of 61 wild or cultivated plants spanning vegetable, spice, oil and fruit as well as other species. These are employed to make 70 remedies, some of which call for other ingredients like salt and sugar. All but 10 of the 70 prescriptions employ only a single botanical. Modes of preparation generally involve one or two of the following: decoction, infusion, chopping, pounding, crushing, drying, roasting, carbonizing and expelling juice or sap. Routes of administration listed are oral (drenches, feed additives) or topical (plasters, rubs, washes and baths). Examples of general health conditions treated are: respiratory, gastrointestinal, urinary, dermatological and udder disorders; fevers, sprains and muscular fatigue; endo- and ecto-parasitoses; wounds; agalactia, anorexia and dehydration. More specific diseases noted are swine erysipelas, swine and fowl pox and vitamin C deficiency. The handout was elaborated and disseminated to HPI-trained paravets in order to supplement their arsenal of modern veterinary treatments with local ones reported to be effective. [See also Catchero and Orprecio n.d.]

Hsia, L.C. and J.H. Lee. 1989. Inducing oestrus by acupuncture. *Animal Husbandry and Agricultural Journal* Apr: 18,20,21.

Acupuncture, moxibustion, aqua-acupuncture and electro-acupuncture can all be used for various livestock ills. In Taiwan, acupuncture is employed to induce oestrus in pigs. It is simple, cheap, natural and effective. The animal comes into oestrus a week after treatment.

Huanca, Teodosio. 1985. Sanidad de alpacas. *Minka* 16(Mar): 24–25.

This article describes 12 parasitic and infectious diseases that commonly attack alpaca in the Andes. Although the author offers only standard Western veterinary advice on treatment and prevention, he gives the indigenous disease name both in southern Peruvian Quechua and local Spanish for some of the ailments, including: *qarachi* (mange, Spanish *sarna*), *wiksa kuru* (verminous gastroenteritis), *ichu kuru* (verminous bronchitis), *bolsa* or *qocha* (hydatidosis), *q'echa* (coccidiosis), *k'utu* (sarcocystosis), *q'echa* (diarrhoea) and *q'oto* (osteomyelitis of the lower jaw).

Hughes, Ian. 1977. *New Guinea Stone Age Trade: The Geography and Ecology of Traffic in the Interior.* Terra Australis 3. Department of Prehistory, Research School of Pacific Studies, Australian National University, Canberra, Australia.

Pages 112–114 describe New Guineans' trade in an edible earth known as *mondono*. They mix *mondono*, a whitish powder, with sweet potatoes and feed it as a tonic to their pigs to fatten them. *Mondono* is probably the natural weathering product of the local rock, granodiorite.

Hunter, A.G. 1986. Urine odour in a camel suffering from surra (*T. evansi* infection). *Tropical Animal Health and Production* 18: 148–156.

Probably the most serious infection of camels is surra, i.e. trypanosomosis caused by *Trypanosoma evansi*. Bedouin in North Africa and camel keepers in Sudan and India's Punjab have all long been known to diagnose surra by smelling suspect animals' urine. Recent observations by veterinarians in Sudan and Somali confirm camel owners' ability to do so accurately. The author notes that this is an example of how 'scientific workers' can overlook valuable clinical knowledge developed by stockraisers themselves.

Hunter, Archie. 1992. Mission to Somaliland. *Vetaid News* 7(Summer): 1.

During his visit to the Sanaag Region of eastern Somaliland, the author noted pastoralists' vast veterinary knowledge, as evidenced by their accurate accounts of the pathology and epidemiology of local livestock diseases such as trypanosomosis, camel pox, haemonchosis and many more. The author and his colleague agreed that parasitic problems appeared to be the most pressing among the sheep and goats that formed the bulk of the animals exported by the pastoralists and so decided that assistance should be concentrated on these diseases.

Hunter, Archie. 1996. Taking the piss. In: Peter Fry (ed.). *Vetaid Book of Veterinary Anecdotes.* Vetaid, Edinburgh, UK. Pp. 104–105.

This brief anecdote notes Somali and Sudanese pastoralists' age-old ethnodiagnostic test for trypanosomosis in camels: a dark, stinking urine. Pastoralists detect the stink either by running their hands down the urine-stained tails of camels or by picking up sand where camels have urinated and then sniffing their palms.

Hussein, Mohamed Ali. 1984a. Summary of discussions and recommendations. In: Mohamed Ali Hussein (ed.). *Camel Pastoralism in Somalia: Proceedings from a Workshop held in Baydhabo, April 8–13, 1984.* Camel Forum Working Paper No. 7. Somali Camel Research Project, Mogadishu, Somalia and Stockholm, Sweden. Pp. 147–148.

This summary of the discussions at a workshop attended by both researchers and Somali camel herders notes that ' ... since diseases are the major problems in camel husbandry, the veterinary aspects of the research dominated the discussions. The elders ... placed great emphasis on the disease problems ... What struck us most was their knowledge and distinction of the different diseases and the practical and very effective ways of disease control and treatment practised by the pastoralist camel herders' (p. 147).

Hussein, Mohamed Ali. 1984b. Traditional systems of camel management and husbandry. In: Mohamed Ali Hussein (ed.). *Camel Pastoralism in Somalia: Proceedings from a Workshop held in Baydhabo, April 8–13, 1984.* Camel Forum Working Paper No. 7. Somali Camel Research Project, Mogadishu, Somalia and Stockholm, Sweden. Pp. 37–48.

Features of traditional Somali systems of camel management described in this paper include: differential grazing strategies for dry and pregnant female camels versus the dairy and pack animals; dietary supplementation with salt, salty earths, or water from salty wells; for studs, extra rations of *ghee* and sesame oil to enhance virility; genetic selection for productivity, endurance, drought resistance and other factors through strict pairing, culling and castration, the last performed by opening the scrotum, removing the testes and then treating the wound with antibiotics or medicinal plant preparations; controlled age of breeding; assistance in calving and colostrum suckling; and weaning methods such as tying off the dam's teats with softened bark or inserting a small stick in the calf's tongue.

Hussein, Mohamed Ali. 1987. Traditional practices of camel husbandry and management in central Somalia. *Camel Forum Working Paper* No. 19. Somali Camel Research Project, Mogadishu, Somalia and Stockholm, Sweden. 15 pp.

Unavailable for review.

Hyde, John L. 1980. Animal Health. In: Jacob A. Hoefer and Patricia Jones Tsuchitani (eds). *Animal Agriculture in China: A Report of the Visit of the CSCPRC Animal Sciences Delegation.* Committee on Scholarly Communication with the People's Republic of China Report No. 11. National Academy Press, Washington, DC, USA. Pp. 142–151.

A team of American scientists touring some of China's veterinary institutions and farms noted various diseases of swine, chicken, ducks, geese, cattle and horses; but they were struck by the absence of shipping fever in cattle, presumably due to the practice of off-loading and watering animals during transport by rail. The team also noted the extensive use of herbal medicine and, especially as an anaesthetic, acupuncture throughout the country.

Ibrahim, Mamman Aminu. 1984. *Evaluation of the Activities of Some African Traditional Anthelmintic Herbs against* **Nippostrongylus braziliensis** *in Rats.* MS thesis, Department of Veterinary Physiology and Pharmacology, Ahmadu Bello University, Zaria, Nigeria. 119 pp.

About 300 medical plants are reportedly used in the traditional control of human and animal helminthosis in Africa. For this study, 30 of these plants were selected on the basis of their availability in Kaduna state, Nigeria, and tested for their anthelmintic activity against *Nippostrongylus braziliensis* in rats. Six of these plants produced deparasitation between 58% and 92%, and six others between 33% and 49%. [Annotation based on thesis abstract.]

Ibrahim, M.A. 1986. Veterinary traditional practice in Nigeria. In: R. von Kaufmann, S. Chater and R. Blench (eds). *Livestock Systems Research in Nigeria's Subhumid Zone. Proceedings of the 2nd ILCA/NAPRI Symposium held in Kaduna, Nigeria, 29 October–2 November, 1984.* ILCA, Addis Ababa, Ethiopia. Pp. 189–203.

Traditional veterinary medicine could offer solutions to Nigeria's problem of the increasing cost of veterinary care. This paper reports some aspects of traditional veterinary practices among the Fulani in Kaduna state, Nigeria. In contrast to traditional healers for people, there are no 'professional' veterinary healers. The knowledge of diseases and their treatment is instead tied to group occupations such as herder and hunter. Within occupational groups, the knowledge is allowed to circulate freely, resulting in more uniformity in practices and less secrecy and mysticism than with traditional human medicine. Another difference between traditional human medicine and veterinary medicine is that human healers rely on disease symptoms and sorcery for diagnosis, while herders also have knowledge of the gross pathology of some diseases. The author discusses the importance of a standardized translation for indigenous disease terms. He describes the Fulani definition for seven forms of helminthic infection, for neurological diseases, streptothricosis, brucellosis and trypanosomosis, as well as aspects of traditional disease control. He also outlines how to collect indigenous veterinary knowledge.

Ibrahim, Mamman Aminu. 1990. Indigenous agro-veterinary knowledge system: An alternative development resource for Africa. Paper presented to the Closing Conference on Human Life in African Arid Lands, Uppsala, Sweden, 5–9 September 1990. 19 pp.

Modernization does not necessarily mean Westernization, as this paper sets out to show with examples drawn mainly from poultry raising in Nigeria. First, the paper discusses 'techno-grafting', on analogy with tissue grafting in medicine, as a more appropriate concept than technology transfer when it comes to sharing knowledge and techniques across cultures. A graft may be accepted or rejected, depending on its compatibility with the rest of an organism – or in this case, with an ethno-agro-veterinary knowledge system. Technografts of exotic chickens, for instance, were roundly rejected by rural Nigerians. For one thing, the exotics lacked culturally acceptable feather colours. For another, the birds were offered to farmers as day-old chicks. But Nigerians believe it is 'wicked' to take such young animals away from their mothers, because the chicks will (and do) die without a mother hen's care. Second, this paper discusses the need for developing countries to place more emphasis on 'indigenous research'. By this is meant research conducted by African scientists working in Africa, taking into account local knowledge, practices, and preferences, and sharing their findings with peers in their own and other developing nations. In poultry breeding, for instance, African scientists should take greater account of the hardiness and popularity of local guinea fowl; and in their work on chickens, they should attend not only to Western standards of performance, such as egg size and output, but also to local ones. An example of the latter is rural Nigerians' concern with hens' overall mothering abilities as these pertain to the total number of chicks that a hen is able to raise successfully to adulthood. The third point discussed in this paper is the need to customize Western science education curricula to African realities, where magical secret societies that 'engage in brutal magico-ritual ceremonies' (p. 9) flourish today even in science and technology universities and polytechnic schools. The author argues that ER&D and other arenas of local knowledge and belief offer one way to make science curricula more relevant to students' beliefs and life experiences. Indeed, an understanding of students' cultural backgrounds is imperative to the educational process. For instance, some may refuse to conduct certain experiments in poultry health and husbandry for fear of supernatural reprisals for what is, by traditional lights, cruelty to animals. At the same time, since a substantial proportion of African knowledge relates to animals, diseases, medicinal herbs and the environment, these subjects 'can serve as sources of materials for scientific illustration and teaching ... even for outrageous claims' (p. 11). For instance, Hausa believe in a group of evil *Inna* spirits that drain away their victim's bone marrow, thereby causing a condition known as *shan Inna*, which is characterized by paralysis and muscular atrophy. In essence, this is an apt description of the polio viruses that correlate with *shan Inna* cases. 'There is no reason why such associations should not be made in teaching' (ibid.). Fourth, the author notes the many benefits of ethnoagroveterinary research for improving livestock health and production, drawing upon examples Africa-wide. Fifth, however, are the difficulties of conducting ER&D, at least in Nigeria. These span, for example, the lack of national scientists interested in the topic; scientists' resistance to the interdisciplinarity required in good ER&D; the paucity of funding for such research; the disappearance of EVK, as its most expert but elderly holders die without heirs to their knowledge; and the challenge of collecting, cataloguing, analysing and returning to stockraisers the vast amount and diversity of information involved in ER&D. In conclusion, the author informs that the Department of Veterinary Physiology and Pharmacology of Nigeria's Ahmadu Bello Univeristy has established an exhibition garden of medicinal and poisonous plants for livestock. Also, it has introduced an elective course entitled Ethnoveterinary Medicine, which is open to third-year veterinary and sociology students.

Ibrahim, Mamman A. 1996. Ethnotoxicology among Nigerian agropastoralists. In: Constance M. McCorkle, Evelyn Mathias and Tjaart W. Schillhorn van Veen (eds). ***Ethnoveterinary Research & Development.*** Intermediate Technology Publications, London, UK. Pp. 54–59.

Little is known of indigenous knowledge and concepts of materials considered poisonous to livestock and humans, or of their traditional antidotes or other treatments and control. Yet poisonous materials abound in the environments of many rural communities in developing countries. This chapter discusses toxicological principles and knowledge among settled Fulani and Hausa agropastoralists of Nigeria. Toxic agents are divided into four categories by origin: vegetable, animal (snakes, wasps, bees, scorpions, etc.), manufactured (e.g. paraffin) and non-physical (e.g. hexes, curses, spirits). Nigerian stockraisers are generally well-aware of the medicinal value, as well as the poisoning dangers, of toxic plants (especially forages) in their environment. For poisoning, they have several effective antidotes. However, ethnoscientific and scientific understandings of toxic substances can vary in important ways, particularly when it comes to manufactured items with which local people are unfamiliar, such as imported commercial medicines and pesticides. To take one example, people often overdose with commercial Western treatments like dips or drenches, on analogy to the larger quantities required in their traditional botanical medicines, which are relatively lower in potency, toxicity and persistence. The author suggests how ethnotoxicological information may provide clues for a variety of development efforts in, for example, veterinary and human medicine, anthropology, agriculture, biology, pharmacology and the environmental sciences.

Ibrahim, Mamman A. and Paul A. Abdu. 1996. Ethno-agroveterinary perspectives on poultry production in rural Nigeria. In: Constance M. McCorkle, Evelyn Mathias and Tjaart W. Schillhorn van Veen (eds). **Ethnoveterinary Research & Development.** Intermediate Technology Publications, London, UK. Pp. 103–115.

Rural Nigerians maintain about two poultry units for each of the country's 100 million people, at no foreign-exchange cost to the nation in terms of imported birds, drugs, equipment, feed, or alien and inappropriate management techniques. In contrast, even at its peak in the early 1980s, the entire 'exotic' poultry industry represented no more than a tenth of a chicken per Nigerian. Yet this industry accounts for huge import bills and absorbs almost all the nation's poultry research efforts. Nigeria's present economic slump has kindled some interest among national scientists in developing local chicken production using local materials. Unfortunately, if the indigenous agroveterinary knowledge system is not first thoroughly understood, it is still all too easy to design breeds and technologies that are just as alien to the local human and physical environment as those imported from elsewhere. This chapter describes Nigerian Hausa and Fulani perspectives on their local poultry enterprises and products. Folk concepts have direct implications for rural development programmes and extension. Even such notions as the belief that hens have invisible breasts from which chicks suckle invisible milk make sense when viewed within the context of the local knowledge and animal-management system as a whole. Hausa and Fulani consider it cruel to procure day-old chicks to raise, as recommended by the extension service; they believe that without a mother's milk, the chicks will die. Indeed, in villages there is no such thing as an orphan chick. Chicks of any breed hardly ever survive the rigours of the indigenous free-range management system without a mother hen to guide them to good forage and shelter; fight off snakes, hawks and dogs; keep the chicks warm and dry under her wings, and via exposure to low levels of pathogens that the hen has experienced, build disease resistance in the chicks. Other beliefs may provide useful clues for appropriate avian R&D. For example, although scientists recognize only one type of local chicken in the country, farmers distinguish at least 12 different varieties by name. Some of these are linked to certain spirits that reflect desirable traits such as aggressiveness, broodiness and good mothering. Such spirit links may provide clues for geneticists and breeders searching for fresh germplasm. Likewise for the low clinical incidence in local chickens of certain diseases prevalent in exotic breeds, which can be explained by deliberate as well as natural selection, as well as the use of indigenous prophylaxes and pharmacotherapies. Still other elements of local knowledge have obvious practical value. For instance, people know the correct incubation periods for chicken, guineafowl and duck eggs; using foster hens, they apply this knowledge to equalize clutch and chick distributions, increase hatching rates, and more. Thus, systematic study of indigenous knowledge systems may help guide agroveterinary practice, research policy, extension efforts, and even educational curricula in developing countries in more appropriate directions.

Ibrahim, M.A., N. Nwude, Y.O. Aliu and R.A. Ogunsusi. 1983. Traditional concepts of animal disease and treatment among Fulani herdsmen in Kaduna State of Nigeria. *Pastoral Development Network Paper* No. 16c. Agricultural Administration Unit, ODI, London, UK. 6 pp.

These observations derive partially from a study among Fulani herders in Nigeria. There are no 'professional' veterinary healers but the knowledge of animal diseases and remedies is tied to group occupation. Traditional concepts of disease and treatment often come close to those of orthodox veterinary medicine. Herders sometimes know the route of infection and have some knowledge of vectors and the diseases they transmit. Traditional disease control includes deworming and management practices against insects such as fumigating animal housing and camps. Fulani use herbs for treatment and prophylaxis and know which plants are toxic for their livestock. Interdisciplinary teams should work out more accurate translations of indigenous disease terms.

Ibrahim, M.A., N. Nwude, R.A. Ogunsusi and Y.O. Aliu. 1984. Screening of West African plants for anthelmintic activity. *ILCA Bulletin* 17: 19–22.

This paper reviews literature on studies of indigenous African anthelmintics. It then describes the screening of 18 medical plants traditionally used by Fulani herders in Kaduna state, Nigeria, for activity against *Nippostrongylus braziliensis* in rats. Six of the plants – *Aloe barteri, Terminalia avicennioides, Annona senegalensis, Cassia occidentalis, Anogeissus leiocarpa* and *Diospyros mespiliformis* – showed significant activity and gave deparasitizations of 92%, 89%, 73%, 69%, 60% and 58% respectively compared to untreated controls.

Ichikawa, M. 1987. A preliminary report on the ethnobotany of the Suiei Dorobo in northern Kenya. *African Study Monographs of the Center for African Area Studies of Kyoto University,* Supplementary Issue No. 7.

The Dorobo in northern Kenya have a well-developed ethnobotany, including many ethnomedical botanicals for humans and livestock. One example of the latter is the [unspecified] use of the sticky latex of *Euphorbia* spp. as a remedy for calf hepatitis and for livestock skin diseases (p. 30).

Idrisu, Alhaji. n.d. Common problems in horses around Zaria. *Journal of the Association of Veterinary Medical Students, Ahmadu Bello University, Zaria, Nigeria* volume and issue numbers not available: 42–48.

This article mentions a combination of modern and traditional methods for tick control among horses in which commercial acaricides are coupled with daily manual removal of ticks. Also, to ward off nocturnal insects, smoky fires are lit in the stalls when horses are stabled in the early evening. Traditional methods are also employed in cases of lameness. Bowed tendons can be treated with plenty of rest and firing. Shoulder lameness is thought to be due to 'bad blood', which is expelled by stabbing the shoulder muscle and then dressing the wound with sheanut butter. However, the author comments that the latter technique can exacerbate the lameness if the wound becomes infected.

Ihiga, M.A., M.J.N. Thairu, L. Bebora and S. Mbugua. n.d. *Indigenous Knowledge on Livestock Health and Production Systems: A Food and Agriculture Organization (FAO) Funded Study with the Kenya Women Veterinary Association End of Project Report.* Kenya Branch of the Women World Veterinary Association, Nairobi, Kenya. 22 pp.

This report is a slightly revised version of Ihiga et al. 1995. It adds an appendix listing veterinary medicinal plants by their scientific as well as local names.

Ihiga, M.A., M.J.N. Thairu and S. Mbugua. 1995. *Food and Agriculture Organization (FAO) Funded Study on Indigenous Knowledge on Livestock Health and Production Systems: End of Project Report.* Kenya Women Veterinary Association, Nairobi, Kenya. 21 pp.

The research described here was part of a series of similar studies carried out in several countries under the auspices of the World Women Veterinary Association and FAO. In the Kenya study, data on EVK, local husbandry practices, and related social institutions and socioeconomic factors were collected and compared for three production systems: pastoral (Maasai), agropastoral (Luhya) and mixed farming (Akamba). Interviews were held with a total of 44 women's focus-groups in the three areas, plus 10 key-informant herbalists identified by the women. Research revealed that all three groups make extensive use of ethnoveterinary botanicals in caring for their cattle, sheep, goats, donkeys, poultry, and for Luhya, pigs. But their local ecologies influence the range of plants available. Akamba have the widest range, followed by Maasai and then Luhya. The most frequently occurring animal disorders have the most specific herbal remedies. Practices such as the manual removal of ectoparasites are widespread. ECF is generally treated by firing the enlarged lymph nodes symptomatic of this disease, but an alternative treatment is to incise the nodes. Dehorning is performed using hot metal bars and a mallet. Knowledge and use of various husbandry practices vary in predictable ways across the three ethnicities. For instance, only Maasai systematically relate the need for foot trimming to footrot; Akamba farmers do not even bother with this operation. Also, Maasai include seasonal information in their diagnoses far more than the other two groups. In general, people prefer traditional to modern drugs because they feel that, if diseased animals die, it is safer to eat the meat of those treated traditionally. However, animals put down by vets are also often eaten. The main

252 *Ethnoveterinary medicine*

disadvantage reported for traditional medicines is the lack of precise dosage information, which necessitated trial-and-error applications.

IIRR. 1994. *Ethnoveterinary Medicine in Asia: An Information Kit on Traditional Animal Health Care Practices.* IIRR, Silang, Cavite 4118, Philippines. 400 pp.

This kit is comprised of four volumes: one each on general information, ruminants (cattle, sheep, goats), swine and poultry. Compiled during an intensive 14-day workshop involving 20 veterinarians, pharmacologists, botanists and stockraisers from eight countries, the kit details botanical remedies and other ethnoveterinary practices used by stockraisers and healers in south and southeast Asia. Workshop participants rated each treatment according to whether it was widely used in the field or had been validated scientifically; only those remedies that the participants were confident would prove useful were written up in the kit. The first booklet addresses cross-species topics: identification, collection, preparation and application of medicinal plants; units of measure for prescriptions; methods for estimating live weight; selected surgical techniques; an ethnoveterinary question list; and glossaries of more than 200 medicinal plants, their English and Latin names, and technical terms in veterinary medicine. The other three booklets cover common disease problems like inappetence, coughs and colds, bloat, wounds, diarrhoea, fever, internal parasites and skin diseases, plus selected management practices like feeding and housing – all by livestock species. Infectious diseases are addressed only briefly because they are less important in smallholder production systems in Asia. For each health problem, its signs, causes, prevention and treatments are listed. Treatments are described in a simple, recipe-like format to enable non-veterinarians to prepare and administer them correctly. Also, the countries in which each treatment is used are noted.

IIRR. 1996. *Recording and Using Indigenous Knowledge: A Manual.* IIRR, Silang, Cavite, Philippines. 211 pp.

This manual discusses various aspects of indigenous knowledge and its use in development work. More than 30 different recording and assessment methods are described, drawn from participatory appraisal, and anthropological, sociological and community-organizational approaches. For each method, the manual gives a brief definition and purpose, lists the materials needed, provides step-by-step instructions on how to implement it, describes its value, and lists some do's and don'ts based on practical field experience with the method. Ten mini-case studies illustrate how development efforts can build on the indigenous knowledge thus gathered. Question guides for more than 20 development fields provide an idea of what to look for when recording local beliefs, practices and technologies. Examples of fields discussed are health, water and sanitation, and different agricultural sectors. Finally, key publications and pertinent resource institutions worldwide are listed. For EVM, the following sections or topics in the manual are especially relevant: the general discussion and most recording methods; examples of using Western scientific methods to assess indigenous knowledge of animal production and healthcare (p. 127); a mini-case study on the traditional system of animal dispersal in Cavite, Philippines; and a question guide on animal husbandry and healthcare.

IIRR/DENR/FF. 1992. *Agroforestry Technology Information Kit* (6 volumes). IIRR, Silang, Cavite, Philippines. 650 pp.

This information kit on agroforestry in southeast Asia is a revised version of DENR/IIRR/FF 1990. Volume 4 focuses on livestock and poultry production, including a list of 12 tree species of veterinary value for ruminants and poultry (pp. 26–32): banana, betelnut, bitter gourd (*Momordica charantia*), coconut, five-leaves chaste tree (*Vitex negundo*), *Gliricidia sepium*, guava, horseradish tree (*Moringa oleifera* L.), *Lantana camara*, Ngai camphor (*Blumea balsamifera*), *Premna odorata* and star apple (*Chrysophyllum cainito*). Animals with diarrhoea are drenched with a decoction of guava leaves. The leaves can also be pounded into a poultice for skin irritations, infested wounds and castration wounds. The leaves of the horseradish tree are fed to lactating sows or cows to stimulate milk production.

Iles, Karen. 1990. *Oxfam/ITDG Livestock Project Samburu. Report of Base-line Study, and Implications for Project Design.* In-house report [draft version, annotated with permission]. ITDG, Nairobi, Kenya. *Ca.* 100 pp.

Baseline research for a livestock development and healthcare training project among Samburu and Turkana pastoralists in Kenya's Baragoi District covered a number of EVK topics. One is the existence of a variety of traditional healers: diviners (Samburu *laibon*, Turkana *emorong*) who predict outbreaks of livestock disease; other healers who specialize in obstetrics and/or bonesetting; and camel castration experts. Also, women often treat small and young stock for simple problems like fleas, ticks and wounds. Another topic is the formation of 'stock friend-ships' in which animals are exchanged between households in order to balance herd compositions or bring in new blood (although breeding among cattle is not controlled except by castration). Examples of health-related management techniques include: as an explicit control on ectoparasites like fleas and ticks, periodically relocating household corrals, burning the old corrals, and sweeping out corrals in use; ensuring that neonates suckle colostrum; housing calves in separate huts or raised barns for the first 2 weeks of life, and thereafter in a calf herd on special pastures near the house; seeing that weak calves suckle more milk, and diarrhoeal ones less; keeping sickly animals at the home camp, where women can feed them on high-quality cut-and-carry forages; making sure all stock receive salt in one form or another; insofar as household labour is available, generally subdividing herds according to age, species, health and reproductive status; depending on household wealth, managing same-species herd segments in different locales so as to ward against epidemic losses and better exploit forage resources. Some ethnoveterinary practices are as follow. To force out certain kinds of endoparasites, infested animals may be denied water for 4 days. Turkana bleed barren or slow-growing stock, as well as animals with FMD. For cattle [and presumably camels] and sheep, respectively, this operation is performed on the jugular vein and between the eyes; either site is used for goats. Overall, both Samburu and Turkana displayed considerable agreement and clarity on disease signs. They were less clear on aetiologies, recognizing God or 'coming from the sky' as distal causes of disease, along with more proximal causes such as ticks or poisonous plants for some ills. This report also presents pastoralists' assessment of the importance of different diseases by local and, where identifiable, scientific names. A survey revealed that people's choice of traditional or modern treatments depended on the species, the disease, and place of residence, the last in relation to where modern drugs could be bought. In general, cattle are more likely to be given modern drugs (38%) than smallstock (24%) or camels (14%). Donkeys are 'animals of scorn and ridicule' (p. 35) that receive virtually no veterinary or other special care. No one in the survey reported calling in a vet or an animal health assistant. Pastoralists' use of modern drugs was often innovative. They mixed cocktails of different ones like terramycin and novidium, inserted novidium tablets under the skin, drenched with novidium for trypanosomosis, and sometimes used it as an eyewash. Extensive appendices to the study detail 84 Samburu terminological categories for species and classes of livestock plus about 40 species-specific disease names each for Samburu and Turkana.

Iles, Karen. 1994. *The Role of Ethnoveterinary Work in the ITDG/Oxfam Animal Health Programme, Baragoi, with Reference to Pastoralists' Perceptions of Helminths.* In-house report. ITDG, Nairobi, Kenya. 101 pp.

This is a focused case study of Samburu and Turkana pastoralists' perceptions of one Western-defined category of livestock disease: helminthosis. The study goal is to recommend how ITDG/Kenya can better fit EVK into its decentralized animal health training efforts. This health problem was selected because it is one that pastoralists commonly treat themselves. To study it, the author sketched out a tri-partite conceptual model of: factors influencing the disease – environment/climate, socioeconomic considerations, ethnoveterinary perceptions, both traditional and modern treatments/controls, management/husbandry, herding strategies, and live-stock species; scientific and ethnoscientific sources of information on all the fore-going; and possible problem solutions – e.g. none, husbandry changes, plant medicines, targeted use of commercial drugs, some combination of solutions and training. An understanding of ethnoveterinary perceptions is key to this whole process in order to determine what people already know about a disease and to develop workable solutions with them. For example, training can build upon Samburu and Turkana perceptions that dirty water or 'something in the grass' causes helminthosis, but adding more precise information on how this is so. Or, as among Turkana, their understandably incomplete diagnoses of ECF – which is relatively new to the area – can be refined so they do not waste their money on buying contra-indicated drugs. To discover such perceptions, the study employed multiple methodologies: participant observation and researcher visits to different herding and watering sites; participatory mapping and group necropsying; disease ranking exercises; and in-depth individual interviews applying a question-list for each type of helminth problem identified by the pastoralists, ideally administered with infested animals present to make interviews less abstract. Pastoralists most frequently cited intestinal worms, probably referring to the tapeworms *Moniezia expansia* or *M. benedeni*. There was little agreement on the exact cause of this problem, although many interviewees vaguely linked it to contaminated grass, soil or water, while others pointed to certain plants. Local notions of *Moniezia* life cycles differed considerably from Western ones. And with one exception, people did not feel that any management practices worsened the problem. The exception was one man who said not moving campsite for a long time does so. Treatments included: mainly during the rainy season, leading infested animals to areas with salty soils; grazing herds on certain plant species; or administering modern drugs. In the last regard, people advised that such drugs should be avoided during the dry season as they can kill the then-weak and -emaciated stock; at the very least, dry-season dosages should be smaller, they said. Equivalent perception data were gathered for other helminth problems that people cited, e.g.: *Taenia hydatigena* and *T. multiceps*; worms of the abomasum (mostly *Haemonchus contortus*); other roundworms; and an unidentified but non-fluke 'liver worm'. Some findings of interest follow. Mainly only women recognized *H. contortus* because – although men slaughter and butcher healthy animals – women do these jobs for sick animals and those dead of disease; also women naturally clean out the abomasum before cooking it. Pastoralists generally considered *T. hydatigena* harmless, and they recognized it only by its characteristic cysts, which they believed were formed by melting fat inside emaciated stock. Unfortunately the cysts from slaughtered animals are fed to dogs. Interviewees reported a number of management practices that may affect the incidence of helminthosis. For instance, until weaning, nursing stock are kept in raised structures except when they are let out to suckle. Although this practice is designed to ward against fleas and lice, it probably reduces exposure to *H. contortus* too. On the other hand, herds are often watered at muddy and permanently damp dams and wells. And while herd movements towards the end of the rainy season may bring the animals to 'fresh', less infested pastures, the annual mustering of the whole herd at the beginning of the rainy season increases crowding and favours rapid parasite multiplication and pasture contamination. Based on findings such as these, the author suggests specific ways to target training topics, to build upon useful local beliefs and practices, and to fill gaps in EVK during healthcare training for Samburu and Turkana. She also gives in-depth guidance on applying the methodologies used in this study. Finally, a series of appendices present all raw data collected.

Iles, Karen and John Young. 1991. Decentralized animal health care in pastoral areas. *Appropriate Technology* 18(1): 20–22.

In describing ITDG/Kenya's paravet programmes for pastoralists, the authors note that it is important for training to build on herders' existing knowledge and perceptions of disease and its treatment, both traditional and modern. Pastoralists seem to have clear ideas of disease signs, but not always of aetiologies. ITDG training has therefore de-emphasized disease recognition in favour of concepts of causation where these are necessary for furthering pastoralists' understanding of animal health problems and available prevention and treatment options. Throughout, however, people are encouraged to continue using traditional treatments they have found to work, and not to abandon them in favour of modern drugs.

ILRAD. 1985. Scientists explore resistance to trypanosomiasis. *ILRAD Reports* 3(2): 1–5.

Trypanotolerant livestock in West Africa include the N'Dama and West African Shorthorn breeds of cattle, Djallonké sheep and dwarf West African goats. These animals have undergone a rigorous process of natural [and anthropogenic] selection over thousands of years, and their genetic value is increasingly recognized. For example, N'Dama cattle are being imported by Central as well as West African countries to form a nucleus for livestock development programmes in tsetse-infested areas.

Iskandar, S.D., S. Karo-Karo and A. Ressan. 1983. Pengaruh biji pinang (*Areca catechu*) terhadap parasit cacing ternak. In: *Simposium Ikatan Sarjana Farmasi Indonesia, 20–22 Januari 1983, Jakarta.* Pp. 120–122.

Arecanut (*Areca catechu*), known in Indonesian as *pinang*, traditionally is made into a popular anthelmintic for small ruminants. This two-week-long study investigated its efficacy against *Haemonchus* sp., *Oesophagostomum* sp. and *Trichostrongylus* sp. in goats. Faecal egg counts were made before and after the treatment. *Areca catechu* proved effective against the nematodes under study, but the effective dose differed for each parasite.

Issaka, Youssao Abdou Karim. 1998. La transhumance des petits ruminants dans la sous-prefecture de Karimama (Benin). *Le N'Dama: Journal du Sous-Réseau PRELUDE Santé, Productions Animales et Environnement* 11, 12(1&2): 32–33.

This brief article describes the annual transhumance patterns and practices of Fulße pastoralists of Benin and their small ruminants. Movements are divided into the 'little transhumance' circuit of January–March, which is restricted to a single department of the country, and the 'big' May–October cross-border transhumance, which spans parts of Burkina Faso, Mali and Niger. These collective tribal travels are often organized by a specialist (*garso*) knowledgeable in where and when to find good water and forage, salt- and potassium-rich soils and plants, and so forth. Reportedly, the moves act to prevent respiratory ills in the flocks. Also noted are special training techniques and cries that Fulße employ to guide the animals and keep them together while on the move.

Issar, R.K. 1981. Traditionally important medicinal plants and folklore of Uttrakhand Himalayas for animal treatment. *Journal of Scientific Research in Plants and Medicines* 2(3): 61–66.

The Ayurvedic *materia medica* of India comprise over 2000 items, of which 90% are plants. This article cites 14 prescriptions involving 16 plants of Ayurvedic veterinary interest from the Uttrakhand Himalayan region. The prescriptions address alimentary disorders, fractures, contusions, eye problems, heatstroke and wounds from wild animals.

ITDG and IIRR. 1996. *Ethnoveterinary Medicine in Kenya: A Field Manual of Traditional Animal Health Care Practices.* ITDG and IIRR, Nairobi, Kenya. 226 pp.

Compiled by a team of 40 veterinarians and traditional healers through a 14-day intensive workshop, the manual documents animal healthcare practices among several Kenyan pastoral and farming communities including Gabbra, Gikuyu (Kikuyu), Kamba, Kipsigi, Luhya, Luo, Samburu, Somali and Turkana, to name those most frequently mentioned. The manual covers more than 60 of the most important health problems faced by stockraisers for camels, cattle, chickens, donkeys, goats and sheep. It is organized into 11 chapters on: preparing and using traditional medicines; nutrition and management; breeding and reproduction; surgery and injuries; skin and eye problems; external parasites; internal parasites; diseases carried by ticks; lung diseases; constipation and diarrhoea; and other infectious diseases. For each disease, the manual lists the signs, causes, preventive measures, and a range of traditional treatments. Notes at the end of each treatment indicate which societies use it on which species, plus a score between 1 and 3 depending on whether it is a practice recognized by conventional veterinary medicine (score 1), a common traditional practice supported by scientific knowledge (score 2), or a common traditional practice known to animal healers in general and believed by them to work (score 3). Treatments are presented in simple recipes to enable readers to prepare and use the remedies themselves. An appendix lists animal, disease and plant names in several local languages as well as local names for different animal age groups. It also gives approximate metric equivalents for commonly-used folk measures for medicines in Kenya; thus, the metric units in the recipes can be readily converted to local standards for ease of application by stockraisers.

ITDG/Kenya. n.d. *Summary of RAPP's Programme Objectives and Longer Term Plans for ELK Work.* In-house report, ITDG, Nairobi, Kenya. 5 pp.

In addition to its on-going work on EVM plant remedies, disease classifications and paravet programmes, this report notes ITDG plans to: pay more attention to traditional husbandry and range-management knowledge and techniques; involve traditional healers in more active roles, rather than just exploiting their knowledge in animal healthcare delivery – perhaps by helping them organize into associations along the lines of the *miti ni dawa* clinics for traditional healers of humans in Kenya; and study the social dynamics of EVK – who holds and uses such knowledge, how is it valued, how can its use be increased? Also noted are plans to disseminate ITDG EVK findings more widely and to collaborate in EVK R&D with a greater diversity of partners, such as national museums, labs and agricultural research institutes.

ITDG/Kenya. 1989a. *Kenya Livestock Programme: A Review of the First Three Years of Operation 1986–89.* In-house report. ITDG, Nairobi, Kenya. 91 pp.

This external evaluation reviews five of the KLP's major projects. In the process, it notes that ITDG/Kenya has developed a 'minimum dataset' protocol for collecting information preparatory to designing decentralized animal healthcare programmes. The dataset section on livestock covers local knowledge about diseases and treatments among average stockraisers and 'experts' and about the type, mode of access, and frequency of use of 'indigenous vet services'. Among other things, the reviewers conclude that ITDG needs to do more intensive analysis of ethnoveterinary data, the overall level of EVK, relations between local EVK experts and ordinary stockraisers, and gender roles in EVK.

ITDG/Kenya. 1989b. *Traditional Healers Workshop: Intermediate Technology Development Group Utooni Development Project.* In-house report, ITDG, Nairobi, Kenya. 13 pp.

A workshop of veterinary and ITDG/Kenya personnel was convened with more than half a dozen traditional livestock healers from a WaKamaba farming area in southeastern Kenya. The goal was to explore and exchange healers' EVK plus opinions about healers' present and future roles in development. Healer participants were all long-time practitioners; some had begun their training as early as age 7 years. They had entered their profession by being taught by their mother or father, inspired by a spirit, or simply having an innate talent for or interest in healing. They named 25 animal health problems they treated, and gave diagnostic, aetiological, prophylactic and therapeutic details for 12 of them. Treatments spanned: herbal medicines [no Latin names given], sometimes prepared with other ingredients such as salt water, animal fat and urine; non-herbal medicaments; habitat and hygiene prescriptions, such as clearing brush, cleaning or moving animals' sleeping places, roofing sheds, and burning plastic bags around the home; management recommendations, such as isolating sick animals, grazing later in the morning, changing grazing sites, and modifying watering times; ritual acts; and commercial drugs and dips. For example, to treat footrot, healers recommend spreading ashes across corral entrances. To prevent fluke infestations, they suggest washing watering points and/or watering animals from basins in places known to promote the disease. Payment for healers' services was highly varied, whether in cash, kind, or nothing at all. Their clients today tend to be the poorest people because 'herbal treatments ... are cheaper than modern *dawas*' (p. 8). 'Richer people call the vet first and if he fails they sometimes call the traditional healer' (p. 4). In such cases, said healers, the animal may have been sick for so long that traditional treatments have little chance of success. Such cases erode people's faith in EVM. Healers ascribed dwindling demand for their services since 'the old days' to many additional factors, however: free medicines from the veterinary department, fewer numbers of animals due to decreased access to traditional grazing grounds, formal education, and Christianization. Healers also felt that vets and animal health assistants have an advantage in that they hold certificates and are not subject to problems such as delayed treatment due to having to go gather herbs after diagnosing an animal. Because of all these factors, said workshop participants, EVM was dying out; and few of their sons or daughters were interested in learning the profession. Their suggestions for improving the situation included, e.g.: development of better storage methods for botanical *materia medica*; organization of, and information exchange among, livestock healers; collaboration rather than competition between themselves and veterinary personnel, for example, with the latter treating more complex diseases referred to them by healers; government recognition for livestock healers like that vouchsafed traditional healers for humans in Kenya; also like the latter, recordkeeping by livestock healers of their cases (treatments, outcomes, testimonials), to give a clearer understanding of their work. Despite the present situation, workshop participants felt that, on the whole, demand for herbal medicines will increase as new diseases develop in both humans and animals, as the price of modern drugs continues to increase, and as people become aware that many such drugs had their origins in traditional medicines.

ITDG/Kenya. 1992a. A process of partnership. *Appropriate Technology* 19(2): unpaginated.

When asked to rank cattle diseases in order of importance, Samburu pastoralists of Kenya put anaplasmosis and ECF at the top of their lists. Although interviewees had not seen cases for several years, they explained that these killer tick-borne diseases prevented them from utilizing the high plateaux pastures that could otherwise save many of their livestock from starvation during droughts and dry seasons. Modern responses to tick-borne disease have centred on dipping animals in toxic chemicals. But this expensive and unsafe technique is not appropriate to Kenya's arid lands. In an effort to seek alternative methods of control, ITDG/Kenya has linked Samburu stockraisers and national veterinary scientists together in a research partnership to combine their knowledge of ticks and their habitats and of possible alternative solutions to the tick problem. The pastoralists are collecting ticks according to their own classification system, and bringing them to the scientists for translation into Western taxonomic systems. In addition, together they are mapping the sites where ticks are found.

ITDG/Kenya. 1992b. *Report on Discussions with Traditional Healers – Mtito Andei October '92.* In-house report, ITDG, Nairobi. 4 pp.

In planning for a follow-on workshop to one hosted earlier [ITDG/Kenya 1989b], ITDG staff canvassed potential healer-participants in another region on a variety of issues. Discussions revealed differing mechanisms by which healers had taken up their work. A majority learned it from their grandfathers; in some cases, their EVK had been passed down through their lineage for generations. Women healers in particular acquired their skills following marriage into a household where a livestock healer lived; but one woman won her knowledge through dreams. In general, healers said they limited their practice to relatives, friends and neighbours known to them. They treated a wide variety of livestock diseases using mainly herbs but also other ingredients such as soda and oil, and, among younger healers, sometimes commercial drugs. Interestingly, most healers occasionally had recourse themselves and/or referred clients to animal health assistants trained in modern veterinary medicine. Opinions as to the future of EVM were mixed. Some healers said they themselves and their medicines were viewed as 'dirty' and that young people were no longer interested to learn about EVM. But others were more optimistic, and had already begun training their children and wives in the work. In terms of workshop content, healers were most keen to exchange information with one another and with project personnel, especially to learn more about disease identification (especially of less familiar diseases), new herbs, and effective dosage rates for both new and old herbal medicines.

ITDG/Kenya. 1993. *Marsabit Prereview Document.* In-house report. ITDG, Marsabit, Kenya. 7 pp.

In discussing ITDG work among Gabbra camel pastoralists of Kenya's Northern Frontier, this document makes reference to the inclusion of EVK into participatory, practical training for paravets, based on an on-going survey of Gabbra EVK. Among traditional treatments so far identified, two merit greater attention and validation: deworming, and a mange preparation that uses parts of the *obe* (?) tree.

ITDG/Kenya. 1996. *Ethnoveterinary Research and Development Project.* Project Outlines. Intermediate Technology, Nairobi, Kenya. 2 pp.

This short document outlines IT Kenya's EVM project which aims to: validate some of Kenya's traditional veterinary treatments; combine them with modern scientific knowledge and techniques to develop more effective ones that use local resources; make EVK an integral part of community-based animal health projects; and influence other institutions to use and promote EVK in their work.

ITDG/Kenya. 1997. Traditional knowledge explored. ***Appropriate Technology*** 23(4): 4.

This update on the ITDG/Kenya team's work in EVK among Samburu pastoralists emphasizes the need for scientific validation of local treatments' efficacy and safety if sceptical development agencies are to be encouraged to take up and disseminate such treatments. The article also notes the team's plans to give training sessions and to work with local schools so as to feed back its findings on ten confidently-used herbal, non-herbal and manipulative treatments to the communities who originally provided the information.

Iyyappan, V.R. 1997. Scent ripens bananas and ragi improves soil texture. ***Honey Bee*** 8(2): 7.

Based on traditional veterinary recipes written in Tamil on palm leaf manuscripts collected by his grandfather, the elderly Mr Iyyappan here shares the treatments he uses on his own animals, drawing upon these manuscripts. He makes a general tonic for cattle by pounding together one mature coconut kernel, 100 g of salt, 50 g of *Tephrosia purpurea* leaves, and 50 g of turmeric rhizome, all mixed in 1 l of fermented rice water and given daily for a week. For inappetence, he administers a handful of pounded bottle-gourd leaves (*Lagenaria sciceraria*) in fermented rice water under the same regime. For indigestion and fevers, he feeds a bolus of 10 g each of garlic, fresh ginger, dried ginger, asafoetida and pepper in 50 g of jaggery. Infertility is treated daily for a week with a handful of *Aristolochia bracteolata* leaves and three *Cyperus rotendus* rhizomes ground together with 10 g of salt, and water is withheld for half an hour after each such feeding.

Jagun, A.G. and P. A. Abdu. 1998. Socioeconomic implication of using (or ignoring) ethnoveterinary medicine: The Nigerian experience. In: E. Mathias, D.V. Rangnekar and C.M. McCorkle, with M. Martin (eds). ***Ethnoveterinary Medicine: Alternatives for Livestock Development – Proceedings of an International Conference Held in Pune, India, 4–6 November 1997. Volume 2: Abstracts.*** BAIF Development Research Foundation, Pune, India. P. 25.

Beginning with colonialism in Nigeria, the introduction of modern medicine for both humans and animals greatly eroded Nigerians' belief in their own, ethnomedical practices, which until recently were looked down upon as primitive or inferior. Still today, most traditional practitioners go about their practices secretly or rely increasingly on modern techniques. Consequently, many indigenous practices previously passed on orally by elders from generation to generation are being lost. But in 1980, in tandem with the worldwide re-awakening to the importance of indigenous knowledge and perhaps also as a 'child of necessity' due to the national economic squeeze and the high cost of the few available veterinary drugs, ethnoveterinary R&D in Nigeria started in earnest. This paper presents the results of a recent field survey on EVK conducted in 11 states of Nigeria by the National Animal Production Research Institute of Ahmadu Bello University. A total of 167 farmers were interviewed, located in 58 towns and villages scattered over 22 of the country's 500 Local Government Areas. Some 82 health problems of cattle, sheep, goats, pigs, poultry and rabbits were identified, and information was obtained on 629 local remedies used by stockraisers in these areas. The authors note the need for more in-depth study of ethnoveterinary practices now, so that Nigeria can overcome its dangerous dependence on foreign veterinary drugs.

Jain, Parmod K. 1994. Local treatment for FMD in UP. *Honey Bee* 5(2): 13.

This article recounts FMD treatments used by local healers and farmers from two villages in India's Uttar Pradesh State. One traditional veterinary practitioner applies 15 to 20 g of *Butea* sp. resin inside the infected animals' mouths thrice daily for several days. As both a prophylaxy and a therapy, another healer feeds a paste made from an aquatic grass (*chopattia*) that grows on pond surfaces, to which barley flour and water or merely water has been added; when he performs this treatment at a stockraisers' home, he must not eat or drink anything from that farmstead. Also, he accepts no payment for his work. A farmer of the same village instead washes the hooves and the inside of the mouths of affected animals with a lukewarm filtrate of *Acacia nilotica* bark boiled in water, sometimes with a little alum added. Another man simply cleans the hooves and anoints them with *Brassica campestris* oil. However, a great many people prefer to pour hot salt water over the hooves, twice a day for several days. Another popular treatment is to make animals with FMD walk in hot sand and then mud twice a day. Some new folk remedies for FMD are to rub the inside of the mouth with a certain plant gum, with alum or with roasted *Euphorbia* sp.

Jain, S.K. and C.R. Tarafder. 1970. Medicinal plant-lore of the Santals (A revival of P. O. Bodding's work). *Economic Botany* 25: 241–278.

Based on Bodding's 1927 volume, this article records 377 medicinal plants that, as of the 1960s, were still employed by Santal tribespeople of India's Bengal-Bihar border. Of the 377, 76 are of veterinary value in treating cattle disorders such as anthrax, FMD, fractures, haemorrhagic septicaemia and rinderpest.

Jalby, R. 1974. *Sorcellerie et Médecine Populaire en Languedoc.* Ed. de l'Aygues, Nyons, France. 183 pp.

Unavailable for review.

Jallo, Yero Dooro. 1989a. **The Life of the People of Ferlo. Vol. 1: Their Social System, Their Strategies of Herding, Their Knowledge about Agriculture** [in Fulfulde]. Goomu Winndiyankoobe Demde Ngenndiije (Groupe d'Initiative pour la Promotion du Livre en Langues Nationals), Ndakaaru (Dakar), Senegal. 170 pp.

This socioeconomic study in the Fulfulde language describes the social system, herding practices, and agriculture of the Fulße in Ferlo, Senegal. The description of herding practices includes sections on survival strategies such as grazing and healthcare and on milk production. [Annotation based on English outline by Sonja Fagerberg-Diallo.]

Jallo, Yero Dooro. 1989b. *The Life of the Fulße in the Ferlo. Vol. 2: Cattle Diseases.* [in Fulfulde]. Goomu Winndiyankoobe Demde Ngenndiije (Groupe d'Initiative pour la Promotion du Livre en Langues Nationals), Ndakaaru (Dakar), Senegal. 92 pp.

This book in the Fulfulde language provides insight into the knowledge and beliefs of Fulße herders about cattle diseases. It is divided into four parts: contagious diseases; non-contagious illnesses; problems that affect only certain classes of animals; and fractures, wounds, etc. The author describes the clinical signs, seasonal occurrence, causes, contagion, treatment, and prevention for each disease. [Annotation based on English outline by Sonja Fagerberg-Diallo.]

James, Arlington A. 1986. *Cabrits Plants and their Uses.* Forestry and Wildlife Division, Ministry of Agriculture, Commonwealth of Dominica. 48 pp.

In this survey of plant use in the Cabrits area of Dominica, four species of veterinary use are noted: *Capraria biflora*, ground with lime juice and administered to sheep with colds; *Cassia occidentalis* seeds, used in unspecified ways for external disorders; *Chenopodium ambrosioides*, crushed and spread in chicken coops to eradicate lice; and *Lantana camara* leaves, used to wash foul-smelling bucks (cf. pp. 3, 5, 7).

Jani, R.G. and P.R. Patel. 1998. Ethnomedicinal effect of whey feeding on ascarid infection in buffalo calves. In: E. Mathias, D.V. Rangnekar and C.M. McCorkle, with M. Martin (eds). *Ethnoveterinary Medicine: Alternatives for Livestock Development – Proceedings of an International Conference Held in Pune, India, 4–6 November 1997. Volume 2: Abstracts.* BAIF Development Research Foundation, Pune, India. P. 26.

A study of parasitic diarrhoea in neonate buffalo from villages in one district of India's Gujarat State revealed high levels of *Neoascaris vitulorum* infection. Using McMaster's technique, counting the number of eggs per gram of faeces (epg) of 144 calves with diarrhoea showed that calves fed whey and salt had significantly fewer parasite eggs in their faeces than calves not so fed. The reduced epg counts might be due to purgative and laxative actions of whey and salt.

Jani, R.G., S.K. Raval and P.R. Patel. 1998. Ethnomedicine for ectoparasites in buffaloes: A clinical study on mange dermatitis. In: E. Mathias, D.V. Rangnekar and C.M. McCorkle, with M. Martin (eds). *Ethnoveterinary Medicine: Alternatives for Livestock Development – Proceedings of an International Conference Held in Pune, India, 4–6 November 1997. Volume 2: Abstracts.* BAIF Development Research Foundation, Pune, India. P. 26.

Ectoparasitic skin diseases in livestock cause annoyance, uneasiness, itchiness and hide damage; and they reduce milk production and the total sale value of animals. During clinical camps organized in villages near Anand, India, 42 buffalo with clinical dermatitis were presented. Their skin lesions were examined and recorded, and skin scrapings were collected and processed for microscopic examination. Examination revealed that 28 buffalo were infested with *Sarcoptes* spp. mites, ten with *Psoroptes* spp. mites, and four with both. These buffalo were used to study the efficacy of a traditional treatment for ectoparasites consisting of bathing the animals on alternate days with a decoction of neem (*Azadirachta indica*) and tobacco

(*Nicotiana tabacum*) leaves with camphor, followed by a topical application of *karanja* (*Pongamia glabra*) oil to the lesions. Microscopic examination of skin scrapings on days 7, 14 and 21 post-therapy revealed complete absence of developmental stages of both mites by day 21; by this time, too, the lesions were also completely cleared. Overall the present findings suggest that the treatment is useful.

Jayasuriya, M.R.T. and T. Jayatileka. 1992. Sri Lankan community livestock care and production programme (CLCP). In: John Young (ed.). *A Report on a Village Animal Health Care Workshop – Volume II: The Case Studies.* ITDG, Rugby, UK. Pp. 58–65.

As part of baseline data collection for the above-referenced programme, the authors note their intent to collect information on non-conventional feed resources to improve animal nutrition and on 'local or traditional practices that could be adopted for the treatment and control of diseases including the use of medicinal herbs' (p. 63).

Jayatileka, T.N. and M.N.M. Ibrahim. 1998. Indigenous animal health practices in Sri Lanka: Extracts from an ancestral palm leaf manuscript. In: E. Mathias, D.V. Rangnekar and C.M. McCorkle, with M. Martin (eds). *Ethnoveterinary Medicine: Alternatives for Livestock Development – Proceedings of an International Conference Held in Pune, India, 4–6 November 1997. Volume 2: Abstracts.* BAIF Development Research Foundation, Pune, India. P. 27.

Through trial and error down through history, people have devised various means of alleviating their animals' ills. In Sri Lanka, the indigenous knowledge thus generated is highly specialized and differs from that found in formal Ayurvedic texts on veterinary science. In the light of the progressive erosion of indigenous knowledge among modern-day peoples, it is all the more important to recapture and re-apply as much historically documented EVK information as possible – such as that set down in the ancient palm-leaf manuscripts of Sri Lanka. This paper reports on one such 146-year-old manuscript authored by two indigenous physicians. Written in simple Sinhala language, the manuscript contains more than 1000 prescriptions for cattle diseases. It also differentiates cattle into breeds/varieties or name groups and notes their relative susceptibility to disease. For example, Raja cattle are believed to be more prone than other breeds to a syndrome known as *adappan*, which is characterized by nasal discharge and tremors. Such information can provide useful clues to researchers seeking disease-resistant germplasm. The manuscript also details how traditional diagnoses relied not only on clinical observation but also on in-depth knowledge of animal husbandry and on the establishment of human–animal psychic bonds. Bloodletting from certain blood vessels and the tip of the tail also figured in ethnodiagnoses and prognoses for some health problems. The manuscript details disease signs, along with their corresponding treatments based on medicinal herbs and other ingredients commonly available at farm level, such as ant-hill mud, milk products, eggs, bonemeal, bat excreta and human urine. The *materia medica* were usually combined in a carrier liquid such as ginger essence, betel juice, *Piper nigrum* or lemon juice, water, and coconut milk or water. The most frequent route of administration was oral, but nasal, aural, anal and transdermal routes were also taken. For example, moxibustion is a popular technique. Akin to acupuncture, it consists of burning medicines into the skin at vital body points according to specific patterns. In fact, moxibustion can stimulate an immune response. Another common technique was manual manipulation to relieve constipation, dystocia and retained placenta. A striking feature of most traditional Sri Lankan treatment regimes was (and today still is) the integration of visible, material elements with invisible, spiritual ones such as spells, blessings and vows and offerings to the gods that oversee livestock. Sri Lankans feel that a satisfactory cure will not be forthcoming without such spiritual reinforcements.

Jayshree, V.L., T.K. Narainswami and B.K. Narainswami. 1998. Ethnoveterinary medicine for domestic animals. In: E. Mathias, D.V. Rangnekar and C.M. McCorkle, with M. Martin (eds). ***Ethnoveterinary Medicine: Alternatives for Livestock Development – Proceedings of an International Conference Held in Pune, India, 4–6 November 1997. Volume 2: Abstracts.*** BAIF Development Research Foundation, Pune, India. P. 28.

Many common livestock diseases can be cured using ethnoveterinary treatments instead of allopathic medicine, which is not only costly but also often has adverse side-effects. This paper presents a variety of such treatments collected from local animal healers in India. To take one example, dogs can be dewormed by feeding them a paste of 1 teaspoonful of powdered papaya seeds in milk and jaggery for taste, given twice a day for 3 days and repeating the treatment after 14 days. This medicine has been found to work well against all sorts of worms except tape-worms, which can instead be treated by feeding 5 to 6 powdered betel nuts boiled in 100 ml of milk until the liquid is reduced by half. The cooled liquid is given as a single dose in the evening for 4 days; and the treatment should be repeated after 6 months. As an on-going prophylaxis for gastrointestinal worms, also feed dogs turmeric and two cloves of garlic daily.

Jean, Maurice. 1984. Le berger Provençal et son troupeau. ***Exposition 'Quand les Plantes Guérissaient les Moutons'.*** Muséum d'Histoire Naturelle de Toulon, France. Pp. 1–22.

This extensive treatise on transhumant sheep management in France's Provence describes how shepherds' duties include preventing rams from servicing ewes. An apron is tied around the ram's abdomen, thereby providing a barrier form of con-traception. Sixteen sheep ailments are also cited, ranging from indigestion from eating grapes to mastitis, which is thought to be caused by spider bites. Likewise for 42 healing plants. These include, e.g., elderberry (*Sambucus* sp.), which can be administered as a diuretic infusion, as a smoke treatment for mastitis, or as a poultice for snake bite. *Helleborus* spp. is used topically for the relief of mange. To facilitate parturition, ewes on the point of giving birth receive a decoction of *Iris germanica* L.

Jiménez J., Salustio, Adelma Troncoso de Jiménez, Abel Muñiz V. and César Gonzales M. 1983. Los alcaloides del lupinus como pesticidas en el control de ectoparásitos. ***Ciencia y Pueblo: Revista de los Institutos IIUN-IIDSA-NUFFIC*** 1: 107–125.

This journal article represents a partial summary of the final report for the 'Proyecto Pesticidas del Lupinus' carried out in southern Peru between 1980 and 1982. The project constituted a systematic investigation of the use of *tarwi*

(*Lupinus mutabilis*) preparations to combat pests of both plant and animal crops. A guiding project principle was 'scientific and social relevance, based on the existing knowledge possessed by the study communities about the traditional use of pesticides' from *tarwi* (p. 122). The focus here is on the use of such alkaloidal compounds to combat ectoparasites of herd animals. Through a series of both laboratory and interdisciplinary field experiments, various *tarwi* preparations were demonstrated to be non-toxic and highly effective against sarcoptic ectoparasites of alpaca and *Boophilus microplus* (Spanish *garrapata*) in cattle. The authors comment on the fact that indigenous knowledge of *Lupinus* parasiticides is being lost. They attribute this in part to numerous official veterinary campaigns that, poorly and irregularly conducted, have led to the disuse of traditional medicines at the same time that they have created distrust and dissatisfaction with Western ones.

Jiménez J., Salustio, Adelma Troncoso de Jiménez, Abel Muñiz V. and César Gonzales M. 1985. *Manual de: Cultivo, Precoesamiento y Aplicaciones del Tarwi.* Proyecto 'Pesticidas del Lupinus', Instituto de Investigación UNSAAC-NUFFIC, Cuzco, Peru. 11 pp.

This short manual discusses how to grow the Andean foodplant *tarwi* (*Lupinus mutabilis*) and then process and utilize its many pesticidal properties. All the *tarwi* products presented here can be confidently used, based not only on formal scientific research but also on Andean consumers', farmers' and housewives' centuries-long use of them. For use as a pesticide, the water in which *tarwi* grains have been cooked for human consumption is used, as it contains as much as 1.2% alkaloids. This liquid can be stored indefinitely. A proven prescription for treating ectoparasites of livestock is to mix 1 bucket of this *tarwi* water with 5 spoonfuls of laundry detergent and half a glass of kerosene. Applied once and then again after 7 days, this mixture is effective against: ticks on cattle; keds on sheep; lice on both the foregoing species plus camelids; sarcoptic mites on camelids and horses; and fleas on dogs and guinea pigs or rabbits. For sheep and sheared alpaca, total immersion of the animal is recommended. For cattle and for sarcoptic mange, topical application with a rag is preferred. The total cost for treating one sheep or one head of cattle with this mixture is calculated to be only US $0.03 and $0.10, respectively, at the time of writing. By comparison, for commercial pesticides these figures are $0.10 and $0.35. In other words, this modified traditional remedy can cut stockraisers' outlays for livestock insecticides by more than two-thirds. Further, cooked *tarwi* grains serve as an excellent ingredient for inclusion in inexpensive but protein-rich homemade rations for fattening pigs and broiler chickens and for increasing milk production in cows. The article details recipes and costs for each of these purposes. In general, *tarwi* can replace the higher-priced and alien soya bean in livestock rations, with no loss in nutritive value. Also noted is a prescription for making a plant-crop pesticide from *tarwi*. The authors suggest that an artesanal industry in *tarwi* products might prove a viable development initiative.

Jirli, Basavaprabhu, Prabhat Kumar Jha and Madhukar Chugh. 1999. Cognitive domain and acceptance of ethnoveterinary medicine by animal scientists. In: E. Mathias, D.V. Rangnekar and C.M. McCorkle, with M. Martin (eds). *Ethnoveterinary Medicine: Alternatives for Livestock Development – Proceedings of an International Conference Held in Pune, India, 4–6 November 1997. Volume 1: Selected Papers.* BAIF Development Research Foundation, Pune, India. Pp. 233–242.

Interviews were conducted with 30 veterinarians and animal scientists in one veterinary college and one dairy research institute of India in order to gauge their awareness, perceptions and acceptance of EVM. Findings revealed that a majority of such scientists were aware of EVM, but many were unwilling to accept it 'as is', without systematic research to validate techniques before recommending them widely. However, most scientists had a positive attitude towards the possible scientific validity of EVM, and many opined that ethnoveterinary medicines could be adopted. The scientists were also asked how they came to know about EVM. Responses indicated that natural/indigenous communication channels – as among parents, grandparents, farmers, friends, neighbours, etc. – played a greater role in this regard than formal ones like magazines, journals, booklets and texts. A subset of respondents also rated 21 out of a list of 34 ethnoveterinary practices and medicines as harmless. The majority of the scientists felt that EVK and other indigenous technical knowledge in India is being eroded, and they indicated their willingness therefore to advocate for scientifically proven EVM resources. More than half stated that they have recommended ethnoveterinary treatments for certain cases of animal health problems. Although scientists were only somewhat aware of NGO work on EVK and other kinds of local technical knowledge, they said they stand ready to assist NGOs in researching and conserving such resources; and the scientists unanimously agreed that these resources should receive legal protection. The authors conclude that the scientific community is becoming increasingly aware of the drawbacks and dangers of unprecedented technological advances that have caused ecological and other problems, and so are willing to explore indigenous-based alternatives for sustainable development. To this end, governments and NGOs should make increased and concerted efforts to tap into the national pool of scientific expertise.

Jirli, Basavaprabhu, Ram Kumar and N.R. Gagadharappa. 1999. Popularising ethnoveterinary medicine by animal scientists. Paper presented to the International Seminar on Integrated Approach for Animal Health Care, 4–6 February 1999, Calicut, Kerala, India.

For many years EVM researchers worked alone. Recently, however, there has been an increase of interest in the subject and a realization of its potential in sustainable, environmentally-friendly livestock production. Previously farmers using traditional practices were looked upon as being superstitious; now they are the focus of attention in the quest for documentation and dissemination of indigenous knowledge. The authors offer a step-by-step guide to popularizing ethnoveterinary practices. The steps are: the research, documentation and classification of ethnoveterinary knowledge; field trials of economically promising practices; economic, technical and social feasibility studies of EVK; training of extension workers in transferable EV practices; dissemination of promising EV practices to farmers through demonstrations; evaluation of results; and refinement of objectives.

Jode, A. de., L. Reynolds and R.W. Matthewman. 1992. Cattle production systems in the derived savannah and southern Guinea savannah regions of Oyo State, southern Nigeria. *Tropical Animal Health and Production* 24: 90–96.

N'Dama cattle and their crosses in Nigeria are reported to have good disease resistance, especially to trypanosomosis. In Oyo State, 59% of herds that had been settled in a single location for 10 years were found to include these trypanotolerant breeds. In herds settled for less than 5 and 1 years, respectively, this figure was 22% and 0%. These findings indicate that settled cattle-raisers clearly recognize the health advantages of the N'Dama breed.

John, Akkara J. 1999. Alternate systems for village animal healthcare using ethnoveterinary medicines. In: E. Mathias, D.V. Rangnekar and C.M. McCorkle, with M. Martin (eds). *Ethnoveterinary Medicine: Alternatives for Livestock Development – Proceedings of an International Conference Held in Pune, India, 4–6 November 1997. Volume 1: Selected Papers.* BAIF Development Research Foundation, Pune, India. Pp. 155–161.

Working in partnership with 65 NGOs in 11 states of India, between 1993 and 1997 the New Delhi-based NGO AFPRO (Action for Food Production) trained unemployed but educated village youth (429 male, 79 female) to become barefoot technicians (BFTs). The goal was to deliver useful, cost-effective veterinary services to stockraisers in remote tribal areas. For AFPRO, this meant combining ethno- with modern veterinary medicine. Trainees were selected by groups of five to ten adjacent communities, whom the BFTs afterwards served in livestock and other development arenas, with remuneration from their clients. AFPRO's BFT training was conducted at the veterinary dispensaries of the Animal Health Department in each state. Training spanned not only conventional topics – such as disease symptoms, commercial treatments, vaccinations, sterilization protocols and zoonoses – but also the use of all herbal medicines from the M/s. Indian Herbs Company, plus Ayurvedic and indigenous Indian medicines for humans that can also be applied to animals. For each disease addressed during training, the relative benefits and costs of herbal/traditional versus modern medicines were discussed, supplemented by audio and visual instructional materials not only from conventional sources but also from the Indian Herbs Company and the Catholic Health Association of India. All BFTs were provided with a tool kit that included alternative as well as modern medicines. BFTs were required to send AFPRO monthly reports on (among other things) the diseases they identified, the number of cases they treated, the choice of treatment type, and recovery and mortality rates. Analysis of these reports indicated that, overall, BFTs [and thus presumably their clients] preferred the cheaper herbal/traditional medicines whenever possible, especially for [unspecified] minor ills; but modern treatments were preferred for highly contagious diseases or [also unspecified] particular cases or patients. Interestingly, drawing upon BFTs' training in alternative livestock medicines, BFTs and their farmer-clients themselves began independently to search out and prepare herbal ingredients in their home locales. Stockraisers in three of the 11 states seemed particularly appreciative of non-conventional alternatives. The author concludes by urging that the most successful of such treatments, as defined by reported farmer demand for them, be meticulously documented and validated.

Jones, Bryony. 1996. At the sharp end in south Sudan. *Vetaid Newsletter* 14(Spring): 3.

While visiting Bor and Aliap Dinka in southern Sudan, Vetaid workers noted that cattle camps are composed of 20 to 50 small herds (*gols*) of 20 to 50 cattle each. At night, each of the animals in a *gol* is tethered by a peg in the ground to form a circle around a dung fire. The acrid smoke of the fire provides an effective deterrent to biting flies and mosquitoes that would otherwise attack the animals.

Jones, David Keith. 1984. *Shepherds of the Desert.* Elm Tree Books/Hamish Hamilton, London, UK.

This illustrated volume on Kenyan pastoralists contains some information on ethnoveterinary practices and beliefs. Turkana incise the tails of live fat-tailed sheep and remove the fat for their own use (p. 39). Samburu break the skulls of their bulls with special ritual stones in order to manipulate the angle of the horns (p. 81). They also train the horns into pleasing shapes by tying them with a rope. Gabbra believe that the 'evil eye' brings misfortune to animals as well as to people (p. 145).

Jones, Karen Elizabeth. 1994. *Legislation affecting the Delivery of Animal Health Services by Paraveterinary Personnel.* MSc thesis, CTVM, University of Edinburgh, Edinburgh, UK. 68 pp.

In a brief discussion of local livestock knowledge in relation to the main theme of this thesis, the author suggests that governments and donors could make greater use of indigenous healthcare knowledge and institutions to extend and reinforce both traditional and modern veterinary services by: granting them greater respect; formally recognizing traditional healers; and by mobilizing healers under customary rather than constitutional law.

Joshi, Durga D. 1979. Role of indigeneous [sic] drugs in veterinary medicines. *Journal of the Nepalese Pharmacological Association* 7(Special Issue): 57–59.

This article lists 37 plants of veterinary importance in the Himalayas of Nepal. There, ancient herbal medicines are still commonly used today by veterinarians, medical officers, Ayurvedic physicians, and local *vaidya* healers. Although none is sold commercially for the veterinary market, the Nepali firm Royal Drugs Ltd markets some herbals for humans. Nepalese veterinarians prescribe these human-oriented drugs for small animal diseases to great effect. Also available and used in Nepal are veterinary herbals made and sold by Indian pharmaceutical houses such as Bhartiya Bootee Bhawan and the Indian Herbs Research and Supply Company. To further the manufacture and availability of such medicines, the author recommends: feasibility and economic studies of indigenous herbal drugs; research, evaluation, improved production techniques, rigorous testing and quality control for herbals selected for commercialization; training of technical personnel in their use; and establishment of commercial and technical links between existing herbal farms and Royal Drugs Ltd.

Jost, C.C., D.M. Sherman, E.F. Thomson and R.M. Hesselton. 1996. Kamal (*Mallotus philippensis*) [sic] fruit is ineffective as an anthelminthic against gastrointestinal nematodes in goats indigenous to Balochistan, Pakistan. *Small Ruminant Research* 20: 147–153.

Single-dose oral treatments of *kamala* – the dried, powdered fruit of *Mallotus philippensis* – were compared with a single dose of fenbendazole (Panacur^{TM}) to determine the relative effectiveness of each against selected gastrointestinal nematodes in goats. Twenty-eight castrated male goats were made parasite-free and then inoculated with mixed cultures of infective, direct life-cycle nematode larvae. Across 26 days, faecal epg counts for the groups treated with *kamala* did not drop significantly ($P > 0.05$) from their pre-treatment values. In contrast, fenbendazole effected a significant decrease ($P < 0.001$) in only 5 days. Although interviews with farmers conducted in Quetta, Pakistan indicated that *kamala* is widely used as a general anthelmintic in the area, research shows it does not eliminate direct life-cycle gastrointestinal nematodes in goats. Therefore, the authors recommend it not be used as the sole treatment for nematode infections of the gastrointestinal tract.

Jost, C., C. Stem, M. Ramushwa, E. Twinamasiko and J. Mariner. 1998. Comparative ethnoveterinary and serological evaluation of the Karimojong community animal health worker program in Uganda. *Annals of the New York Academy of Sciences* 849: 327–337.

The Karimojong Community Animal Health Worker (CAHW) programme in Uganda was evaluated using participatory ethnoveterinary techniques. These techniques revealed that stockraisers considered anaplasmosis, CBPP, ECF and rinderpest to be the main causes of cattle mortality. Also, people said they preferred to own animals that had been conventionally vaccinated against rinderpest. They thought that approximately 40% of their cattle had been so vaccinated, but serological tests showed this figure to be as low as 10%. This discrepancy suggests that ethnoveterinary interviews do not provide numerically accurate data concerning disease protection. However, the authors suggest that such cost-effective techniques are adequate for gathering basic indications of disease patterns.

Jovellanos, Mariano Ll. 1992. Veterinary herbology. Paper presented to the PVMA-Ilocos Chapter's convention, San Fernando, La Union, Philippines, 18 September. 7 pp.

The author discusses the best way to prepare and administer veterinary botanicals. Plants may be given in animal feeds or simply by allowing stock to graze medicinal species in pastures and hedgerows. Ideally, plants should be collected at the onset of the rainy season, in the early morning, and when the leaves are just unfurling, because their medicinal properties are at their peak under these conditions. Methods of dosage, treatment and preservation are described. The last category includes making tinctures, essences and brews.

Kabaija, E. 1989. Non-conventional indigenous mineral supplements used for cattle feeding in the pastoral rangelands of Ethiopia. *Tropical Animal Health and Production* 21: 256–262.

Ethiopian pastoralists provide their livestock with indigenous mineral supplements via rock salt, soil licks and water from saline wells. This study sampled indigenous supplements from different regions in Ethiopia and analysed them for calcium, copper, iron, magnesium, manganese, phosphorus, potassium, sodium and zinc content. Most licks had low solubility in both water and acid and were alkaline, which may reduce their palatability. Also, most licks were high in iron and sodium but low in all other elements, especially phosphorus and copper. The author recommends supplementing cattle that receive traditional licks with phosphorus. All water sources studied were considered satisfactory except for one, where its 8500 mg of solutes per litre exceeded safety limits. Cattle drinking this water got diarrhoea; but herders believed the diarrhoea helped eliminate stomach worms.

Kajjak, Nancy, Hernando Bazalar and Luis F. Coronado. 1989. Manejo de la salud animal en una comunidad campesina de Junín. In: Hernando Bazalar and Constance M. McCorkle (eds). *Estudios Etnoveterinarios en Comunidades Altoandinas del Perú.* Lluvia Editores, Lima, Perú. Pp. 53–67.

The first half of this chapter describes 38 home remedies for ailments of cattle, sheep, horses, donkeys and swine employed in a peasant village studied by the SR-CRSP in Peru's Mantaro Valley. Remedies are organized according to six categories of ailments (ectoparasitism, endoparasitism, infectious diseases, obstetrical problems, nutritional deficiencies and other signs and conditions, including supernatural ills). Each category is further broken down into more precise subtypes. Based on both firsthand field observations and a review of Peru's ethnopharmacological literature, the authors offer their general assessments of the actual or potential efficacy of the remedies described. The chapter's second half details the results of a year's tracking of the incidence of livestock diseases among ten families' herds of cattle and sheep (180 and 1760 cases, respectively) and of the types of therapies stockowners chose in each case. Therapies are classed as: Andean, i.e. apparently indigenous; syncretic, i.e. a mix of Andean and Western; and exogenous, i.e. commercial pharmaceuticals. Parasitism is the most pervasive problem. The chapter concludes by noting that Andean peasants are open to trying whatever options are available in order to protect one of their most 'critical resources – their livestock'.

Kambewa, Bizaliel Muvetsa Daimon. 1996. *Identification of Indigenous Veterinary Remedies for Livestock Health Problems in Malawi: A Case Study in Mzuzu Agricultural Development Division (ADD).* MSc Thesis in Animal Science/Animal Production, Bunda College of Agriculture, University of Malawi, Lilongwe, Malawi. 89 pp.

A survey of 53 farmers in seven of the 13 non-dipping areas of the Mzuzu Agricultural Development Division in Malawi was conducted to identify what veterinary remedies farmers used. Interviewees reported treating a range of ailments in ruminants, pigs and chickens. Two plants widely cited by interviewees as ectoparasiticides were subsequently subjected to pharmacological screening. These were *Tephrosia vogelii* and *Physostigma mesoponticum*. Likewise for

Vernonia adoensis and *Sema didymobotrya*, which farmers said combat worms in goats. Preliminary results confirmed *P. mesoponticum* as a potential acaricide, but the other plants showed no significant anti-parasitic action.

Kambewa, B.M.D. 1999. Integration of indigenous veterinary remedies in farming systems in Malawi. Paper presented to the International Seminar on Integrated Approach for Animal Health Care. Calicut, Kerala, India. 9 pp.

This paper reviews the need for an integrated approach to animal healthcare in Malawi. Malawi's government ministries are unable to support the large livestock sector of the country, so farmers continue to make good use of their indigenous knowledge when treating their animals. The author calls for greater efforts to promote the integration of indigenous remedies in livestock and crop production into the household, in conjunction with protection of natural resources such as forests. For example, *Tephrosia vogelii* is already being planted to improve soil fertility, so it would be relatively easy to promote its use as an animal acaricide and maize pesticide at the same time.

Kambewa, B.M.D., M.W. Mfitilodze, K. Hüttner, C.B.A. Wollny and R.K.D. Phoya. 1999. The use of indigenous veterinary remedies in Malawi. In: E. Mathias, D.V. Rangnekar and C.M. McCorkle, with M. Martin (eds). *Ethnoveterinary Medicine: Alternatives for Livestock Development – Proceedings of an International Conference Held in Pune, India, 4–6 November 1997. Volume 1: Selected Papers.* BAIF Development Research Foundation, Pune, India. Pp. 60–66.

This case study identified Malawian smallholders' indigenous veterinary remedies and also evaluated the preparation (mainly extractions), handling (especially storage time) and effectiveness of certain ethnomedicines. In five non-dipping and two dipping rural areas, a total of 53 farmers were iteratively interviewed across 1.5 months in 1995. The farmers also assisted in collecting samples of the medicinal parts of 69 plants they used; species were identified botanically based on literature searches and information from the National Herbarium in Zomba. Besides plants, animal parts, salt, soil and dung figured in the ethnoveterinary pharmacopoeia, and common ethnoveterinary treatments included bloodletting, wound care, cauterization and obstetrics. Farmers said that they had learned about the remedies from ancestors (93%) and through dreams (6%) and they noted that the medicines sometimes worked and sometimes not. Under controlled conditions, a selection of remedies was screened. These included treatments for tick, flea and roundworm infestations in cattle, chickens and goats, respectively. Findings confirmed farmers' own assessment that some of the medicines were highly effective (those for ticks and fleas) while others were not (those for worms). An evaluation of handling practices was conducted on the extract of *Physostigma mesoponticum* Taub tubers, used to treat *Rhipicephalus appendiculatus* ticks, in a larval packet method. Results showed that the local tuber paste could be used effectively twice and that its extract could be stored and used for 2 weeks between 22°C and 30°C and at 85% to 98% relative humidity. The author notes that the survey's findings are only illustrative of the extent and effectiveness of ethnoveterinary remedies in Malawi because this was a case study and tests were done under controlled conditions. Next steps needed are more comprehensive research coupled with field trials.

Kariuki, D.P. 1992a. *Visit to Turkana District 6–10 August 1992.* In-house report. ITDG, Nairobi, Kenya. 21 pp.

A participatory ITDG/Oxfam study with Turkana pastoralists of Kenya explored the latters' ethno-entomological and -veterinary knowledge of ticks and tick-borne livestock diseases in their environment. Pastoralists themselves identified ticks as a problem, not only because they transmit disease but also because, coupled with lice and fleas, a heavy tick burden can kill camel foals, calves, lambs and kids weakened by the dry season. Ticks also cause abscesses and significant economic losses due to hide damage. In this study, pastoralists collected what they deemed different types of ticks and sent them to a scientist for formal taxonomic identification. The scientist later returned the preserved insects to their collectors and discussed tick ethnotaxonomies and locally recognized disease factors with them. Pastoralists knew that ticks suck blood and inject 'poison' into the bloodstream. They said ticks cause heartwater, which Turkana term ruminant 'madness' and relate specifically to the *Amblyomma* genus. And rightly or wrongly, they blamed ticks for many other ills, including anthrax, rinderpest, fever (in some cases possibly ECF), abscesses, footrot, teat injuries, ear swellings (possibly an allergic reaction?) and yet other conditions such as difficult breathing and photosensitization. People were astute at distinguishing the genus, but not always the species, of ticks. However, they could not differentiate among male and female nor, except for one elder, between adults and nymphs. Study participants noted that they manually pick ticks off their livestock or, in the case of camels, shave them off with the hair. After removing ticks from the britch of sheep, stockowners may also lightly cauterize the wounds, sprinkle them with ash and then dress them with loose goat faeces. People further mentioned that they sometimes used a certain chemical (staladone). But because it is expensive, they often dilute it. Also, they had noticed the beginning of resistance to the chemical in that 'the *dawa* is not killing the ticks' anymore. In discussions with the scientist, pastoralists learned of cheaper alternatives such as pyegrease and tick and flea powders, which are also far less toxic to human handlers than staladone. The scientist further recommended that chewn tobacco could be rubbed over animals to remove ticks, since Turkana are always chewing tobacco and they already use the juice to treat scorpion bites. Participants and scientist alike agreed that conventional tick control measures like dips and sprays, which require a lot of water, were infeasible in the Turkana's arid environment.

Kariuki, D.P. 1992b. *Visit to Turkana District 5–10 December 1992.* In-house report. ITDG, Nairobi, Kenya. 4 pp.

In a follow-up study on Turkana knowledge of tick biology and ethology, the author engaged pastoralists from Kakuma Division in a participatory mapping exercise. The exercise revealed local knowledge about the habitat distribution of the three major tick genuses in the area. Participants noted that *Ambylomma* spp. are mostly found in the hills and along river bends, where they attack all species and cause abscesses and heartwater. They said *Hyaloma* spp. live mainly in the hills and in river beds and attack all but donkeys. *Rhipicephalus* spp. were said to cluster along a single river and to favour areas of sisal vegetation; this genus was blamed for livestock ear infections and swellings.

Karo-Karo, S. 1990. *Effectivitas Nikotin Ekstrak daun Tembakau Terhadap Cacing Lambung* (Haemonchus contortus *Rudolphi) pada Kambing* (Capra hircus *Linn.*). MSc thesis, Fakultas Pascasarjana, Bogor Agricultural University, Bogor, Indonesia. 54 pp.

The efficacy of nicotine extract from tobacco leaves against *Haemonchus contortus* was tested in 27 goats. The animals were divided into nine groups. One group served as control while the other eight received between 27.2 mg and 465.8 mg of nicotine extract per animal orally. At a dosage of 310.5 mg/goat or 24.8 mg/kg body weight, the faecal egg count declined by 78%, although the number of parasites remained constant. Dosages below 310.5 mg/goat reduced egg numbers in the faeces by only 35.7%, and 465.8 mg/goat produced signs of toxicity.

Karunathilakaratne, T.A.R.W.M.M. 1986. Indigenous methods of treatment for some common conditions of cattle in the N.C.P. *Sri Lanka Veterinary Journal* 34(1/2): 69–70.

Traditional Sri Lankan prescriptions for four cattle and one buffalo disease are given in this article. FMD is treated with a drench of tamarind leaves and gingelly oil. Lesions are coated either with copper sulphate and margosa oil or with these two ingredients mixed with pig dung. Haemorrhagic septicaemia is treated by feeding a mixture of copper sulphate, sodium sulphate and alum, which is placed inside an orange and roasted. Placed in a cloth, the roasted orange mixture can also be hung around the animals' necks as a prophylactic. A drench for bloat consists of gingelly seed and garlic in coconut juice. Worm infestation prescriptions for cattle and buffalo calves consist of, respectively, mixtures of ground margosa-leaf juice and margosa oil and woodapple juice with coconut.

Kasonia, Kakule. 1997. *Une Reconnaissance des Savoirs Paysans: Plantes Médicinales et Médecine Vétérinaire Traditionnelle d'Afrique Centrale.* Vol. I: Pharmacopée Vétérinaire Traditionnelle d'Afrique Centrale (375 pp.); Vol. II: Mise a l'Epreuve d'Extraits de Plantes Utilisées en Afrique comme Antiasthmatiques et Antitussifs (37 pp.); Vol. III: Annexes (223 pp.). Doctoral dissertation, Faculty of Veterinary Medicine, University of Liege, Belgium.

This doctoral dissertation draws upon the PRELUDE Network's extensive databank of (as of August 1996) 1166 plants and 5000 prescriptions used in traditional veterinary medicine in 14 countries of sub-Saharan Africa. The dissertation presents a preliminary, tripartite analysis of such plants for the Great Lakes region of the Central African nations of Burundi, Rwanda and Zaire. Analysis asks: which botanical families and genera are most often used by traditional veterinary doctors and reported by them or others (coherence), with what consistency in their application to specific livestock diseases (convergence) and with what overlaps in human ethnomedicine (concordance)? The overarching hypothesis is that the higher a plant scores across these three parameters, the more likely it is to be biomedically effective. This hypothesis is tested and largely borne out, by subjecting high-scoring plants to review in the global phytochemical, biological and pharmacological literature; plants for which such literature is lacking constitute prime candidates for follow-on research. As a more definitive test of the hypothesis, some of the high-scoring materials (those used to treat respiratory ailments) were also subjected to confirming laboratory analyses. The author makes the important point that the obverse of the hypothesis does not necessarily hold. This is because traditional healers who depend upon 'trade secrets' to earn their reputations and livelihoods may refuse to reveal particular plants. Thus, 'popular' plants must be distinguished from 'secret' ones, because the latter will likely be underreported in the field, in data-banks, etc. So the absence of report data attesting to a plant's broad-based familiarity and use cannot necessarily be taken to imply its inefficacy. Nevertheless, the author recommends his methodology as one, cost-effective way to approach the validation of ethnomedical pharmacopoeia and/or to choose promising avenues of research for new drug discovery. The dissertation as a whole is structured in three volumes. The first explores such topics as: EVM in Africa; contributions from, and problems between, ethno- to orthodox veterinary and human medicine; ethnomedicine's relationship to the maintenance of biodiversity; and the importance of inter-disciplinarity in ethnomedical research at the level of botanists, pharmacologists and pharmacognosists, but also anthropological and sociopolitical aspects of stockraising and EVM. The latter point is illustrated by reference to two Great Lakes groups, the Wa-Nande and Ba-Hema. Findings also suggest that natural definitions of disease are more prevalent in EVM, while supernatural ones are more common in human ethnomedicine of the area. Volume II presents both published and unpublished results of the laboratory tests performed on the respiratory phytotherapies [see above]. Volume III consists of seven data annexes dealing with the statistical and other manipulations performed for the coherence/convergence/concordance analysis, for which all raw data are also presented.

Kasonia, K. and M. Ansay. 1996. Demarche du Sous-reseau PRELUDE: Santé, Productions Animales et Environnement en matière d'echanges des savoirs et de recherche endogene. In: Karl-Hans Zessin (ed.). *Livestock Production and Diseases in the Tropics: Livestock Production and Human Welfare. Proceedings of the VIII International Conference of Institutions of Tropical Veterinary Medicine held from the 25 to 29 September, 1995 in Berlin, Germany.* Volume II. Deutsche Stiftung für Internationale Entwicklung, Zentralstelle für Ernährung und Landwirtschaft, Feldafing, Germany. P. 474.

A university research and liaison programme, the SPAE subnetwork of PRELUDE has as its overarching objective the improvement of animal health and production via intercultural dialogue about the re-valuing and, where feasible, re-application of traditional veterinary and husbandry techniques. The subnetwork focuses on three tasks: joint identification by stockraisers and researchers/developers of EVK; interdisciplinary 'valorisation' of this knowledge, whether via field, clinical or laboratory studies; and feedback of all resulting findings into the dialogue between bearers of traditional and conventional veterinary knowledge.

Kasonia, K. and M. Ansay. 1999. A recognition of rural knowledge: Medicinal plants and traditional veterinary medicine of central Africa (testing the traditional veterinary pharmacopoeia). In: E. Mathias, D.V. Rangnekar and C.M. McCorkle, with M. Martin (eds). *Ethnoveterinary Medicine: Alternatives for Livestock Development – Proceedings of an International Conference Held in Pune, India, 4–6 November 1997. Volume 1: Selected Papers.* BAIF Development Research Foundation, Pune, India. Pp. 67–72.

The work reported here describes a feasible and cost-effective way to pre-screen medicinal plants from 'old knowledge' for possible use in new medicines, whether for livestock or people. This method was tested on the phytopharmacopoeia of the Great Lakes region of central Africa via searches and statistical measures using the PRELUDE databank. The product of an international network based in Belgium, this databank is devoted to traditional veterinary medicine of sub-Saharan Africa. To test the internal coherence – and by implication, the validity – of rural people's veterinary knowledge, consistencies among the botanical characteristics of medicinal plants, their particular veterinary usage and cognate uses in human ethnomedicine were computed. In the process, plants were coded as 'popular remarkable', 'secret' or 'commonly used in veterinary and human medicine'. This ancestral knowledge was validated (or invalidated) by documentary research and investigation of the plants' pharmacological and phytochemical properties. In this way, for example, 50% of all the 'popular remarkable' plants employed by traditional practitioners for gastrointestinal diseases were confirmed effective. Based on such cross-evaluation of multiple data, the authors recommend this as a feasible bioprospecting method for pointing researchers to sources of new molecules as a starting point for designing new modern medicines. Equally important, however, is the fact that the knowledge captured in such databanks is the unique medical resource for more than 80% of the world's population. Research such as that described here can be applied to informing the holders of this knowledge, like rural peoples and healers, of the activity or inactivity of certain plants in their ethnopharmacopoeia. With this added information, people may be more interested to preserve the biodiversity of their environment, e.g. by cultivating gardens of validated medicinal plants. This method also opens the way to the standardization of demonstrably beneficial indigenous phyto-treatments. In short, the method offers a way to begin evaluating ethnopharmacological knowledge and making it more homogeneous, more efficient, less mysterious and more profitable to its present holders and its future users worldwide.

Kasonia, K., M. Ansay, M. Baerts and J. Lehmann. 1996. Regard comparatif sur l'usage des plantes medicinales en médecine vétérinaire et humaine et sauvegarde de la biodiversité Africaine. In: Karl-Hans Zessin (ed.). *Livestock Production and Diseases in the Tropics: Livestock Production and Human Welfare. Proceedings of the VIII International Conference of Institutions of Tropical Veterinary Medicine held from the 25 to 29 September, 1995 in Berlin, Germany.* Volume II. Deutsche Stiftung für Internationale Entwicklung, Zentralstelle für Ernährung und Landwirtschaft, Feldafing, Germany. P. 380.

This conference poster-paper notes that, although many studies of ethnobotanicals for both veterinary and human medicine have been conducted in central Africa's Great Lakes region, rarely do such studies find 'concordances', i.e. the use of the same plant by multiple traditional practitioners for treating the same symptom(s) within and across patient species. The authors' statistical analysis of the data from such studies suggests that the lack of concordance may be linked to the fact that approximately 80% of all the plants reported are used to treat psychosomatic ills. For more purely somatic ills, patient and practitioner reports attest to a corpus of effective botanical febrifuges, tonics, galactagogues and vermifuges. Higher levels of concordance can perhaps be expected within this corpus. Drawing upon the PHARMEL and PRELUDE databanks, the authors examine this question, pointing up some concordances they have thus discovered between the use of certain plants in both veterinary and human ethnomedicine in the Great Lakes region.

Kasonia, K., M. Ansay, N. Basegere, P. Gustin, S. Kaba, M. Katsongeri and M. Matamba. 1991. Note d'ethnopharmacologie vétérinaire en cas de verminoses, diarrhée, coprostase et météorisme au Kivu et Kibali-Ituri (Zaïre). *Tropicultura* 9(4): 169–172.

In stockraising in intertropical Africa, worm infestations and diarrhoea are important and ubiquitous health problems. But African stockraisers have various botanicals to combat these and other conditions like coprostasis (faecal impaction) and meteorism (tympanites). This article reports the results of a survey of pertinent plant-based medicines among peoples of central Zaire. A total of 32 plant species belonging to 22 families were found to be employed singly or in combination in 34 home remedies, divided as follows: 11 for worms, 12 for non-specific diarrhoea, 4 for haemorrhagic diarrhoea, 2 for neonatal diarrhoea, 4 for coprostasis and 1 for meteorism. Plant parts used spanned leaves (59%), fruits or seeds (12%), the whole plant (12%), stem bark (9%), roots, rhizomes or tubers (5%) and root bark (3%). Pharmaceutical procedures included maceration (51% of remedies), decoction (25%), infusion (2%), no modification (20%) and other (2%). The preferred mode of administration was overwhelmingly oral (90%), followed by rectal (10%). All these data are summarized in a table by plant species. A second table outlines similar uses for 11 of the 32 species in other African countries, as reported in the pharmacological literature. Such overlaps suggest that these species are good candidates for further investigation. Moreover, review of the literature reveals that a number of the plants identified have demonstrable antimicrobial properties. Thus, with perhaps only a little further study of their mode of preparation and administration, they could likely be recommended for treating such conditions as bacterial diarrhoeas. The authors further note that in 80% of cases the plant parts used in Zairian home remedies surveyed grow aboveground, where animals can simply graze on them. This suggests possibilities for pasture improvements to combat basic animal health problems. Such improvements would be cheaper than pharmaceutical synthesis of the active ingredients or even just commercial packaging of crude botanicals.

Kasonia, K. and K.M. Yamalo. 1994. Ethnologie des traitements vétérinaires dans la région du Nord-Kivu (Zaire). In: Kakule Kasonia and Michel Ansay (eds). *Métissages en Santé Animale de Madagascar à Haïti: Actes du Séminaire d'Ethnopharmacopée Vétérinaire 'KAGALA', un Partage de Savoirs Burkina-Faso, Ouagadougou, 15–22 Avril 1993.* Presses Universitaires de Namur, Namur, Belgium. Pp. 275–286.

A survey of ethnoveterinary practices in North Kivu, Zaire, revealed no veterinary equivalents of traditional human healers in the region. However, along with veterinary field agents, herders themselves were able to point researchers to 61 healing plants used for local cattle, small ruminants, swine, poultry and rabbits. These are listed by both Latin and local names in Table 1. Of the 61, 19 are employed specifically for livestock ailments; and the authors judge that at least another 9 of the remaining 42 plants used in human ethnomedicine would have practical veterinary applications. Table 2's 'Summary of Pathological Cases Covered by Traditional Veterinary Cures in North Kivu, Zaire' presents 27 pathologies for livestock and, in some cases, also humans, along with their phytotherapies. The latter consist overwhelmingly of single-plant preparations, sometimes accompanied by one or two other ingredients like seasalt or cooking oil. Modes of administration are mainly oral (drenches and feed additives) and topical (direct applications and sprays). But eye and nose drops are also used, along with still other modes. For instance, to drive off lice and fleas, tobacco leaves are placed beneath poultry nests or are powdered and sprinkled on the nests. A cure for rabbit bloat consists of adding chopped *Thymus vulgaris* L. leaves to the feed. Contagious ecthyma in small ruminants may be treated in a variety of ways: washing the lesions with a decoction of pounded *Hibiscus surattensis* L. leaves and drenching with the same decoction; moistening the sores with lemon juice; or rubbing the lesions with heated tobacco leaves or with a decoction of green *Basella alba* L. leaves. For varying kinds of diarrhoea in varying species, 13 different remedies are presented. The list continues.

Katsuyama, O. 1994. Veterinary folk remedies in Japan. *Revue Scientifique et Technique de l'Office International des Épizooties* 13(2): 453–463.

Starting from the earliest-known references in A.D. 595 and continuing through an ethnoveterinary survey in the 1970s, this article reviews folk remedies for livestock in Japan. The traditional veterinary pharmacopoeia comprises incantations, charms, herbal medicines, bloodletting, acupuncture and moxibustion. This last treatment involves thermal stimulation of the acupuncture points by burning a cone of *Artemisia moxa* at the prescribed point on the patient's skin. In the past, sandal-like straw shoes were fashioned to protect the hooves of cattle and horses. Horse doctors known as *hakuraku* or *bakuro* performed bloodletting and hoof-trimming. Several treatments for canine diseases are cited: a meal of boiled adzuki or soya beans for wounded dogs; topical application of camphor for ectoparasites; and a drench of boiled soya-bean water as an antidote to shrimp poisoning. Also noted is the modern-day registration and commercialization of at least ten veterinary drugs based on traditional herbal preparations. At the same time, various prophylactic charms obtained from temples are still in use – many of them as items to be hung in the entranceways to animal quarters. Once such is bamboo grass that has been blessed, hung in an ailing horse's stable and then later fed to the horse.

Kaufmann, Brigitte. 1998. *Analysis of Pastoral Camel Husbandry in Northern Kenya.* Hohenheim Tropical Agricultural Series No. 5. Margraf Verlag, Weikersheim, Germany. 194 pp.

Camels' unique adaptation to arid and semi-arid areas enables pastoralists to survive in these high-risk environments. Though rare, studies on camel pastoralism often view this species' productivity as low, blaming pastoralists' poor management. This thesis presents a rapid analysis methodology for identifying interventions that might increase the sustainability of pastoral systems of camel husbandry. The methods combine questionnairing and bioeconomic modelling. Three standardized question-naires were applied to 50 herders from each of three pastoral groups (Gabbra, Rendille, Somali) in Marsabit District, Kenya in order to assess and compare camel reproduction, management and production. In addition, the 1908–1995 life histories of 287 Gabbra, 476 Rendille and 416 Somali she-camels and their offspring were recorded. The resulting data were used to calculate inherent fitness and production parameters, which were then fed into a bioeconomic model for assessing herd productivity and doing *ex ante* evaluation of possibly helpful interventions. The appropriateness and feasibility of proposed interventions were also discussed with the 150 herders. For all three groups, the thesis briefly outlines herding strategies, watering and mineral supplementation, breeding practices, disease prophylaxes and therapies, calf care, milking regimes, the use of castrates and reasons for offtake. Most herders knew various disease signs and treatments. Appendix 5 briefly describes the following ills and their traditional and Western treatments: swollen glands, septicaemia, purulent conditions, skin necrosis, navel ill, *saam* and *ilgoff* (two unidentified calf diseases), trypanosomosis, paralysis, pneumonia, swollen neck, diarrhoea, orf and tick infestation. Only a few herders used dewormers, usually only for camels with diarrhoea or poor growth. Dewormers included extracts of *Albizia anthelmintica* bark and *Acacia brevispica*. Somalis separate diseased animals from healthy ones, while Gabbra and Rendille herders do not. (Gabbra said separation requires too much labour.) But pregnant camels are usually separated for careful observation. And all interviewees considered calf care especially important. Calves receive sufficient milk and good pasture; a 'special man' is nominated to milk their dams; and ticks are regularly removed. However, most herders reported restricting newborns' intake of colostrum in the belief that excess colostrum causes diarrhoea or other digestive problems. The thesis notes that some management practices represent specific adaptations to the harsh environment, e.g. splitting herds into milking versus mobile units and feeding salt. Other practices go beyond mere adaptation to enhance production. These include, e.g., certain birthing measures, specific milking and suckling regimes, selective breeding and disease prevention and control strategies. In some areas, however, pastoralists did not seem to appreciate management impacts on production and productivity. For example, they did not always recognize the connections between calf mortality and limited colostrum intake, between poor production and irregular mineral supplementation, between inbreeding and prolonged use of the same studs, or between contagion and disease treatments. Shortening the calving interval, modifying milk offtake and price, reducing calf mortality and controlling mastitis were identified by analysis as interventions that could increase productivity. However, the effect of each such intervention will vary across pastoral groups because of their differing management systems and goals. Moreover, analysis showed that recommendations based on performance indicators alone are inappropriate. For example, if only outputs are compared, the Somali system appears superior to the Gabbra and Rendille systems by about 50%. But when the greater fodder requirements of the Somali system are taken into account, it proves only 10% more productive than the Rendille's; and it is 7% less productive than the Gabbra's. The thesis concludes by recommending the combined assessment of management, production and productivity in order to arrive at system-specific analyses of, and interventions for, camel pastoralism.

Kaufmann, Brigitte A. and Christian G. Hülsebusch. 1998. Camel calf losses in pastoral systems in northern Kenya: Importance, causes and traditional remedies. In: E. Mathias, D.V. Rangnekar and C.M. McCorkle, with M. Martin (eds). *Ethnoveterinary Medicine: Alternatives for Livestock Development – Proceedings of an International Conference Held in Pune, India, 4–6 November 1997. Volume 2: Abstracts.* BAIF Development Research Foundation, Pune, India. Pp. 31–32.

Dromedaries are uniquely adapted to the arid or semi-arid Horn of Africa, where camels' contribution of milk and transport is critical for pastoralists' survival. This study investigated causes of camel calf losses, which are a key factor in herd productivity, in three pastoral systems (Rendille, Gabbra and Somali) of northern

Kenya, along with ethnoveterinary knowledge of calf diseases. Mortality rates and causes were calculated based on progeny histories of 1506 Rendille, 789 Gabbra and 1206 Somali camel calves born during 1980–1995. Mortality up to weaning at 12 months of age was 27%, 22% and 31%, respectively; and diseases accounted for 59%, 71% and 82% of these losses. Other causes were drought, predation and accidents. In each camel population, three major ailments were responsible for about two-thirds of all calf losses to disease: Rendille – diarrhoea (33%), septicaemia (18%) and tick intoxication (15%); Gabbra – diarrhoea (21%), septi-caemia (24%) and orf (25%); and Somali – diarrhoea (23%), skin necrosis (23%) and *ilgoff* (28%). Pastoralists' assessment of important calf diseases was estab-lished, along with their importance ranking, symptom description and different traditional treatment methods. Since only a few diseases account for the bulk of losses, interventions targeted at these diseases are likely to have a high positive impact on animal health and productivity. Findings further revealed that herders' perception of disease importance matched well with the actual losses to disease experienced in the past. Thus, stockraisers' own knowledge and assessment of disease importance are valuable resources for planning interventions, whether in extension, healthcare delivery services, or epidemiological research.

Kaye, G. Arthur. 1992. Deworming with papaya seeds. *Footsteps* 12(Sep): 14.

Ghanaians use papaya seeds to make a homemade remedy for intestinal worms in livestock, including roundworms in ruminants and other worms in both ruminants and poultry. The seeds are soaked in water to remove their outer covering. After straining and sun-drying, they are ground into a powder, which can be stored for a long time in an airtight container. When deworming is indicated, a drench of 1 tea-spoon of the powder in 4 l of water is mixed up.

Keilbach, N.M., M. Larios and L. Saez. 1996. Training with farmers in northern Nicaragua. In: Karl-Hans Zessin (ed.). *Livestock Production and Diseases in the Tropics: Livestock Production and Human Welfare. Proceedings of the VIII International Conference of Institutions of Tropical Veterinary Medicine held from the 25 to 29 September, 1995 in Berlin, Germany.* Volume II. Deutsche Stiftung für Internationale Entwicklung, Zentralstelle für Ernährung und Landwirtschaft, Feldafing, Germany. Pp. 527–531.

As part of its low-input agriculture mandate, the northern Nicaraguan NGO Universidad Campesina or 'Peasant University' (UNICAM) has instituted an animal health and husbandry programme to provide training in both traditional and modern veterinary medicine. Transmission of EVK in this programme is based on a farmer-to-farmer methodology, supported by practicals. UNICAM technical staff act mainly as facilitators, supplementing local knowledge with some scientific information or ideas where necessary. However, the author notes that it is not always easy to communicate 'about things that cannot be seen, like bacteria, defence mechanisms or vitamins' (p. 530). UNICAM has encouraged farmers to systematize their EVK by recording dosages, so they can share more precise information among themselves. In addition, a major study of herbal remedies for livestock [not reported here] has been carried out in the region. UNICAM has found that Nicaraguan farmers have different levels of EVK and that their livestock savvy is generally less than their cropping expertise. People with greater-than-normal cattle knowledge are much respected and frequently consulted by other cattle-raisers. Even so, stockraisers do not always put into practice health measures already known to them. Many women have a good understanding of cattle behaviour and problems, but are not confident of this knowledge because cattle work has traditionally been a male prerogative. Most women keep poultry, however; but they have problems dealing with poultry diseases. In contrast, local knowledge of fodder trees is high and farmers experiment on their own with different ways to use this resource more extensively.

Kelawala, N.H. and Amresh Kumar. 1998. Analgesic and therapeutic effects of electroacupuncture in dogs. In: E. Mathias, D.V. Rangnekar and C.M. McCorkle, with M. Martin (eds). ***Ethnoveterinary Medicine: Alternatives for Livestock Development – Proceedings of an International Conference Held in Pune, India, 4–6 November 1997. Volume 2: Abstracts.*** BAIF Development Research Foundation, Pune, India. Pp. 32–33.

Electroacupuncture (EA) is an improved, techno-blended version of the ancient Chinese medical/veterinary technique of acupuncture. This paper reports on a series of studies conducted in India to observe EA's analgesic and selected therapeutic effects in dogs. In one study, the animals were divided into two groups and respectively subjected to EA stimulation at acupoints BL-23, GV-6, ST-36, SP-6 and GV-26 (Group I) or acupoints ST-36, SP-6, TW-8, GV-6, LU-1 and TW-8 (Group II). Then, each group was tested for analgesic effects after experimental abdominal pelvic surgery. Muscle relaxation and analgesia was greater for Group II. After EA, in both groups heart rate and respiration rate significantly increased ($P < 0.05$). Increases in rectal temperature and decreases in tidal and minute volume were insignificant ($P > 0.05$). In both groups, recovery was quick, smooth and uncomplicated. Another study tested the therapeutic effect of EA in 16 dogs in which paresis was experimentally induced through injuring the sciatic nerve (axonotmesis). The animals were randomly divided in an experimental and a non-treatment control group of eight each and all were subjected daily to neurological examination. The treatment group were given EA at acupoints ST-36, ST-32, BL-30, BL-67, GB-30 and GB-34, after which they showed better wound conditions and no post-operative infection compared to controls. By day 30 after induction of paresis, dogs in the treatment group regained a near-normal state and showed no signs whatsoever of paresis, whereas the control animals remained abnormal up to day 60. Results indicate that EA is an effective treatment for paresis in the absence of spinal cord disorders. The paper concludes by discussing the advantages and limitations of EA for analgesia and treating paresis.

Kelawala, N.H., Rajesh Tripathi and Amresh Kumar. 1998. Resuscitation of dogs by electroacupuncture at nasal philtrum point (GV 26). In: E. Mathias, D.V. Rangnekar and C.M. McCorkle, with M. Martin (eds). ***Ethnoveterinary Medicine: Alternatives for Livestock Development – Proceedings of an International Conference Held in Pune, India, 4–6 November 1997. Volume 2: Abstracts.*** BAIF Development Research Foundation, Pune, India. P. 33.

Twelve dogs were divided equally into a control and treatment group and in the latter the resuscitation effects of electroacupuncture (EA) at the nasal philtrum (GV 26) point were studied at 10 minutes after induction. All animals were anaesthetized with 30 mg/kg bw of thiopentone sodium intravenously. Cardiopulmonary parameters such as heart rate, respiration rate, tidal volume, minute volume and mean arterial blood pressure were recorded for both groups. The EA treatment group showed a significant decrease in the duration of anaesthesia and in the time taken to achieve complete recovery.

Kemparaja, B.K. Narainswami and Vidya Kulkarni. 1998. Effective ethnoveterinary practices for treating affections of skin and limbs in large animals. In: E. Mathias, D.V. Rangnekar and C.M. McCorkle, with M. Martin (eds). *Ethnoveterinary Medicine: Alternatives for Livestock Development – Proceedings of an International Conference Held in Pune, India, 4–6 November 1997. Volume 2: Abstracts.* BAIF Development Research Foundation, Pune, India. Pp. 33–34.

This paper describes a number of treatments employed by Indian stockraisers and traditional healers (*nati vaidyas*) for skin and limb problems in large animals. These treatments were tried on several animals and found to be quite effective. Allergic oedema, malignant oedema and eczema can be cured by local application and oral feeding of *Aristolochia indica, Clerodendrum inerme* and *Andrographis paniculata* leaves. Mange and fungal skin infections respond to topical applications of *Argemone mexicana* seed paste, *Azadirachta indica* decoction or *Thespesia populnea* tree latex. Likewise for ectoparasites and crushed *Annona squamosa* and *Leucas aspera* leaves. Haemorrhages are controlled by applying any of the following: juice extract from the stem core of *Musa paradisica*, the leaf juice of *Tridax procumbens*, turmeric powder, or coffee. Udder oedema can be reduced by piercing the skin with *Coix lacryma-jobi* thorns. Abscesses are made to mature by applying finely ground white stone in butter or warm salt water. Firing is used to treat chronic joint affections and, in young animals, to increase disease resistance. Fractures are immobilized with a strip of cloth soaked in red soil paste, with bamboo splints, or with fresh *Dodonaea viscosa* sticks. All these practices look promising, but they should be tested vis-à-vis conventional ones; and only proven ethnoveterinary practices should be advocated.

Kenyon, Simon J. and Susan M. Kenyon. 1991. The importance of attitudes to animal health and production in development assistance projects. Paper presented to the American Anthropological Association session on Ethnoveterinary Research and Development: Applications for Theory and Practice. Chicago, Illinois, USA. 11 pp.

Ethnoveterinary medicine provides a new perspective from which to view the successes and failures of livestock development. In this paper, three types of livestock production systems are discussed and illustrated: the intensive stockraising system of the United States, nomadic pastoralism of Sudan and smallholder farming of West Java. The ethnoveterinarian or veterinary anthropologist is a useful asset when it comes to evaluating the technical as well as the social implications of livestock development programmes.

Kerharo, J. and J.-G. Adam. 1964. Plantes médicinales et toxiques des Peul et des Toucouleur du Sénégal. *Journal d'Agriculture Tropicale et de Botanique Appliquée* 11(8–9): 384–444.

Always attentive to the health and nutrition of their herds, Peul and Toucouleur pastoralists of Senegal 'know perfectly the virtues and noxiousness of the vegetation in their region . . . these herders are capable of designating almost all the plants . . . by their common name and of indicating their usages' thanks to '. . . observing, comparing, reflecting and ultimately attaining a remarkable level of knowledge about the properties of the vegetation' (p. 392). Based on extensive interviews with native curers, this article lists 100 plants, their Latin, common and local names, their appearance and their uses in every conceivable aspect of human physical, mental and magical health. While the introduction notes that this 'treasure' of knowledge has equal application in animal and human ethnomedicine, unfortunately, the authors are less specific about the former. However, they do note veterinary treatments for stomach ailments (*Acacia senegal*, p. 399), colics (*Carica papaya*, p. 419), enhanced fertility and lactation (*Annona senegalensis*, p. 406; *Borreria verticillata*, p. 413; *Calotropis procera*, p. 416; and *Feretia apodanthera*, p. 442), wounds (*Combretum glutinosum*, p. 427), unthriftiness (*Crossopteryx febrifuga* combined with salt, p. 433) and vaginal problems (*Ficus glumosa*, p. 443), plus the use of purgatives (*Acacia seyal*, p. 399) and a plant-based substance to spread around animal quarters to drive off snakes (*Afrormosia laxiflora*, p. 403). Flora toxic to livestock are also mentioned, like *Cissus quadrangularis* (p. 425). Presumably, many of the human health measures described also apply to animals, e.g. anthelmintics, plasters and antitoxins for snakebite.

Kern, J.R. and J.H. Cardellina. 1983. Native American medicinal plants: Anemonin from the horse stimulant *Clematis hirsutissima*. *Journal of Ethnopharmacology* 8(1): 121–123.

This article notes the effective use of *Clematis hirsutissima* as a horse stimulant among the Nez Percé, Sioux and Teton tribes of North American Indians.

Kerven, Carol and Christopher Lunch. 1998. Routes to privatisation for livestock collectives in Kazakstan and Turkmenistan. *AgREN Newsletter* 38: 10, 15–17.

With the breakup of the USSR, the new Central Asian Republics are now privatizing their previously collectivized and intensive stockraising systems. Along with other factors, the loss of Soviet inputs and markets has led to a return to more traditional breeds, species mixes and production systems and goals in some parts of the former USSR. In Kazakstan, for instance, many stockraisers have gone back to the local fat-tailed sheep, which are heavier and hardier than the alien crossbreeds introduced under Russian hegemony. The fat-tails are better able to forage under snow, for example; and their tails carry an 'extra' supply of energy for the winter. Kazaks have also increased their holdings of meat horses and downy goats in place of cattle, which have difficulty surviving on the sparse winter ranges. Likewise, Turkmeni stockraisers have shifted back to local meat breeds of sheep. It is fortunate that such indigenous genetic resources were still available.

Khan, Sulaiman. 1986. *Case Study of Md. Dhanu Mia of Kasinathpur Village.* OFRD, Comilla, Bangladesh.

Four ethnoveterinary treatments are cited in this Bangladesh case study (cf. pp. 1–6). For controlling FMD in cattle, farmers wash the animals' mouth with potash and hot water. FMD lesions of the feet are painted with a mixture of sugar paste and naphthalene. The names of several local plants used in curing diarrhoea and rheumatism in cattle are given. For rheumatism, the plant leaves are mixed with cow dung. [Abstract based on Gupta et al.'s 1990 annotated bibliography.]

Khandelwal, Sitaram and Yogesh Shrivastava. 1997. The ethnobiology of pest management, veterinary care, storage and fishing amongst the tribes of western India. In: Anil Gupta (ed.). *International Conference on Creativity and Innovation at Grassroots for Sustainable Natural Resource Management, January 11–14, 1997: Abstracts.* Indian Institute of Management, Ahmedabad, India. Pp. 100–101.

This paper notes some of the most common feeding, digestive, lactation, breeding and injury problems of dairy cattle among western Indian tribes and describes some of the local treatments for these problems [not detailed in the abstract, however].

Khanna, B.M. 1967. *A Study of the Indigenous System of Veterinary Medicine as Practiced by the Farmers of Hissar I Block.* MSc thesis, Haryana Agricultural University, Hissar, India.

This thesis lists numerous ethnoveterinary practices in one part of India (cf. pp. 89–96). Among them are: 16 kinds of poultices; a dressing for myiasis consisting of 12 ingredients, including powdered camphor, peacock feathers and a lizard boiled in oil; bandages of human hair to mend cattle's broken horns; an eyewash of saline for minor opacity of the cornea; and 16 other treatments for more serious eye problems, including liquids and dusting powders. [Abstract based on Gupta et al.'s 1990 annotated bibliography.]

Khanna, B.M., Y.P. Singh and R.P. Singh. 1978. Veterinary therapy in Hissar villages: 1. Digestive and respiratory disorders. *The Haryana Veterinarian* 17(1): 42–51.

Based on a field survey, this article describes remedies used by Hissar farmers to cure digestive and respiratory disorders in their buffaloes and cattle. The farmers treat tympany by putting a fistful of tobacco in the animal's mouth to chew or by drenching with the following preparations: *Calotropis gigantea*; sarson and other oils; decoctions of various plants such as *Citrullus colocynthis* and *Trigonella foenum*; and a mixture of milk, *gur* and *desi ghee*. If other treatments fail, some farmers puncture the rumen of sick animals. Similarly, a wide spectrum of herbal and non-herbal preparations is used to cure impaction of the rumen, indigestion, diarrhoea and colic. Few farmers treat bronchitis in their livestock, but most take measures to cure pneumonia. They burn cow dung and rub the ashes on the animal's body for 15 minutes every day until it recovers. Other treatments for pneumonia include keeping the animals close to a fire; drenching with decoctions; incising the tip of the ear; and dipping a piece of cloth in kerosene oil, tying it to the horns and igniting it.

Khanna, N.D. and U.K. Bissa. 1998. Indigenous knowledge of camel production and ethnoveterinary practice among Indian pastoralists. In: E. Mathias, D.V. Rangnekar and C.M. McCorkle, with M. Martin (eds). *Ethnoveterinary Medicine: Alternatives for Livestock Development – Proceedings of an International Conference Held in Pune, India, 4–6 November 1997. Volume 2: Abstracts.* BAIF Development Research Foundation, Pune, India. P. 34.

In arid areas of India, the camel plays an integral role in family, society, religion and economics. Across generations, pastoralists have developed and transmitted great intrinsic knowledge of both extensive and intensive camel production, along with ethnoveterinary pharmacology and ethnobotany. All camel-rearing peoples of India rely heavily on EVM to prevent and treat their animals' diseases and injuries, although ethnomedicines are limited nearly entirely to locally available flora. Such flora includes plants with antitoxin, lactogenic, fungal and balanced-feeding properties. Also, surgery is practised for abscesses, wounds, fractures and obstetric problems. In sum, the spectrum of EVM in drylands is wide. But detailed research on the identity and efficacy of local treatments is lacking. This paper also notes gender divisions of labour in camel management and discusses the effectiveness, sustainability and sociocultural acceptability of local production systems.

Khedut Anubhav Vani. 1992. Innovative practices contributed by readers of local versions. *Honey Bee* 3(1): 7–8.

This article describes several traditional veterinary practices as originally reported in *Khedut Anubhav Vani*, the Gujarati version of the *Honey Bee* newsletter. To control early-stage rabies, Gujarati tribals drench with an aqueous mixture of two unspecified items or they brand the afflicted animal's head; they say the branding is the more effective technique. Fractures and dislocations are splinted with fresh *Butea monosperma* wood cut to the length of the fractured part; meanwhile the patient is fed *Diospyros melanoxylon*, a tree fodder believed to encourage bone healing. Broken horns are dressed with a paste of *Eleusine coracana* grain-flour and/or of the pulp of the *modlu* (?) tree; these pastes help heal and harden the broken horn edges. Before milking, bovines are given alum dissolved in fresh water; this is believed to stimulate milk flow.

Kidd, Randy. 1995. Who needs vaccines? *The New Farm* (Feb): 6–9.

In developing countries today, there is a move away from vaccines, antibiotics and steroids toward more natural or biological means of promoting cattle health. For instance, instead of vaccinating cattle, they can be cross-bred with disease-tolerant animals. Just as pest control has shifted its emphasis from eradication towards more integrated methods of pest management (IPM), so should the prevention of infectious disease. The author puts forward the suggestion that there should be a move away from vaccine use and towards improving the gene pool for disease tolerance in the USA.

Kimball, Linda Amy. 1985. Brunei Malay traditional ethno-veterinary practices. *Borneo Research Bulletin* 17(2): 123–150.

Kimball defines 'ethno-veterinary' as 'all traditions of medical and healthcare for animals other than that of modern Western scientific medicine'. She describes the

Brunei sociocultural setting, the role animals play in it and the care they receive. Brunei Malay believe that most diseases are caused by evil *hantu* spirits. Amulets and smoke from burning garlic, onion skins or wood from old rice-pounding mortars are used to prevent *hantu* attacks. Other techniques for coping with veterinary problems are few. The people recognize parallels between human and animal ailments and apply many of the same treatments to both. The author also discusses slaughtering and control of pests such as monkeys and wild pigs.

King, F.H. 1927 [1911]. *Farmers of Forty Centuries or Permanent Agriculture in China, Korea and Japan.* Edited by J.P. Bruce. Harcourt and Brace, New York. 379 pp.

On pages 157–161 of this classic work on Chinese, Korean and Japanese agriculture, the author describes incubators for chicken, duck and goose eggs in Hangzhou, China. The incubators are constructed of outer and inner earthenware jars. Live charcoal is placed in the outer jar, while the eggs are stored in a basket in the inner jar. After several days in the incubator, the eggs are examined and those that are infertile are removed and sold. The remaining eggs are turned five times in 24 hours. Depending on the species, after 11 to 16 days the eggs are transferred to woven shallow trays installed above the incubators, where the eggs continue to benefit from the warmth of the incubators. There the chicks hatch and stay until they are sold. Careful regulation of the temperature is a crucial factor in the hatching process.

Kirsopp-Reed, Kate. 1992. *Rural People's Knowledge: Its Role in Livestock Development in the Tropics.* MSc thesis, CTVM, University of Edinburgh, Edinburgh, UK. 51 pp.

The worldwide use of multi-purpose botanicals such as aloe, garlic, *Cassia* and *Solanum* spp. plus other basic *materia medica* such as urine, ash and salt in rural peoples' care of their animals' health suggests the concept of a universal ethnoveterinary pharmacopoeia. Based on a literature review, the author marshalls other shared examples of ectoparasite and pest control, surgery, traditional vaccination, fertility enhancement, herding strategies to prevent disease and knowledge of contagion and infectious disease generally. Taken together, it may be possible to define a common global corpus of rural peoples' ethnoveterinary know-how.

Kisamo, Wilson M. 1998. Ethnoveterinary bioprospecting and conservation. In: E. Mathias, D.V. Rangnekar and C.M. McCorkle, with M. Martin (eds). *Ethnoveterinary Medicine: Alternatives for Livestock Development – Proceedings of an International Conference Held in Pune, India, 4–6 November 1997. Volume 2: Abstracts.* BAIF Development Research Foundation, Pune, India. Pp. 34–35.

Every longtime stockraising group around the world has its own healthcare and husbandry traditions. But the author fears that the knowledge embodied in such traditions among (especially minority) ethnic groups may be disowned due to a number of increasingly unfavourable factors. In order to sustain EVK, in particular, bioprospecting and conservation of valuable traditional plant medicines are imperative lest useful knowledge be discarded.

Ki-Zerbo, Joseph. 1994. Savoirs, savoir-faire, faire savoir et développement endogène en Afrique. In: Kakule Kasonia and Michel Ansay (eds). *Métissages en Santé Animale de Madagascar à Haïti: Actes du Séminaire d'Ethnopharmacopée Vétérinaire 'KAGALA', un Partage de Savoirs Burkina-Faso, Ouagadougou, 15–22 Avril 1993.* Presses Universitaires de Namur, Namur, Belgium. Pp. 31–39.

This keynote address from the first pan-African conference on EVK raises many fundamental issues concerning approaches to the study and practice of EVM. A sampling of the author's observations are as follow. There has been a polarization between high-tech livestock development – such as the importation of US breed-stock to Senegal, where the animals could survive only with very sophisticated veterinary inputs – and the fast-disappearing low-tech knowledge of African livestock producers and especially healers. What is needed is a middle-tech layer, so to speak, that can negotiate between and interlink the poles. The author sees two hopes for fostering such a layer. One is African-born veterinary scientists, who have a foot in both worlds and are thus well-placed to mediate between them and, in the process, to correct the false Mannichean dichotomy between modern and traditional. The other hope is healers themselves. If taught to read and write, there could be 'an enormous multiplier effect' (p. 36) that would stem the alarming loss of their knowledge. Descriptions of livestock treatments written by healers themselves would also obviate the problem of researchers' and developers' missing out on substantive information or treatment details during oral interviews and surveys with healers. Further, literacy would benefit healers' clients. They could refer to clear written directions, with more precise posologies, for self-administered livestock treatments prescribed by healers. The author devotes considerable discussion to the relative advantages and disadvantages of exogenous and endogenous know-how and to the ideal relationship between modern and traditional medicine. He sees the latter as one of dialectical synthesis between, respectively, 'the universal and the particular' rather than one of simply 'mixing African bark decoctions into . . . chemical products' (p. 38).

Klima, George J. 1985 [1970]. *The Barabaig: East African Cattle-Herders.* Waveland Press, Prospect Heights, Illinois, USA. 114 pp.

Several medico-religious veterinary practices among East Africa's Barabaig are described in this ethnography, as well as common husbandry methods. For example, a powder believed to promote cattle health and fertility is sprinkled across the entrances to cattle kraals and to the huts in which calves, sheep and goats are housed. The homestead is then quarantined for 2 days to allow the powder to take effect. If a head of cattle dies suddenly, it is carefully examined for outward signs of disease, but no autopsy is performed. If no signs are detected, sorcery is diagnosed and counter-magic is performed. If there are any new deaths thereafter, the family decamps to a new area with its herds. To encourage or restore the fertility of a barren cow or one that miscarries, a strip of hyena or eland hide is tied around the cow's neck. This technique of sympathetic magic is based on the belief that hyenas and eland always give birth successfully, with no neonate mortality. Thus, reason Barabaig, these species' hides can impart the same characteristics to problem cows. The author terms such beliefs 'fractured genetics'. Barabaig use the hide of a deceased calf in another, more naturalistic way to ensure that its dam continues to give milk. The hide is stuffed with straw to make a dummy of the dead calf and, when milking time nears, the dummy's back is sprinkled with salt and presented to the dam. When she licks the dummy, lactation re-commences. To ini-tiate normal milk letdown, the woman doing the milking holds the calf's head between her legs as she stands near the cow; in this way, the dam thinks the calf is at the udder. During the day, calves and dams are kept apart; at night, all are cor-ralled together at night but separate from other classes of stock. Blood for human consumption is harvested from bulls by tying a leather tourniquet around the animal's neck and then shooting a blocked arrow into the jugular vein; after about 1 gal of blood is extracted, the tourniquet is removed and the vein is pinched shut by finger pressure. Cattle urine is used as an all-purpose antiseptic. Barabaig reg-ularly drive their stock to salt lakes or organize caravans to bring blocks of salt from the lakes to the animals.

Knight, C. Gregory. 1974. *Ecology and Change: Rural Modernization in an African Community.* Academic Press, St Meinrad, Indiana, USA.

This text reviews livestock production in Tanzania. Calves are generally infected with ECF early in life; thus adult cattle are the immune survivors of this early exposure. Ventilation or air quality may be responsible for initiating health prob-lems, but these can be easily corrected (cf. pp. 114–125).

Koenen, Eberhard von. 1996. *Heil-, Gift-, u. essbare Pflanzen in Namibia.* Klaus Hess Verlag, Windhoek, Namibia. 336 pp.

This book brings together the results of interviews conducted throughout Namibia on the uses of local plants. The plants are mostly of human medicinal value or poi-sonous. However, one species with veterinary applications is mentioned. Himba cattle herders use *Tapinanthus oleifolius* (mistletoe) to stimulate expulsion of the placenta.

Köhler-Rollefson, Ilse. 1992. The Raika dromedary breeders of Rajasthan: A pastoral system in crisis. *Nomadic Peoples* 30: 74–83.

Also known as Rebaris or Dewasis, the sedentary Raika pastoralist caste of India's Rajasthan State herd sheep, goats and camels. Since the 14th century, Raika have pursued large-scale breeding of camels to sell the males to princes for pack animals and mounts for desert warfare and, today, to farmers as draught animals. Raika control breeding, selecting for the best sires and changing them every 4 years while avoiding inbreeding in other ways as well. Given that Raika believe the sire is mainly responsible for calf traits, numerous factors figure in sire selection, includ-ing strength, temper, coat colour, female relatives' milk yields and ability to father many male calves. Raika keep careful track of their camels' pedigrees, memoriz-ing each one's ancestry as far back as eight generations. They know their herds of 100 to 200 head so well that they can identify each individual animal's footprints. Certain famous bloodlines are known region-wide. Since Raika do not buy camels, the main mechanism for exchange of breedstock is via dowry upon marriage. Since Raika marry only among certain villages, these reciprocal animal transfers have consolidated the gene pool and led to the development of several quite distinct breeds, e.g.: the red-coloured multipurpose Bikaneri, the swift and long-limbed Jaisalmeri, the dark-brown Marwari and the heavy-boned white Mewari. There is an absolute taboo against killing or eating camels. Raika milk their camels for own-household consumption, however; and camel manure is used for fertilizer, which is sometimes also sold. The sheared hair is given to a weaver caste to manufacture various domestic items for the pastoralists' use. Raika's two main camel health problems are trypanosomosis and mange. By herders' own confession, there is no effective traditional treatment for the former, as it rarely occurred in their traditional rangelands, although one man recommends an aqueous drench of salt and *Colocynthis* sp. ashes. Trypanosomosis reared its ugly head only as grazing pressures from land reform and irrigated cultivation forced herders to take up long-distance migration, including into more humid zones. Unfortunately, trypanocides are not available in Rajasthan. Pastoralists have several remedies for mange, however: burned diesel oil; a mixture of DDT and whey; or the pounded bark of *Tecomella undulata* mixed with whey. They find commercial insecticides are too expensive. The third most frequently mentioned disease is ringworm, to which they apply cow dung and then ghee. Abortion is also a major problem. There are camel healers; and worship at the shrine of local deities is a universal response to camel disease.

Köhler-Rollefson, Ilse. 1995a. Camels in the land of kings. *Natural History* 3: 54–61.

Raika are members of a Hindu caste in India's Rajasthan State that specializes in breeding livestock, especially camels. Raika have detailed knowledge about camel breeding, management and healthcare. In the latter regard, they diagnose trypanosomosis by the smell of the suspect animal's urine and they vaccinate against camel pox by soaking a bit of blistered skin from an infected animal in water and then rubbing the solution into shallow incisions in the nose of healthy animals. For chronic diseases, a hot iron is applied to the affected or other, prescribed areas. Originally bred as military transport, camels became an important source of draught power in many parts of western India after the feudal system dissolved in 1947. However, because of shrinking grazing lands, camel numbers have dramatically decreased across the last 50 years. Traditionally, Raika do not use the meat or hides of their camels and when travelling they milk only a few animals. However, exploiting their camels for increased milk production might help maintain Raika's camel culture and improve their living standards.

Köhler-Rollefson, Ilse. 1995b. Tierhaltung bei den Hirtennomaden: Zeit der Tiere – Zeit der Menschen. In: Manuel Schneider, Karlheinz A. Geissler and Martin Held (eds). *Politische Ökologie. Sonderheft 8: Zeit-Frass: Zur Ökologie der Zeit in Landwirtschaft und Ernährung.* Pp. 71–75.

Entitled 'Animal Production of Nomads: Time of Animals – Time of People', this article explores how pastoralists have adapted to difficult ecological conditions and, via stockraising, successfully exploit marginal lands otherwise unsuited for agriculture. Camel-keeping, for example, allows people to survive in areas with less than 200 mm annual rainfall. After describing some characteristics of camels and their nomadic keepers (particularly Raika in India), the article concludes that despite all the hardship and uncertainty they experience, nomads are probably more satisfied with their work than are stockraisers in modern, intensive production systems who no longer have any personal relationship with their animals. Perhaps there is a lesson to be learned from nomads in this regard for modern animal husbandry.

Köhler-Rollefson, Ilse. 1996a. Kamele im Land der Könige. *AvH Magazin* 67: 27–32.

Published in the Germany's Alexander von Humboldt Journal, this is a German-language version of Köhler-Rollefson 1995a.

Köhler-Rollefson, Ilse. 1996b. Traditional management of camel health and disease in North Africa and India. In: Constance M. McCorkle, Evelyn Mathias and Tjaart W. Schillhorn van Veen (eds). *Ethnoveterinary Research & Development.* Intermediate Technology Publications, London, UK. Pp. 129–136.

The camel has been sorely neglected in Western veterinary research and teaching. Many colonial and post-colonial professionals in animal health have acknowledged that camel pastoralists are the real experts on camel diseases. Located mainly in northern Africa (e.g. Bedouin and other Arabs, Hausa, Twareg, Rashaida, Somali) and India (e.g. Rebari, Punjabi), these peoples have complex classifications of up to 600 categories or terms per ethnicity for camel diseases, anatomy, body parts and ages, plus rational ethnoveterinary practices. Based mainly on a review of the colonial literature, this chapter discusses ethnotherapies for the three most economically important camel diseases: mange, pox and trypanosomosis. It also mentions a variety of other astute camel-care techniques, such as: training camels not to eat toxic plants, splinting fractures, removing persistent *corpus luteum* by rectal manipulation, inducing abortion, vaginal suturing of prolapsed uteri and protecting camels' eyes and feet with leather blinkers and shoes. For mange, a wide variety of *materia medica* is prepared and administered topically: plant tars, oils, leaves, fruits and seeds; animal fats, oils, milk, marrow and urine; sulphur, charcoal, mud and sea water. For pox, young camels are immunized at climatically favourable times of the year, using crude vaccines prepared from the scabs from infected animals. Trypanosomosis treatments centre on prevention – whether by avoidance of the tsetse-fly vector via varied grazing and watering strategies, smudge fires and topical fly-repellents; by special rations and rest; and possibly by controlled breeding to increase genetic resistance to trypanosomosis. There are also numerous phyto-prophylaxes and -therapies. The latter focus on increasing overall good health and thus disease resistance. Ethnodiagnostic methods for trypanosomosis are many and often they are as accurate as Western laboratory analyses. Indigenous prophylactic and therapeutic measures are of great significance for the development of camel husbandry, given that: Western R&D on these animals has been so limited; pharmaceutical companies have stopped manufacturing drugs of known efficacy against certain camel diseases due to limited markets for the drugs; and local treatments are often more environmentally friendly than the Western ones that do exist.

Köhler-Rollefson, Ilse. 1996c. Where have all the camels gone? 'CHIP' is trying to find the answers. *Pastures: The Newsletter about Pastoralists and Livestock Development in Asia* 1: 13–14.

The plight of Raika camel pastoralists in India's western Rajasthan State is a familiar one: shrinking access to traditional grazing grounds, making for chronic livestock undernourishment, a concomitant increase in animal disease and thus an overall decline in herd sizes. Raika camels are experiencing increased incidences of mange, trypanosomosis and especially abortions, which now strike up to 50% of pregnant camels. In response to these problems, two NGOs have initiated a participatory action/research effort known as the Camel Husbandry Improvement Project. CHIP is now researching the medical and cost effectiveness of different healthcare interventions using a test herd of Raika families' own camels and working with field assistants drawn from among the Raika community itself. As part of this effort, traditional Raika disease classifications and veterinary treatments are being recorded.

Köhler-Rollefson, Ilse. 1997a. Between burning irons and antibiotics: The significance of ethnoveterinary medicine. *Reports of the DFG: German Research* 2/3: 4–6.

This is an English version of Köhler-Rollefson 1997c.

Köhler-Rollefson, Ilse. 1997b. Hone the homemade. *Down To Earth* 6(11): 40–41.

EVM can be defined as 'the knowledge possessed by non-literature cultures with regard to animal health and disease that is passed on in an oral tradition down the generations' (p. 40). EVM's oral transmission distinguishes it from other kinds of non-Western medicine like Ayurveda and acupuncture. This article overviews the kinds of techniques, *materia medica* and health problems characteristically treated by EVM generally, illustrating from Raika camel pastoralists and other stockraising groups of India. For example, one Raika livestock healer helps bovines give birth using a preparation of roasted, ground wheat and sesame seeds. Raika in general use the oil of a certain tree as an effective remedy for camel mange. Another popular traditional treatment is careful firing and branding, which can sometimes cure camel ills that modern veterinary medicine cannot [see Köhler-Rollefson 1997a&c]. In the hands of expert local healers, many indigenous botanical, mechanical and surgical techniques are quite effective. When Raika and other traditional stockraising groups turn to modern veterinary drugs, however, they often stumble. For instance, sheep breeders in India use the antibiotic tetracycline indiscriminately, believing that it alleviates as many as 13 different diseases. Other producers have exchanged their homemade mange oil for plant pesticides like malathion and BHC (benzene hexachloride), which are highly toxic to livestock, people and the environment. In sum, stockraisers may place too much faith in modern drugs and agrochemicals; and unfamiliar with such medicaments' proper indications and posology, they may seriously misuse them. Drug labels do not help much, in that many people in the developing world are illiterate. In any case, the labels are often in English! But rarely would Raika and other groups consider consulting a veterinarian. They have little trust or confidence in vets, who come from very different social and educational backgrounds and may not even speak their language. Part of the solution to such problems may lie in the validation and wider dissemination of useful ethnoveterinary medicines, perhaps via packaged commerical preparations. India already has a model for this approach, in its manufacture of traditional Ayurvedic medicines.

Köhler-Rollefson, Ilse. 1997c. Zwischen Brenneisen und Antibiotika. Zur Bedeutung der Ethnotiermedizin. *Forschung* 1: 24–26.

Entitled 'Between Firing and Antibiotics', this article addresses the importance of EVM illustrating from animal healthcare practices of Raika camel pastoralists in the arid west of India. The Raika are a caste of herders who in pre-colonial times tended the breeding herds of the maharajahs' war camels. During colonization, British military veterinarians noted the profound EVK of Raika herders (see Köhler-Rollefson 1996b). Even today, Raika prefer to doctor their animals themselves rather than use the free treatments offered by the government veterinary service. Raika distinguish at least 30 to 40 fodder plants, along with different plants' importance for such factors as milk production and fertility; and most herders are familiar with 20 to 30 camel diseases. For camel healthcare, Raika rely on a mixture of sound management (e.g. grazing strategies that largely duplicate camels' natural patterns of behaviour), plant remedies and other treatments. A particularly popular treatment is firing, the scars from which write a medical record into the animals' hides. A complex technique with possible parallels to acupuncture, firing calls for expert skills in terms of the anatomical location of the operation, the temperature of the hot iron employed and the duration of the burn. For especially difficult health problems, herders call upon specialized Raika animal doctors, many of whom also treat humans. Healers say their veterinary knowledge is learned from their fathers and uncles and/or is 'God given', by which they mean they acquired it empirically through their own efforts. Along with traditional medicines, surgery and manipulation, healers sometimes resort to magic and to modern drugs such as antibiotics. Found in nearly all villages, these individuals form a network of specialists that operates parallel to the state veterinary service system. Because they speak the local language and are familiar with the local ethnoveterinary system, such healers' integration into conventional health services could help improve local veterinary care and animal production. This may prove difficult, however, because healers come from a much lower caste than most veterinarians, making for serious communication problems; furthermore, government vets tend to view Raika herders and healers as stupid.

Köhler-Rollefson, I. and J. Bräunig. 1998. Anthropological veterinary medicine: The need for indigenizing the curriculum. Paper presented to the 9th International Conference of Institutions of Tropical Veterinary Medicine, Harare, Zimbabwe. 4 pp.

The League for Pastoral Peoples (LPP) is a German organization devoted to technical support and advocacy for pastoralists. Provision of animal health services to such groups is an important part of technical support strategies. But in its work as a mediator and moderator between pastoralists, on the one hand, and project-based and academic scientists in animal production and veterinary medicine on the other, LPP has observed a serious lack of articulation and communication between these two groups. This lack is essentially due to the fact that they inhabit totally different cultural as well as techno-ecological realities. In much of the South, animals are still kept under traditional systems. They are raised mainly on natural graze, not fodder or formulated feed; they spend the night in pens or open fields, not stables; they are managed in such a way as to minimize risks and ensure long-term survival for their keepers, not maximum performance and short-term financial gain; and they are viewed as vital elements in human social and cultural life, indeed almost as family members, not as biological machines. This situation contrasts sharply with dichotomous Western views and veterinary practices that divide pets as fulfillers of emotional needs from farm animals as mainly just a food source. These fundamental differences are not spelled out in textbooks. But they need to be, along with the inherent values, ecological and economic appropriateness and valid ethnomedical treatments and practitioners in traditional husbandry and healthcare systems. For example, many anthropologists, animal geneticists, range managers and veterinary scientists have demonstrated that, rather than being primitive or backward, traditional pastoral systems can: make optimal use of extremely harsh and unpredictable ecosystems; generate and steward invaluable biodiversity, in the form of exceptionally resilient, disease-resistant and even productive breeds; control numerous effective yet inexpensive and often quite sophisticated techniques of disease treatment, prevention and control, sometimes along with a centuries-old ethnoscience of veterinary medicine; and by almost any measure, surpass industrialized societies' scores on animal welfare. Such considerations must be explicitly acknowledged in veterinary education, at the very least for students genuinely concerned to serve the animal health and welfare needs of people in such systems. Educators need to teach respect and understanding for plural traditions of livestock management so their students can better deal with clients from other cultures in finding context-specific solutions to such clients' veterinary problems.

Köhler-Rollefson, Ilse, Babiker E. Musa and Mohamed Fadl Achmed. 1991. The camel pastoral system of the southern Rashaida in eastern Sudan. *Nomadic Peoples* 29: 68–76.

The Rashaida are a fully nomadic Saudi-Bedouin group who migrated from Saudi Arabia to eastern Sudan in the mid-1800s. They raise sheep, goats and especially camels. The household herd of 50 to 70 camels provides the transport necessary to a nomadic lifestyle and the milk that is the mainstay of Rashaida diets. Even for camels that become sterile after calving, Rashaida know how to make them keep giving milk for many years. Male camels not kept for transport or stud are slaughtered for meat at ritual occasions or sold for commercial slaughter, usually to Egypt. Recently, Rashaida have also entered the lucrative business of breeding racing camels, which they may sell for as much as US $80 000 for a prize racer. They raise two distinct breeds: one for racing and riding, on which they keep mental pedigrees for seven generations; and another smaller and stockier one for milk and meat, whose pedigrees they do not track. They have also begun to buy bigger and stronger-boned camels from another tribe to cross with the second breed in order to produce a better meat animal. Purposeful selection is restricted to male camels, which are chosen from for their good temper and conformation from high milk-yielding female lines. Interestingly, they do not worry about mating a she-camel to her own sire. Rashaida have a varied veterinary pharmacopoeia for their camels. Mange is treated with a topical application of salt with either sesame or cottonseed oil, or another homemade ointment. Nowadays, however, pastoralists consider these salves too much work to make; they prefer to buy Western drugs such as Ivermectin instead. *Acacia arabica* is administered for endoparasites. A neck disorder of unknown aetiology is treated by making incisions under the eye with a sharp knife; if this does not work, the neck is punctured and cauterized with a hot nail. Lameness is also dealt with by incising the affected area. Various surgical procedures are used for mouth, throat and nose conditions, such as hypertrophy of the papillae, enlargement of the soft palate or the hyoid bone and *Cephalopsis tintillator* infections. Contagious skin necrosis is treated with cauterization. In the rare case of dystocia, a malpositioned foetus is corrected manually. If this is not possible, the foetus is killed and dissected *in utero* with a straight shaving knife. To correct prolapse of the uterus, a slope is dug to elevate the hindquarters of the animal; the organ is washed with soap and water, then lubricated with oil and pushed back into place; and finally, the vulva is sutured with bark fibres and a needle. Rashaida are astute when it comes to aetiologies and diagnostics. For example, they attribute trypanosomosis to biting flies; and they accurately diagnose it from an animal's general condition plus the smell of the urine (although they have no effective traditional treatment). Endoparasites are diagnosed by a combination of signs that includes swelling over the supraorbital ridges, oedema under the neck, decreased milk production and failure to stand up after drinking.

Köhler-Rollefson, I. and H.S. Rahore. 1996. Ethnoveterinary medicine: A 'new' perspective for livestock services. *Pashudhan* 11(10): 1, 8.

This article provides a brief case study of EVK among India's Raika pastoralists (see Köhler-Rollefson 1992, 1995a, 1996a&c). Raika will sometimes contact a *vaid* – a traditional healer of animals and humans – for severe cases of livestock disease. Some *vaid* treat all animals, while others are restricted to certain animal species or have developed specialized skills such as obstetrics or firing. Raika have particularly elaborate techniques of firing, the scars from which write an animal's medical history directly into its hide. Raika livestock experts can read this history much as Western doctors read a human patient's case file.

Köhler-Rollefson, Ilse, with Hanwant Singh Rathore. 1998. *NGO Strategies for Livestock Development in Western Rajasthan (India): An Overview and Analysis.* League for Pastoral Peoples, Ober-Ramstadt, Germany. 39 pp.

In overviewing livestock development strategies for sheep, goats, camels, buffalo and donkeys among 10 NGOs working in Rajasthan, India, this study found that, with one exception, 'Currently, NGOs do not place any significant emphasis on the research and revitalization of livestock related indigenous knowledge and institutions, even though Rajasthan has a particularly strong tradition in this respect. In some cases, awareness about the value and even the existence of [such] traditional knowledge is lacking among NGO staff' (p. vii). This despite the fact that, according to a survey in one district, people prefer to draw on their own animal healthcare resources and experience, consult a traditional healer or, if all else fails, a spirit medium – even when official veterinary services are available in their area. In part, this is due to the fact that for certain animal health problems, the earnings from livestock are insufficient to defray the costs of modern treatments. This is the case for the two paramount diseases of camels, for instance (mange and trypanosomosis). The study also found that, again with one exception, the NGOs sampled did not deal with nomadic pastoralists [who often control more extensive and/or profound EVK]. However, one NGO was concerned to revive human ethnomedicine and to promote nurseries of associated plants. The authors suggest that many aspects of such human-oriented activities are also relevant for the improvement of animal health services. In planning for paravet training, NGOs failed to integrate their efforts with local healthcare systems, e.g. by including traditional healers and practices. Instead, NGOs 'presume that animal owners are all but ignorant and have no useful knowledge of their own. They focus one-sidedly on "westernised" knowledge, without utilising the existing traditional knowledge that in some communities is quite extensive' (p. 29). Finally, the study notes that NGOs do little by way of conserving indigenous breeds. In sum, NGO strategies fly in the face of the fact that 'Rajasthan's rural people have developed an extensive body of traditional knowledge on all aspects of animal husbandry, management and breeding' (p. 33). The authors add that the existence and significance of this knowledge needs to be projected not only to NGOs but also to professors and students of animal science and veterinary medicine in academia.

Köhler-Rollefson, I., H.S. Rathore and R.R. Dewasi. 1996. The Camel Husbandry Improvement Project in Rajasthan (India): Towards the development of extension services for camel pastoralists. In: Karl-Hans Zessin (ed.). *Livestock Production and Diseases in the Tropics: Livestock Production and Human Welfare. Proceedings of the VIII International Conference of Institutions of Tropical Veterinary Medicine held from the 25 to 29 September, 1995 in Berlin, Germany.* Volume II. Deutsche Stiftung für Internationale Entwicklung, Zentralstelle für Ernährung und Landwirtschaft, Feldafing, Germany. P. 591.

Among other topics, this conference poster-paper summarizes findings on the nature and scope of EVK from a League for Pastoral Peoples' project to improve camel husbandry in Rajasthan, India. On-going research there sheds doubt on the potential of modern veterinary care to enhance economic outputs from camel raising, instead underscoring the efficiency of traditional animal healthcare. The resulting data provide valuable pointers for the development of a cost-effective extension service for camel pastoralists.

Konate, Tiemoko and Colleagues. 1994. Synthèse des fiches sur la pharmacopée traditionnelle au Burkina-Faso. In: Kakule Kasonia and Michel Ansay (eds). *Métissages en Santé Animale de Madagascar à Haïti: Actes du Séminaire d'Ethnopharmacopée Vétérinaire 'KAGALA', un Partage de Savoirs Burkina-Faso, Ouagadougou, 15–22 Avril 1993.* Presses Universitaires de Namur, Namur, Belgium. Pp. 179–180.

This tabular synthesis of findings from a survey of traditional medicines in Burkina Faso lists some 20 ailments of herd animals and poultry and, where known, the Latin names of plants observed to be used in treating these ailments in the country.

Koney, E.B.M. and A.N. Morrow. 1990. Streptothricosis in cattle on the coastal plains of Ghana: A comparison of the disease in animals reared under two different management systems. *Tropical Animal Health and Production* 22: 89–94.

An investigation of streptothricosis in cattle on the coastal plains of Ghana found that the incidence of this disease was greater in traditional production systems than in cattle kept under improved management. But it also found that N'Dama breeds were more resistant to streptothricosis than N'Dama crosses. West African Shorthorn cattle also proved resistant to streptothricosis.

Kopczynska-Jaworska, B. 1961. Das Hirtenwesen in den polnischen Karpaten. In: László Földe (ed.). *Viehzucht und Hirtenleben in Ostmitteleuropa: Ethnographische Studien.* Akadémiai Kiadó, Verlag der Ungarischen Akademie der Wissenschaften, Budapest, Hungary. Pp. 389–438.

Shepherds in the Polish Carpathians typically diagnose sheep diseases by visible clinical signs. As a result, very different diseases that have similar clinical signs are treated with the same remedies. Shepherds drench sheep afflicted by liver flukes with sauerkraut juice or a decoction of juniper berries; and they cover wounds with a mixture of resin, wax and sheep butter. The herders are skilful bonesetters. To treat and prevent snake bites, they use magical techniques.

Kuit, H.G., A. Traore and R.T. Wilson. 1986. Livestock production in central Mali: Ownership, management and productivity of poultry in the traditional sector. *Tropical Animal Health and Production* 18: 222–231.

A survey of small-scale poultry production in Malian urban and agropastoral systems noted one traditional health intervention: the use of ground red pepper for unspecified ills.

Kumar, A., S. Kumar and M.P. Yadav. 1981. Antirickettsial property of *Allium sativum* Linn. *in vivo* and *in vitro* studies. *Indian Journal of Animal Research* 15(2): 93–97.

Antirickettsial properties of garlic were demonstrated in studies with chickens. This paper was unavailable for review.

Kumar, Dinesh. 1999. Indigenous technologies for health coverage in sheep. In: E. Mathias, D.V. Rangnekar and C.M. McCorkle, with M. Martin (eds). *Ethnoveterinary Medicine: Alternatives for Livestock Development – Proceedings of an International Conference Held in Pune, India, 4–6 November 1997. Volume 1: Selected Papers.* BAIF Development Research Foundation, Pune, India. Pp. 73–77.

Five sheep farmers interviewed in each of 30 villages of Rajasthan State cited a total of 189 indigenous ovine healthcare practices. The percentage of interviewees who reported using each technology was calculated. In addition, 25 scientists rated the technologies for their soundness from a veterinary-scientific perspective on a scale of 0 (unsound) to 1 (wholly sound). More than 50% of the farmers used 71 of the 189 technologies, indicating that they have considerable faith in quite a number of their traditional practices. Scientists gave 27 technologies a score of > 0.5, indicating their scientific relevance. Some examples of the range of indigenous treatments, the percentage of farmers using them and their relevance score (Pi) are: for inducing heat in sheep, sesame oil (45% of farmers, Pi = 0.38); for retained placenta, a boiled mixture of *ber* bush, milk and *gur* (87%, 0.50); for diarrhoea, barley flour mixed in rice starch (73%, 0.54); for jaundice, a talisman tied to the tail (78%, 0.00); for mastitis, burning dried red chillies after passing them over the sheep (51%, 0.02); for indigestion, castor oil (76%, 0.70); for enterotoxaemia, cutting the ear and tail of the affected sheep (92%, 0.14); for FMD, burning pig excreta in the sheep paddock (58%, 0.16); and for itching, a topical paste of *gandraph*, salt and oil (17%, 0.64).

Kumar, Dinesh, H.C. Tripathi, S. Chandra, S.K. Tandan and J. Lal. 1998. Spasmolytic effect of alcoholic extract of *Dalbergia sissoo* leaves – An anti-diarrhoeal ethnoveterinary drug. In: E. Mathias, D.V. Rangnekar and C.M. McCorkle, with M. Martin (eds). *Ethnoveterinary Medicine: Alternatives for Livestock Development – Proceedings of an International Conference Held in Pune, India, 4–6 November 1997. Volume 2: Abstracts.* BAIF Development Research Foundation, Pune, India. P. 36.

This paper reports on an experiment to test the validity of rural Indian and Nepali stockraisers' use of *Dalbergia sissoo* leaves to treat non-specific diarrhoea in their animals. An alcoholic extract was prepared from mature leaves and tested on the isometrically mounted isolated rabbit ileum. Alcohol (40%) and tannic acid (1%) served as controls for the carrier medium and the leaves' high tannic-acid content, respectively. The extract caused dose-dependent reduction in the amplitude of rhythmic contractions of the intestine. At 300 μg/ml and above, the extract inhibited pendular movements of the intestine within 5 minutes. The effect persisted until the tissue was washed several times, whereupon the rhythmic motility revived slowly and completely within 15 to 30 minutes. A similar effect was observed with an extract from fresh macerated *D. sissoo* leaves. Neither control induced any observable change in the rhythmic motility of the ileum. To investigate further the possible inhibitory mechanism, various spasmogens such as acetylcholine (ACh), histamine and barium chloride ($BaCl_2$) were administered to the batch in the absence and presence of *D. sissoo* alcoholic extract. Exposure of the tissue to 300 μg/ml of extract for 10 minutes caused 71.0 ± 4.7%, 69.0 ± 6.0% and 82.0 ± 3.4% reduction in the contractile responses induced by submaximal concentrations of ACh (10–7 M), histamine (10–5 M) and $BaCl_2$ (10–4 M), respectively. These observations indicate that the effectiveness of *D. sissoo* leaves for non-specific diarrhoea in animals could be due to the leaves' non-specific spasmolytic effect.

LaBarre, Weston. 1948. The Aymara Indians of the Lake Titicaca Plateau, Bolivia. Memoir Series of the American Anthropological Association No. 68. *American Anthropologist* 50(1, Part 2): 1–247.

Pages 70–76 of this ethnography on Aymara Indians in Bolivia describe animal husbandry practices. The Aymara believe that llama and alpaca cannot copulate without human aid and therefore always help them when mating. *Karachi* is an endemic disease in alpacas. It is contagious and infectious and causes pustules, especially in the genital region. The Indians say that it is a form of syphilis and treat it with a pomade of lard, sulphur and mercury oxide.

Lakhabhai, Becharbhai Khatana. 1997. Lakhabhai: Indigenous veterinary expertise getting eroded. *Honey Bee* 8(2): 15.

This brief article profiles a traditional Rabari livestock healer who treats many animal ailments, all *gratis*, based on his 60 years of herding and his experiments in curing himself and his own animals. He is particularly adept at difficult births and he has a unique treatment for FMD that consists of fumigating the affected stock with smoke from burning hedgehog spines. Mr Lakhabhai is keen to train young people in his ethnoveterinary skills, but no one is interested because the work earns no money.

Lal, Jawahar, Suresh Chandra, S. Gupta and S.K. Tandan. 1998. Pharmacological effects of *Tinospora cordifolia*. In: E. Mathias, D.V. Rangnekar and C.M. McCorkle, with M. Martin (eds). ***Ethnoveterinary Medicine: Alternatives for Livestock Development – Proceedings of an International Conference Held in Pune, India, 4–6 November 1997. Volume 2: Abstracts.*** BAIF Development Research Foundation, Pune, India. Pp. 36–37.

Ayurvedic medicine ascribes many medicinal properties to *Tinospora cordifolia*, a large climbing plant of the tropics. The stem, in particular, has been reported to possess expectorant, antipyretic, antidiabetic and blood-purifying activities. This study investigated the anti-inflammatory, analgesic and anticonvulsant effects of an alcoholic extract of *T. cordifolia* stem, employing oral doses of 100, 300 and 1000 mg/kg bw in rats and mice. As studied in carrageenin-induced hind-paw oedema in rats and compared with aspirin, anti-inflammatory activity of the extract was nil. Its analgesic activity was tested by Randall-Selitto assay in rats, acetic-acid-induced writhing in female mice and tail clip and hot plate tests in mice. In the assay, the extract produced significant analgesic activity; the writhing test suggested peripheral analgesic activity; and no central analgesic effect could be detected in the tail clip and hot plate tests. The extract was also devoid of anti-convulsant activity during maximum electroshock and chemoshock tests in mice. In sum, this study confirms the medicinal value of *T. cordifolia* stem for pains due to inflammation.

Lam, Dasho Shinkhar. 1994. A view from the top of the world! *Honey Bee* 5(2): 19.

In Bhutan, to dislodge leeches from inside the nostrils of livestock (and humans), the animal is stood in hot sun to make it thirsty; a bowl of water is then placed under its nose and the nose is wetted. This causes the leeches to emerge partway, where they can be pulled out using a noose of horse tail-hair. Bhutanese livestock poisoned by toxic plants are fed molasses; and hot herbal baths are prescribed for several [unspecified] livestock ills.

Lans, Cheryl. 1996. ***Ethnoveterinary Practices Used by Livestock Keepers in Trinidad and Tobago.*** MS thesis, Department of Ecological Agriculture, Wageningen Agricultural University, Wageningen, The Netherlands. *Ca.* 220 pp.

The first systematic study of EVK in the Caribbean, this thesis covers a wide front. Chapter 1 describes the marginal agriculture of Trinidad and Tobago (T&T) and the importance of EVM in view of the faltering national economy and government exchequer and hence the need for agricultural technology that is appropriate for low-resource farmers. The author finds it ironic that, while T&T farmers cannot afford expensive imported veterinary inputs, the equivalent traditional medicines from which such inputs often were developed are in danger of being lost due to lack of R&D interest. An example is an aloe-based US product to boost chicks' immune response, versus the pure *Aloe vera* that T&T farmers have long used for the same purpose. Chapter 2 turns to theoretical perspectives on the social construction of knowledge in an actor-network context. It discusses the formulation and status of scientific versus local knowledge and how the latter can become marginalized by power networks (e.g. of scientists or government veterinarians) or, conversely, revitalized by new types of networks that may or may not include power elites. Also discussed are intellectual property rights issues in relation to 'common knowledge' such as EVK. Chapter 3 describes the multi-ethnic origins of T&T EVK in European, Latin American, Indian, Amerindian and African folk medicine, with admixtures of Western-scientific medicine. For instance, European influences are reflected in T&T beliefs in the law of signatures, as when yellow-coloured plants are used to combat jaundice. Latin American influences are evident in hot/cold theories of disease. Indian (mainly Ayurvedic) medicine is represented in the clinical practices of *ojha* healers, who use magico-religious techniques and masseurs or 'vein pullers', who manually correct supposedly overlapping or twisted veins. Also, Hindu priests provide spiritual healing, as do various Christian spiritualists. Amerind contributions to T&T EVK mainly take the form of certain medicinal plants indigenous to the Americas, plus the putatively Mayan sacred number, '9' – the quantity in which drops of medicine or the days to take it are often formulated. African traditions predominate in T&T EVM, however. These include both naturalistic and personalistic/supernatural components. An example of the latter are illnesses like evil eye; presumably caused by human envy or ill-will, these are treated by the herbal and magical skills of *obeahmen*. Western-scientific medicine may be mixed with naturalistic 'bush' medicines of African or other origins, as when people prepare a *tisane* (medicinal 'tea') out of local plants plus drugstore products such as Epsom salts. Chapter 3 also overviews the post-1950 English-language scientific literature on T&T plant medicines. The plants used fall into three categories: wild, domesticated and partner species, with the last defined as plants that are not cultivated but are actively protected and nurtured. All three are available from women street and market vendors. However, some species are in danger of extinction due to urbanization and the increased use of weed-killers. Also presented in Chapter 3 is research on correlations between phases of the moon and plant growth, animal reproduction and sudden livestock deaths, plus the considerable congruency between T&T beliefs and scientific findings on lunar influences. Chapter 4 describes the philosophical and methodological approach taken in the author's firsthand field studies of T&T EVM [see Lans and Brown 1988b]. The results – which include many overlaps between livestock and human ethnomedicine – are presented in tabular and listing formats in Chapter 5, by informant/interviewee sources in Chapter 6 and as draft booklets on poultry and ruminant EVM in Appendix 4. Sources were of many types: plant vendors, herbal-ists, school students and their parents, veterinarians, Ministry of Agriculture employees, a Spiritual Baptist preacher and of course stockraisers themselves. Overall, naturalistic remedies based on 76 and 32 plant and non-plant *materia medica* respectively were identified, along with 2 personalistic and 20 lunar-related treatments. Examples of non-plant materials used to treat livestock include: various dairy and petroleum products; bleach, clay, lime, alum; ants' nests and cobwebs; soft candles and cattle tail-hair; and comestibles like coffee, sugar, flour-water, vinegar, pickle salt water, salted fish and beef, molasses and Guinness stout. One surgical treatment – bleeding pigs' ears – is mentioned for mastitis, along with one man's secret knowledge of indigenous vaccinations for chickens. [For examples of plant-based remedies see Lans and Brown 1988a&b.] Chapter 6 also summarizes some of the author's general observations plus informants' answers to broad ques-tions about EVM. For instance, plant names vary by ethnic group. Older people know more polyprescriptions than do younger people. There is a particular plethora of medicinal or obstetric treatments surrounding animal reproduction, birthing and lactation – perhaps because of the diffusion of such knowledge for and among women. For people living near the ocean, seawater is a frequent ingredient in traditional medicines. Farmers who keep rabbits know of no available commercial remedies for this species and thus must have recourse to EVM. Neither is there much EVM for pigs, for a variety of reasons: Hindus and Moslems do not raise them; small farmers have been forced out of hog-raising by the concentration of this industry on a handful of large, agribusiness-oriented farms; and aside from swine fever, few diseases affect small-scale pig production, which is characterized by rapid offtake and turnover of hardy local breeds. Also documented in Chapter 6 are modes of EVK acquisition. The primary one is grandparent → parent → child or, in a generational skip, grandparent → grandchild. Old 'aunties' are also commonly cited sources of EVK. Another frequent mode of EVK acquisition was own-observation and -experimentation. In addition, people pick up knowledge from herbalists, midwives, employers, local medical doctors, etc. and in idiosyncratic ways. In the latter regard, one man described how he looked at the pictures in a book on human gynaecology and then applied what he saw to calves; another said he obtained his EVK indirectly, from the widow of a farrier (i.e. a local animal healer). However, quite a few informants noted that healers may selfishly take their EVK with them to the grave. Chapter 7 continues the discussion of actor networks, but now focusing on T&T veterinarians' use of and experiences with EVM plus their highly varied views of local versus scientific knowledge vis-à-vis maintenance of their elite power position. Chapter 8 introduces the concept of 'memory banking', re-engaging issues of intellectual property rights, publication and other modes of EVK dissemination, the role of formal education in EVK maintenance and diffusion and more. Chapter 9 critically overviews all the foregoing issues and findings. Four appendices follow, on: media and cultural aspects of EVK; T&T plant lists and livestock health statistics; workshop participants; and draft extension booklets on EVK for poultry and ruminants. Two overarching conclusions of this study include the following. First, farmers' choice between traditional and modern medicines or between competing traditional medicines 'is pragmatic, based on past successful . . . use; if it is not working, it will be changed after checking neighbours and friends' (p. 39). Second, the author urges investment in R&D on EVK in order to stimulate 'the . . . confidence needed to resist a market that extracts indigenous knowledge, adds value to it, claims intellectual property rights and then resells it to the original owners' (p. 23), lest even more smallholder stockraisers be driven into penury [and into urban areas] by their inability to access such expensive, imported inputs.

Lans, Cheryl and Gabriel Brown. 1998a. Ethnoveterinary medicines used for ruminants in Trinidad and Tobago. *Preventive Veterinary Medicine* 35: 149–163.

The twin-island Caribbean republic of Trinidad and Tobago is 100% self-sufficient in pig and poultry products, but for ruminants this figure hovers around only 20%. Thus the government is concerned to support ruminant production. Yet at the same time, the Ministry of Agriculture has experienced a marked reduction in resources, pressuring it to reduce its efforts. In the face of such needs and constraints, research was undertaken to see how EVM could help. Indeed, Trinidad and Tobago farmers employ a variety of EVM practices eclectically drawn from the African, European, Indian and Latin American traditions that have met and mingled on the islands.

Using an equally eclectic methodology [see Lans and Brown 1998b], the authors collected information on 30 ruminant health problems for which 25 botanical and other (e.g. sugar, molasses, flour, coconut oil, paraffin, whale oil, charcoal, cotton bolls) *materia medica* are employed therapeutically or prophylactically. These materials are fed or grazed directly or, more often, prepared as decoctions, teas (hot infusions), or wound poultices. Drenching equipment consists of bamboo joints, old shoes, or thin-necked bottles. The plants are used in both mono- and poly-prescriptions and often for more than one ailment. For instance, prescriptions for retained placenta and 'bruised blood' (haematomae and clotted blood after birth) span: drenching with a decoction or tea of wild coffee leaves or a tea of turmeric rhizome; or simply feeding a few branches of *Spondias mombin*, or a handful of bamboo leaves, or 3 lbs of paddy rice. An infusion of *Stachytarpheta jamaicensis* is believed to increase milk production, as is turmeric tea. To 'clean out the womb' and induce oestrus, a decoction of *Ruellia tuberosa* or *Petiveria alliacea* root may be given, both of which also serve as dewormers. An alternative 'womb cleaner' is a shotgun prescription of the roots and leaves of *P. alliacea*, wild coffee and *Achyranthes indica*, the roots of turmeric and *Mimosa pudica*, garlic and salt. *Aloe vera* gel is used for the same purpose as well as a laxative and a treatment for internal injuries. A tea of *Laportea aestuans* serves for urinary problems. Animals are encouraged to graze *P. alliacea* as a natural anthelmintic. There is a whole galaxy of wound and burn treatments, which are distinguished by different methods of plant preparation (mainly crushing, grating and scraping) and by their oily ingredients. Throughout the article, preparation and dosage details are given where available. But the authors note that the latter are 'vague' or, put another way, 'case and context specific' and thus difficult for informants to describe in the abstract. Also, the quantity of plant leaves used and the days in dosing regimens are often keyed to odd numbers and/or phases of the moon. One supernatural ill, evil eye, is noted. As per the literature on African ethnotoxicology, the authors class evil eye as a type of poisoning by distance. It is combatted by tying a red string around the neck of the threatened animals, painting a blue spot on them, or in the case of valuable cows in Trinidad, consulting certain Indo-cultural specialists such as 'vein pullers', masseurs or Hindu priests who offer up prayers. In concluding, the authors make several provocative points. One is the importance of studying cultural and religious aspects of ER&D so that resources are not wasted on trying to validate treatments given only for extra-medical reasons. Another is recognition that, where there has been extensive cross-cultural exchange, EVK may not have been borrowed intact, which may help explain the existence of ineffective treatments. Overall, however, good candidates for validation are treatments that are widely used in a given society, documented as being similarly used in other countries and supported by the phytochemical and pharmacological literature. In the latter regard, the article includes a table of such literature pertinent to the uses claimed for 17 of the 25 plants identified.

Lans, Cheryl and Gabriel Brown. 1998b. Observations on ethnoveterinary medicines in Trinidad and Tobago. *Preventive Veterinary Medicine* 35: 125–142.

In Trinidad and Tobago, most poultry production inputs are imported; but because of imported pharmaceuticals' high cost, even large-scale poultry operations also use traditional medicines wherever possible. To identify and validate EVM practices for poultry, the authors devised a stepwise methodology. First, teenage students from nine schools nationwide were asked to interview family, friends and neighbours on poultry EVM and then to report their findings in essay or written question/answer form. The schools were selected to represent Trinidad and Tobago's rural/urban, ethnic, gender and regional diversity. From students' reports, common practices and 28 key informants for more in-depth interviewing by the authors were identified. Meanwhile, for the same purposes semi-structured interviews were conducted with Ministry of Agriculture (MOA) field officers and extensionists reputed to be knowledgeable in EVM. As a final, participatory form of data validation and verification, focus-group workshops were held with a total of 55 participants selected from among the key informants and MOA personnel. They reviewed a draft booklet on poultry EVM produced by the first author from the data gathered to that point, refining and correcting the information, e.g. by clarification of dosages. Results revealed a variety of treatments, several of which were used on small and large poultry farms alike. Treatments involved mostly fresh plant materials administered in birds' food or drinking water. For inappetence, for instance, crushed garlic is sprinkled on the feed or coconut milk is put in the drinking water. Lime, lemon or sour-orange juice is added to the water to combat respiratory problems and heat stress; in addition, perforated bags full of citrus peelings may be placed in the water tank. Also for respiratory ills, for a flock of 10 000 chickens a decoction of 908 g of *Momordica charantia* stems and leaves with 20 *Pimenta racemosa* leaves in 4 l of water may be administered in the drinking water, along with some molasses for palatability. To reduce vaccination stress and to promote survival and growth generally, chicks in their first 2 weeks of life may be given *Aloe vera* in one of two ways: for 4000 chicks, 1 large aloe leaf cut in half is administered in the same way as citrus peels; or aloe gel may be put directly into the water tank. An alternative is adding *Bryophyllum pinnatum* juice to the tank for 5 days after vaccination. To repel ectoparasites of ducks and chickens, farmers may sprinkle any of a variety of leaves on the birds' litter or in their nest boxes. Plants used for this purpose are *Azadirachta indica*, *Cedrela odorata*, *Cordia curassavica*, *Petiveria alliacea* and *Renealmia alpinia*. Some informants also described how, after dipping their fingers in wood ash, they twist off a gristly membrane that sometimes grows over the tongues of backyard chickens. Others noted that chickens' picking through cashew shells produces sores on the beak (probably from the cardol and acacardic acid in the pericarp). The authors further describe several self-initiated, farmer-managed research trials on poultry ethnomedicines. These involved *B. pinnatum* extract, *M. charantia* extract and ground garlic in lime juice to combat, respectively, vaccination and debeaking stress, aspergillosis infections and respiratory reactions to Newcastle-disease vaccination. The farmer conducting these experiments reported good results with all the treatments. The article's conclusion overviews findings from the pharmacological literature on all the plant species mentioned. It also discusses pros and cons of the participatory research methods employed. Additional observations of interest are that: on-farm EVM experiments with poultry are highly feasible and fast because of ethnomedicines' low cost and rapid flock turnover; and trials on ethnobotanicals generally should be designed to focus on effectiveness while still maintaining high methodological standards – perhaps via cohort studies with defined populations rather than clinical assays.

Larrat, R. 1939. Le vétérinaire indigène. *Bulletin des Services Zootechniques et des Épizooties de l'Afrique Occidentale Française* 2(2).

Unavailable for review. However, based on Dupire 1962, pages 55– 60 of this publication present a number of indigenous curing techniques among stockowners of Senegal, Sudan and Mauritania.

Larrat, R. 1940. Médecine et hygiène indigènes. *Bulletin des Services Zootechniques et des Épizooties de l'Afrique Occidentale Française* 2(4): 45–58.

According to the author, all stockraisers agree that hygiene, exercise and good nutrition are the key to healthy animals. Fulani of French West Africa are no different. They believe livestock should bathe daily and that horses should be fed sufficient quantities of millet, hay and salt. Traditional vaccination methods against CBPP are described for Fulani in Sudan, Ivory Coast and Niger. A calf suffering from CBPP is slaughtered and its lungs are harvested. The lung is dried with some bark and root tannins and then a piece the size of a bean is incised into healthy livestock.

Larrat, R. 1941. Origine et évolution de l'art vétérinaire en Afrique occidentale Française. *Bulletin des Services Zootechniques et des Épizooties de l'Afrique Occidentale Française* 4(Sup): 253–259.

The author notes that the first healer must have been the first herder and that cattle medicine must have preceded horse medicine. This article reviews the history of stockraising in Francophone Africa. Treatments were discovered through empiricism and observation of animals in the wild and were often enhanced with religion and magic.

Larrea, Imanol. 1993. *Ethnoveterinary Medicine: Practices for the Prevention and Control of Diseases.* MSc thesis, CTVM, University of Edinburgh, Edinburgh, UK. 44 pp.

This thesis reviews some of the ethnoveterinary literature up to 1993. Ethnosemantics, ethnotaxonomy, pharmacology and manipulative techniques are described. The potentials for combining and extending ethnoveterinary with modern veterinary medicine are discussed. The thesis uses Mathias-Mundy and McCorkle (1989) as its basis.

Lattimore, Owen. 1941. *Mongol Journeys.* Doubleday and Doran, New York, USA.

In the breeding season, Mongols fit their rams with an apron of felt. They remove the apron at intervals of about 10 days and allow the rams to mate. As a consequence, lambs are born in batches about 10 days apart and the risk of losing animals in spring storms is greatly reduced.

Lavine, Sigmund A. 1974. *The Horses Indians Rode.* Dodd and Mead, New York, USA.

Page 51 mentions that among American Plains Indians members of the horse cult had secret formulas to cure sick horses. They also prepared potions 'that assured warriors their mounts would never falter'.

Law, Donald. 1973. *The Concise Herbal Encyclopedia.* Saint Martin's Press, New York, New York, USA. *Ca.* 266 pp.

Entitled 'Herbs for Veterinary Purposes', Chapter 7 of this volume lists a wide variety of treatments for caged birds, cats, dogs, cattle, horses and sheep. [The author is British and most of the treatments appear to be based on temperate-zone plants.] A few examples for each species are as follows. For birds with colds, put fennel, fresh chickweed and 1 to 2 drops of aqua camphor in the drinking water; feed more fresh greens daily, plus herbs with iron; and check the room for draughts. Dogs and cats with worms can be dosed twice with ground areca nut (60 grains for small dogs and cats, 120 for large dogs). Also thoroughly clean the animals' sleeping quarters. Dress and tightly bandage sores, cuts and wounds with a paste of slippery elm and honey. Adding a little apple-cider vinegar to cattle and horse feed will help keep these species free of infection. A good conditioner for horses consists of aniseed or of 2 tsp daily of the following mixture: 2 oz each of fenugreek, capsicum and serpentaria with 4 oz each of ginger and gentian, all in 1 lb of flaxseed meal. For mange, apply a paste of sulphur and creosote to the affected areas and soak all harnesses and blankets in creosote. A homemade sheep dip can be made by boiling 20 fluid oz of oil of clove and 1 lb of soap in water and then mixing this with 50 gal of water. Turning herd animals out onto fresh grass usually cures constipation. The author provides a brief list of plant and other ingredients (e.g. whisky) commonly used in veterinary work. He opines that often people spend considerable sums on medicines they could instead make for themselves 'for next to nothing' (p. 10); and he warns against 'the total unwillingness of some graduates to believe that anybody without a university education is capable of intelligent thought and observation' (p. 23). In general, however, he emphasizes the importance of allowing animals to be freed as much as possible to seek out plants on their own, as sick creatures will self-medicate and healthy ones will naturally add variety to their diets.

Law, Robin. 1980. *The Horse in West African History: The Role of the Horse in the Societies of Pre-colonial West Africa.* Oxford University Press, Oxford, UK.

Chapter 3 deals with historical and contemporary aspects of husbandry, health and training of West African horses. Potash is often mixed into horses' feed as an all-purpose medicine or tonic. In Yorubaland horses were washed with a soap mixed with scrapings from the root of the violet tree, as a fly-repellent. A tobacco-based ointment was used for the same purpose in northern Nigeria.

Lawrence, Elizabeth A. 1982. Cultural perspectives on human–horse relationships: The Crow Indians of Montana. Paper presented to the Third International Symposium on Veterinary Epidemiology and Economics. Arlington, Virginia, USA, 6–10 September 1982.

Veterinarians who work in a stock-owning society other than their own must understand its attitudes towards animals. Otherwise, the veterinary services may have disastrous consequences for both animals and people. To illustrate the problems that arise when two diverse cultures come into conflict, this paper describes the relationships between Crow Indians and their horses and marked differences between Crow views of animals and those of the dominant White culture.

Lawrence, Elizabeth A. 1985. The horse in the Crow Indian history and culture. Paper presented to the Annual Meeting of the American History Society. Las Vegas, Nevada, USA, July 23, 1985.

This is a slightly revised version of Lawrence 1982.

Lawrence, Elizabeth A. 1987. The heritage of American Indian horse doctors. Paper presented to the Annual Meeting of the American Veterinary Society. Chicago, Illinois, USA, July 20, 1987.

This paper is a condensation of Lawrence 1988.

Lawrence, Elizabeth A. 1988. 'That by means of which people live': Indians and their horses' health. *Journal of the West* 27(1): 7–15.

After its acquisition early in the eighteenth century, the horse became an integral part of the culture of many American Indian societies. As a result a system of veterinary care developed that included health maintenance, preventive medicine and treatment for sick and injured animals. Because native Americans typically did not separate the sacred and the secular, religion was a powerful force in equine medicine. It influenced health-related aspects of the animals' daily care, horse racing and the protection and multiplication of the herds. Ethnoveterinary practices included ceremonies with songs and prayers, blessing rites, witchcraft, herbal and other medicines and surgical techniques such as castration and bloodletting. Certain treatments and techniques such as gelding required horse specialists and shamans. Many Indian societies, especially the equestrian tribes of the plains, developed a horse medicine cult, membership of which was restricted to small numbers of men. Some health measures, such as hoof care, were carried out by the horses' owners. Examples from different Indian tribes illustrate how the health and well-being of Indians and their horses were intimately intertwined.

Lawrence, Elizabeth Atwood. 1991. Relevance of social science to veterinary medicine. *Journal of the American Veterinary Association* 199(8): 1018–1020.

The veterinary profession and the social sciences are connected in many ways. EVM bridges both, contributing socially and economically valuable knowledge to conventional veterinary knowledge and practice. Certain folk treatments have been proven scientifically and are now used daily by physicians as well as veterinarians.

Also noted is the fact that humans and animals are subject to similar diseases and transmit certain diseases from one to the other. Thus both human and animal health may benefit from ethnoveterinary research.

Lawrence, Elizabeth Atwood. 1996. I stand for my horse: Equine husbandry and healthcare among some North American Indians. In: Constance M. McCorkle, Evelyn Mathias and Tjaart W. Schillhorn van Veen (eds). ***Ethnoveterinary Research & Development.*** Intermediate Technology Publications, London, UK. Pp. 60–75.

Plains Indians of North America placed great value on their horses. Native systems of equine care were developed that included health maintenance, preventive medicine and therapeutic measures for sick and injured horses, as well as for special racing, war and hunting mounts. Owners often treated their horses themselves, paying attention to such husbandry and healthcare needs as adequate supervision and quartering, nutrition (including knowledge of poisonous forages), reproduction, overall conditioning (including exercise and rest) and behaviour modification/training. But many tribes also had 'horse doctor' specialists whose treatments utilized a varied mix of herbal medicines, surgery (bloodletting, bonesetting and especially gelding), firing, baths, sweats, smoke treatments, exercises, rituals, songs, chants, prayers, amulets, designs painted on the hide and light blows to the body. In some tribes, doctors were the same for horses and humans. The literature attests that both owners and horse doctors enjoyed considerable success in treating a number of equine problems, notably blind staggers, gunshot and other wounds, distemper, coughs, sores and lesions of various kinds and broken bones. Widely-used botanicals included alumroot (*Heuchera* sp.) baneberry root (*Actea rubra*), *Clematis* root, big turnip, bitter-root, a variety of buckwheat, *camote-de-monte*, creosote, datura, fir needles, juniper, milkweed, peony root, pinyon pitch, ponderosa pine, several species of sage, smellfoot, snakeweed, spruce and yarrow. Other *materia medica* were: buffalo fat, horn and sinew from wild animals, salt, sea coral, turquoise, red ochre, mud and gunpowder. Considerable attention was paid to hooves. Certain roots applied to hooves supposedly made horses more sure-footed or reinvigorated them after a hard run; other medicines increased fleetness and endurance. For tenderfooted horses, Apache applied grease and gunpowder to the hooves and then blew fire from a live coal on them; Comanche instead led their horses back and forth through a slow fire of wild rosemary-artemisia. For worn hooves, Apache, Blackfoot, Cree, Crow and Navajo all fashioned moccasin-like shoes of buffalo, cattle, deer, or horse hide in the form of a pouch secured with a rawhide drawstring. The moccasins were always packed with fresh manure, which was renewed from time to time; beforehand, they might be soaked in water. Also of note, many tribes slit their horses' nostrils in order to make them long-winded. Because horses were considered sacred, virtually every pragmatic treatment was accompanied by ceremonial acts. In every Amerind horse-keeping group, these sacred creatures formed an integral part of people's social and spiritual existence, reflecting the traditions and worldview characteristic of each culture and the highly personalized, lifelong and medically reciprocal, relationships between horses and their masters.

Lawrence, Elizabeth A. 1998. Human and horse medicine among some native American groups. *Agriculture and Human Values* 15(2): 133–138.

Plains Indians and other Native Americans perceived people and animals as closely related and all a part of Nature. Thus therapeutic and prophylactic regimes in Amerind human and veterinary medical practice were often the same or similar within and across tribes. For example, among Plains Indians generally, *Juniperus virginiana* remedied coughs in both horses and people. *Echinacea angustifolia* was a universal antidote for snakebite as well as a popular fumigant for relieving distemper in horses and headaches in humans. Alum was used to treat sore mouths and sore throats in the two species. Potawatomi preparations of alder (*Alnus incana*) bark cured skin diseases, such as ponies' galled spots and people's itchy patches. The boiled buds and bark of the birch tree (*Betula nigra*) were used respectively by Catawba and Alabama Indians to treat ringworm and skin lesions in humans and sore hooves in horses. Navajo horse chants served to promote human as well as equine fertility. Likewise for Ogalala Sioux horse dances to treat *loco* 'craziness'. Bonesetting techniques were everywhere essentially the same for both species. Indeed, the same medical practitioners often attended all patients as a matter of course. This was the case among, e.g., Assiniboine, Blackfoot, Cheyenne, Piegan and Sioux. For example, Blackfoot horse doctors treated humans and horses alike with botanicals, horse parts and secret dances, songs and rituals. Finally, not only did people heal horses; according to a number of tribes' beliefs (e.g. Apache, Crow, Navajo), horses also helped heal people. These animals were also said to transmit useful obstetric and other ethnomedical knowledge to favoured individuals. Conversely, mistreated horses were believed to be able to cause illness, injury or misfortune for their tormentors.

Leakey, L.S.B. 1977. *The Southern Kikuyu before 1903.* Vol. 1. Academic Press, London, UK.

Pages 207–254 of this historical ethnography deal with animal husbandry. The Kikuyu believed that small ruminants' ingestion of dew-covered leaves caused stomach trouble while rain-wet grass was less harmful. Bucks (but not rams) were usually castrated by biting, cauterizing or beating the seminal cords. In cattle the testes were removed through a small incision and the wound closed with fresh cow dung. Dung was also used to cover the wounds after bleeding an animal. With a special bow and arrow, the Kikuyu bled goats, sheep and cattle to obtain blood for human consumption or to treat ailing animals. Other treatments consisted of the application of herbal remedies and substances such as wood ash and branding with a hot iron. Kikuyu specialists aided cows with birth difficulties and performed embryotomies. For goats and sheep, the author describes 11 disease conditions and their treatments and 12 for cattle. An example of a remedy for growth between the hooves of goats and sheep is the following: an awl is stuck into the base of the growth to hold it firmly, then the skin around the growth is cut with a sharp knife. The whole growth is pulled out, the wound is then washed with hot water blown into it through a castor oil stem. Animal fat is applied to the wound to keep out dust and dirt.

Leao, Chheng Heat. 1994. Cambodian ethnoveterinary medicines. Unpublished manuscript presented to the IIRR Workshop on Ethnoveterinary Medicine in Asia. IIRR, Silang, Cavite, Philippines. 2 pp.

The author conducted interviews with some 20 Cambodian refugees in California to record their EVK. Twenty-two traditional remedies are noted for the treatment of worms, coughs, colds, conjunctivitis, diarrhoea, bloat, flatulence, constipation, wounds and snakebites. Most of the 22 are plant-based mono-prescriptions. To take one example, infected wounds are treated with watered-down lime juice or with the ground leaves and flowers of *Rosa sinensis*.

Lebbie, S.H.B. and P.R. Mustapha. 1985. Goat production in the Swaziland middleveld. In: R.T. Wilson and D. Bourzat (eds). *Small Ruminants in African Agriculture.* ILCA, Addis Ababa, Ethiopia. Pp. 225–234.

A survey of farmer practices was carried out in Swaziland's Middleveld. 150 farmers responded to the survey as did veterinary extension workers. The latter treated a lot of goat disease that farmers attributed to pneumonia or evil.

Leeflang, Paul. 1993. Some observations on ethnoveterinary medicine in northern Nigeria. *Indigenous Knowledge and Development Monitor* 1(1): 17–19.

Nigerian Fulani pastoralists' knowledge of contagious diseases is highlighted in this short article. For such diseases, Fulani separate sick from healthy animals and also water them separately. Traditional vaccinations against FMD and CBPP are mentioned. Fulani appreciate the role of insects in the spread of disease; therefore they apply home-made fly repellents, light smudge fires to drive off pests and avoid grazing areas and shade trees infested with ticks. They also feed their animals salty plants to make ticks fall off; pick ticks off cattle by hand; and burn infested rangeland.

Legbagah A. Régine. 1983. *De la Thérapeutique Traditionnelle en Médecine Vétérinaire: Cas de la Republique Populaire du Bénin.* These, Option Production Animale, Departement des Techniques de Sciences Naturelles, College Polytechnique Universitaire Abomey-Calavi, Coutonou, Bénin. 107 pp.

The rural population of Benin 'is hardly touched by modern medicine' (p. 6). In 1978, the government of Benin thus inaugurated an international seminar on African Pharmacopoeia and Traditional Medicine in Service of the General Masses, with the aim of recognizing this resource and of organizing traditional practitioners. This initiative dealt only with human ethnomedicine. This thesis seeks to add balance with a discussion of the EVK of Fulani (Peul) stockraisers in Benin. In detecting and diagnosing animal health problems, Fulani attend not only to visible clinical signs of disease, but also to their animals' social behaviours, posture, gait, other movements, respiration, weight and so forth. On these bases, Fulani are adept at accurately diagnosing a great many parasitic, bacterial and viral diseases of ruminants and poultry. Treatments may be magical and/or medical. The former are known only to a select group and are jealously guarded. The latter rely heavily on plants, which may be prepared in decoctions, hot and cold infusions or 'torrifications' (cooked to ash). The main modes of administration are oral and topical (e.g. baths, unguents and fumigation). Fulani have a standard measure for oral dosing of cattle, the *hodear*. It consists of one drinking-calabash-ful (about 125 ml), which quantity is varied by animal weight. Poultry are dosed in drops equalling about 15 cc. Medicines are generally given in the morning or evening, once or twice daily, until symptoms disappear. Pages 17 to 59 of the thesis detail scores of plant remedies for common diseases of cattle and poultry in Benin. There are potions not only for diseases but also for regularizing oestrus cycles (said to be quite effective) and for increasing the probability of having female offspring. Besides plants, other ingredients in the veterinary pharmacopoeia are stove-ash, clay, potash, salt, animal fat, milk, butter, eggs, honey, freshly killed vipers, gasoline and diesel fuel. Firing and branding with red-hot irons are favourite Fulani treatments. Also noted are obstetric operations for retained placenta and prolapsed uterus. In the latter, after the uterus is replaced, the vulva is pinched closed with two sticks for a week. Before any such operations, Fulani wash their hands in a solution of *Cochiospermum tinctorium*. They are careful about sweeping out poultry quarters, periodically wetting them down with petroleum products or burning them over with straw and sprinkling the area with *Manihot caculenta* and *Tridas procumbens* leaves – all to control parasites and pathogens. Overall, however, the author believes that most of Fulani EVM is therapeutic rather than prophylactic. Somewhat in contradiction to her earlier remarks about diagnosis, she attributes this to stockraisers' lack of means for determining prodromes. In assessing the efficacy of Fulani EVM, she opines that traditional treatments often outstrip modern ones when it comes to skin problems and wounds. In particular, the control of ectoparasites in poultry is 'very effective' (p. 57), as are treatments for many reproductive conditions. Pages 65 to 76 recap 13 conditions for which the author considers EVM helpful. However, EVM is less successful with certain viral and bacterial diseases; and it is largely at a loss when it comes to epidemics. With regard to the future of EVM, the thesis argues that traditional medicine, which since colonial times has been criminalized in Benin, needs to be 're-valued' and the barrier between it and modern medicine lifted. It should be rescued, supported and given an official character akin to that of conventional praxis; protections should be put in place to conserve the necessary plant resources; and traditional preparations and dosages should be codified. Three annexes offer details on the plant species cited in the text.

Lehane, Robert. 1998. Key to more productive livestock in the tropics: Distribution of *Fasciola gigantica*. *Partners in Research for Development* 11(May): 8–9, 12–14.

The tropical liverfluke, *Fasciola gigantica*, is the most costly of all bovine health problems in Indonesia. About a third of the nation's 10 million cattle and buffalo are infected, making for production losses conservatively estimated at 110 million Australian dollars annually. This problem persists in part because of the high price of commercial flukicides. Indonesian and Australian scientists are therefore exploring non-drug, biological and management control alternatives. They are only now discovering some of the parasitic life-cycle mechanisms behind southeast Asians' age-old practice of keeping ducks along with bovines. It turns out that ducks carry another fluke, *Echinostoma revolutum*, whose larval stage infects the same aquatic snail as *F. gigantica*. However, the two types of larvae cannot co-exist in the snail host. Briefly put, the duck-fluke larvae crowd out those of the ruminant fluke, thus breaking *F. gigantica*'s life cycle. Based on this finding, researchers have devised and disseminated modifications on farmer practices that can dramatically reduce fluke infestations in ruminants. Modifications include: siting duck cages directly over the drains running out of ruminants' pens to the rice fields, which are grazed post-harvest by bovines; or for people who cart, rather than drain, ruminant faeces onto the fields, carting their duck litter to the fields at the same time. However, these procedures have raised a new human-health problem in the form of schisto-some dermatitis, for which scientists must now seek 'alternative' alternatives [so to speak]. One possibility is substituting chicken for duck droppings. Another [albeit more labour-intensive] option is to store duck faeces in a container of water for 2 days before depositing them on fields. Simultaneously, researchers are experi-menting with varying the seasonal timing of turn-out of ruminants onto post-harvest paddy fields, coupled with only once-annually but carefully-timed drenching with commercial flukicides.

Leidl, K., F. Jere, G. Wanda, K. Hüttner and M. Stange. 1996. Establishment of a basic animal health service programme in northern Malawi – Dimensions of activities through field work prior to implementation. In: Karl-Hans Zessin (ed.). *Livestock Production and Diseases in the Tropics: Livestock Production and Human Welfare. Proceedings of the VIII International Conference of Institutions of Tropical Veterinary Medicine held from the 25 to 29 September, 1995 in Berlin, Germany.* Volume II. Deutsche Stiftung für Internationale Entwicklung, Zentralstelle für Ernährung und Landwirtschaft, Feldafing, Germany. Pp. 550–558.

Malawian farmers are used to coping with livestock health problems themselves. In part, this is because government and other outsider veterinary services do not accept farmers' assessment of what the principal problems are. While the former view outbreaks of epidemic disease as paramount, farmers are far more concerned about recurring endemic diseases and parasitism.

Leonard, Pamela J. n.d. Extension services and the role of the government in Ya'an City dairy goat development. Unpublished manuscript. HPI/China, Sichuan Province, China. 12 pp.

During her research on extension services and the role of government in dairy-goat development in Sichuan Province, China, the author of this personal communica-tion stumbled across a few ethnoveterinary practices relating to goats. Kids were usually not able to take advantage of their dam's colostrum, as they were not allowed to nurse until the afterbirth had been expelled. A local midwife gave a mastitic doe a warm-water massage; the midwife also knew how to handle breach births of kids. Local barefoot doctors applied acupuncture and Chinese medicine based on yin/yang principles to animals.

Leparc, Jacques-Robert-Arthur-Justin. 1947. *La Médecine Vétérinaire Populaire au Bocage Normand.* Doctoral thesis, Veterinary Medicine, Faculté de Médecine de Paris, France. 61 pp.

This thesis ostensibly seeks impartially to describe folk veterinary practices and practitioners in one region of France, based on field interviews. Chapter 1 deals with beliefs, terminology, remedies, incantations, magical manipulations and other ethnoveterinary aspects, organized alphabetically by the name of the ailment within species: cattle, horses, sheep, swine, domestic carnivores, rabbits, poultry and bees. Chapter 2 briefly describes the work of three kinds of folk veterinary specialists: bonesetters, healers and sorcerers. Chapter 3 details the origin, iconography and ceremonies associated with six 'veterinary saints' believed to cure and protect livestock. The author notes that contemporary French stockowners pragmatically combine both folk and scientific, natural and supernatural practices. In an otherwise interesting work, however, the thesis bizarrely concludes with 19th-century psychologizing about the inferior 'brains' of rural French as versus 'the elite', farmers' miserliness in not calling upon professional veterinary services, their 'almost morbid curiosity' (p. 57) in inventing home remedies and their love of mysticism.

Leperre, P. and J.R. Claxton. 1994. Comparative study of trypanosomosis in zebu and N'Dama cattle in the Gambia. ***Tropical Animal Health and Production*** 26: 139–145.

An experiment was conducted in the Gambia to compare trypanosomosis incidence between zebu and N'dama cattle. The two breeds were compared under identical management conditions and animals were maintained together at three locations, traditionally managed and under a range of tsetse challenges. Results show trypanosomosis incidence was significantly higher in zebu than N'dama ($P < 0.001$).

Levesque, Louis. 1991. ***Les Traditions Guérisseuses des Animaux en Basse-Normandie.*** Presses de la Renaissance le Bessin, Bayeux, France. 47 pp.

In discussing aspects of past and present EVK in Normandy, France, the author divides traditional practices into three types: religious, magical and empirical. Historical examples of all three are given for horses, cattle, sheep, pigs, dogs, cats and poultry. Even today, however, horseshoes are hung in chicken houses to guard against lightning; and holly and dog-rose bouquets are suspended in calf sheds to ward off contagious fungal infections. Many rural Normandy families kept bees in straw hives; and such was the association between people and beekeeping that a death in the family was announced by placing a black veil over the hive. Reportedly, *sorciers-guérisseurs* 'sorcerer-healers' still practise in Normandy, resisting the pressures of modern agricultural and veterinary services.

Leyland, Tim. 1994. Planning a community animal health care programme in Afghanistan. In: Kate Kirsopp-Reed and Fiona Hinchliffe (eds). ***RRA Notes Number 20: Special Issue on Livestock.*** IIED, London, UK. Pp. 47–51.

Using participatory rural appraisal techniques, a Vetaid CBAH project surveyed sedentary farmers and Koochi pastoralists in Afghanistan's Daye Chopan District in order to discover (among other things) their EVK concerning livestock disease recognition, feeding and coping strategies and other animal-health-related practices and beliefs. Findings were used in designing a training programme for selected stockraisers as Basic Veterinary Workers. The final curriculum built upon trainees' existing livestock knowledge and useful traditional beliefs and practices as recorded during the survey, as well as training in basic commercial drugs, Western treatment techniques, management of a revolving fund and more. The survey employed a simple disease-ranking tool. It revealed 5, 6, 3 and 2 diseases consistently viewed by stockraisers as significant for their small ruminants, cattle, camels, equines and poultry, respectively. The Pushtu names for these diseases were recorded along with emic details of their symptoms, occurrence and local treatment and control measures. The ranking exercise helped people clarify their top disease problems and potential solutions available to them. The author notes that ranks were quite consistent across different wealth strata of interviewees, but that translating Pushtu disease names into scientific terms was a challenge. This was because people's description of symptoms fit a variety of possible pathogens. He concludes that 'Western-trained vets face a language and communication barrier which can only be partially solved by using participatory methodologies' (p. 48).

Li, Ann-si. 1999. Practising veterinary medicine in a developing country using acupuncture, traditional Chinese medicine and allopathy. In: E. Mathias, D.V. Rangnekar and C.M. McCorkle, with M. Martin (eds). ***Ethnoveterinary Medicine: Alternatives for Livestock Development – Proceedings of an International Conference Held in Pune, India, 4–6 November 1997. Volume 1: Selected Papers.*** BAIF Development Research Foundation, Pune, India. Pp. 206–210.

Veterinary medicine is often an art as much as it is a science. In developing countries where animal owners may not always be willing or able to return repeatedly for lab tests and on-going pharmacotherapy, or where no labs and medicines are available, optimal (rather than maximal) single-visit diagnostic and treatment methods are often needed. In such circumstances, the veterinary practitioner is obliged to try to render the best care she/he can, given her/his clinical experience and based solely upon the physical examination and history. Cases may be presented that require conventional approaches such as antibiotics or surgery; but simultaneous use of traditional Chinese medicine can sometimes aid or speed recovery. Younger patients commonly respond to herbal tonics to boost their immune systems, as in upper respiratory infections in kittens; and post-surgical acupuncture in older patients often enables them to become ambulatory more quickly, as in ruptured anterior cruciate repair. The combination of treatment modalities can be mutually compatible and more rapid and beneficial for the patient. Thus, the veterinary practitioner, the client and the patient all experience greater outcome satisfaction than they would with a monomodal treatment under constrained circumstances.

Li, Cai and Gerald Wiener. 1995. ***The Yak.*** RAP Publication No. 25. FAO Regional Office for Asia and the Pacific, Bangkok, Thailand. 237 pp.

Chinese documents from the 8th century B.C. testify to the multiple vital roles of the yak (*Bos grunniens* or *Poephagus grunniens*) for Himalayan peoples. They rely on this miracle animal for: milk and milk products; meat; bone, fibre and hides plus the innumerable household, clothing, tenting and other items fashioned from these materials, such as bags, slingshots, saddles, ropes, bridges, boats; human medicines that utilize yak penises, bladders and bezoar stones; draught and threshing power; transport and riding; dung for fuel, fertilizer and construction materials; and cash income from sales of trained and untrained animals and, in some areas, of tourist crafts and services. Nor is this to mention the yak's contributions to local entertainment (racing), to art and religion (e.g. huge butter sculptures and sacred tail whisks), or their use as 'biological snow ploughs'. Recently, yak have been introduced outside the Himalayas. An example is the Caucasus Mountains where, at 3500 to 4000 m, per-unit liveweight production costs are a tenth that for cattle and even a bit lower than for sheep. Today there are perhaps 14 million domesticated yak. They are mostly owned and managed by transhumants, who raise them on open ranges year-round, directing the herd by throwing or slingshooting small stones at them. Thus, a single herder can handle up to 150 animals. Among most yak-raising peoples, at least during the many warm-season movements, the animals of several families or a whole village are pooled and then divided into four sub-herds of dairy, dry-cow, stock-replacement and steer/pack animals. Bulls live alone except during mating time. When the subherds are returned at night to the group encampment, each family calls their own animals to its tent by name or by special cries or songs. In most areas, breeding is uncontrolled and, for pure-breds, unassisted. This is probably because natural selection for sheer survival is the single most important genetic consideration. Tibetans in particular rarely castrate or cull for breeding or productivity reasons, because herd numbers are valued over herd quality. The more yak a family owns, the richer and stronger it is. Consequently, some animals may live as long as 24 years, although the average is closer to 16. An exception to this rule is found in China's Sichuan Province. There, herders have elaborate traditional systems for selecting breeding bulls based on sires' copious hair and large numbers of progeny, dams' milk performance and numerous characteristics of the candidate bulls, including horn conformation, shape of multiple body parts and coat colour. All-black or black animals with white speckles are the normal choice, because dark colour resists the intense solar radiation of high altitudes; but in a few other localities, herders prefer white yak. Rejects are castrated, usually with no post-operative problems, using various open surgical methods and dressing the wound with iodine and a powder. The castrates become meat or work animals. (Interestingly, pack yak can walk for up to three days without food or water and for up to a month with only night-time grazing.) For at least 3000 years, Chinese have crossed yak with local *Bos taurus* to reap the benefits of hybrid vigour and produce better milk and draught animals for lower altitudes. Likewise for yak × *Bos indicus* crosses in Bhutan, India and Nepal. Usually, yak females are bred to *Bos* bulls; and crosses are perforce back-crossed as F1 males are sterile. Humans assist only at crossbreed births since dystocia is rare in pure-breds. To induce a cow to accept a foster calf, herders have several strategies: smearing the calf with the cow's own milk; covering it with the hide of her dead calf; or sprinkling salt on the calf so the cow will sniff, lick and adopt it as her own. Calves that cannot be fostered are fed using a hollow yak horn with a yak-hide nipple. Dams typically are not milked until a month after parturition, thus ensuring calves a good start in life. Weaning is achieved by subdividing herds (see above) or in recalcitrant cases by inserting a piece of wood sharpened at both ends through the calf's nasal septum. All husbandry activities are geared to the seasons. Throughout China, a typical annual schedule is: early summer – supervise births, protect calves, adjust and subdivide herd, castrate; mid-summer – comb out the down fibres and shear the hair, dip against external parasites, vaccinate (usually only for rinderpest and only in areas where it has not been eradicated, and sometimes for anthrax); late summer/early autumn – milk, arrange mating, harvest and store grass for winter supplements; early winter – cull, slaughter, count herd and repair pens, enclosures, dipping pits, etc.; mid-winter – stop milking, shelter herd;

spring – provide supplemental hay, silage and maybe a little grain to females and weak, ill or plough yak. Herders know all the species of pasture plants on their lands, along with the feed and medicinal properties of each. In alpine areas, there is a separate grazing area for each season: swampy lands in early spring, followed by grasslands with *Ophiopogon japonica*, which herders say acts as a dewormer and stimulates oestrus (the latter is detected, albeit imperfectly, by the use of teaser bulls); summer bog-meadows with *Kobresia*, *Trollius* and *Caltha* spp., which increase milk yield and colours butter a rich orange; seeded grasslands in autumn, to build up body condition for the winter; and sheltered south-facing slopes rich in wilted grasses in winter. Coupled with periodic intra-seasonal herd movements every 10 to 40 days during warm weather, this system is equivalent to so-called 'modern' ones of rotational grazing; and it is 'enshrined in local proverbs and sayings which tell succinctly what to do and when' (p. 127). One such saying encodes the daily grazing principle of 'early out and late back in summer and autumn, late out and early back in winter and spring'. Where altitude permits, mixed-species grazing with small ruminants is the norm, as they exploit different forages from yak. There is great variation in milking procedures and timing within and across yak-raising groups. However, a few practices of note include: offering a little barley powder mixed with salt to tempt cows into the milking stall; in the absence of a stall, hobbling the forelimbs; and lubricating the teats with butter. With regard to diseases, yak are subject to most of the same ills as cattle world-wide. With the exception of some vaccinations (mainly in areas where the government provides them *gratis*), however, there is little recourse to formal veterinary medicine due to the remoteness of yak territory and the extremely high cost of conventional treatments. Diseases for which ethnoveterinary responses are mentioned include: FMD, for which affected animals are quarantined; and liverfluke, for which herders restrict springtime swamp grazing to only half a day at a time, do not graze swamp and marshlands after a rain and burn over such lands in the winter. Herders recognize the clinical signs of anthrax and its danger to humans and they do not eat the meat of affected animals. Most people also know to boil milk before consuming it or processing it into other products. Some variant husbandry and healthcare practices noted for non-Chinese yak-raising regions include the following: Mongolians generally de-horn their yak and they say that winter pastures that look brown from a distance are more nutritious than whitish-coloured ones; Indians provide virtually no shelter for their yak and in winter they must make greater use of lichens, dry leaves and tree loppings for fodder; in many parts of the former Russian federation, yak are left unsheltered and survive with little difficulty, even in the deep snow of winter. Other countries that raise significant numbers of yak are Afghanistan, Bhutan, Nepal and Pakistan. No matter where, however, the culture, religion and social life as well as the economic livelihoods of all yak-raising peoples are closely tied to this unique animal. The authors warn that the spread of modern concepts of feeding, management, breeding, etc. plus pressures from technical advice can erode traditional values and knowledge and with them yak numbers and thus the productive exploitation of otherwise unproductive environments. Consequently, any proposed interventions must first be carefully analysed in the context of the production system as a whole and of the multiple goods and services yak provide their keepers. To illustrate this point, various examples of where and why yak development efforts have sometimes gone wrong are adduced.

Ligers, Z. 1958. Comment les Peuls de Koa castrent leurs taureaux. **Bulletin de l'I.F.A.N.** Series B(1–2): 191–204.

In the Malian village of Koa, on the banks of the Niger River, Fulani stockraisers castrate all but one or two of their bulls to make them grow faster, larger, taller, meatier, stronger and, in Fulani eyes, handsomer. All these features add up to a bigger price upon earlier sale of steers as versus bulls. Another reason for castration is that steers are less fierce than bulls. Their presence dampens within-herd fighting, which can lead to weight loss among the whole herd as a result of increased movement, stress and lost grazing time. Nor is this to mention injuries to animals and their masters. Steers also make superior lead animals on long migrations. They will readily guide the rest of the herd into river crossings, will respond promptly to their master's call and, because of their distinctive lowing and bellowing, are easy to locate. All these characteristics greatly simplify the herder's job. According to Koans' Bambara, Bozo, Rimaibe and Somono neighbours, Fulani were the original inventors, many generations ago, of the excellent idea of castration. The procedure normally takes place in the early morning or in the evening at two times of the year: when the millet first sprouts; and in the middle of the cold season, when the herds return to Koa from their transhumance and when wounds heal more readily. At the latter time, too, animals need not move far from the village. However, young bulls may be castrated any time they begin to cause problems in the herd. Certain men are recognized as expert castrators (Fula *dérango*, Bambara *kóbo*) according to their experience and talent. But castration is a group effort, surrounded by various proscriptions and prescriptions on behaviour and dress. First, young men throw and tie the bull, using one of three techniques. Next is the operation itself, performed by the expert using a sharp knife to extract the testes and cut the 'nerves' close to the body. He follows this by reciting a short Islamic verse and 'spitting' three incantations over the wounds. The animal is then loosed to run into the bush, where it may remain alone for as many as 5 days. The expert throws the testicles into the Niger River as a gift to the god of the river. In return for their services, the young men and the expert are feasted on a bull or a steer from the owner's herd and given kola. Bulls exempted from castration in order to become studs are selected with great care, the paramount criterion being a dam outstanding for her milk production.

Lin, J.H., Y.Y. Lo, N.S. Shu, J.S. Wang, T.M. Lai, S.C. Kung and W.W. Chan. 1988. Control of preweaning diarrhea in piglets by acupuncture and Chinese medicine. **American Journal of Chinese Medicine** 16(1–2): 75–80.

Experiments in Taiwan to determine the effectiveness of acupuncture and a traditional Chinese polyprescription for diarrhoea in unweaned piglets found that aqua-acupuncture, using jets of water, had no prophylactic value but did cure 79% of diarrhoea cases. The traditional polyprescription of pueraria, coptis, scute and liquorice showed anti-pyretic, anti-inflammatory and anti-microbial activity. Piglets given this preparation experienced a lower incidence of diarrhoea and a higher average weight gain than untreated controls. In fact, 85% of the treatment group were cured in the space of a 4-day observation period.

Lin, J.H. and R. Panzer. 1994. Use of Chinese herbal medicine in veterinary science: History and perspectives. ***Revue Scientifique et Technique de l'Office International des Épizooties*** 13(2): 425–432.

Veterinary acupuncture has become increasingly accepted as part of orthodox medicine. The authors suggest that Chinese herbal medicine deserves similar recognition because there is great potential for more agile or powerful combinations of traditional and modern medicine and of medicine and agriculture. In these regards, they identify five areas for immediate research. First are clinical trials to investigate topics like the following in livestock and/or humans: the substitution of medicinal herbs for the antibiotics, preservatives and steroids currently added to feed rations to avoid infections and enhance animal growth; the millennia-old Chinese herbals for correcting reproductive failure, which has become a costly concern in both stockraising and human infertility; the many alternatives in Chinese medicine for more cheaply treating common diseases like colds, fevers, indigestion and diarrhoea, or for doing so with fewer side effects; and the use of animal models for the herbal treatment of human disease, like modelling enzootic bovine leukosis or canine hepatitis for the corresponding diseases in humans. Second and related is research to validate and explain the utilization of well-known natural plant and animal tissues for specific medical conditions, such as blood from slaughtered animals to treat anaemia. Third is understanding the pharmacological action of medicinal herbs and then using them in new forms like injections. The latter may allow for a more efficient deployment of especially rare and expensive herbs. Fourth is the cultivation of medicinal plants, which might prove more profitable than other crops for some farmers. Moreover, increased information on cultivation could help standardize herbal production and thus improve quality control. Fifth and finally is the development from Chinese herbal medicine of new and more benign pesticides for crops. To all these ends, the authors recommend: increased financial investment by governments on research into herbal medicine; the creation of university courses and training programmes; the formation of societies, organizations and journals on herbal medicine; greater cooperation between human and veterinary doctors and researchers; and personal efforts on the part of interested parties to diffuse more information about traditional Chinese medicine.

Lindo Revilla, Jesús. 1982. Como curar la hinchazón. ***Minka*** 8(Aug): 8.

With graphic illustrations, this one-page article presents an Andean home remedy for bloat in cattle based on drenching with an infusion of *tullway* (*Trichocereus* sp.).

Linquist, B.J. and David Adolph. 1992. ***A Look at the ITDG Marsabit Project: A Short Sojourn with the Yaa Galbo.*** In-house report. ITDG, Marsabit, Kenya. 76 pp.

Gabbra pastoralists of northern Kenya indicated that their number-one development needs lay in the domain of animal health. To begin to address this need, using an ethnoveterinary question list [see publications by Grandin and Young], the authors surveyed Gabbra about the most important diseases in their area plus present and preferred treatments, both modern and traditional. Preliminary results produced 42 disease names, 13 of them specific to young animals. Annex 5 of this report presents the raw data on 31 diseases, which spanned anthrax, CBPP, CCPP, 'craziness' (probably coenurus cerebralis), FMD, haemorrhagic septicaemia, poxes, manges, ringworm, swellings, trypanosomosis and a number of unidentified conditions in Gabbra cattle, sheep, goats and camels. Traditional veterinary *materia medica* include animal fats and oils, honey, charcoal, tobacco and other botanicals. These are administered topically, orally, intra-nasally or as fumigations. Non-pharmacological therapeutic techniques include branding/firing, bloodletting, incising or scarifying the skin, controlling drinking-water intake and permitting only well-water rather than ground-water. Prophylactic measures include, again, branding, plus herd movements and subdivisions and avoidance of infested or contaminated areas. For craziness, Gabbra simply slaughter. Some gender differences in disease names and rankings emerged during research. For instance, women cited two camel ailments of which men appeared unaware; and women's responses tended to centre on problems of young and small stock, for whom they have primary responsibility. At all three milking times of the day, women carefully examine these stock and, if necessary, treat them with potions, brands, eyewashes of salt water and milk and so forth. Indeed, in any discussion of small ruminant ills, men always referred researchers to their wives. Elderly women may also treat camels, although the survey uncovered the existence of male healers (*chires*) mainly for camels. *Chires* tend to specialize in reproductive and infertility problems, orthopaedics, or chronic diseases. Reportedly, they are skilled diagnosticians who prepare and administer both traditional and modern treatments or recommend such treatments to other stockowners. They may or may not charge for their services. Excerpts from interviews with two such healers are reproduced in this report. In addition to many traditional therapies, these two men noted a number of diseases for which they 'and even God' had no response (e.g. anthrax) or for which modern medicine was the preferred (e.g. trypanosomosis) or only (coughs) recourse. In the process, they expressed considerable concern about ectoparasites, along with an ability to differentiate between adult and nymph stages of ticks and their effects. Thus, the first ITDG paravet training package elaborated for Gabbra focused on ectoparasites. Other observations of interest include the following. While Western scientists rank trypanosomosis as the most important disease of camels, Gabbra do not share this assessment, although they do take care to avoid areas where the biting fly that vectors tryps abounds. Pastoralists see haemorrhagic septicaemia in camels as a more-often fatal disease; yet they withhold both drinking water and feed from camels with it.

Linquist, B.J., David Adolph and Stephen Blakeway. 1996. *Dinka Ethno-Veterinary Knowledge – A Resource Manual: Findings of a Preliminary Study.* UNICEF Operation Lifeline Sudan Southern Sector Livestock Programme, Nairobi, Kenya. 100 pp.

This manual records Dinka local knowledge as it relates to livestock, recapitulating the information presented in Adolph 1996 et al.and Blakeway et al.1996. The authors stress that this manual should be regarded as a first draft.

Lira, Jorge A. 1985. *Medicina Andina: Farmacopea y Ritual.* Centro de Estudios Rurales Andinos 'Bartolomé de las Casas', Cuzco, Perú. 189 pp.

Although the focus of this book is human ethnomedicine of the southern Peruvian Andes, it frequently refers to local veterinary practices as well. Examples include the use of: '*karkka* cane in smoke cures for herd animals suffering from equine adenitis; another smoke cure for this same condition plus rhinitis (Spanish *moquera*) based on burning *kkayara* cactus; a multiple-plant recipe or alternatively an *ajenjo*/maize-beer cure for the ubiquitous liver fluke; a unique root for fattening swine; toasted *maych'a* leaves to drive out ear ticks; baths with a decoction of *mokko mokko* or of *alhucema* in liquor to combat bloat (Spanish *sopladera*); washes with *tarwi* water [see also Avila Cazorla et al.1985a&b] combined with the ash from burnt cow manure to remove ectoparasites of ruminants; a dampened sheep skin applied to the rump of an animal with a urinary blockage; *willka willka* seeds in dog food to make the creatures more fierce and burying these seeds in herd animals' corrals to ward off disease and rustlers; and topical applications of ground *yanawarmi* leaves with maize-beer residue to treat burrowing ectoparasites of swine. The author also offers a description of the annual cattle marking festival.

Llanque Chana Andrés. 1989. *Médecine Vétérinaire Traditionelle dans la Société Aymara des Hauts-plateaux du Pérou.* Diplome d'Étude Avancé, Ecole des Hautes Etudes en Sciences Sociales, Université de Paris, Paris, France. 68 pp.

Among Aymara Indians of the Andes, the traditional veterinary pharmacopoeia is comprised of animal, vegetable and mineral *materia medica*. This thesis describes livestock diseases with both natural and supernatural ethnoaetiologies, along with their local remedies. Examples of plant therapies are: *Artemisia absinthiul* decocted and administered to expel intestinal worms; when pounded with salt it is applied to wounds; when finely powdered and boiled in water it is mixed with a little almond oil and used for enemas. *Buddleia longifolia* can be pounded and mixed with honey and used to reduce inflammation due to dislocations. Tick diseases can be treated by applying paraffin to affected parts. An animal that has suffered a fright is believed to lose its soul and thus sicken. In such cases, its owner and a *p'aqo* (ritual healer) pray to certain spirits and give them offerings of a mixture of coca leaf, incense and llama fat while circling the patient with perfumed vapours and chanting for the animal's soul to be returned to it.

Loculan, Ma. Dinah R. 1985. *The Utilization of Medicinal Plants for Animal Health Care in Lipa City.* BSc thesis in Agriculture with a major in Animal Science (Animal Health), University of the Philippines, Los Baños College, Laguna, Philippines. 54 pp.

With a view to increasing livestock production among Filipino smallholders at a lower cost by substituting local for imported drugs, this thesis sets out to provide baseline information on medicinal plant preparations commonly used for specific animal ailments. It is based on interviews by a random sample of 100 backyard stockraisers (97% male) in 22 rural neighbourhoods of Lipa City, Batangas Province, Philippines. There, people keep cattle, water buffalo, swine, goats, horses, poultry and dogs. The interview protocol consisted of four parts. Part I gathered social, economic and cultural data about the interviewees. They ranged in age from 21 to 76 years, with a mean of 47. The vast majority were married and Catholic. Part II focused on plant information – i.e. common name, parts used, ailments and animals treated, age of animals, method of preparation, mode of administration, dosage, recovery time and results. In response to Part II, interviewees reported 45 plants they use in prophylactic as well as therapeutic treatments for the animal species noted above. The plants are listed in Table 2, along with the number and percentage of interviewees mentioning each one. A 12-page Table 3 gives treatment details for each plant, along with its Latin name. Treatments involved both mono- and polyprescriptions prepared and applied in numerous standard ways. To take just a few examples, treatments applied to all species include: a decocted drench or drink of *Premna odorata* leaves and flowers or its sap/juice relieves fevers and colds or coughs, respectively; the sugared water of young coconuts combats the dehydration that accompanies various ills; and an infusion, decoction, or plaster of *Jasminum sambac* flowers applied as an eyewash, eyedrops or eye-patch cures sore, infected or wounded eyes, respectively. [For preparation and treatment details, see the thesis itself.] Part III of the interview protocol consisted of the following questions and answers. Where did the interviewee get his/her medicinal plant(s)? Answer: from farms (60% of interviewees) and their own backyards (40%). Who recommended them? Answer: mostly non-relatives (53%), excluding veterinarians and traditional healers known as *arbularyo* and relatives (28%). Has the interviewee found them to be effective and why? Answer: yes (99%). Is he/she still using conventional medicines? Answer: yes (84%) or sometimes in severe cases (11%). Part IV was left open for additional remarks. In this regard, some interviewees explained how they take into account disease severity and patient weight and size in calculating dosages. Others commented that plant remedies are most effective if used in the early stages of a disease. A number felt that such remedies produce no side effects. And many emphasized their extremely low cost. The author concludes that greater 'Efforts to continuously tap this resources [sic] could definitely provide farmers with readily available, effective and economical medicines for their animals and eventually stop if not reduce [the] present high degree of dependency on costly imported medicines' (p. 49).

Loculan, M.D.R. and C.D. Mateo. 1986. Utilization of medicinal plants for animal health care. *Philippine Journal of Veterinary and Animal Sciences* 12(3–4): 1–7.

In the Philippines, a study of 100 backyard stockraisers in 22 neighbourhoods of Lipa City revealed that 91% of them had used medicinal plant treatments for their cattle, carabao, goats, horses, swine, poultry and dogs for anywhere between 1 and 50 years. Moreover, 99% claimed that the treatments were effective regardless of patient age. In total, 45 medicinal plants were identified, of which 60% are found on people's own farms and 40% right in their backyards. Typically chopped, ground or pulverized in fresh, dried or roasted form, the plants are prepared as decoctions, infusions, poultices and plasters, and are given as feed additives, drenches, drinks, baths, washes, rubs or eyedrops.

Lonergan, David J. 1985. Personal communication (letter) to C.M. McCorkle of 15 April 1985. 3 pp.

These notes are based on a study of Sard shepherds of Sardinia, Italy. Sards inject an all-purpose antibiotic into any sickly sheep; if the animal does not respond, then it is bled by making incisions on the muzzle beneath each eye. Sards believe that illness is caused by changes in the weather rather than extremes in weather or the persistence of inclement conditions.

López Buendía, Gerardo. 1988. Aproximación histórica al uso de las plantas medicinales en veterinaria a través de la tradición oral. In: Luz Lozano Nathal and Gerardo López Buendía (coordinators). *Memorias: Primera Jornada sobre Herbolaria Medicinal en Veterinaria.* Universidad Nacional Autónoma de México, Facultad de Medicina Veterinaria y Zootecnia, Coordinación de Educación Continua, México DF. Pp. 8–11.

Urban as well as rural peoples have recourse to home veterinary remedies – as attested in this report of a Mexico City survey of market vendors and their clients, stable owners, operators of other animal enterprises, herbalists, students and professors of the university veterinary school, and other urban sources. The author enumerates 38 treatments based on some three dozen local plants for curing or preventing diseases and injuries in dogs, cats, horses, ruminants, swine, poultry and rabbits and for training these species. All this information has been preserved and passed on orally. Yet many veterinarians have incorrectly deprecated these home remedies, to which people turn first before they decide to consult a veterinarian. Far from being an obstacle to the practice of veterinary medicine, this knowledge represents an important, centuries-old legacy that veterinary science should conserve, study and enrich.

López Buendía, Gerardo, Luz C. Lozano Nathal and Ivonne Aubert de la P. 1988. Proyecto HERVET 10: Aspectos teórico-práctico para el desarrollo de una base de datos relacional sobre plantas medicinales para uso en medicina veterinaria. In: Luz Lozano Nathal and Gerardo López Buendía (coordinators). *Memorias: Primera Jornada sobre Herbolaria Medicinal en Veterinaria.* Universidad Nacional Autónoma de México, Facultad de Medicina Veterinaria y Zootecnia, Coordinación de Educación Continua, México DF. Pp. 144–155.

The importance of efficiently systematizing data about medicinal plants cannot be overemphasized because the information exists largely in oral and/or fragmentary form and is fast disappearing. HERVET 10 is a computerized, IBM-PC-compatible and menu-driven database elaborated specifically to organize, standardize, store, update and rapidly retrieve and synthesize such information for veterinary medical use. Moreover, the diskette system can be easily and inexpensively shared among veterinary schools and practitioners. The system encodes 24 variables per plant, including: family, genera, species and variety or subspecies; common names and regional synonyms; physical description; biological type (herb, bush, tree, etc.); geographic distribution; habitat; uses, both medicinal and non-medicinal; methods of collection and conservation; animal species that utilize the plant; therapeutic indications; contraindications and collateral effects; known pharmacological action; plant parts utilized; mode of preparation; chemical composition of the different parts; chemical taxonomy of biologically active components; reliability of information, classed as oral only, confirmed in multiple regions and/or historical sources, noted in various scientific or clinical studies, or researched in completed formal studies; toxicity; historical antecedents and sociocultural context; and bibliographic references. All variables can be cross-indexed and searched. The programme also provides for users to input new data in a special format which is later verified and integrated into the larger database.

López Miranda, Arnaldo. 1971. Contribución al mejor conocimiento de la histología floral de tres especies de Ranunculáceas, utilizadas en medicina popular. ***Boletín de la Sociedad Botánica de la Libertad*** 3(2): 119–136.

This study states that mixing flowers of *Laccopetalum giganteum* Wedd. in with livestock feed will stimulate animal fertility.

López Villafranco, Edith and Abigail Aguilar Contreras. 1989. Experiencias en el estudio etnobotánico y la herbolaria medicinal en veterinaria en la región de Mecapalapa, Pantepec, Puebla. In: Gerardo López Buendía (ed.). ***Memorias: Segunda Jornada sobre Herbolaria Medicinal en Medicina Veterinaria.*** Universidad Nacional Autónoma de México, Facultad de Medicina Veterinaria y Zootecnia, Coordinación de Educación Continua, México DF, México. Pp. 27–39.

This conference paper reports ethnobotanical and ethnozoological findings from field studies conducted among traditional healers (curers, bonesetters, midwives) and residents (Totonac, Nauhuatl, Otomí, Tepehua and mestizo) of Mecapalapa Community in Mexico's Puebla State. Findings are organized into six tables. The first enumerates five plants and their use as inhalations, drenches or drops in treating equine, canine and poultry ills. The second table lists four plants interviewees cited as toxic to domestic animals. The third describes the use of live animals (e.g. cattle, sheep, pigs, birds, iguanas, snails, bees, worms, snakes) or their body parts and products (e.g. milk, blood, wool, lard, fat, eggs, nests, internal organs, honey and even bath-water) in livestock ethnomedicines, often in combination with other items like sulphur, zinc, tobacco and sherry. The remaining three tables respectively list: animals that cause sickness; those that figure in local myths and ceremonies; and plants named after animals.

Loutan, L. 1984. Veterinary auxiliaries. In: Jeremy Swift (ed.). ***Pastoral Development in Central Niger: Report of the Niger Range and Livestock Project*** (NRLP). Ministère du Développement Rural, Service de l'Élevage and USAID, Niamey, Niger. Pp. 763–781.

Orthodox veterinary services cannot reach far-flung pastoralists, especially in the dry season when herds are most widely dispersed and animals are greatly weakened. A solution is creation of veterinary auxiliaries or 'paravets', themselves herders living in the bush. This has the advantages of saving on service personnel, vehicular and other expenses; enhancing direct herder participation and self-reliance in the care of their animals' health; increasing two-way communication between pastoralists and the government; and serving as a disease intelligence network. This chapter details and critically evaluates an NRLP pilot paravet programme. Topics covered are: the paravets' tasks – i.e. treating simple diseases with a limited number of effective medicines, with a focus on reducing mortality among classes of animals particularly at risk, such as young animals and pregnant or lactating females; and promoting systematic prophylactic healthcare; selection of trainees – herders should participate in the selection; and natural areas of operation should be defined, e.g. around a veterinary post, market or major water point; training issues – including location, timing and length of training, use of native language, pedagogic materials and approaches, instructors and the needs to emphasize prevention, provide training in outreach work and schedule periodic re-training;

types of drugs and equipment to distribute to paravets; supervision and re-supply of the paravet corps; remuneration of trainees – achieved by a 5% mark-up on the medicines they buy and then dispense, and by the respect they win from their peers; definition of the relationship of the paravet to the livestock service and to his peers (this can be problematic because the former may consider the paravet a subordinate labourer and the latter may see him as merely a dispenser of 'government' drugs and advice); general infrastructural and organizational issues. The chapter provides many sensitive insights into each of these topics. Quantitative analysis of the pilot programme demonstrated that paravets reached herders with no other access to veterinary services; for many such clients, this was their first contact with Western-type treatments. Thus, the author concludes that paravets '. . . play a complementary role, acting as an extension of the veterinary service without competing with it' (p. 766).

Lozano Nathal, Luz C. 1988. La tesis de licenciatura sobre plantas medicinales en la Facultad de Medicina Veterinaria y Zootecnia, UNAM (1916–1987). In: Luz Lozano Nathal and Gerardo López Buendía (coordinators). *Memorias: Primera Jornada sobre Herbolaria Medicinal en Veterinaria.* Universidad Nacional Autónoma de México, Facultad de Medicina Veterinaria y Zootecnia, Coordinación de Educación Continua, México DF. Pp. 23–33.

This paper overviews 24 theses from UNAM's College of Veterinary Medicine and Animal Science (FMVZ) that deal with medicinal plants. The theses are listed and, where information was available, abstracted under five categories: studies of the effects of a single plant (13 theses); of a combination of plants (2); comparisons of traditional treatments using one (3) or more (3) plants with their commercial equivalents; and library-based studies (3). Despite the facts that approximately 3000 medicinal plant species exist in Mexico and that many are used to treat animals, FMVZ theses on these resources have been few. They amount to only 0.4% of the 5700 theses produced between 1916 and 1987. The author thus urges more research on the wealth of medicinal plants in Mexico.

Lozano Nathal, Luz C. 1989. La etnoecología y la herbolaria medicinal en veterinaria. In: Gerardo López Buendía (ed.). *Memorias: Segunda Jornada sobre Herbolaria Medicinal en Medicina Veterinaria.* Universidad Nacional Autónoma de México, Facultad de Medicina Veterinaria y Zootecnia, Coordinación de Educación Continua, México DF, México. Pp. 156–161.

Chronicles dating from 1579 suggest that native peoples of Mexico rapidly transferred much of their ancient human and animal ethnomedicine to the new livestock species introduced by the Spaniards, while also adopting European medicinal plants. All this was done within a unique cultural matrix that located local fauna and flora in both spiritual and utilitarian contexts. With regard to EVM, the author gives contemporary examples of both. For instance, a healer attending a sick dog should avoid sex, work and sun if his cures are to take effect. A string tied around the necks of young donkeys and mules will protect them from the evil eye. To prevent fowl cholera, put the plant *mayorga* in the birds' drinking water; to ward off fowl pox in chicks, fumigate them with dried *chancarro* leaves. To make turkeys grow rapidly, feed them elder or other greens (e.g. *árnica, bejuco colorado*). For birds showing incipient signs of illness, place them in water for a moment to 'cool them down' and then give them a Sulfathiazol pill. Treat infected or fly-blown wounds in pigs with ground tobacco leaf and lime. But, how should Western-trained veterinarians and zootechnicians confront such constellations of spiritual and utilitarian practice and belief? A common reaction has been summarily to reject anything they did not learn in their formal studies as wrong or super- stitious. In Mexico, this has led to numerous fiascos in livestock development. One case from the Lacandon jungle was the substitution of inappropriate technology packages for traditional yet more productive farmyard methods of pig and chicken raising. Another was the introduction of Rambouillet and Merino sheep into the Chiapas highlands, where local textile technologies are not adapted to process the wool of these breeds. The answer lies in multidisciplinary approaches that combine local with modern scientific knowledge attuned to the particular cultural-ecological setting. Some examples are: searching for new forage possibilities among native rather than alien species; extending perhaps lower-producing but hardier breeds like the naked-neck chicken or the hair pig; designing livestock structures that employ only readily available construction materials; and, of course, using herbal medicines. In the last regard, however, the author emphasizes that the study of EVM cannot be limited only to phytotherapy; it must take into account *all* elements figuring in stockraisers' cultural sensibilities and ecological realities, plus the historical processes that led to these.

Lozano Nathal, Luz and Gerardo López Buendía. 1988. Prólogo. In: Luz Lozano Nathal and Gerardo López Buendía (coordinators). *Memorias: Primera Jornada sobre Herbolaria Medicinal en Veterinaria.* Universidad Nacional Autónoma de México, Facultad de Medicina Veterinaria y Zootecnia, Coordinación de Educación Continua, México DF. Pp. 1–3.

This prologue to the Proceedings of the First Conference on Herbal Veterinary Medicine in Mexico introduces 20 papers presented in the conference. The authors of the prologue note that, while herbalism has recently received a great deal of attention in Mexico, its study has been largely limited to human health. But herbal- ism in veterinary medicine has a long history in the country too, particularly among rural smallholders. The authors ascribe its origins and persistence to three factors: rural people's empirical observation of natural phenomena; an oral tradition which transmits these observations from generation to generation; and the extrapolation and application of ethnomedical concepts and practices for humans to animals. The authors urge that, along with its magico-religious, cultural and socioeconomic context, this folk veterinary wisdom receive more scholarly attention. They also emphasize that research on this subject must be interdisciplinary. Finally, they note that important 'therapeutic resources' are rapidly being lost due to the disappear- ance or acculturation of ethnic groups who control this knowledge and to the extinction of many species of flora. The authors hope that the conference proceed- ings will stimulate veterinary scientists and veterinarians to better appreciate, preserve and utilize these resources.

Lukefahr, S.D. 1992. *A Trainer's Manual for Meat Rabbit Project Development.* HPI, Little Rock, Arkansas, USA. 103 pp.

An effective home remedy for mange in rabbits is topical application of mineral, engine or vegetable oil, all of which effectively drown the mites that produce the mange. In Cameroon, farmers mix a cup of red palm-oil with a few drops of kerosene and apply the solution to the mangey rabbit's ears and skin (p. 52).

Lundborg, Gun. 1994. Protecting pasture. *African Farming* (Jul/Aug): 29–30.

Sheep and goat production is everywhere on the rise. While this means more meat, milk and fibre for families and markets, it has also meant expansion of stockraising into marginal lands and consequent overgrazing. Overgrazing can be prevented by applying phosphates and seeding forage species on the land. *Medicago* spp. are particularly productive, since they yield a large quantity of biomass and tolerate cold well. These advantages were demonstrated in a study conducted in the mountains of Syria.

Lupton, James Irvine. n.d. The diseases and treatment of cattle, sheep and pigs. In: W.J. Miles (ed.). *Modern Practical Farriery, a Complete System of the Veterinary Art as at Present Practised at the Royal Veterinary College, London.* William Mackenzie, London, UK. 96 pp.

Before the 19th century, veterinary medicine in England was traditionally the domain of farriers, i.e. blacksmiths. As universities expanded their curricula, smiths' empirical knowledge was gradually incorporated into formal schooling. This chapter describes the state of English veterinary knowledge for cattle, sheep and pigs as of this transitional period. Examples of *materia medica* of the time are: castor and linseed oil, Epsom salts, ammonia, ginger, powdered myrrh, tinctures of arnica and opium, and port wine. A few examples of treatments are: for mastitic cows, bloodletting and/or a poultice of linseed meal, bran and belladonna applied to the udder and held in place by tying a towel over the loins; a sheepdip for lice and ticks made of dilute carbolic acid; a fomentation of camphor, goose grease and spirits of wine, applied to the udders of mastitic ewes; an emetic of white hellebore, ipecacuanha and potassic-tartrate of antimony for quinsy (a throat infection), strangles or malignant sore-throat in swine; also for sore throats, hot 'blisters' [poultices?] or rugs wrapped around the neck.

Ly, Boubakar Sadou and Sabine Schenk. 1986. *Glossaire des Termes Principaux de l'Élevage Peul Français/Français-Peul.* FAO, Rome. 142 pp.

This glossary lists livestock terms in the native Pulaar dialects of Fulani in two regions of Burkina Faso. Its goals are to increase development planners' and national extensionists' appreciation of livestock concepts, practices and their rationales, and constraints and potentials among Fulani pastoralists of the African Sahel so that all these groups can better communicate about pastoral development needs. Differing terms are distinguished by locality, by singular/plural forms, by connotations and nuances and by changes in usage or frequency over time, as the reality they encode shifts. As per Fulani's own production emphases, here the focus is on cattle and small ruminants, with lesser attention to equines, camels, poultry and pigs. While the glossary does not pretend to be exhaustive, it covers 12 semantic categories in as many chapters, with summary remarks on the implications of findings in each. For example, the Fulani lexicon on 'herd acquisition' signals a shift to growing monetarization in that herds are now more frequently built up through purchase rather than traditional modes such as raiding, rustling, appropriating strays, shareherding, inheritance, tithing, familial charity, gifting and endowment (i.e. gifting of animals to a child upon her/his birth). Also evident in this lexicon is a shift to hired herders and a corresponding impoverishment of independent herders. Analysis of terms in the second category, 'herd composition', reveals an acceleration of sales of young male animals and, in general, an over-exploitation of stock to the detriment of herd continuity. Category 3 deals with genetic, reproductive and productive terms. It reveals a 'strong selection of both male and female breed stock', especially for their milk-producing properties. Category 4's anatomical and physiological vocabulary documents Fulani's by-and-large detailed savvy in these arenas; but it also reveals a lacuna in Fulani knowledge of glands and glandular secretions and effects. Category 5 deals with coat colours and configurations, the genotypic properties Fulani ascribe to these phenotypic characteristics, and the way herders purchase, cull, or bred stock accordingly. An interesting observation is the loss of considerable earlier phenotypic knowledge, beliefs and expressions due to the spread of Islam in Africa. In other words, not only Western but also Arab culture has contributed to the erosion of truly indigenous livestock knowledge and practice. Category 6 tackles pasture types and fodder plants, trees and shrubs. It notes their seasonal availability and palatability to different animal species; their reported toxic or other negative effects, if any, on animal health; in one case, their status as an indicator of overgrazing; and their their additional uses as hays, human food, market commodities, live or dead fences, craft and construction materials, and medicines. In the last regard, specifically mentioned are *Citrus quadrangularis* as a fumigant to enhance livestock birth rates and *Ipomoea vagans* as a galactagogue. This chapter also comments on the negative effects on these invaluable botanical resources from immigration, cropping, drought and nomads' permanent sedentarization. Also noted are native plants that the authors consider especially good candidates for further development attention. Category 7 deals with crop and agro-industrial byproducts and minerals along much the same lines as Category 6 but with particular attention to byproducts provided to special classes of livestock such as milk cows, feeder sheep and sick or aged animals. Terms for watering sources, for diurnal, nocturnal and seasonal watering schedules and for associated structures and paraphernalia are the subject of Category 8. Of interest here are special watering arrangements for weak or ill stock and for individual animals infamous for fouling water. Category 9 addresses health, disease and disease treatments, and predators. Besides listing terms for animal ills, clinical signs, disease-bearing pests, reproductive statuses and herbal, surgical, magical and other treatments, this chapter offers observations like: the lack of any traditional therapies for brucellosis or rinderpest; immediate slaughter of tubercular animals; Fulani's exceptional skills at correcting dystocia; and eagles' preferred predation of neonate calves, jackals' of small ruminants and hyenas' of newborn, sick and aged animals. Category 10, the lengthiest, covers terms for: herders; herd management techniques, e.g. for corralling, handling, hobbling, taming, tracking, belling, weaning, subdividing herds, calling to animals, loading them, controlling predators and strays, etc.; movement schedules, directions, trails, routes and reading the stars for same; climatic conditions; pastoral labour-sharing arrangements; associated items of material culture; livestock ethology, including vocalizations; and much more. Of note is the Fulani custom of soothingly addressing and caressing their animals so as to reduce stress and increase production. Category 11 deals mainly with terms pertaining to the production, harvesting, processing, consumption and marketing of animals and their products. Category 12 does likewise for herders' 'socio-professional environment', which includes the term *dokotoro na'i* 'cow doctor' and a variant on the French for 'veterinarian'. In general, the authors find that the introduction of modern veterinary medicine has led to great losses in Fulani's empirical veterinary knowledge and practice. Now, only very elderly persons in very remote areas still control much of such know-how and skills. However, supernatural practices remain widespread, notably in the form of magic, talismans and incantations. The authors further comment that differential diagnostic abilities among Fulani they interviewed were limited. Overall, this study underscores the point that semantic investigations provide a good indicator of the importance of animals to a given people's livelihoods and lifeways, as well as of the extent of people's EVK. In addition, semantic research provides an excellent entré into and appreciation of stockraising societies, which can in turn usefully inform the design of livestock development interventions.

Maeda-Machang'u, A.D., S. Mutayoba, G.H. Laswai, R.V. Kurwijila and E.S. Kimambo. 1995. *Local knowledge in animal health and production systems: Gender perspectives.* Final Report of an FAO-funded project. Sokoine University of Agriculture, Morogoro, Tanzania. 126 pp.

This FAO-sponsored study interviewed 60 households in each of three livestock production systems (pastoral, extensive agropastoral and intensive agropastoral) in Tanzania focusing on local knowledge in animal health and production systems. Pastoralists made the greatest use of EVM in treating problems such as abortion, bloat, impaction and mastitis. But modern veterinary drugs were preferred for anaplasmosis, anthrax, babesiosis, CBPP, ECF, heartwater, trypanosomosis and worms. For diarrhoeas, 48%, 43% and 9% of the pastoralists interviewed employed traditional treatments, modern drugs and management techniques, respectively. Management techniques were also popular for ephemeral fever, heartwater and tick control. Also mentioned for the agropastoral systems were the treatment of FMD sores with a solution of urine and lukewarm salt water and the mechanical removal of retained placenta. Across all three production systems, 75% of interviewees employed some form of EVM.

Mag-Uumad Foundation. 1995. POs form barefoot veterinarians. *The Mag-Uumad Newsletter* 4: 182.

This brief article notes that, with support from the Mag-Uumad Foundation, People's Organisations in the Philippines have begun to establish volunteer paravet programmes to help support livestock distribution schemes there (cattle, carabao and pigs). In at least one such programme, paravets have taken it upon themselves to test out herbal remedies for livestock as an alternative to chemical ones.

Mahendrarajah, E.S. 1997. Crows multiply champaca trees: Innovations from Sri Lanka. *Honey Bee* 8(3): 10.

Some farmers of Sri Lanka strengthen and rapidly fatten a sheep by confining it in a ten-foot deep, 10-by-6-foot pit, where it is intensively fed until it reaches the desired state of health or weight. Similar practices are followed for ducks in China and camels in Kutch.

Majok, Aggrey Ayuen and Calvin W. Schwabe. 1996. *Development Among Africa's Migratory Pastoralists.* Bergin and Garvey, Westport, Connecticut, USA. 285 pp.

This volume reprises and significantly expands on topics introduced in other, earlier publications by its authors, but now from an overarching development standpoint. The authors note that pre-World War II studies focused on African pastoralists' subsistence systems were rare. Beginning in the late 1950s, a few anthropologists linked this topic to ecological issues. But even by the 1970s, there was little attempt to relate such information to the provision of services or amenities to pastoralists. Among other things, this book argues for drawing upon traditional healers as a source of travelling animal health auxiliaries and assistants in national livestock and epidemiological surveys. Among the Dinka of Sudan, for example, traditional veterinary doctors (*atet*), themselves herd owners, are expert at such procedures as basic surgery, bonesetting, obstetrics and herbalism. Their presence in migratory cattle camps and transhumant home-bases makes veterinary services readily available to pastoralists. Via collaboration with formal-sector veterinary personnel, they could extend even more, decentralized services to their co-ethnic clients. Given the facts that, among pastoralists, practitioners like *atet* treat humans as well as livestock and that zoonoses are widespread, the authors also argue for an intersectoral approach to healthcare delivery, adducing examples and models to this effect and discussing appropriate institutional and educational structures. Another topic in this volume is daily cattle care among the Dinka (who also keep small ruminants and poultry). One practice is the nightly pegging-down of each head of cattle in a crescent-moon arrangement within the home-base byre and the building of dung fires, especially near stud and song bulls and prize cows, to drive off flies. Men sleep near the door of the byre, ready to fight predators and other threats to the death. The authors also offer an overview of animal diseases among African pastoralists in historical and socioeconomic context. The discussion of hydatidosis (also known as echinococcosis) is illustrative. This 'big belly' ailment is a parasitic zoonosis in which certain tapeworm larvae encyst themselves in the organs of people who swallow the parasite's eggs, which are passed in the faeces of infected canines. Many African pastoralist groups recognized the cysts in their livestock but traditionally did not associate them with the disease in humans. While some groups (e.g. Maasai) thought such cysts were harmful, others (e.g. Turkana) thought they were livestock's means of storing water during drought. In some areas, such as Turkanaland, the zoonosis is endemic as a result of practices like: feeding the cysts from livestock to dogs; keeping pet dogs in the hut, where they lick babies clean of vomit and faeces and women of menstrual blood; and eating jackals. Turkana healers traditionally treated human hydatidosis with hot iron cautery. The authors surveyed *atet* of one Dinka subtribe as to their differential diagnosis, treatments and beliefs for major livestock diseases. On the basis of clinical and post-mortem signs, these healers by and large correctly diagnosed anthrax, CBPP, rinderpest, FMD, fasciolosis, trypanosomosis, blackleg, and diarrhoea as versus dysentery. However, their diagnoses of tuberculosis, certain diarrhoeal conditions and something they called 'tick disease' were less astute in that they embraced multiple conditions. For certain diseases they recognize as highly contagious, Dinka institute controls in the form of forcing owners of infected stock to flee with their animals (CBPP), separating sick from healthy animals (rinderpest, diarrhoea) and not eating affected parts of the carcass (tuberculosis). For rinderpest, Maasai noted early on that cattle who contracted a milder form of this disease from wild eland were protected from more virulent forms of it. They also observed that cattle caught malignant catarrh from wildebeests during the latter's calving season. Only much later did Western veterinary medicine make the same observations for these two viral diseases, i.e. that eland rinderpest is naturally attenuated for cattle and that grass contaminated by wildebeest uterine blood and placental fluids can infect cattle who graze it with malignant catarrh.

Málaga, C.E. 1988. *Yerbas Medicinales Peruanas: Plantas que Curan.* Editorial Litográfica La Confianza for Editorial Mercurio, Lima, Perú. 232 pp.

The focus of this popular publication is human ethnomedicine. It also mentions a few ethnoveterinary practices, however. One is mixing seeds of *beleño negro* into horse feed to fatten the animals. Another is drenching horses with olive oil to relieve stomach ache. A number of plants that are poisonous to animals are also noted (pp. 57–59, 136, 142).

Malik, J.K., V. Raviparakash and A. Ahmad. 1998. Research and development of ethnoveterinary pharmacology in India – An overview. In: E. Mathias, D.V. Rangnekar and C.M. McCorkle, with M. Martin (eds). *Ethnoveterinary Medicine: Alternatives for Livestock Development – Proceedings of an International Conference Held in Pune, India, 4–6 November 1997. Volume 2: Abstracts.* BAIF Development Research Foundation, Pune, India. Pp. 37–38.

Traditional medicines occupy an important place among the remedies employed to treat different ailments of livestock in India. The wealth of knowledge on EVM was originally confined to a few individuals and transferred from generation to generation, mainly as a family tradition. Subsequently, researchers started compiling information on EVM; but such information was often difficult to access and offered no scientific proof of the benefits attributed to the various *materia medica*. Later, materials were evaluated based on modern pharmacological procedures. Recently, there has been a surge of interest worldwide in R&D in ethnoveterinary pharmacology and especially in the scientific validation of ethnobotanicals. A large number of native medicinal plants have been screened for various pharmacological properties, mainly to develop products for human diseases; but little such attention has been paid to ethnobotanicals for the control and treatment of livestock diseases. Nevertheless, the research on age-old ethnobotanical remedies for humans has paved the way for the development of a number of preparations for treating diseases and enhancing productivity in domestic animals. Veterinary drug formulations have been developed for ectoparasites, worms, wounds, bacterial infections and inflammations; for reproductive, gastrointestinal, urinary-tract and respiratory disorders; and for greater milk and egg production. The outcome has been therapeutically improved traditional remedies that are still easily accessible and cost-effective. The future for ethnopharmacology to enhance the health and production of Indian livestock is bright. However, more concerted and coordinated efforts are needed that take a multifaceted approach, involving traditional physicians, medical chemists, veterinary pharmacologists and clinicians and veterinary pharmaceutical industries. These should address issues of quality control and standardization of herbal pharmaceuticals.

Malik, Jitendra K., Aswin M. Thaker and Allauddin Ahmad. 1996. Ethnoveterinary medicine in Western India. In: Constance M. McCorkle, Evelyn Mathias and Tjaart W. Schillhorn van Veen (eds). *Ethnoveterinary Research & Development.* Intermediate Technology Publications, London, UK. Pp. 148–157.

India boasts a wide range of effective traditional veterinary and animal-husbandry practices. This chapter provides an up-to-date overview of such practices in Gujarat State spanning management techniques, breeding strategies, feeds and ethnoveterinary prophylaxes and therapies focusing on the most common and economically important disorders of farm animals. Stockowners use herbal, non-herbal and drug-free techniques because of their safety, inexpensiveness and effectiveness. In India, herbal treatments are particularly popular. The chapter features a table of 66 plants commonly used in prescriptions, also described here, for external injuries, eye disorders, ectoparasitism, gastrointestinal ills, reproductive and related disorders, dietary deficiencies and other health problems of cattle, buffalo, camels and goats. It also summarizes general information on the preparation of botanical medicines for livestock, plus current scientific knowledge of India's ethnoveterinary pharmacopoeia. In addition, a number of surgical operations are noted. In cases of horn cancer, the horn is surgically removed, the cavity is packed with red lead and a pinch of mercury and is bandaged. A cataract operation entails surgically removing part of the brow above the eye and applying kern oil of the marking-nut tree to the eye with a bit of cotton. For several diseases (e.g. tympany, CCPP), the tips of the ears are amputated. Cauterization is a common, multi-purpose technique.

Maliki, Angelo B. 1981. *Ngaynaaka: Herding according to the WoDaaße.* Rapport préliminaire – Discussion Paper No. 2. Ministry of Rural Development, Niger Range and Livestock Project, B.P. 85, Tahua, Niger. 181 pp.

This study describes livestock raising as practised by the WoDaaße. The first chapters outline the nomadic year, herd composition and herd management (including information on genetics and salt feeding). Pages 34–63 relate directly to EVM. The WoDaaße have a good knowledge of the reproductive cycle and heat symptoms of their animals. They observe their cows during pregnancy; they know the signs of approaching birth and cut the cervix with a razor blade if the birth channel is not wide enough. The author describes still other practices regarding birth and the care of the newborn calf. He also lists 70 forage plants and indicates their medical and other uses. The WoDaaße classify diseases affecting their livestock into two major categories: 'hot' and 'cold'. The former are more dangerous. The animal stops grazing, its body is 'on fire' and it dies quickly. 'Cold' diseases are less severe. Animals continue grazing but do not gain weight. Contagious diseases are placed in an extra category. The author lists 65 WoDaaße disease terms and describes clinical signs and folk treatments for many of these ills. The pastoralists cure and prevent diseases with cauterization, bleeding, indigenous medicines and vaccination. Pages 65–66 explain magical beliefs about fertility and illness. The report concludes with a discussion of herding strategies and of proverbs about livestock herding.

Maliki, Angelo and Mahamat Saley Bahram. 1988. *Projet Ishtirak: Le Programme de Formation d'Auxiliaires Vétérinaires (AV).* In-house report. Oxfam, N'Djaména, Chad. 4 pp.

In this update on the Ishtirak Project's paravet programme in Chad, the authors note that the ideal trainee is someone who is already locally recognized and respected as a livestock healer. They also describe how the first day of Ishtirak training is given over to an open discussion with trainees about their opinions of the livestock health picture in their region and the impact of different diseases on animal production, plus trainee presentations and self-critiques of their principal ethnoveterinary prophylaxes and therapies.

Mammerickx, M. 1994. Les anciennes méthodes de prophylaxie des maladies animales en Belgique. *Revue Scientifique et Technique de l'Office International des Épizooties* 13(2): 487–498.

This article reviews the history and control of bovine plague (contagious typhus) in Belgium. In the early 18th century, the principles of hygienic prophylaxis, based on an astute understanding of contagion, were set out and incorporated into Belgian law. But they were not applied effectively until the second half of the 19th century. Control methods consisted of, e.g.: denying sick animals access to communal grazing grounds and water sources; disinfecting mangers and troughs with lime; herders' washing their hands and faces with vinegar after handling infected animals; burying the milk from sick cows so that people would not consume it; circumscribing animal and herder movements; forbidding therapeutic measures; and more. The most drastic step was to slaughter all cattle suspected of disease, in which case government subsidies were paid to the owners.

Manandhar, N.P. 1989. Ethno veterinary [sic] medicinal drugs of [the] central development region of Nepal. *B.M.E.B.R.* 10(3–4): 93–99.

This botanical survey in Nepal uncovered 35 plants used in treating cattle, buffalo, sheep and goats. The article details the plants' mode of preparation and administration by disease. *Asparagus racemosus* W., for example, is fed to cattle to cure milking disorders. *Azadirachta indica* A. leaf paste is applied to wounds, particularly of horses' backs. Powdered *Cannabis sativa* L. leaf is fed to relieve diarrhoea in cattle.

Manandhar, N.P. 1991. Medicinal plant-lore of [the] Tamang tribe of Kabhrepalanchok District, Nepal. *Economic Botany* 45(1): 58–71.

Jhankries 'healers' of Nepal's Tamang tribe use as many as 95 wild and domestic plant species in their ethnomedicine for humans and livestock. Ethnoveterinary applications noted in this article include the following [apparently oral] plant medicines: to prevent miscarriages, root juice of *Scutellaria scandens* Buch.-Ham.; for coughs, a paste of *Spermadictyon suaveolens* Roxb. bark; and for liverfluke disease, the squeezed-dry bark of *Schima wallichi* (DC.) Korth. Tamang reportedly attribute most ills to spirits. So they also employ magic, religion and sacrifices to dispel disease. But they never fail to employ plant treatments as well. Thus *jhankries* 'are faith healers on the one hand and herbalists on the other' and these 'traditional healers are still the only medical practitioners available to the Tamang tribe living in remote parts' (p. 69).

Manandhar, N.P. 1992a. Ethno veterinary [sic] drugs: Reported use from the central development region. In: IIRR (ed.). *Regenerative Agriculture Technologies for the Hill Farmers of Nepal.* IIRR, Silang, Cavite, Philippines. Unpaginated (3 pp.).

Based on an ethnobotanical survey undertaken by the author, this three-page article lists 45 plant species used in Nepali EVM. The plants are organized alphabetically by their Latin names, followed by a one-sentence description of their ethno-veterinary use in cattle, sheep, horses or dogs. The plants are administered in a variety of ways for, e.g.: diarrhoeas, diptheria, parasites and gastrointestinal, urinary and ocular problems, intoxication; muscle swelling, fractures and dislocations; wounds, myiasis and internal injuries from a fall; snakebite; milking problems; infertility ease of parturition; and strength, vigour and warmth.

Manandhar, N.P. 1992b. The use and conservation of traditional medicine plant resources. In: IIRR (ed.). *Regenerative Agriculture Technologies for the Hill Farmers of Nepal.* IIRR, Silang, Cavite, Philippines. Unpaginated (4 pp.).

This three-page paper mentions the use of the leaf juice of *Cannabis sativa* L. as an anti-diarrhoeal for cattle. The juice is given the cattle to drink; and *Cannabis* leaves are mixed into their feed.

Mane, P.M. 1989. *Study of Traditional Agricultural Practices.* Aga Khan Rural Support Programme, Ahmedabad, India.

Lucerne, barley and methi seeds are sown together as a winter crop in Saurashtra, India. This mix of forages is extremely palatable to cattle and enhances their digestion. [Abstract based on Gupta et al.'s 1990 annotated bibliography.]

Mane, P.M. 1992. Branch of *Euphorbia* sp. *Honey Bee* 3(2): 20.

This paragraph-long article describes how one Indian tribal man has kept a small bouquet of *Euphorbia* sp. branches hanging at the gate of his animal byre for the past 2 years, as an FMD prophylaxis. He says that his stock have thus remained free of FMD even though those of his co-villagers are infected. The man learned of this treatment from relatives of his in another village in India.

Manjunatha, B.P. 1999. Therapeutic efficacy of a herbal preparation in dermatological conditions of animals and its influence on wound healing. In: E. Mathias, D.V. Rangnekar and C.M. McCorkle, with M. Martin (eds). *Ethnoveterinary Medicine: Alternatives for Livestock Development – Proceedings of an International Conference Held in Pune, India, 4–6 November 1997. Volume 1: Selected Papers.* BAIF Development Research Foundation, Pune, India. Pp. 120–125.

This paper reviews research on Himax, a commercial herbal ointment that contains *Sida veronicaefolia, Tagetes erecta, Berberis aristata* and oleum picis liquidae. *In vitro* studies showed Himax to be effective against pathogenic bacteria like *Streptococcus, Staphylococcus* and *Pseudomonas* spp. and of fungi like

Trichophyton and *Microsporum*. The therapeutic efficacy of Himax in different species of domestic animals was evaluated in approximately 1800 clinical dermatological conditions caused by pathogenic species of bacteria, fungi, mites and virus or by trauma and other non-specific causes. Himax proved highly efficacious in completely curing all such cases. Histological and biochemical studies on Himax's influence on wound healing revealed fast and excessive deposition of granulated tissue with high concentrations of hexosamine and hydroxyproline, increased mitotic activity, early wound contraction and re-epithelialization. In sum, this review confirms the therapeutic efficacy of this herbal preparation in treating various dermatological conditions of domestic animals.

Mapatano, Sylvain Mulume. 1997. Farmer-research brigades in Zaire. In: Laurens van Veldhuizen, Ann Waters-Bayer, Ricardo Ramírez, Debra A. Johnson and John Thompson (eds). ***Farmers' Research in Practice: Lessons from the Field.*** Intermediate Technology Publications, London, UK. Pp. 139–151.

In Zaire, farmers cannot count on formal scientific research to solve their agricultural problems because such research is defined largely by internationally-linked canons and institutions. As farmers themselves point out, they cannot afford the expensive 'modern' agricultural techniques and inputs generated and promoted by these institutions. Instead, people must resort to self-help. In this regard, 'local research brigades' can be instrumental. This chapter reports on several such brigades organized by NGOs in eastern Zaire. A number of the brigades focused on animal nutrition, housing, reproduction and genetic improvement, as well as EVM. In order to make their own and other communities' EVK more widely available, brigade farmers compiled information from community members (especially the elderly) about common animal diseases and their local treatments. They also devised methods to conserve herbal medicines locally. Brigade farmers disseminate these findings through exchange visits to view one anothers' experiments, intra- and inter-community meetings and workshops and self-organized or government agricultural fairs. The community, NGO and formal R&D inter-linkages such events stimulate can lead to the design of specific, farmer-oriented livestock R&D projects, as well as to technical and financial support for farmers to analyse problems or obtain basic equipment like jars for storing dried herbs. 'Pros' of this research-brigade approach include, above all, assurance that research generates research products relevant to the problems farmers themselves consider most urgent. Also, events publicizing farmers' own findings lend value and recognition to their local knowledge and achievements, thereby encouraging not only the preservation of existing skills and techniques, but also the creative generation of new local knowledge. At the same time, such events 'gradually efface the social barriers between farmers and other stakeholders in agricultural R&D' (p. 148) and give the former an opportunity to make complaints, demands and suggestions to the latter. Another positive outcome of the brigade approach has been the evolution of some innovative research methodologies. Likewise for networking across brigades addressing similar problems. 'Cons' include the fact that information flows tend to be slow, asystematic and geographically and sometimes linguistically limited. But these 'cons' can perhaps be overcome by the use of rural radio and technical brochures in local languages. Nevertheless, 'The more appropriate the innovation for a wide spectrum of farmers, ... the quicker news of it seems to spread from person to person' (p. 149). Ethnoveterinary examples of this principle in action included the various ways Zaire farmers induce oestrus in goats, as well as effective plant medicines for livestock.

Mapatano, M. and K. Chifundera. 1993. Dynamique paysanne et usage de la pharmacologie dans l'élevage au Bushi. Unpublished manuscript.

Unavailable for review.

Mapatano, M. et al. 1995. L'élevage de petits ruminants au Bushi: Une démarche et des actions participatives. *Capricorne* 8(2): 11–16.

Unavailable for review.

Marchand, A. 1984. Médecine vétérinaire populaire et maladies parasitaires. *Ethnozootechnie* 34: 19–23.

This brief article presents numerous examples, both historical and contemporary, of ethnoveterinary practices to combat parasitism worldwide. Techniques are grouped into five categories: mechanical and physical therapies, chemical treatments, nutritional controls and herd management, hygienic measures and 'mystical' (i.e. magico-religious) actions. Perhaps of particular note is the widespread and long-standing therapeutic or prophylactic use of such items as salt, garlic, tobacco, tar and, in present-day France, motor oil. The author concludes by noting that '. . . the observations made and the experiences acquired through generations and generations are dominated by good sense. They offer us a great lesson in humility' (p. 23).

Marcus, S. 1992. *A Preliminary Study on the Anthelmintic Properties of* **Terminalia glaucescens** *in Cattle in the Northwest Province of Cameroon: An Ethnoveterinarian Approach.* DVM thesis. University of Utrecht, Utrecht, The Netherlands. No. of pages unknown.

Unavailable for review, but see Toyang et al. 1995.

Mares, R.G. 1951. A note on the Somali method of vaccination against contagious bovine pleuropneumonia. *The Veterinary Record* 63(9): 166.

CBPP is a well-recognized disease among Somali cattle owners. They combat it with a form of indigenous vaccination that consists of inserting minced pieces of lung from an animal dead of CBPP into an incision on the bone of the face, halfway between the eyes and nostrils. After the tissue reacts, it is radically excised and its debris removed from the area which is then cauterized flush to the bone. Infected vaccinations are treated by line firing. The vaccination is unquestionably effective but may cause swelling and inflammation.

Mares, Robert G. 1954a. Animal husbandry, animal industry and animal disease in the Somaliland Protectorate. Part I. *The British Veterinary Journal* 110(10): 411–423.

Somali pastoralists keep camels, small ruminants and some cattle. Horses have virtually vanished because the land has become too barren to support them. Pastoralists regularly feed salt to their herds. They are experts on forage plants and readily recognize salty and toxic plants. The author describes watering, breeding, calf-rearing and castration practices for the different species. The latter include striking the seminal cord with a light mallet, destroying the testicular tissue with a hot needle and open surgery.

Mares, Robert G. 1954b. Animal husbandry, animal industry and animal disease in the Somaliland Protectorate. Part II. *The British Veterinary Journal* 110(11): 470–481.

The first part of this article describes Somaliland's livestock industry during the Protectorate years. The author views the slaughtering arrangements then current as the most hygienic practicable. The second part deals with animal disease. A branding iron and a sheep-head soup are the mainstays of Somali therapeutics. Also, the latex of *Euphorbia somaliensis* and camel urine are used as mange remedies. Somali vaccinate cattle against CBPP [see Mares 1951], rinderpest and sometimes CCPP. The author also discusses anthrax and trypanosomosis; and he provides a comprehensive list of diseases encountered in Somaliland along with their local names, plus a glossary of Somali words relating to animal husbandry and EVM.

Mariner, J.C., D.M.O. Akabwai, J. Toyang, N. Zoyem and A. Ngangyou. 1994. Community-based vaccination with thermostable vero cell-adapted rinderpest vaccine (Thermovax). *The Kenya Veterinarian* 18(2): 507–509.

In describing two pilot, community-based vaccination programmes among Fulani of Cameroon and Karamajong of Uganda, the authors note that training for community vaccinators integrated selected Western veterinary concepts with EVK. For example, pastoralists' every-day healthcare and husbandry experience provided analogies for course discussions on the concept of infection, the difference between treatment versus vaccination and the scaling of drug dosages. Discussions also made it evident 'that pastoralists have a highly developed knowledge of disease identification' (p. 508).

Mariner, J.C., G.G.M. van't Klooster and A. Berhanu. 1996. Rinderpest control in Ethiopia: Participatory approach to vaccination in remote pastoral communities. In: Karl-Hans Zessin (ed.). *Livestock Production and Diseases in the Tropics: Livestock Production and Human Welfare. Proceedings of the VIII International Conference of Institutions of Tropical Veterinary Medicine held from the 25 to 29 September, 1995 in Berlin, Germany.* Volume I. Deutsche Stiftung für Internationale Entwicklung, Zentralstelle für Ernährung und Landwirtschaft, Feldafing, Germany. Pp. 324–329.

PRA with Afar pastoralists in Ethiopia found that they have 'a remarkable understanding' of rinderpest epidemiology. Correctly noting that older Afar cattle are essentially immune as a result of having survived previous outbreaks, participants stressed that in their herds rinderpest is largely a disease of young cattle. Pastoralists added that this disease is mainly a problem in the one grazing area, the Rift Valley escarpment. There, their herds mix with the more susceptible highland cattle. Further, they noted the role of warthogs in the early stages of outbreaks. Elders described a traditional but now-abandoned rinderpest vaccine made by mixing the faeces and urine of an animal dead of the disease with unspecified plant extracts. After standing overnight, a few drops of the mixture were administered intra-nasally to young calves in the morning. Elders said this crude vaccine protected most calves by giving them a mild case of the disease, although some did die. Today, Afar prefer a commercial vaccine. But they say it is difficult to obtain because veterinary service personnel rarely come to their area. Indeed, parts of Afarland have not been visited by the service in living memory. Where service personnel do appear, often it is at a time of the year when many cattle are in distant grazing grounds and personnel do not remain long enough for pastoralists to bring these animals in for vaccination. Informants from the veterinary service confirmed all these statements, citing the lack of crushes as an excuse. During PRA, Afar also accurately defined a number of other clinical entities, including CBPP, anthrax, blackleg and surra.

Marinow, Wasil. 1961. Die Schafzucht der nomadisierenden Karaktschanen in Bulgarien. In: László Földe (ed.). *Viehzucht und Hirtenleben in Ostmitteleuropa: Ethnographische Studien.* Akadémiai Kiadó, Verlag der Ungarischen Akademie der Wissenschaften, Budapest, Hungary. Pp. 147–196.

Pages 182–184 of this chapter describe the nine most important sheep diseases and their treatments among nomadic Karakatshan shepherds in Bulgaria. Sheep with coenurosis, a parasitic disease, are sometimes treated by perforating the skull with a hot iron rod to drain the pus or by opening the skull with a small knife to remove the parasitic cysts. When an animal has eaten poisonous plants, the shepherds bleed it by piercing blood vessels above its eyes. To avoid infection with liver flukes, sheep are not allowed to graze when the grass is wet with dew. The nomads treat mange by rubbing a decoction of tobacco on the lesions. In general, the Karakatshan sheep are quite healthy; fewer die from diseases than from predation by bears and wolves. Herders also supplement their sheep with salt where necessary.

Marlborough, Lindsay. 1997. *Ethno-veterinary Knowledge of the Latuka in Southern Sudan: A Study for the German Agro Action Livestock Programme, Torit County.* German Agro Action, Nairobi, Kenya. 48 pp.

The first part of this report describes the way in which ethnoveterinary information was gathered and used in CAHW workshops among Latuka agropastoralists in war-torn southern Sudan. Interviewees included members of different male age-grades in agropastoral communities, women's groups and primary schools. Methods spanned: PRA evaluations and rankings, e.g. of disease importance and local versus modern treatment effectiveness; semi-structured interviews; direct observation of management practices and clinical cases; and description and sampling of clinical materials and plants and other items used in local veterinary plus human-medical treatments. The researcher classed treatments as plant-based, non-plant-based and rituals/blessings. Examples of the second type are: applying cow dung, spent battery acid or 3-day-old urine to wounds; using snake skin, ground clam shells and a fine red soil for eye ailments; firing lymph nodes; and bloodletting, sometimes performed by slashing a muscle affected by a blackquarter-like ill. The author wonders if this latter treatment might be helpful via admitting oxygen into areas of anaerobic bacterial infection. The goals of the research were to identify valuable healthcare and husbandry practices, reconfirm their utility to CAHW trainees and then focus the remainder of training on non-traditional remedies for diseases for which few or no useful traditional treatments can be identified. Indeed, when compared with the pastoral Dinka and Nuer of the region [see the companion UNICEF studies by Adolph et al. 1996, Blakeway et al. 1996 and

Linquist et al. 1996], Latuka agropastoralists appear to control less and less effec-tive EVK, although it circulates freely. For example, Latuka knew of few tick-prevention techniques and they generally failed to mention ticks as a source of disease. Contrarily, they believed that colostrum causes worms. But the majority of ethnoaetiologies were cited as 'caused by God' or simply 'unknown'. On the other hand, there are skilled Latuka specialists for livestock obstetrics and for the open castration used on cattle and herding and hunting dogs. For sheep and goats, owners themselves perform bloodless castration. But there is no class of herbalists; and particularly among younger Latuka, disease names are sometimes confused and their ethnodiagnostic abilities are shaky. For instance, they apply the same term to rinderpest as to diarrhoeas of other origins. In all age groups, disease descriptions were sometimes so incomplete that some of the conditions discussed during interviews could not be scientifically identified. In other cases, disease names are assigned by symptoms, in such a way that a single term can denote several scientifically different diseases. For example, *aruson* 'nodules' can mean dermatophilus, lumpy skin disease, or oesophagostomosis. In part, this multiplicity of meanings arises from the fact that there are five distinct dialects of Latuka. Thus the author emphasizes the importance of seeing clinical cases and being present at necropsies whenever possible during ethnoveterinary information collection. The study paid particular attention to women, noting that they are often involved in preparing plant and other treatments for ruminants and that they have an excep-tional knowledge of and confidence in traditional poultry treatments. Treatments of chilli or cannabis or *Ziziphus* spp. were said to be effective against diarrhoea in poultry and *Ziziphus* also for coughs. Women further noted that they smoke and dry the meat of poultry dead of disease. The second part of the report consists of a 'Resource Manual' that records all the information collected from Latuka inter-viewees, including a lexicon of diseases of cattle, sheep, goats and poultry. The author makes numerous recommendations for future ER&D. In particular, she emphasizes that EVK studies and findings should form an automatic, start-up and on-going activity to provide input into CAHW programmes. Besides clinical observation and sampling [above], she also notes the need to collect more precise and/or systematic baseline information about: plant identification, in both local and scientific terms; doses, toxicity, etc. and human-medical uses of traditional treat-ments; and people's assessment of the relative efficacy of treatments.

Martin, Marina. 1996. *The Use of Rural Appraisal Methods in the Study of Ethnoveterinary Medicine.* MSc thesis, CTVM, University of Edinburgh, Edinburgh, UK. 65 pp.

This study describes participatory methods to gather ethnoveterinary information among Fulani pastoralists in the village enclaves of Gashaka-Gumpti National Park, Nigeria. Such information was not readily disseminated to outsiders when an informant's peers were present, as Fulani guard prescriptions and techniques within the family. The thesis lists approximately 40 plants in the local ethno-pharmacopoeia, some 30% of which were applied to both livestock and humans. Techniques for the preparation and administration of many prescriptions are noted. One is to add plant materials to homemade mineral mixes that herders prepare and present to stock on rocks or in wooden troughs. Islamic priests (*malam*) practise medico-religious healing. In one case, a *malam* chalked Koranic verses onto a slate which he then washed, conserving the chalky water in a bowl. To this liquid, he added the ground bark of ten plants and some salt, all of which was then administered orally to cattle as a protection against diseases and evil spirits.

Martin, Marina. 1997. The use of rural appraisal in the study of ethno-veterinary medicine. *Indigenous Knowledge and Development Monitor* 5(1): 23.

This is a condensed summary of Martin 1996.

Martin, Marina. 1998. Ethnoveterinary medicine and Edinburgh. *The Bush Telegraph* 26: 29–30.

This communiqué summarizes contributions by the University of Edinburgh's CTVM to the First International Conference on Ethnoveterinary Medicine, held in Pune, India. There, six past or present CTVM students and faculty participated [see corresponding abstracts by Ashdown, Blakeway, Catley, Fielding, Padmakumar and Martin] with papers on African, Asian and global EVK. The article also notes the completion of nearly a dozen MSc theses on EVK at the University of Edinburgh [not all referenced here, however]. CTVM faculty and graduates are now poised to recoup valuable traditional veterinary practices in the UK and other parts of Europe based on the lessons they have learned from their study of continuing, albeit endangered, EVK in the South.

Martin, Marina. 1998. Participatory appraisal and ethnoveterinary medicine. In: E. Mathias, D.V. Rangnekar and C.M. McCorkle, with M. Martin (eds). *Ethnoveterinary Medicine: Alternatives for Livestock Development – Proceedings of an International Conference Held in Pune, India, 4–6 November 1997. Volume 2: Abstracts.* BAIF Development Research Foundation, Pune, India. P. 39.

To collect and disseminate ethnoveterinary information, researchers employ various methods adapted from the technical/biological and social sciences to suit the needs of the particular R&D thrust. Anthropologists, agronomists, veterinarians, extensionists, etc. generally record information based on observations and interviews. The latter may involve formal or informal, oral or written interview guides, questionnaires and surveys or, alternatively, participatory appraisal tools. This paper focuses on the latter, overviewing how such tools can facilitate researchers' ethnoveterinary R&D and extensionists' communication with stockraisers while at the same time empowering stockraisers. These tools are suitable for use with stockraisers everywhere in the world, whether they are literate or illiterate, rural or urban, male or female, old or young. Tools presented here include mapping, matrices, ranking, role playing and seasonal calendars. A specific example is given of 'body mapping', in which participants silently and independently sketch the body of an animal they own (or have recently seen, treated or know of) and then depict its ailments by body part and by the type of ethnoveterinary or other medical response they used (or would/might use). The 'artist' then shows her/his drawing to the researcher/extensionist (or another stockraiser), explains the ailment and treatment in her/his own words and thereafter engages in free and open-ended discussion back and forth with the interlocutor. This exercise demonstrates the strength of even the simplest participatory techniques for increasing rapport and mutual technical but inter-cultural understandings of animal healthcare.

Martin, Marina. 1999. Integrated approaches to animal healthcare: case studies from Tanzania and Mozambique. Paper presented to the International Seminar on Integrated Approach for Animal Health Care, 4–6 February 1999, Calicut, Kerala, India.

This paper demonstrates how traditional and modern animal healthcare can be combined to produce an optimum level of healthcare delivery for livestock. Case studies from the British NGO Vetaid illustrate this concept. Community animal health workers (CAHWs) play an essential role in delivering veterinary services to remote rural areas of Tanzania and Mozambique. The paper highlights CAHW selection and training methods plus the choices open to CAHWs for treating livestock with an appropriate conventional or traditional therapy.

Martin, Marina and Evelyn Mathias. 1998. International conference on ethnoveterinary medicine: Alternatives for livestock development. *Indigenous Knowledge and Development Monitor* 6(1): 25.

The above-referenced conference brought together some 200 delegates from 20 nations of Africa, Asia, Europe and the Americas. Delegates included government authorities, PVO and NGO staffers, representatives of pharmaceutical firms, practising veterinarians, scientists and academics of many disciplines, extensionists and traditional livestock healers. Together, they discussed the merits and drawbacks of EVM and how best to deploy it in development efforts. In addition, traditional healers demonstrated some of their practices; and participants as a whole identified 46 EVK research and field projects underway worldwide. Examples of conference topics addressed were: the ethnobotany, pharmacology, clinical validation and commercialization of ethnoveterinary treatments; homeopathy and acupuncture for livestock; methods of EVK R&D; and future directions for the field. In this last regard, participants generated the following recommendations for validating and applying EVM. Promising ethnomedicines and practices should be tested both in the laboratory and the field. Raw materials and finished products should be standardized to make them more reliable and thus appropriated for wider commercialization. Clear and informative materials need to be prepared for extensionists to be able to promote EVM. Also, EVM should be integrated into mainstream veterinary curricula at all levels. Finally, policymakers' and development professionals' awareness of EVM and its potentials should be increased, so they can bring it to bear in improving stockraisers' livelihoods. Further outcomes of the conference included: Indian scientists' proposal to mount a national EVM project as well as a nationwide network of veterinary colleges, labs and PVOs/NGOs; and plans to institute an electronic EVM network worldwide.

Martínez A., Miguel A. 1988. Investigaciones multidisciplinarias en la sierra norte de Puebla: Aspectos metodológicos. In: Luz Lozano Nathal and Gerardo López Buendía (coordinators). *Memorias: Primera Jornada sobre Herbolaria Medicinal en Veterinaria.* Universidad Nacional Autónoma de México, Facultad de Medicina Veterinaria y Zootecnia, Coordinación de Educación Continua, México DF. Pp. 156–163.

'Nature, Science, and Culture' is an on-going research project in the northern sierra of Puebla State that, in its integration of 16 different disciplines, provides a possible model for ethnoveterinary research and development (R&D). The author outlines 15 basic methodological steps for collecting, evaluating and documenting such information. Noteworthy among these are: searching out and working with traditional specialists in veterinary medicine; taxonomizing local classifications of plant and animal species, diseases, etc.; and learning the ritual, mythological, symbolic, social, cultural and historical significance of the plants, animals and diseases involved so as to better understand ideological aspects of indigenous management of animal health. The necessity and richness of a multidisciplinary team approach to this kind of research is emphasized, as are its more socially and economically appropriate outcomes in comparison to laboratory-based 'high-tech' R&D.

Martínez, Maximino. 1959. *Las Plantas Medicinales de México.* Editorial Botas, México DF, Mexico.

In colonial Mexico, *Eysenhardtia polystachya* was placed in the drinking water of poultry as an all-purpose prophylaxis. *Euphorbia lancifolia* was known as an excellent galactagogue for both livestock and humans; and scientific reports from the 1980s recount cases in which [unstipulated treatments] of *E. lancifolia* tripled milk production in cattle.

Marucchi, Jacques. 1950. *Psychologie Paysanne: Empirisme et Médecine Vétérinaire.* Doctoral thesis, École Nationale Vétérinaire d'Alfort, France. 70 pp.

Reprising the same themes as Leparc (1947), the aim of this thesis is to elucidate 'the peasant mentality' and contemporary ethnoveterinary practice among French stockowners so that professional veterinarians can better 'attack' peasant 'routinism, ignorance and credulity' (p. 10) in this area. Leaving aside such psychologizing, however, the chapter entitled 'Empirical Procedures' describes and assesses numerous folk practices, natural as well as supernatural, effective as well as in-effective, by species and ailment. In contrast, the chapter on 'Empirical Practitioners', while noting their 'excellent' skills at such operations as embryo-tomies and castrations, devotes itself thereafter to anecdotes 'demonstrating their incompetence' (p. 55).

Marusi, Aurelio and Ada Bocchi. 1983. Le piante officinali in medicina veteri-naria. *Veterinaria* 5: 111–114.

Despite the advent of modern chemotherapeutics, medicinal plants continue to be used with positive results in veterinary as well as human medicine. This article reports on three such plants employed among rural Italians and especially moun-tain people of the Appennines, where human–livestock contact is still daily and direct. There, owners take a more affectionate attitude toward their animals and some consider plant medicines to be less harmful than modern ones such as anti-biotics and synthetic hormones. Indeed, the long-term effects of such drugs in live-stock are as yet little studied, given that most animals go early to slaughter. The traditional uses of the three plants in question are described in light of current pharmacological and physiological knowledge. First is *Artemisia vulgaris* L., which is widely employed to cure digestive problems, diarrhoea and retained placenta in cattle. The latter practice may have derived from its use during medieval times to regulate women's menstrual cycles. Documented in both French and Swiss pharmacopoeia, *A. vulgaris* has been shown to contain many beneficial elements that, among other things, act as a vermifuge and a gastrointestinal and uterine anti-inflammatory. Second is hellebore rhizome of the *Viridis* and *Niger* varieties [for unspecified ills]. The root is inserted using a large needle into the musculature of cattle, horses and mules. This technique [known in English as pegging] provokes inflammation and oedema at the point of insertion and a successive reaction of the whole organism, as 'an aspecific stimulant therapy' (p. 113). In addition, the rhizome is presumed to have beneficial pharmacological effects due to its alkaloid and glucoside content. A drawback to this technique, however, is that it is difficult to control the effects. Third is orobanche [no Latin name given], a genera of parasitic non-chlorophyll plants reputed to induce oestrus in cows, possibly by delivering oestrogens or progesterone-like steroids. Definitive scientific evidence of this effect is lacking, however, because so many different nutritional and environmental factors impinge upon oestrus. The authors note that many modern drugs were originally derived from plant medicines and that commercialized herbals are still widely used in dairy animals to increase lactation and equilibrate the composition of milk. Especially in view of concerns about drug residues in animal products and growing human chemoresistance to antibiotics, they conclude that there is still a place for phytotherapies in modern veterinary medicine.

Marx, Walter. 1984. Traditionelle tierärztliche Heilmethoden unter besonderer Berücksichtigung der Kauterization in Somalia. *Giessener Beiträge zur Entwicklungsforschung: Beiträge der klinischen Veterinärmedizin zur Verbesserung der tierischen Erzeugung in den Tropen*, Reihe I, Band 10: 111–116. Wissenschaftliches Zentrum Tropeninstitut, Justus-Liebig Universität, Giessen, Germany.

Somali nomadic pastoralists widely practise traditional veterinary medicine. They know about the contagiousness of certain infectious diseases and have developed prophylactic management measures against these and other, non-infectious diseases. Traditional Somali therapies can be divided into two main types: magico-religious practices, such as reciting the Koran, to combat internal and 'psychological' diseases; and herbs, bloodletting and cauterization, to treat other diseases. Cauterization in particular is used for a great variety of diseases. In cases of lameness, sprains and muscle strains, the success of this treatment is patent. In other cases, however, its effectiveness is more difficult to assess. For infectious diseases, cauterization's stimulation of non-specific defence mechanisms may be offset by its depression of antibody production through the release of histamines [see also Marx and Wiegand 1987].

Marx, Walter and Dietrich Wiegand. 1987. Limits of traditional veterinary medicine in Somalia – the example of chlamydiosis and Q-fever. *Animal Research and Development* 26: 29–34. Institute for Scientific Cooperation, Tuebingen, Germany.

Tick control and cauterization are important elements in Somali EVM. Disease surveys of Somali livestock have shown that chlamydiosis and Q-fever are prevalent in the lower Juba region and in the Central Rangelands. Pastoralists call chlamydiosis *qange* and treat it with cauterization. According to Western experts this treatment may be harmful because cauterization induces the release of histamines resulting in a decrease of antibodies. Because Q-fever caused by *Coxiella burnetii* in livestock is often asymptomatic, pastoralists do not know that their animals are infected. Traditional tick control methods in southern Somalia are effective only for camels, which have a significantly lower prevalence of *Coxiella burnetii* than do other livestock.

Maryanto, Ibnu and Dwi Astuti. 1992. Pemanfaatan tumbuhan dalam etno-veteriner masyarakat Alor dan Pantar. In: *Prosiding Seminar dan Lokakarya Nasional Etnobotani. Bogor, Indonesia, 19–20 February 1992.* Pp. 90–96.

Based on observations made during field research on the Indonesian islands of Alor and Pantar, this conference paper lists some 45 local treatments, based on 24 plant species, for diseases of herd animals and poultry.

Ma'sum, Komarudin. 1990. *Bahan Obat dan Pengobatan Tradisional Untuk Ternak di Jawa Timur.* Sub Balai Penelitian Ternak Grati, Jalan Pahlawan, Grati, Pasuruan, Indonesia. 75 pp.

The first part of this report on traditional medicines and treatments for livestock in East Java constitutes an earlier, Indonesian-language version of Ma'sum 1991. However, this earlier report boasts the following four appendices not available in English: cultivation instructions for 35 medicinal plants; a table of the medical uses of 108 plants; a list of plant names in different local languages; and pictures of selected medicinal plants with their Latin, Indonesian and English names.

Ma'sum, Komarudin. 1991. Traditional veterinary medicine for ruminants in east Java. In: E. Mathias-Mundy and Tri Budhi Murdiati (eds). *Traditional Veterinary Medicine for Small Ruminants in Java.* Indonesian Small Ruminant Network, SR-CRSP, Central Research Institute for Animal Science, Agency for Agricultural Research and Development, Bogor, Indonesia. Pp. 29–37.

A score of farmers interviewed in East Java provided approximately 60 traditional veterinary prescriptions for treating 24 common health problems of ruminants, classified as cattle, calves, buffalo, sheep and goats. Salted fish and tamarind are fed to fatten animals. Some prescriptions combine commercial and natural ingredients. For example, kerosene, sulphur and naphthalene are mixed with coconut oil to treat scabies. For chronic wounds, a commercial insecticide mixed with limestone and turmeric rhizome is applied.

Mateo, Carmencita D. 1986. Medicinal plants for animal healthcare. *Animal Production Technology* 2(1): 26–32.

After reviewing Loculan's 1985 work in Lipa City, the Philippines on urbanites' use of medicinal plants for animal healthcare, this article goes on to describe a study at the University of the Philippines-Los Baños to determine the efficacy of feeding *Momordica charantia, Moringa oleifera* and *Portulaca oleracea* to prevent anaemia in piglets. The plant mixture was found to be as successful as iron injections in this regard.

Mateo, Carmencita D. 1987. Use of herbal medicine in disease control and prevention in livestock. *Animal Husbandry and Agricultural Journal* 21(1): 14–17.

This article covers much the same material as Mateo 1986.

Mathias, Evelyn. 1996. How can ethnoveterinary medicine be used in field projects? *Indigenous Knowledge and Development Monitor* 4(2): 6–7.

This article summarizes the definition, use, drawbacks and potentials of EVM based on an analysis of the literature, discussions at conferences and workshops and the author's own experiences. In discussing the present state of the art of ER&D, the author touches on: field research, validation and testing, publications, applications, commercialization and women's roles in EVM.

Mathias, Evelyn. 1998. Implications of the one-medicine concept for healthcare provision. *Agriculture and Human Values* 15(2): 145–151.

In both veterinary and human medicine, developed countries are currently witnessing a trend towards alternative medical practices based partly on traditional ones. This article debates the advantages and disadvantages of combining modern and traditional medicine, and human and veterinary medicine in a truly 'one medicine' approach to healthcare delivery for both people and animals. Such an approach could: enhance biomedical progress; especially in remote areas, improve medical/veterinary outreach; offer greater treatment choices for patients; make for culturally more appropriate healthcare; and save money. On the other hand, a one-medicine approach would call for generalists rather than specialists, meaning that rare diseases might go unrecognized; and current educational systems, administrative structures, legislation and 'status thinking' militate against intersectoral collaboration, not to mention the integration of traditional with modern medicine. The author concludes that there are no instant recipes for such an approach. Rather, by drawing from each of these four 'baskets' of medical options, governments and developers should devise fine-tuned, location-specific and cost-effective 'hybrids' of healthcare solutions. Advocacy, changes in educational curricula, new institutional linkages and legal reforms could help overcome obstacles to this more flexible and pragmatic approach.

Mathias, Evelyn. 1999. Farmers' knowledge and integrated livestock healthcare. Paper presented to the International Seminar on Integrated Approach for Animal Health Care, 4–6 February 1999, Calicut, Kerala, India.

The different veterinary-medical traditions, such as allopathy, homeopathy, Ayurvedic medicine, phytotherapy and ethnoveterinary medicine, each have different strengths and drawbacks. Integrated approaches to animal healthcare select and combine the most appropriate options from all these alternatives. Ethnoveterinary medicine refers to farmers' and herders' knowledge and approaches to livestock healthcare and production. It is not restricted to the use of medicinal plants but also includes: stockraisers' knowledge of animal diseases, grazing grounds, fodder plants and many other things; producers' management, prevention and treatment practices; and their many tools and technologies for implementing all the foregoing. However, EVM has its limitations. Medicines are often cumbersome to prepare. The necessary plants may not be available in all seasons. There are few treatments against infectious epidemic diseases. Treatment schedules are often vague and herbal medicines are difficult to standardize. And some practices are harmful. On the other hand, EVM is locally available, cheap and readily understood by its users. Its strengths lie in treating common, basic health problems like wounds, skin diseases and parasites and in working to prevent these and other health threats through management, feeding and herbal and other prophylaxes. When integrating EVM into animal healthcare programmes, it is important to recognize this whole spectrum of practice, not just stockraiser knowledge of treatments. This paper provides a checklist of, and selected methods for implementing, steps to facilitate EVM integration.

Mathias, Evelyn and Constance M. McCorkle. 1996. Animal health. In: Joske Bunders, Bertus Haverkort and Wim Hiemstra (eds). ***Biotechnology: Building on Farmers' Knowledge.*** MacMillan Education Publishing, London and Basingstoke, UK. Pp. 22–51.

This chapter examines EVM as a form of biotechnology. The production of traditional vaccines and other drugs can be characterized as *in vitro* biotechnologies, while the management of disease-causing organisms within the host animal's body or the manipulation of the patient's cells and tissues qualify as *in vivo* biotechnologies. These two treatment categories can be further parsed by whether their intent is preventive, promotive, or therapeutic. Vaccination, for example, is a preventive measure. Sometimes, immunization is accomplished indirectly, simply by controlled exposure of healthy animals to sick ones. This technique signals considerable local knowledge of disease transmission and epidemiology. An interesting example of a useful and harmless *in vivo* technique that can be applied preventively, promotively, or therapeutically is feeding ruminants a penny. The coin slowly decomposes in the stomach, thus releasing copper and forestalling or ameliorating hypocupraemia. This trick – originally part of British stockraisers' ethnoveterinary toolkit – is now recommended by clinical veterinarians. For aphosphorosis, some stockraisers cleverly graze their stock on fields recently spread with fertilizers containing phosphates. An example of a promotive *in vivo* technique is improvement of pH imbalances in the rumen by giving special feeds or drinks. These may include vinegar or clays and soda-pop, depending on whether acidifying or alkalizing effects are sought. A related traditional practice, also employed by Western vets, is to feed the cud of a healthy head of cattle to one that has indigestion, has ceased to ruminate, or has just received antibiotics. The cud rehabilitates the patient's rumen ecology. Besides oral and intranasal administration, other modes of homemade medicines' delivery attested in the literature include: anal and vaginal suppositories; in parts of Africa, injections effected via a hollow straw or by spitting chewn medicaments into the patient's eyes; and especially in France, hanging up bouquets of medicinal flora and fauna. The authors observe that often there are cultural preferences or emphases in ways of manipulating plant materials and livestock cells and tissues. Although most cultures use virtually all techniques, many Asian peoples favour complex polyprescriptions of plant-based medicines; Native Americans are fond of smoke cures, based on smouldering medicinal plants; and a universally popular treatment in Africa is firing and branding to prevent or cure innumerable livestock ailments. African pastoralists are also partial to bloodletting. While there are few culturally unique practices, one might be certain Brazilian groups' cauterizing by sprinkling gunpowder on the affected body part and igniting it! Yet this is a helpful treatment for the ill to which they apply it (footrot lesions). Most longtime stockraising groups manipulate animal germplasm through selective breeding, often via open or bloodless castration. Some camel raisers insert a stone into a she-camel's uterus to prevent conception. Conversely, they may remove a persistent corpus luteum from the camel's ovary so as to induce heat (also a common Western practice). Taiwanese use acupuncture to bring their sows into heat. And so forth. Beyond ethnoveterinary technique, this article discusses the cultural and socioeconomic context of EVM at some length, including: indigenous disease classification and causation theories; the generation and transfer of EVK and its differential distribution among varying biosocial groups across societies; relatedly, different such groups' roles and rationales in veterinary decision-making; and the scientific testing and commercialization of EVM. The chapter concludes with a discussion of the limitations, potentials and future directions for ER&D in terms of research, technology transfer, development, policy-making and EVM's relation to conventional veterinary medicine.

Mathias, Evelyn, Constance M. McCorkle and Tjaart Schillhorn van Veen. 1996. Introduction: Ethnoveterinary research and development. In: Constance M. McCorkle, Evelyn Mathias and Tjaart W. Schillhorn van Veen (eds). *Ethnoveterinary Research & Development.* Intermediate Technology Publications, London, UK. Pp. 1–23.

The 20th century has witnessed spectacular advances in medicine and agriculture. However, they have been accompanied by staggering population growth, environmental degradation and sometimes negative health effects. Moreover, the positive benefits of these advances have reached only a fraction of the earth's people. For medical services, for example, some 85% of the world's population still rely mainly on local/traditional treatments and practitioners for themselves and their livestock. Given current demographic, economic and other trends, most of this 85% are unlikely to gain affordable and sustainable access to high-tech Western-style medicine in the foreseeable future. This is perhaps particularly true at the interface between medicine and agriculture, i.e. livestock healthcare. For all these reasons, there is a growing need for alternative medical paradigms and options. Hence the burgeoning interest in ethnoveterinary R&D as introduced in this, the first published volume on the subject. The 22 chapters that follow the introduction span 10 major species of animal domesticates raised by more than 80 ethnic groups in some 40 nations of Africa, Asia, Europe and the Americas. Together, the book mentions nearly 100 livestock diseases plus more than 300 medicinal plants or other traditional *materia medica* used to combat them. This introductory chapter overviews: the background and rationale for ER&D, including its potentials and limitations in both First and Third Worlds; ER&D's complex relation to multiple social, biological/technical and of course biomedical disciplines; basic principles, approaches, methods and topics within ER&D; and the many different development needs it addresses and supports. The latter are not confined solely to animal healthcare. They also span rural enterprise development, primary education, environmental protection, public health and the delivery of human medical services. Illustrating from the other chapters in the volume, discussion is organized by: ethnoveterinary knowledge systems (ethnosemantics and taxonomics, ethno-aetiologies and diagnostics, ethnoepidemiology); ethnoveterinary practices (pharmacology, toxicology, immunization, surgery, manipulative and mechanical techniques, husbandry and herding strategies, reproduction and genetics, pest control, product harvesting and handling, medico-religious practices); and above all, practical applications of ER&D findings in guiding development interventions, influencing relevant policies and institutions and re-shaping academic research and training. Also discussed are methodological issues in ER&D. The chapter concludes by outlining key R&D needs for the future. Most notably, these include increased attention to: non-pharmacological prevention and treatment options suggested by traditional practices; improved ER&D methodologies and training materials; and critical analysis and reform of healthcare-related policies and institutions in light of ER&D findings.

Mathias, Evelyn and Raul Perezgrovas. 1999. Application of ethnoveterinary medicine: Where do we stand? In: E. Mathias, D.V. Rangnekar and C.M. McCorkle, with M. Martin (eds). *Ethnoveterinary Medicine: Alternatives for Livestock Development – Proceedings of an International Conference Held in Pune, India, 4–6 November 1997. Volume 1: Selected Papers.* BAIF Development Research Foundation, Pune, India. Pp. 133–143.

Indigenous livestock management and healthcare offer great potential for livestock and also human development. Some indigenous technologies and services are cheaper, more appropriate and more readily available than those brought in from outside. Others can be improved or blended with outside know-how, often also very cheaply and appropriately, so as to contribute to the development of locally-based and therefore more sustainable solutions to livestock health problems. Still, livestock development programmes and projects have been slow to integrate ethnoveterinary information and practices. This paper discusses where EVM is actually put to good development use, how widespread this use is, what groups and organizations are involved in ER&D, what factors determine the extent of use and which problems need to be overcome in order to increase the use and impact of ER&D. Overall, hands-on applications of ER&D findings to development efforts in the field seem to have been rather limited to date. Research projects by far outweigh the number of development activities promoting or building on selected indigenous practices, perhaps because the 'R' and the 'D' in ER&D are so often separated from each other. This means that research recommendations are seldom implemented and experiences from field application are not documented, making for a distressing loss of valuable information on the efficacy or shortcomings of ethnoveterinary options. The different groups involved in ER&D are: farmers; healers; healthcare providers such as extension services, development projects and private practitioners (traditional as well as modern); instructors of veterinary training courses, colleges and universities; and government officials, decision-makers and development planners. The paper discusses factors influencing the use of ER&D by each group. These include remoteness of a project's location; the community's way of life (e.g. settled or nomadic, agropastoralist or pastoralist); environmental conditions; the availability of veterinary alternatives; characteristics of the local versus introduced healthcare systems in terms of efficacy, costs, availability and cultural feasibility; economic value and purpose of the animals kept; social, psychological, religious, etc. aspects of the human/animal relationship; proof (or lack thereof) of the efficacy of ethnoveterinary treatments; incentives to promote local rather than conventional approaches; status thinking; and even merely the awareness of the existence of ethnoveterinary medicine. Because of the dearth of written information on all the foregoing questions and variables, however, the authors warn that many of the generalizations made in this paper should be treated as hypotheses still requiring verification. Nevertheless, it seems clear that for ER&D to be applied, the following are needed: packages of proven ethnoveterinary practices and remedies that can be integrated into conventional veterinary service systems; methodologies to document, select and disseminate ethnoveterinary practices at the field level; links among research, education and extension; and initiatives to convince key players in livestock development of the value of EVM.

Mathias, E., D.V. Rangnekar, C.M. McCorkle and M. Martin. 1998. Preface. In: E. Mathias, D.V. Rangnekar and C.M. McCorkle, with M. Martin (eds). *Ethnoveterinary Medicine: Alternatives for Livestock Development – Proceedings of an International Conference Held in Pune, India, 4–6 November 1997. Volume 2: Abstracts.* BAIF Development Research Foundation, Pune, India. Pp. viii–xii.

The first international conference on EVM, held in India in 1997, was attended by some 200 delegates (about 17% female) from 20 countries of Asia, Africa, Europe and the Americas. Delegates were drawn from NGOs, government organizations, private enterprise and stockraising communities of India. They included veterinarians, animal scientists, veterinary technicians, indigenous healers, pharmacologists, ethnobotanists, economists, anthropologists and sociologists who, in the aggregate, worked as research scientists, professors, clinicians, field practitioners, extensionists, businesspeople and policymakers. This preface to the collected abstracts from the conference outlines the rationale behind the meetings, which was to: promote the use of EVM in livestock development; explore possibilities for developing systems to improve the accessibility and efficacy of livestock health services; foster an exchange of information and experience among individuals and organizations working in EVM and consolidate their knowledge base; and identify priorities and approaches for future research and fieldwork in this area. The first 2 days of the conference featured more than 60 formal presentations on three EVK topics: research and validation, applications and future approaches. A highlight of the event was the presentation by indigenous healers from throughout India of their veterinary practices and prescriptions. On the last day, ten working groups assembled to produce recommendations on a range of specific EVK topics, e.g.: commercializing EVK products, incorporating EVK into educational systems and devising databank and other storage methods for EVK. Volume 1 of the proceedings contains selected conference papers, a summary of the traditional healers' discussions and the workshop recommendations. Volume 2 includes the abstracts of all papers presented, plus additional papers submitted by individuals unable to attend. It also provides contact information for all these participants. [See also Martin and Mathias 1998.]

Mathias, E., D.V. Rangnekar, C.M. McCorkle and M. Martin. 1999a. Annexes. In: E. Mathias, D.V. Rangnekar and C.M. McCorkle, with M. Martin (eds). *Ethnoveterinary Medicine: Alternatives for Livestock Development – Proceedings of an International Conference Held in Pune, India, 4–6 November 1997. Volume 1: Selected Papers.* BAIF Development Research Foundation, Pune, India. Pp. 271–302.

In both map and tabular form, an annex to the above-referenced conference proceedings summarizes attendees' collective knowledge of EVK-oriented projects on-going around the world at the time of the conference. A total of 46 such projects are listed, spanning Africa (14 projects in 7 countries), Asia (26 in 6), Europe (2 in 1) and the Americas (4 in 2). The projects deal with most farm-animal species plus camels, dogs and cats. They are variously implemented by combinations or consortia of: international and national, religious and secular NGOs; government research institutes, livestock services and other agencies; independent research and/or development centres; universities; clinical practices and other private enterprises; and grassroots organizations like dairy cooperatives, breeder groups and tribal associations. The types of projects represented are quite diverse. Likewise for their EVK aims and components. Besides on-farm clinical trials of EVM and documentation and research on EVK generally, their aims span: conservation of medicinal plants, rare animal breeds and habitat generally; cultural conservation of pastoral lifeways; bioprospecting and commercial product development; agricultural development; training for veterinarians, reform or decentralization of veterinary services and vaccination campaigns. Accompanying this annex is another that illustrates the kinds of ethnoveterinary-oriented events that have taken place since the 1997 conference. A few examples are: a summer short course at India's National Veterinary Research Institute on techniques for the scientific validation of ethnoveterinary practices; a PRELUDE seminar in Belgium on local actors in relation to plant, animal and environmental resources; hosted by an Indian dairy union, an international seminar on integrated approaches to animal healthcare; a regional workshop on a similar topic but for NGOs and emphasizing EVM, co-sponsored by a German and an Indian NGO; and an international conference in Italy on medicinal plants in Mediterranean EVM. A third annex offers a compilation of resources for EVM. These include organizations (mainly NGOs), websites, mailing lists, journals, newsletters and key books. The next two annexes catalogue the names, affiliations and contact information for the 233 participants in this first international conference on EVM.

Mathias, E., D.V. Rangnekar, C.M. McCorkle and M. Martin. 1999b. Discussions and recommendations. In: E. Mathias, D.V. Rangnekar and C.M. McCorkle, with M. Martin (eds). *Ethnoveterinary Medicine: Alternatives for Livestock Development – Proceedings of an International Conference Held in Pune, India, 4–6 November 1997. Volume 1: Selected Papers.* BAIF Development Research Foundation, Pune, India. Pp. 253–270.

In addition to the traditional healers' workshop [see Ghotge 1999], ten topic-specific working groups were formed at the above-referenced conference, based on participants' expressed interests. The results of their deliberations are presented here in an Action Plan format, with the following components identified by each group: action/objective, justification, audience/beneficiaries, expected outcome, implementers, locale, resources, timeframe, constraints and assumptions. A sampling of the working-groups' thinking about their various topics and the priority actions/objectives they set is as follows. (1) Pharmacology and ethnobotany: documentation and conservation of ethnobotanicals; evaluation of same, e.g. via establishment of national institutes for veterinary pharmacology and toxicology; quality control and standardization of veterinary herbal drugs. (2) Validation and clinical trials: protocol development, documentation of plants and practices, prioritization and controlled trials. (3) Field applications: a network of ethnoveterinary groups, a textbook on ethnoveterinary practices, inclusion of EVM in veterinary curricula and extension. (4) Education: awareness-raising, student projects, official registration, social science skills, lesson guides, need-based education and farmer contact. (5) Commercialization: standardization of raw materials and finished products, pre-clinical and clinical evaluation of products, restoration of natural habitats and medicinal plants. (6) Acupuncture and homeopathy: awareness-raising; short courses, including distance learning; formal control bodies; standardization of methods. (7) Camels: a column on camel EVK in the *Journal of Camel Practice and Research*, a field manual on same, an EVK network. (8) Community and intellectual property rights: formation of local healers' associations, facilitation of formal agreements among all stakeholders, development and support of appropriate information systems among same, promotion of conservation and sustainable use of biodiversity by ensuring equitable local access to medicinal plants. (9) Integrated animal and disease management: exploit the strong points of different medical systems, widen coverage of production systems, pay attention to husbandry, make institutions more flexible. (10) Documentation and networking: EVM mailing list, website, interactive databank.

Mathias, E., D.V. Rangnekar, C.M. McCorkle and M. Martin. 1999c. Preface. In: E. Mathias, D.V. Rangnekar and C.M. McCorkle, with M. Martin (eds). *Ethnoveterinary Medicine: Alternatives for Livestock Development – Proceedings of an International Conference Held in Pune, India, 4–6 November 1997. Volume 1: Selected Papers.* BAIF Development Research Foundation, Pune, India. Pp. ix–xiv.

Of the 60+ papers presented at the first worldwide conference on EVM, 34 are collected in this volume. They are divided into five categories. First are applied studies of ethnoveterinary systems. Spanning Africa, Asia and Latin America, these papers go beyond just listing and describing medicinal plants and EVM techniques to: analysing local EVK systems and the actors involved; comparing knowledge, attitudes and practices (KAP) across cultures; exploring when people choose traditional versus modern veterinary medicine; and suggesting how local practices can be integrated into extension. Second are papers focusing on mainly non-laboratory methods for validating EVM. Methods include systematically recording EVM treatment outcomes, conducting literature searches and surveying the KAPs of different actor groups. Botanicals employed in EVM are the subject of the third category. Topics here span not only the results of particular pharmacological and clinical tests but also ways of identifying potentially useful EVM plant resources in one region based on comparative research in other regions. Fourth are papers on EVM applications in extension and community-based animal healthcare, as viewed from both global and country-specific stances and from the perspective of complementarity among multiple veterinary traditions. Only two papers fall into the fifth and final category of 'Education', thus signalling the need for greater attention to how to incorporate EVM into on-going training systems of all kinds.

Mathias-Mundy, Evelyn. 1989a. Indigenous knowledge on veterinary medicine. Paper presented to the 66th Annual Meeting of the Central States Anthropological Society, University of Notre Dame, South Bend, Indiana, USA, 10–12 March, 1989. 13 pp.

EVM deals with folk beliefs and practices relating to the healthcare of animals. It is an important resource and can improve the feasibility and sustainability of development projects. Recording indigenous disease classifications requires the cooperation of biological and social scientists. Ethnoveterinary medicine and ethnomedicine share many elements. The author presents examples of ethnoveterinary pharmacology, vaccination, surgery and management practices. She sees limitations to EVM in its lack of treatments against epidemic diseases, the ineffectiveness of some treatments, the incorporation of harmful practices and frequently inadequate ethnodiagnoses. In the Third World a syncretism of local and Western veterinary medicine would likely prove most advantageous.

Mathias-Mundy, Evelyn. 1989b. Techniques and practices in ethnoveterinary medicine. In: D.M. Warren, L.J. Slikkerveer and S.O. Titiola (eds). *Indigenous Knowledge Systems: Implications for Agriculture and International Development.* Studies in Technology and Social Change No. 11. Technology and Social Change Program, Iowa State University, Ames, Iowa, USA. Pp. 79–85.

This paper surveys ethnoveterinary pharmacology, vaccination, surgery and management practices throughout the world. A wide spectrum of herbal and other remedies is used in ethnoveterinary practice. Several African societies have developed methods to vaccinate their cattle against CBPP. Indigenous surgical methods include wound care, cauterization, bloodletting and castration. Management practices generally reflect a sound adaptation to climate, flora and other environmental influences. The author briefly discusses housing, parasite control, breeding and calf rearing. She concludes that EVM contains many techniques and practices that, by Western scientific standards, are indeed effective and thus provide a rich resource for development.

Mathias-Mundy, Evelyn. 1989c. Of herbs and healers. *ILEIA Newsletter for Low External Input and Sustainable Agriculture* 4(3): 20–22.

Researchers can learn from local stockowners' knowledge of animal husbandry and veterinary care. Illustrating with examples, this article overviews practices and beliefs relating to animal health worldwide. Indigenous treatments for skin diseases and certain external and internal parasites, wound care, basic surgery, feeding strategies and many management practices are potentially useful for development programmes, whereas epidemics and fatal endemic diseases are probably better treated with Western-style vaccination and drugs. In addition to promoting selected ethnoveterinary practices, development projects should utilize the skills and knowledge of traditional healers in healthcare delivery.

Mathias-Mundy, Evelyn. 1991. Traditional management practices support sheep and goat health. *Indonesian Small Ruminant Network* 2(2): 3–4.

This article reviews an SR-CRSP study on sheep and goat production in Bogor, Indonesia, in which animals were kept in raised, partitioned barns with slatted bamboo floors. This type of housing helps control disease by reducing the risk of parasitism inherent in free-range grazing; limiting contact, fighting and crowding among animals; ensuring good ventilation of quarters; and providing for hygienic handling of faeces. To improve their condition, the animals are also fed salt, either as salty water sprinkled over the feed or as salty herbal drenches. To reduce fly strike, kitchen ash is rubbed into a newborn's navel and its dam's vulva. Some 50 plants are used to treat over 20 diseases in this area. Shrimp paste and kerosene also figure in the veterinary pharmacopoeia.

Mathias-Mundy, Evelyn and Constance M. McCorkle. 1989. *Ethnoveterinary Medicine: An Annotated Bibliography.* Bibliographies in Technology and Social Change No. 6. Technology and Social Change Program, Iowa State University, Ames, Iowa, USA. 199 pp.

This publication represents an earlier, 'grey literature' bibliography of EVK written by the second and third authors of the present publication. For greater access, the 261 abstracts therein are reproduced in the present bibliography, some in revised or expanded form. However, this first volume is distinguished by a substantive analytic introduction that synthesizes all the technical, cultural and socioeconomic information embodied in the abstracts. Readers may thus find the introduction useful for contextualizing the present volume's abstracts. The introduction is organized as follows: definition and importance of EVM; recording EVK; ethnomedical systems and disease causation theories, including a brief comparison of human and animal ethnomedicine and a discussion of local healers; disease classifications; ethnoveterinary techniques and practices in toxicology, vaccination, surgery, husbandry and magic and religion; the limitations, potentials and applications of EVM; and concluding remarks.

Mathias-Mundy, Evelyn and Constance M. McCorkle. 1990. Ethnoveterinary medicine in Asia: A resource for development. Paper presented to the Second International Congress of Ethnobiology, 22–26 October, Kunming, China. 15 pp.

Based on Mathias-Mundy and McCorkle 1989, this paper provides an overview of the field of ethnoveterinary medicine in Asia, along with examples of ethnoveterinary techniques and practices from the region. Three classical medical systems prevail in Asia: Ayurveda, humoral pathology and the Chinese system. They typically apply to both humans and animals; and healers of human diseases often also treat animals. Asian EVM includes the use of numerous herbal remedies, preparations from non-herbal ingredients, surgical techniques, vaccinations and a wide range of management practices. Not all ethnoveterinary treatments or practices are effective and some may even be harmful. However, many are useful and provide a valuable resource for development. Projects should select promising remedies and promote them. Livestock health problems most likely to be treatable with local remedies include worms, wounds and skin diseases. Epidemics and infectious life-threatening diseases are probably better treated with modern medicine. Projects should also work with local healthcare practitioners, since they constitute a valuable human resource. The appendix lists ethnoveterinary references from Asia by country. The bulk of ethnoveterinary information comes from India, followed by China. Many of the Chinese references, however, were unavailable for review.

Mathias-Mundy, Evelyn and Constance M. McCorkle. 1993. Ethnoveterinary research: Lessons for development. In: IIRR (ed.). *Indigenous Knowledge and Sustainable Development: 25 Selected Papers Presented at the International Symposium Held at the International Institute of Rural Reconstruction, September 20–26, 1992.* IIRR, Silang, Cavite, Philippines. Pp. 218–236.

Ethnoveterinary R&D can be defined as the interdisciplinary study and application of local animal healthcare practices and practitioners. It draws on many different methods and covers topics in more than 20 distinct subject matters as defined by Western science. This conference paper briefly summarizes ethnoveterinary findings from published and unpublished materials for most of these subjects. Concrete examples illustrate how an understanding of local veterinary and husbandry practices, disease concepts, classifications and terminology can provide valuable insights for the planning and implementation of livestock development projects. Among other things, such 'knowledge of local knowledge' can improve communication among project implementors, extensionists and stockraisers. Also, educational curricula that recognize and build on a given nation's or people's own know-how will be more relevant and interesting to students from that country or ethnicity. Similarly, technologies that draw on local know-how will be more familiar to project beneficiaries and often cheaper and more sustainable than wholly alien technologies. Applying indigenous knowledge requires careful recording, documentation and testing and adaption, however.

Mathias-Mundy, Evelyn and Constance M. McCorkle. 1995. Ethnoveterinary medicine and development: A review of the literature. In: D. Michael Warren, L. Jan Slikkerveer and David Brokensha (eds). *The Cultural Dimension of Development: Indigenous Knowledge Systems.* Intermediate Technology Publications, London, UK. Pp. 488–498.

This chapter briefly reviews some of the existing literature on traditional veterinary medicine worldwide. It also indicates several immediate applications of systematic research in this field to international agricultural development. The chapter is a condensation of the information detailed in the first annotated bibliography of ethnoveterinary medicine, by Mathias-Mundy and McCorkle 1989.

Mathias-Mundy, Evelyn and Tri Budhi Murdiati. 1991. Conclusions and recommendations. In: E. Mathias-Mundy and Tri Budhi Murdiati (eds). *Traditional Veterinary Medicine for Small Ruminants in Java.* Indonesian Small Ruminant Network, SR-CRSP, Central Research Institute for Animal Science, Agency for Agricultural Research and Development, Bogor, Indonesia. Pp. 51–52.

A series of surveys of traditional medicine for sheep and goats in West, Central and East Java was supported by the Indonesian Research Institute for Animal Production and the SR-CRSP. Survey findings were reported in a 1990 workshop, which then gave rise to this edited volume. Highlights of the workshop conclusions and recommendations of the volume include the following. Local names for plants vary from place to place and different plants have the same or similar names; thus clear scientific identification and classification of the plants is important. The fact that certain plants are used throughout Java to treat a particular disease suggests these plants may indeed be effective for that disease, although the composition, preparation and dosages of remedies vary according to local conditions and farmers' knowledge and experience. Nevertheless, such plants would be good candidates for scientific study and confirmation. Research of this sort should give priority to the diseases that attack beneficiaries' stock most frequently. Also, the economic costs and benefits of traditional versus modern veterinary medicines require research. Finally, it would be helpful to compile a regularly updated database of information on traditional remedies, for dissemination through a network.

Mathias-Mundy, Evelyn, Sri Wayhuni, Tri Budhi Murdiati, Agus Suparyanto, Dwi Priyanto, Isbandi, Beriajaya and Harini Sangat Roemantyo. 1992. *Traditional Animal Health Care for Goats and Sheep in West Java: A Comparison of Three Villages.* SR-CRSP Working Paper No. 139. Balai Penelitian Ternak, Pusat Penelitian dan Pengembangan Peternakan, Bogor, Indonesia. 20 pp.

This working paper summarizes the results of comparative research on local animal healthcare practices for small ruminants in three villages of West Java. [See also Priyanto et al. 1991 and Wahyuni et al. 1992.] Across the three villages, it compares: management and mating practices; the care pregnant animals and newborns receive; animal condition; the diseases reported and observed; who takes care of and/or treats the animals; local disease classifications and corresponding epidemiological knowledge and practices (such as carcass disposal) and, of course, treatments. Results indicate that the management system clearly influences animal condition. For example, in the village that grazed its goats and sheep under rubber trees, animals were much thinner than in the other two villages, which confined their small ruminants in raised barns under a cut-and-carry system. Therapeutic practices were similar in all three villages and the spectrum of medicinal plants overlapped although there were some differences as to the plant parts used and the ailments to which they were applied. Observations in one village suggest that dosage and treatment regime are weak points in the local system; also, the care of pregnant animals could be improved. Several implications for livestock development projects emerged from this comparative research. For one, although the study villages all lay in the same general area, management practices and disease problems varied. Hence, a different approach to improving local healthcare systems would be required for each village. Any improvements should also consider how, in all three villages, customs and beliefs currently influence livestock management and therapeutics. Another implication is that veterinary interventions should target both sexes because, as research revealed, women as well as men actively participate in animal healthcare. The appendix lists the medicinal plants used in all three villages, along with the plants' applications.

Matthewman, Richard W. 1980. Small ruminant production in the humid tropical zone of southern Nigeria. *Tropical Animal Health and Production* 12: 234–242.

A study of village systems of sheep and goat production conducted in the humid tropics of southwestern Nigeria found that dwarf animals were more resistant to trypanosomosis than larger animals. Thus these smaller, hardier types of small ruminants often constituted the bulk of village livestock in tsetse-infested areas.

Matzigkeit, Uly. 1990. *Natural Veterinary Medicine: Ectoparasites in the Tropics.* Tropical Agroecology No. 6. Verlag Josef Margraf Scientific Books, Weikersheim, Germany (for AGRECOL). 183 pp.

Vast amounts of chemicals have been expended in attempts to eradicate insects and other carriers of livestock diseases. The outcome has been chemoresistance in the targeted insect species and environmental pollution. This book offers an alternative based on local knowledge of plant-derived pesticides and repellents. The first part of the book describes numerous species of ticks, mites, lice and flies that attack livestock. For each species it recommends specific natural control measures, most of which involve local plants, as reported in the scientific literature. The second part focuses on the plants themselves. It details the botanical classification and features, distribution, habitat, propagation and pesticidal properties and uses of 21 plants. The distribution and application of an additional 40 plants are also briefly noted. The book's goal is to benefit small farmers by intensifying their use of cheap local resources, reducing their livestock losses and thereby improving their incomes and diets while at the same time minimizing environmental damage.

Maydell, Hans-Juergen von. 1986. *Trees and Shrubs of the Sahel, Their Characteristics and Uses.* Schriftenreihe der GTZ No. 196. TZ-Verlagsgesellschaft, Rossdorf, Germany.

Pages 69–71 of this book present a table on medicinal uses of trees and shrubs in the Sahel and indicate a number of plant species that are used in veterinary medicine.

Mazars, G. 1994. Traditional veterinary medicine in India. *Revue Scientifique et Technique de l'Office International des Épizooties* 13(2): 433–451.

This article presents a historical review of Ayurvedic veterinary medicine in India. Rooted in sacred Vedic texts written between 1500 and 600 B.C., Ayurvedic EVM deals with horses, elephants, camels, cattle, goats and sheep. Treatments range from surgery to medicinal preparations administered in different modes and routes: powders, snuffs, decoctions, electuaries (pastes) and ointments, plus sweating, cauterization, bloodletting and enemas. Several modern-day Indian laboratories commercially produce preparations based on ancient Ayurvedic prescriptions. Traditional formulations produced on a large scale include tonics, fortifiers, digestives, antiparasitics and antifungals. Many, perhaps most, of these products are polyprescriptions. For example, one veterinary tonic currently on the market is composed of 59 ingredients; and a popular pomade is prepared from nine plant oils plus extracts from seven other plants. Considerable chemical and pharmacological research has been conducted on many of the plants used in Ayurvedic medicine and clinical studies have proliferated in recent years. While the author notes the desirability of more such research specifically for veterinary applications, he also comments that much of the Ayurvedic pharmacopoeia has proved its worth by the simple test of time. More neglected areas of research are Ayurvedic recommendations on animal feeding, disease prevention and cauterization techniques.

Mbaka, Mwenda. n.d. Survey of traditional Akamba skills in handling livestock diseases: Consultancy for ITDG. Unpublished proposal. Machakos, Kenya. 4 pp.

This document constitutes a proposal to ITDG/Kenya to survey EVK among Akamba stockraisers of Kenya. Procedures and outputs anticipated for such a survey are outlined. They include: detailed descriptions of the most confidently applied treatments for common diseases; a list of remedies for other diseases recognized in the area; community members' and expert healers' assessment of treatment effectiveness, the latter as reflected in the frequency and consistency of interviewees' mention of a given remedy; assessment of the extent of remedies' use and of the combined use of traditional and modern medicines; a veterinarian's assessment of possible treatment efficacy, backed by a review of any pertinent literature; small trials on the most promising remedies; and thus the identification of treatments suitable for incorporation into animal health training and extension programmes.

Mbaka, Mwenda. 1989. Ethnoveterinary medicine – who needs it? A focus on Machakos District of Kenya. Unpublished paper, Machakos, Kenya. 11 pp.

In his research among traditional Akamba doctors of both livestock and humans in Kenya's Machakos District, the author found they used plant, animal, mineral and mystical *materia medica* in their treatments, as well as manipulative, orthopaedic and surgical techniques. This report focuses on their plant prescriptions, of which more than 30 are reported here along with their human ethnomedical uses. Some of the livestock ills that healers thus cure include: in all animals, FMD, bloat, constipation, swellings, respiratory problems, flukes, leeches, fungal and other skin problems, otitis, ophthalmia, corneal opacity and eye injuries, wounds (as from castration, dehorning and severed umbilical cords as well as cuts), general infections, post-partum vaginal irritaton, agalactia and snakebite; in cattle, ECF and anaplasmosis; in goats, diarrhoea, colic and pneumonia; and in poultry, respiratory, liver (diagnosed only upon necropsy) and other infections, plus poor doing. Healers also prepare preventive medicines such as: footbaths of ashes for FMD; fly repellents to forestall myiasis; snake repellents for fumigating around houses, camps and corrals; and tonics for convalescent stock. Most plant remedies are monoprescriptions, but healers sometimes prescribe two remedies in succession so that the second offsets debilitating side effects of the first. Modes of preparation of plant parts span: intact or pounded leaves; ground, roasted twigs and roots; dried and powdered barks; juices and saps, either full-strength or diluted in water; suspensions; cold infusions; decoctions; and ashes. Typically, plant parts are first pounded. Routes of administration documented are oral, topical, intra-ocular (eye-drops) and again, fumigation. In his investigations, the author was struck by several differences between older and younger healers. The former would delay treatment until they could obtain all the necessary materials; in the meantime, they gave only an avowed 'first aid'. In contrast, younger healers were eager to administer even sham treatments in order to win prompt tangible remuneration from clients. Neither would younger healers speak with the researcher unless they were paid to do so. In contrast, older healers were happy to share their knowledge freely once they were convinced of the *bona fides* of the author (a BVM) as a colleague; and they then accepted token remuneration only reluctantly.

Mbaka, Mwenda. 1991. Traditional Akamba veterinary skills: Progress report of research carried out at Kibauni Location of Mwalal Division in Machakos District. Unpublished manuscript, Machakos, Kenya. 4 pp.

This report briefly describes the vet-author's visit with various kinds of Akamba healers in Kenya. Besides five licensed herbalists and two 'mystical diagnosticians', he met with one extended family of healers. The grandfather of this family is renowned for his skills at treating both humans and livestock and one of his daughters-in-law has joined his practice. One of his sons specializes in human ethnomedicine in Machakos town while a daughter practises on both humans and animals in the countryside. Meanwhile, one of the man's grandsons has become an Animal Health Assistant with the local livestock service. Another group of healers visited by the author was composed of three women who shared a human/livestock practice. Each specialized in a different range of ailments and thus called in her partners to consult as needed. Most healers interviewed were reluctant to give details of their treatments unless the author paid for the information, for a variety of reasons. One echoed a common complaint among modern physicians, i.e. the high costs incurred during (ethno)medical schooling. Healers explained that, besides the requirement that one receive a calling to practise ethnomedicine in his/her dreams, one must also undergo an expensive ritual initiation ceremony conducted by a certain medicine man. This is necessary in order to secure the bonds with the spirit world that will make healers' remedies safe and effective. Interviewees also recounted stories of healers who had freely shared their traditional knowledge with researchers, only to have the latter enrich themselves by making and selling their ethnomedicines themselves! Also, they pointed out that, just like their human/livestock counterpart healers in cities, they too should be paid for any consultations. However, interviewees were happy to discuss disease descriptions and to give the author test samples of already-prepared remedies *gratis*. Based on all these experiences, the author makes several practical recommendations to future EVK researchers. First, he implies that on the whole it is more worthwhile to work with healers than with ordinary stockraisers if the goal is to identify 'best bet' livestock remedies. Second, he suggests the following order of and type of interviews: (1) with many different healers on general disease topics *gratis*; (2) with stockraisers at large, to determine their opinion of healers' skills and their assessment of the best practitioners; and finally, (3) based on all the foregoing, paid consultations with the most expert livestock healers.

Mbarubukeye, Sylvain. 1994. La recherche sur la médecine vétérinaire traditionnelle au Rwanda. In: Kakule Kasonia and Michel Ansay (eds). *Metissages en Santé Animale de Madagascar à Haïti: Actes du Séminaire d'Ethnopharmacopée Vétérinaire 'KAGALA', un Partage de Savoirs Burkina-Faso, Ouagadougou, 15–22 Avril 1993.* Presses Universitaires de Namur, Namur, Belgium. Pp. 253–274.

This proceedings publication synthesizes the results from an extensive national survey of ethnoveterinary practices among 532 traditional livestock healers [of unspecified sex] in Rwanda in 1991. The survey was followed by a workshop among 53 healers plus researchers from CURPHAMETRA and the National Veterinary Laboratory of Rubirize. The survey found that 62% of the 532 acquired their ethnoveterinary knowledge verbally from their fathers. A further and alarming, finding was that only 10% of the healers were under age 40 years.

Interestingly, all but 18% of the 532 were willing to share their EVK with the researchers. On the other hand, 98% said they would be willing to collaborate on an equal footing with researchers, given their desire to gain official recognition. All but 19% said they charged for their services, with fees varying from US $0.35 to $21.00. In the aggregate, healers recognized 106 animal diseases, although each individual treated on average only three to five diseases. In rank order, the 10 that, as a group, they dealt with most often were: mastitis, three-day fever, theileriosis, anaplasmosis, brucellosis, worms, prolapsed uterus, dystocia, deliveries and mange. Their treatments are exemplified in three prescriptions for mastitis. To take one example, mastitis was treated by rubbing into the udder a mixture of the leaf juices of *Anisopappus africanus*, *Clematis hirsuta*, *Dracaena steudneri*, plus kaolin. In general, healers appeared to favour polyprescriptions in their plant medicines. This paper's conclusion discusses the time- and cost-savings of testing 'whole' traditional medicines rather than focusing on isolating and testing their ingredients. It also underlines the importance of interdisciplinary and international cooperation in the study of EVM. Two tabular annexes present: 50 locally recognized livestock diseases plus the clinical signs and aetiologies known to healers; and a list of plants commonly used in EVM, identified according to both local and scientific diseases to which they are applied.

Mbarubukeye, S., S. Ntegeyibizaza, P. Rutabandama and D. Kaboyi. 1995. Essai de traitement de la théileriose bovine par une méthode traditionnelle au Rwanda. *Lettre du Sous-réseau PRELUDE: Santé, Productions Animales et Environnement* 8: 4.

Trials by Rwandan veterinary scientists on the efficacy of an unspecified traditional treatment for ECF suggested possible beneficial effects in diminishing the clinical signs of the disease.

Mbassa, G.K. 1992. Evidence of natural resistance to East Coast Fever in Sanga zebu cattle in Tanzania. In: G. Tacher and L. Letenneur (eds). *Proceedings of the Seventh International Conference of Institutions of Tropical Veterinary Medicine, Yamoussoukro, Ivory Coast: Volume II.* Pp. 475–480.

This conference paper notes that, in Tanzania, a Sanga × zebu crossbreed of cattle known as *Tarime* is resistant to ECF or suffers only mildly compared to other zebu. As a result of breeding for ECF resistance, herd phenotypes in the Shinyanga region where this cross is found have changed from short, black, thick-skinned and blunt-horned zebu to taller, brown, thin-skinned and sharp-horned animals.

McCabe, J. Terrence. 1985. Livestock disease in south Turkana. In: Rada Dyson-Hudson and J. Terrence McCabe. *South Turkana Nomadism: Coping with an Unpredictably Varying New Environment, Volume II.* Human Relations Area Files, Inc., New Haven, Connecticut, USA. Pp. 366–377.

Based on interviews with Turkana herders of Kenya, pages 366 to 377 (the appendix) of this study details 23 diseases affecting Turkana cattle, sheep, goats and camels. The author also discusses disease intensity and periodicity as reported by the herders, i.e. their ethno-epidemiological knowledge. Differences across informants concerning the precise symptoms of a disease were resolved through group discussions until a consensus was reached.

McCorkle, Constance M. 1982. ***Management of Animal Health and Disease in an Indigenous Andean Community.*** Sociology Technical Report Series No. 4. SR-CRSP, Department of Rural Sociology, University of Missouri-Columbia, Columbia, Missouri 65211, USA. 68 pp.

Based on interviews and participant observation, this study describes sheep and llama diseases and their diagnosis, cause, cure and prevention from the viewpoint of agropastoralists in the Peruvian peasant community of Usi. By comparing these findings with equivalent data from modern veterinary medicine, the author analyses whether local ethnoveterinary beliefs and practices promote productive animal management. Matching ethnoveterinary disease names with their corresponding scientific counterparts is not always easy. Veterinary science classifies diseases by aetiology while indigenous classification primarily utilizes the most visible clinical signs. Moreover, the unit of definition often differs. The author discusses supernatural causes for diseases (evil winds and others), parasitic diseases (diarrhoea, worms and coughing, turning sickness, mange and sleeping sickness), non-parasitic diseases (pink-eye) and plant poisoning. She concludes that Usiño ethno-diagnoses are sometimes accurate or, especially in the case of endoparasitism, often inaccurate for understandable reasons. Ethnoaetiologies, although different from scientific ones, nevertheless may lead to effective treatment and prevention. People from Usi seldom apply modern drugs for various reasons. From a Western point of view, the lack of indigenous preventive measures against parasites and overgrazing seems irrational. However, the author points out that the villagers act rationally with respect to their agropastoral situation and the competing demands of herding and cultivation. Development programmes should be adapted to the particular constraints of agropastoralism.

McCorkle, Constance M. 1983a. ***Meat and Potatoes: Animal Management and the Agropastoral Dialectic in an Indigenous Andean Community, with Implications for Development.*** PhD dissertation, Anthropology, Stanford University, Stanford, California, USA. 453 pp.

This dissertation presents a case study of animal husbandry in an agropastoral community of Quechua Indians in Peru. The theoretical aim of the work is to validate cross-culturally a dialectical model of preindustrial agropastoralism utilizing a New World database, at the same time correcting overly neofunctional analyses of such subsistence systems. The study also emphasizes the real economic importance of herds, no matter how small their numbers, for peasant survival. The first two chapters introduce the theoretical framework and research setting. Chapter 3 outlines indigenous terms and taxonomies pertaining to herd animals. Chapter 4 provides a detailed description of the manifold tasks involved in Andean peasant pastoralism, including shearing, docking, castrating, breeding, feeding, control of predation, maintenance of structures and equipment. Chapter 5 describes the social organization of labour through which these tasks are accomplished. Chapter 6 is devoted to indigenous theories, practices and beliefs concerning animal health. Emic views of 13 ailments spanning supernatural, parasitic, non-parasitic and toxic aetiologies are detailed according to stockowners' description of their clinical signs and diagnosis, cause, treatment, prevention and control [see also McCorkle 1982]. The work concludes with a discussion of the practical implications of a dialectical model of peasant agropastoralism for development programmes seeking to enhance either plant or animal agriculture in such milieu.

McCorkle, Constance M. 1983b. *The Technoenvironmental Dialectics of Herding in Andean Pastoralism.* Technical Report No. 30. SR-CRSP, Department of Rural Sociology, University of Missouri-Columbia, Columbia, Missouri 65211, USA. 103 pp.

This report describes nearly every aspect of herd animal management among Quechua agropastoralists of highland Peru. The annual cycle of pastoral tasks is outlined, beginning with the reproductive and protective rites that open the pastoral year and continuing through breeding, feeding, slaughter, docking, castrating and shearing. With regard to the latter, the author notes that shearing wounds may be soothed with a homemade herbal treatment. Additional management factors discussed are: pastoral structures, designed so that animals are less likely to fight, drown or crush one another and are protected from heatstroke and photosensitization; pastoral paraphernalia, including herd dogs; herd composition by species, sex and age; losses and culls; and the control of predation [see also McCorkle 1983a].

McCorkle, Constance M. 1986. An introduction to ethnoveterinary research and development. *Journal of Ethnobiology* 6(1): 129–149.

Ethnoveterinary research and development (ER&D) is a relatively new interdisciplinary study undertaken by veterinarians and anthropologists. Its core consists of the systematic investigation and application of veterinary folk knowledge, theory and practice so as to better promote livestock productivity through improved management of animal health. In an extensive review of the literature, the author discusses veterinary ethnosemantics and taxonomies; ethnoveterinary pharmacology; cauterization, bleeding, vaccination and other manipulative techniques; magico-religious practices; appropriate methods for extension and veterinary services; and animal health and livestock production systems research. She concludes that folk beliefs and practices should be the starting point for veterinary research, development and extension and that there is a move in ER&D towards analysing veterinary development issues within a holistic but comparative and production-system-specific framework. Out of this comparative approach, some consensus is emerging that educational, managerial, marketing and other such interventions often may be more appropriate, economical and effective development strategies than modern drug therapy. The article concludes by outlining future research needs in ER&D.

McCorkle, Constance M. 1988. *Manejo de la Sanidad de Rumiantes Menores en una Comunidad Indígena Andina.* Editorial Hipatia for the Comisión de Coordinación de Tecnología Andina, Lima, Perú. 77 pp.

This booklet is essentially a Spanish translation of McCorkle 1982.

McCorkle, Constance M. 1989a. Veterinary anthropology. *Human Organization* 48(2): 156–162.

Veterinary anthropology investigates and applies folk veterinary knowledge, theory and practice in order to improve livestock health and productivity. The ultimate goal is increased human well-being. Veterinary anthropology is an interdisciplinary endeavour combining anthropological field methods with the technical skills and laboratory expertise of veterinarians and animal scientists. The author presents two examples of veterinary anthropology from Peru. The first consists of an analysis of *q'icha*, a major category of livestock disease recognized by Quechua Indians. This case illustrates the comparative emic/etic and anthropological/biological approach of this new field. The other example describes how, through participatory on-farm research, the SR-CRSP in Peru promoted the utilization of a traditional wild-tobacco remedy in that region as a dip against ectoparasites. The author discusses the importance of veterinary anthropology for development, emphasizing that it can simultaneously identify not only where indigenous knowledge systems can be improved, but also how these improvements can be brought about.

McCorkle, Constance M. 1989b. Veterinary anthropology on the Small Ruminant CRSP/Peru. In: Constance M. McCorkle (ed.). *The Social Sciences in International Agricultural Research: Lessons from the CRSPs.* Lynne Rienner Publishers, Boulder, Colorado, USA. Pp. 213–227.

This chapter represents a somewhat revised and expanded version of McCorkle 1989a.

McCorkle, Constance M. 1989c. La medicina etnoveterinaria en una comunidad campesina del Cuzco. In: Hernando Bazalar and Constance M. McCorkle (eds). *Estudios Etnoveterinarios en Comunidades Altoandinas del Perú.* Lluvia Editores, Lima, Perú. Pp. 27–50.

This chapter represents a revised, up-dated and greatly condensed version of McCorkle 1988.

McCorkle, Constance M. 1994a. *Ethnoveterinary R&D and Gender in the ITDG/Kenya RAPP.* Report of a Consultancy for the Rural Agricultural and Pastoral Programme. ITDG, Nairobi, Kenya. 54 pp.

For more than 10 years, ITDG's Rural Agricultural and Pastoral Programme (RAPP) has been conducting ethnoveterinary fieldwork in three districts of Kenya. After reviewing the RAPP's research methodologies and findings [see the various Wanyama abstracts for details], this report sketches out a strategic plan for the continuation of RAPP's ethnoveterinary R&D efforts for the next three years (1995–1998) along with one-year objectives for each district. Short-term recommendations are to: locate, consolidate and analyse the wealth of information and local-expert opinion garnered from the many baseline studies and exploratory activities to date; and integrate EVK findings into ITDG veterinary training packages and parlance, as well as university curriculum design. In the longer term, an interdisciplinary team should plan research to validate EVK, including botanicals, mechanical, managerial and preventive techniques.

McCorkle, Constance M. 1994b. *Farmer Innovation in Niger.* Studies in Technology and Social Change No. 21. Center for Indigenous Knowledge and Agricultural and Rural Development (CIKARD). Iowa State University Research Foundation, Ames, Iowa, USA.

This publication is an abbreviated version that presents only the technological findings of the longer, 1988 study by McCorkle, Brandstetter and McClure.

McCorkle, Constance M. 1995. Back to the future: Lessons from ethnoveterinary RD&E for studying and applying local knowledge. *Agriculture and Human Values* 12(2): 52–80.

This article overviews the background, rationale, principles and nine categories of subject matters addressed in ethnoveterinary research, development and extension (ERD&E). Subject matters are further divided into 26 sub-issues. Also noted are 17 concrete lessons learned from such work for the study and application of local knowlege of any kind, plus 16 mini-case studies of types of effective/ineffective, ancient/innovative, environmentally friendly, techno-blended and other kinds of ethnoveterinary practices and understandings from the global literature. Above all, the article underscores the importance of less commonly addressed topics in ERD&E. These span: mixed grazing and the keeping of companion species to reduce disease and predator threats to livestock (and humans and their productive environment), plus other astute animal-health herding strategies; relatedly, two-way concepts of zoonoses and ethnozooprophylaxis; the formation of respected, profitable and therefore sustainable professional associations of traditional veterinary healers drawing upon human ethnomedical models pioneered by governments (as in Kenya's traditional healer associations) or by international pharmaceutical firms and environmental NGOs (such as Shaman Pharmaceuticals' apprenticeships or Conservation International's scholarships for young healers) to stem the frightening loss of local knowledge, of *in situ* biodiversity and of skilled users of *materia medica* for traditional medicine; relatedly, the expanding commercial production of ethnoveterinary pharmaceuticals both nationally and internationally, as long exemplified in Asian countries and, more recently, in First World nations; the joint delivery of animal and human, traditional and modern healthcare; relevant to all the foregoing, socio-organizational structures and mechanisms for implementing both traditional and new approaches to healthcare, plus the place and meaning of medico-religious beliefs and practices; the incorporation of findings from ethnoveterinary R&D in local school and university educational curricula; and methods for first studying and validating findings in a cost-effective and bioethical way that national R&D agencies and NGOs are able to apply. Also introduced is an innovative concept of IDM or integrated disease management, on analogy to IPM (integrated pest management) in cropping research. A highlight of the article is a concluding discussion of six circumstances under which EVK may be harmful, ineffective, insufficient, inappropriate, seemingly only marginally helpful or simply absent.

McCorkle, Constance M. 1998. Ethnoveterinary medicine. In: Allen M. Schoen and Susan G. Wynn (eds). *Alternative and Complementary Therapies in Veterinary Medicine: Principles and Practice.* Mosby, Inc., St Louis, Missouri, USA. Pp. 713–741.

This chapter is a slightly revised reprint of McCorkle 1995, which was included in this volume in order to introduce alternative veterinarians in the First World to on-going research into traditional livestock methods in the Third World.

McCorkle, Constance M. and Hernando Bazalar. 1989. Los estudios etno-
veterinarios del SR-CRSP en el Perú. In: Hernando Bazalar and Constance M.
McCorkle (eds). *Estudios Etnoveterinarios en Comunidades Altoandinas del
Perú.* Lluvia Editores, Lima, Perú. Pp. 13–22.

This chapter introduces what is apparently the first anthology exclusively devoted
to ER&D. The volume as a whole synthesizes a decade of research (1980–1990)
on this subject conducted by the SR-CRSP's Sociology and Veterinary Medicine
Projects in Peru. The chapter describes: the substance, goals and importance of
ER&D; the four high-altitude Andean communities that participated in the SR-
CRSP studies; and the combination of methodologies employed, including anthropological interviews and participant observation, laboratory analyses and
participatory on-farm trials. On-the-ground problems (and solutions) in conducting
such trials are also described, based on the SR-CRSP's firsthand experience.

McCorkle, Constance M. and Hernando Bazalar. 1996a. Field trials in ethnoveterinary R&D: Lessons from the Andes. In: Constance M. McCorkle, Evelyn
Mathias and Tjaart W. Schillhorn van Veen (eds). *Ethnoveterinary Research &
Development.* Intermediate Technology Publications, London, UK. Pp.
265–282.

To date, most ER&D efforts have been of an exploratory, descriptive, bibliographic, or conceptual nature. Actual field trials to validate specific treatments or
techniques have been relatively rare. Rarer still are trials that fully involve producers
themselves under normal on-farm conditions and that employ modest levels of
R&D support akin to those available to developing-country livestock research
agencies. This chapter self-critically overviews the results of several such trials,
conducted by the SR-CRSP on ovine ethnopharmacology in peasant communities
of highland Peru. Backed by literature reviews, preliminary field studies, laboratory investigations and especially farmers' own assessments of major animal health
problems, the trials focused on ovine parasitism as the most prevalent and economically destructive class of diseases among Andean livestock [also see
McCorkle and Bazalar 1996b]. A participatory-action-research approach was
taken; and trials were conducted mainly with women, who bear the bulk of responsibility for stockraising among indigenous peoples of the Andes. All trials shared
the following features. Farm families to whom the test and control animals
belonged were matched for similarity in socioeconomic status and husbandry
regimes, such as grazing areas, livestock housing and inputs used. Also, treatment
and non-treatment control animals were matched for sex, age and reproductive
status (e.g. no pregnant ewes were included). Throughout the trials, all sheep continued to be managed under the normal husbandry routine. That is, they grazed
together with the rest of the flock and with other families' flocks on communal pastures by day; and at night, the sheep were corralled with their herdmates. This
meant that trial animals were constantly exposed to reinfection by the parasites
being treated against. Careful pre-, interim- and post-measurements were made of
parasite burdens and experimental animals' weight; and treatment groups were
monitored for adverse side effects, of which there were none. Only rough comparative costs were calculated for the ethnomedicines tested versus the commercial
equivalents on offer, due to the terrorist murders of the project economist along

with one of the veterinarians. The ethnopharmacotherapies tested were all traditional ones: a topical wild-tobacco treatment originally used for bovines and equines, but reformulated in the trial as an insecticidal dip against sheep keds [see, e.g. Fernández 1991a]; a pumpkin-seed anthelmintic drench; and two traditional flukicides, one a decoction of artichoke leaves and the other a cold infusion of the leaves of a forest shrub, each combined with salt and mineral or cooking oil. Local people had long forgotten the precise traditional prescriptions for the last treatment and for the anthelmintic. But project researchers were able to reconstruct them by searching the Andean ethnomedical literature on the corresponding prescriptions for cattle and humans, respectively. The chapter presents details of: women's (as well as men's and children's) participation in every step of the trials; precise treatment preparation and dipping or dosing regimes tested; parasite knock-down points and, where relevant, faecal-egg and adult-parasite counts; statistical significances; and so forth. All four of the ethnomedicines showed antiparasitic activity, compared to the untreated controls. Moreover, with inputs of modern scientific knowledge to modify the frequency and timing of traditional applications, it was possible to increase this activity for the endoparasiticides. Also, all were far cheaper than their commercial equivalents. The chapter discusses elements that the SR-CRSP found to be important to the success of participatory on-farm trials, notably: establishment of a resident interdisciplinary but mainly-national team of researchers on-site, for tight coordination across disciplines and close 'insider/outsider' collaboration; backstopping of the field team by higher-level national researchers with access to basic laboratory facilities; engagement of producers in every step of R&D, including prior negotiation of a formal accord as to the research priorities and contributions of each of the parties involved; and a stock-replacement plan to permit culling of experimental and control animals for necropsy so as not to expose participating farmers to unfair enterprise risk. The chapter concludes with seven sets of lessons learned for future ER&D. First is that such research gives farmers better-informed and greater quality control, over choice of livestock treatments vis-à-vis non-validated ethnomedicines or the often adulterated or outright fraudulent commercial veterinary products often foisted off on poor, illiterate and ethnically oppressed groups. Second is the virtue of technoblending, such that: new uses for old remedies may be discovered, as in the tobacco treatment reformulated for ovines as well as other species; more efficient routes of administration may be devised, e.g. dipping instead of topical application; or a more effective treatment regimen may be devised for an existing ethnomedicine, as was the case with the artichoke drench. Third is that not all ethnoveterinary know-how is 'indigenous' in the strict sense of the term. The artichoke, for example, is an Old World plant. The point here is that people 'mix and match' from whatever is at hand. Thus, over-zealous proponents of indigenous knowledge must beware of rejecting valuable local treatments merely because of some preconceived unicultural or historical source criteria. A fourth lesson is that sometimes local knowledge may be so eroded that recourse to sources and informed individuals well outside the local area may be necessary in order to reconstruct it [see also Roepke 1996]. A fifth set of lessons centres on the empowering effects of farmer participation. Even where stockraisers still cling to ethnoveterinary treatments, often they do so out of economic necessity while yet believing their traditional ways to be inferior. Participatory R&D can liberate people from such intellectual imperialism, engender a fresh sense of confidence in themselves and their capacity to take greater control over their own development needs and in the process give them new ideas and skills such as those embodied in the scientific method of controlled comparison and systematic observation. An empowerment bonus may also result when women are included in such exercises. For example, one outcome of the SR-CRSP trials was the first-time formation of a local women's organization concerned with agricultural development. A sixth lesson is that ER&D can have positive impacts on other development sectors, such as environment or human health. For example, the success of the tobacco trials started people thinking about how to protect and increase this valuable wild plant resource. A seventh and final set of lessons concerns ways in which, circumstances permitting, trials like those described here might be better designed, e.g. by including: larger sample sizes; double-blind procedures; controls for carrier materials (the salt and oils); establishment of reference points for treatment efficacy on-station; greater attention to parasite burdens by season and life-cycle in interpreting trial results; and depending upon trial goals, steps to prevent reinfestation of experimental animals. A final point is that some kind of credible validation of EVK is often greatly welcomed by the holders of that knowledge, whether via experimental trials or other methods [see, e.g. IIRR 1994 and various articles by Wanyama]. Promoting unvalidated techniques, traditional or modern, is bioethically unacceptable.

McCorkle, Constance M. and Hernando Bazalar. 1996b. Reducing veterinary costs by building on local knowledge: A case with female farmers in Peru. Paper presented to the 16th Annual Agricultural Symposium at the World Bank, Vision to Action, 9–10 January, Washington, DC, USA.

This symposium paper presents findings and experiences from interdisciplinary on-farm R&D in sustainable animal agriculture conducted by the SR-CRSP in tandem with women in a cluster of 14 agropastoral communities of the Peruvian Andes. In such communities, women have primary responsibility for animal husbandry, while men take charge of cultivation. The research focused on parasitism, which the women named as their number-one livestock health problem but for which Western veterinary medicine had proved to be unsustainable under prevailing infrastructural and politico-economic conditions. Moreover, some potent Western treatments posed possible threats to environmental and human health. Thus, the SR-CRSP and its female farmers *cum* co-researchers turned their attention to ethnoveterinary alternatives. Alone or 'techno-blended' with inputs of Western-scientific knowledge, these offered greater promise of yielding technologies that were more 'sustainable' in every sense of the word. This paper briefly introduces the field of EVM and then outlines both the participatory process and the scientific results of the SR-CRSP's on-farm trials to validate five ethnoveterinary treatments for the locally self-sufficient and sustainable control of endo- and ecto-parasitism. Finally, the larger development potentials inherent in a participatory on-farm R&D approach that builds on local knowledge and resources are discussed. Potentials span, e.g.: generation and adoption of productivity-increasing and/or risk-reducing livestock technologies or practices that are truly sustainable because they are locally grounded and therefore usually cheaper, more reliable and certainly more accessible, comprehensible and culturally 'comfortable' than purely alien interventions; impetus to the maintenance of biodiversity, e.g. in the form of valuable medicinal plant species; still other 'bonuses' for both environmental and human health; greater client-responsiveness and cost-savings in national agricultural R&D programmes; and, at a more intangible level, renewed appreciation of own-culture know-how and increased critico-analytic and socio-organizational skills among (especially female) producers, thereby empowering them to play a more dynamic role in addressing their agricultural R&D needs themselves.

McCorkle, Constance M., Robert H. Brandstetter and Gail D. McClure. 1988. *A Case Study on Farmer Innovations and Communication in Niger.* Communication for Technology Transfer in Agriculture Project, Academy for Educational Development, Washington DC. 125 pp.

Researchers in the Communication for Technology Transfer in Agriculture Project studied farmer-to-farmer communication networks in relation to the transfer of farmer innovations in the Sahel of Niger. One ethnoveterinary innovation is cited (pp. 9–10, 47). The roots of a *Ficus* sp. tree are highly sought-after for treating stomach problems in humans and bloat in livestock. Unfortunately, overuse of the root led to the tree's extinction in the area studied. However, one enterprising local farmer re-established the tree in his home herb garden and, through repeated experimentation, created a new leaf-based compound just as therapeutic as the traditional root prescriptions. Thanks to his ethnoscientific efforts, the source of this highly prized medicine is now sustainable and renewable.

McCorkle, Constance M. and Edward C. Green. 1998. Intersectoral healthcare delivery. *Agriculture and Human Values* 15(2): 105–114.

Within a given culture – no matter whether modern or tradition-oriented – essentially the same fundamental medical theories, practices and pharmacopoeia tend to be applied to human and non-human ills and patients. In modern societies, healthcare services and practitioners are sharply divided between human and veterinary medicine; but in more traditional or indigenous medical systems, often the same healers treat all species. Given the spiralling costs and continuing infrastructural, training and drug-supply difficulties of extending specialized modern medicine to all of the world's burgeoning human and livestock population, especially for poorer countries and remote or nomadic stockraising peoples, an intersectoral approach to healthcare is warranted. This approach delivers traditional as well as conventional services to both livestock and humans and thus involves respected local healers as well as formally trained doctors and veterinarians. This approach would greatly increase the number of people with affordable access to a wider choice of healthcare services for themselves and their animals. It would also cut costs on gathering epidemiological intelligence and implementing public health programmes. An example is dual vaccination campaigns for livestock and rural children. With the lure of the veterinary immunizations, even in remote and war-torn rural zones such programmes have achieved child vaccination rates that far outstrip conventional approaches implemented in urban areas of the developing world. Furthermore, people's acceptance of vaccination is promoted by analogy to their homemade vaccines for livestock. Findings from such campaigns suggest that revenues from the veterinary services can significantly defray the expenses of extending basic healthcare to the human owners of the animals. Finally, involving local healers not only encourages increased client recourse to healthcare services of all sorts; it also helps stem the loss of valuable ethnomedical resources, whether in the form of biodiverse, natural *materia medica* or the profession of local healing itself – both of which have long been undermined, or at best ignored, by established Western medical/veterinary science.

McCorkle, Constance M. and Marina Martin. 1998. Parallels and potentials in animal and human ethnomedical technique. *Agriculture and Human Values* 15(2): 139–144.

This article overviews parallels between ethnomedical techniques for animals and humans. Worldwide, treatments are administered in much the same, and in many cases identical, routes and modes; and many of the same animal, vegetable and mineral *materia medica* are employed. Examples of technical overlaps are given for: pharmacology; surgery (mainly general surgery, bonesetting, wound care and obstetrics); traditional vaccinations; mechanical/hydro/physical techniques, e.g. acupuncture/pressure, moxibustion, massage, exercise, rest, baths, sweats; behavioural strategies, including quarantine, movements to avoid disease threat, habitat modification and hygiene, keeping of companion species and behavioural controls on mating; ethnodentistry; and medico-religious practices. The implication of such overlaps for the delivery of intersectoral healthcare are briefly discussed. Examples of implications include: the development of medicaments for humans based on successful ethnoveterinary remedies and vice versa; discouraging versus encouraging and extending both ethnomedical and conventional-medical practices and hygienic measures that are unsound versus sound for humans and animals alike; and thereby maximizing people's access to health services, knowledge and self-help skills.

McCorkle, Constance M. and Evelyn Mathias-Mundy. 1992. Ethnoveterinary medicine in Africa. *Africa: Journal of the International African Institute* 62(1): 59–93.

This article constitutes the first in-depth review of EVM in Africa. The review itself is followed by a critical analysis – from both social-scientific and biological/technical perspectives – of how this valuable but endangered body of knowledge can be put to work in agricultural development. Much of the article draws upon material covered in the first annotated bibliography (Mathias-Mundy and McCorkle 1989).

McCorkle, C.M. and E. Mathias. 1996. Paraveterinary healthcare programs: A global overview. In: Karl-Hans Zessin (ed.). *Livestock Production and Diseases in the Tropics: Livestock Production and Human Welfare. Proceedings of the VIII International Conference of Institutions of Tropical Veterinary Medicine held from the 25 to 29 September, 1995 in Berlin, Germany.* Volume II. Deutsche Stiftung für Internationale Entwicklung, Zentralstelle für Ernährung und Landwirtschaft, Feldafing, Germany. Pp. 544–549.

Based on an overview of approximately 60 paravet training programmes worldwide, the authors note that relatively few such initiatives have included ethnoveterinary treatments in their curricula. Moreover, without prodding, trainees themselves may not remark the existence of such treatments [because they know outsiders often denigrate them]. When it comes to selecting paravet trainees, only a handful of programmes have taken into account an individual's repute as an established local healer. Fewer still consulted traditional healers [e.g. as to disease prevalence, service demand, remuneration, necessary prior skills, etc.] in the course of baseline studies preparatory to programme design.

McCorkle, Constance M., D.V. Rangnekar and Evelyn Mathias. 1999. Introduction: Whence and whither ER&D? In: E. Mathias, D.V. Rangnekar and C.M. McCorkle, with M. Martin (eds). *Ethnoveterinary Medicine: Alternatives for Livestock Development – Proceedings of an International Conference Held in Pune, India, 4–6 November 1997. Volume 1: Selected Papers.* BAIF Development Research Foundation, Pune, India. Pp. 1–12.

Building upon the first author's keynote address to the above-referenced conference, this proceedings introduction briefly overviews the definition and the 20-year evolution of ER&D as a recognized field of study and notes some of the key actor groups and publications therein. It then asks what new directions ER&D should take as the field matures and moves into the new millennium. The answer, say the authors, is toward greater holism via more and/or stronger linkages with a greater diversity of disciplines and actors. Specifically noted are: interdisciplinary linkages, especially between veterinary medicine and animal science and with fields that have so far been little engaged in ER&D, such as economics and policy analysis; intersectoral linkages, notably with the environmental, educational and human-medical sectors; intercultural linkages, here discussed under the categories of techno-blending and conceptual blending; and finally, linkages with more different kinds of institutions – not only UN agencies, universities, research centres, agricultural and livestock extension services, but also zoos, museums, botanical gardens, rare-breeds societies, animal welfare groups, wildlife reserves, alternative as well as conventional veterinary-professional associations and of course stock-raiser and healer organizations. With increased numbers of disciplines and actors behind it, ER&D will have a greater chance of offering valid and cost-effective options to producers everywhere.

Mejia, Mario. 1996. Rebirth of indigenous farming systems after agricultural collapse in Colombia. *Honey Bee* 7(4): 7–8.

In Colombia's Cauca Valley, the system of coffee monocropping collapsed after the crash of coffee prices in the 1980s. This article describes the establishment of model farms to demonstrate alternative agricultural techniques for the small and poor farmers who suffered most severely in the crash. Ten different cropping models (one based on medicinal plants) and three different stockraising models have been installed on the farms, as designed by the author in collaboration with NGOs. Each seeks to provide a minimum subsistence income for peasant families. Three of the livestock models centre on beekeeping, guinea pig production and stall-fed cattle raising. In the latter, ten head are fed on cultivated cut-and-carry fodders such as *Trichanthera gigantea*, *Erythrina edulis* and imperial or king grass (*Axonopus scoparius* and *Pennisetum purpureum*, respectively). In addition, the cattle receive plantain stems, native herbs, salt, molasses and urea. A complementary strategy is farming of red California earthworms, which are fed on the cattle and pig manure collected every 2 and 1 days, respectively. Animal houses are disinfected once or twice a month; piggerys are washed twice a day. Small drainage tanks beside the animal shelters collect the waste water, which is then used to enrich compost. These practices keep livestock quarters clean while making maximum use of livestock byproducts. [Presumably elements of different models can be mixed, e.g. to grow medicinal plants for livestock treatments.]

Mellor, P.S. 1978. Biting flies attacking cattle in the Dhofar Province of the Sultanate of Oman. *Tropical Animal Health and Production* 10: 167–169.

This article describes a visit to Oman to collect biting flies from cattle. Collection was done during daylight hours because local people reported that this is when fly attacks are greatest. In many areas stockraisers grazed their cattle by night in order to avoid the flies.

Merker, M. 1910. *Die Masai: Ethnographische Monographie eines ostafrikanischen Semitenvolkes* (2nd edition). Dietrich Reimer, Berlin, Germany.

Pages 161–179 of this ethnography on the Maasai deal with indigenous husbandry and veterinary medicine for ruminants, donkeys and camels. Maasai herders select stud bulls when these are still young and castrate the remaining male calves by open surgery. Some older bulls unsuited for breeding and other livestock species are castrated by crushing the seminal cords with a cudgel. Treatments for swollen joints and tendons consist of branding the affected parts, commonly in a grid-like pattern. Other swellings are exposed directly to smoke from burning the stems of *Solanum* sp. The author details Maasai perceptions of the causes, signs and treatments for several internal and infectious diseases and he provides Western diagnoses for some of these conditions. The Maasai vaccinate their cattle against CBPP. While their method is successful, it sometimes causes localized swelling and inflammation, occasionally leading to the loss of an eye.

Meserve, Ruth I. 1986–87. A Mongol cure for the rabid horse. *Journal of the Mongolia Society* 10: 89–96.

The same, but more detailed, cure for rabies is described here as in Meserve 1993. A traditional Mongol therapy for a rabid horse was to cut off the tip of its tongue, prick the two ends of the jawbone, beat them with a stone, cauterize the areas and then drench with a broth of ginseng root. Finally, the tip of the tail was docked. A parallel amputation technique to prevent rabies in dogs existed in ancient Rome where, 40 days after a puppy's birth, the tip of its tail was docked. Another technique to prevent rabies as well as inappetence noted by Pliny was to remove a small worm supposedly embedded in pups' tongues.

Meserve, Ruth I. 1992a. Natural calamities. *Altaic Religious Beliefs and Practices. Proceedings of the 33rd Meeting of the Permanent International Altaistic Conference, Budapest, 24–29 June 1990.* Pp. 221–227.

To protect horses, mules and donkeys from being struck by lightning, traditionally Mongols slit the animals' ears and nostrils. If lightning struck nevertheless, a shaman was called in to appease the thunder god and to pour milk over the stricken animal's head and mane, which were then cleansed with incense. In times past, mange was sometimes mistaken for lightning strike.

Meserve, Ruth I. 1992b. Some remarks on the illnesses of horses according to the Ch'ien-lung Pentaglot. In: Bernard Hung-Kay Luk (ed.). ***Contacts between Cultures. Eastern Asia: Literature and Humanities Volume 3.*** The Edwin Mellen Press, Lewiston, Queenstown and Lampeter, UK. Pp. 339–342.

The Ch'ien-lung Pentaglot, written around 1800, lists 23 rhino-laryngeal symptoms of animal illness, ranging from a runny nose to running sores. Certain of these signs may be symptomatic of glanders, also termed farcy, when it advances from the respiratory to the lymphatic system and the skin. Although Mongol horses and camels might suffer from this ill, as of the late 1800s and early 1900s, Mongols did not feel it reached such alarming proportions as in Europe and thus resisted outsiders' urgings to destroy affected herds. Some early European visitors concurred with this assessment, observing that glanders rarely developed fully in animals kept on the open prairie and that stock which tested positively nevertheless continued to work for many years. In addition to general good care of their herds according to the seasons, Mongols employed a variety of folk remedies for glanders-like signs, e.g.: thrusting bound chopsticks up an afflicted camel's nose; smearing various oils in and around the nose; and fumigating the patient by burning sheephorn and wolf's hair. A case is described in which a muleteer, unable to cure colic by putting red pepper up his mule's nostrils, consulted an amateur veterinarian among the lamas at a nearby temple. The lama bled the mule by making incisions just behind the forelegs. After being given a native 'Beecham's pill', food and rest, the mule recovered.

Meserve, Ruth I. 1993a. Additional notes on Mongol treatments for rabid animals. ***Mongolian Studies*** 16: 41–54.

Traditional Mongol cures for rabies were numerous. One consisted of amputating and cauterizing the tip of the rabid animal's tail and tongue and then drenching with a broth of ginseng root. Asparagus, euphorbia, skullcap (*Scutellaria lateriflora* L.) and vinegar all also figured in rabies therapies. Other studies report that spiritual methods were often used to rid animals or people of the evil spirit believed to cause rabies. These methods spanned magic, incantations, spells and conjurations.

Meserve, Ruth I. 1993b. The Bactrian camel: Two Mongolian manuscripts in the Royal Library, Copenhagen. In: Chieh-hsien Ch'en (ed.). ***Proceedings of the 35th Permanent International Altaistic Conference, September 12–17 1992, Taipei, China.*** Pp. 349–359.

Along with ancient camel welfare laws in Mongol China, several 18th and 19th century Mongol treatments for the less-well-studied Bactrian camel of central Asia are described in this conference paper. For sore feet, the tender part of the sole was covered with a sort of temporary shoe consisting of a leather patch held in place by thin thongs drawn through the adjacent callosities of the sole. Blood blisters in the sole were bled to ease and cool the whole foot. The Bactrian's most common ailment, mange, was treated with a drench of goat-meat soup and topical applications of burnt vitriol, snuff or gunpowder; patients might also be fumigated in an enclosed space by burning certain substances sold by Chinese apothecaries. Mongol nomads' *materia medica* included field mice, dried dung, insects, butter, earth, hair, salt and various steppe grasses as well as other botanicals. If a camel evinced a choking cough, tears and black sweats, it was made to swallow a live field mouse. If that did not work, it had to swallow a live black mouse. If both mouse treatments failed, then the four quarters of the two humps were punctured with a thin knife, the swollen gland between the shoulders was pierced and the blood of a black goat was poured into the incisions. Brain concussions were treated by beating the animal on the temples. The manuscripts reported on here also provided detailed instructions for the seasonal care and conditioning of camels. The author notes that no mention is made of any kind of magic or ritual involved in any treatments.

Meserve, Ruth I. 1993c. The traditional Mongolian method of conditioning horses and preventive veterinary medicine. *International Symposium on Mongolian Culture, Taipei, Taiwan, Republic of China.* Pp. 484–501.

Mongol treatment manuals for livestock (horses, camels, sheep, cattle) may be divided into sacred and secular texts. The former can be further divided into texts based in Tibetan religion (a foreign influence) and administered by lamas, versus those based in Mongolian folk religion (more indigenous). Some of the secular texts record herders' everyday treatments based on family traditions while others describe techniques learned from lamas and medicines acquired from Chinese shops or Western passers-by. The texts on preventive medicine show the least foreign influence. Among other things, they describe the traditional Mongolian system of preventive equine care according to the four seasons in relation to individual animal condition. This system focused on judicious selection and protection of different kinds of pasturage, controlled diet and watering, strict exercise and rest/tethering rules, training and saddling techniques and various methods to condition horses to the cold and other environmental stresses. This system appears to have changed little from the 13th century until well into the 20th, as until then modern veterinary medicine was unable to offer few improvements on traditional husbandry and healthcare methods.

Meserve, Ruth I. 1996a. Early Turkic contributions to veterinary medicine. *International Journal of Asian Studies* 1: 128–137.

Judging from the wealth of terminology in manuscripts dating from the 4th century onward, Turkic peoples of Central Asia controlled a wide range of veterinary knowledge. For horses, camels, cattle, sheep and goats, these sources mention: health problems such as stomachache, animal bites, lameness, fatigue, worms, malnutrition, sores, boils, fly worry, bloat; diseases that appear to equate to mange, scabies, glanders, strangles and rabies; and treatments that involve plant materials, grazing regimes and amulets. For example, a Mongol treatment for camel mange was to feed the animal a broth of goat meat and to rub snuff, gunpowder or burnt vitriol into the sores.

Meserve, Ruth I. 1996b. The surgical instruments of the animal doctor in Central Eurasia. In: Giovanni Stary (ed.). *Proceedings of the 38th Permanent International Altaistic Conference (PIAC). Kawasaki, Japan: August 7–12, 1995.* Harrassowitz Verlag, Wiesbaden, Germany. Pp. 243–258.

Local livestock surgeons of inner Asia learned their skills from butchering and from preserving hides, bones and some internal organs for household, religious and recreational uses. With the introduction of acupuncture from China, Central Asian surgeons' already profound knowledge of anatomy was expanded to the nervous and circulatory systems. Their skills were traditionally applied to horses, cattle, sheep, goats and camels; with the recent introduction of pigs, this species was also treated. This published conference paper describes the tools that inner Asian live-stock surgeons used from ancient times well into the 20th century. Knives of all sorts were the most common implement for debriding, incisions, bloodletting and amputations. Awls, needles and nails – made of iron, brass or copper – were used for puncturing, for probing or excavating a wound and for lifting tissue or cartilage. Awls and needles could be wielded cold, heated or red-hot; in the latter case, they were fitted with wooden handles. These implements came in varying lengths for operating on small, medium and large animals. Depending on the treatment, they would be plunged to different depths, as measured in finger-lengths. Afterwards, punctures were generally cauterized using heated stones, bones, green wood, sedge or metal items such as a coin, part of a stirrup, the back of an axe or an iron shovel. In modern times, a special small, flat iron with a narrow triangular surface and a long, raised handle replaced these items, especially in castrations. Tubes and pipes were employed for draining blood, urine, pus and gases. Hollowed animal horns served as funnels, e.g. for drenching. Bellows were used for administering enemas or for forcing powdered medicine deeply into a wound or sore. Wooden clamps were employed in castration, traditionally performed by especially 'gentle-handed' specialists. Pincers and tweezers were helpful in cleaning and excavating sores and wounds and 'shoeing' camels. Leather straps and whips sometimes served for binding or supporting or splinting a limb. A cure for a pony with colic consisted of tying the rope in a clove hitch around the belly and then pulling on it, thus causing the horse to buck violently and break wind. Claws, paws and jaws from a variety of animal species served as currycombs and scrapers, e.g. for scabies. Various medico-magical properties might also be attributed to these items, according to the species from which they came. Leather and cloth patches, shields and bags figured in some surgical and many husbandry procedures. One is the famous practice of shoeing a camel with a sore pad. In this operation, a patch of camel or sheep skin or sometimes felt was sewn over the injured pad after cleaning and doctoring. The patch was stitched to the calloused edges of the pad with camel-hair twine. By the time the stitching wore through, the pad was healed. Flaps of cloth, felt, leather or birch bark were fastened around rams' bellies to prevent mating and over the tender vaginas of she-camels that had recently given birth. To prevent suckling, people put udder guards on cows or wooden muzzles on calves. Newborn animals were placed in leather or felt bags to protect and warm them. For restraint of animals during treatment, all manner of straps, ropes, whips, halters, bridles, hobbles and stakes were employed.

Meserve, Ruth I. 1996c. The terminology for the diseases of domestic animals in traditional Mongolian veterinary medicine. *Acta Orientalia Academiae Scientiarum Hung* XLIX(3): 335–358.

Analysis of manuscript evidence, dictionaries and travel reports can often re-capture a wealth of material on a people's lost or little-known veterinary know-ledge. The richness of such lexical research is illustrated in this article's listing of 156 Mongol disease terms, often accompanied by traditional diagnostic and treat-ment information, drawn from documents only recently made available as a result of the breakup of the USSR. One example is the compilation of documentary information on the term *amarau*, which refers to pustules or cankers in or around camels' and horses' mouths, possibly relating at times to FMD. Documents reveal a wide range of traditional treatments for *amarau*: applying salt and salted tea to the sores; cauterizing or phlebotomizing them; rubbing the tongue with a mixture of scorched deer hair or a horse-hoof plus dried dog faeces, salt and butter; or putting henbane in the patient's food. Another example is *sirki*, which pertains to lice and possibly flea infestations in horses, sheep and cattle. One treatment was to apply butter or tobacco juice. Another was to fumigate the animal, cleanse its body with scum from boiled liquids and then give it a rubdown with ashes.

Mesfin, T. and T. Obsa. 1994. Ethiopian traditional veterinary practices and their possible contribution to animal production and management. *Revue Scientifique et Technique de l'Office International des Épizooties* 13(2): 417–424.

This article overviews traditional veterinary practices and practitioners maintained by different ethnic groups in Ethiopia. The hypothesis is that the variety of ethno-veterinary treatments and healers within a country may provide an index of the potential usefulness of this neglected body of knowledge for national systems of animal healthcare and livestock development. Depending on ethnicity, in Ethiopia ethnomedical practitioners consist of bonesetters (*woghesha*), midwives (*awalag*), holymen (*debtera*), fortune tellers (*tenkuwai*) and spiritists (*kallicha*). All these healers may treat both humans and animals. However, these groups keep their ethnomedical knowledge secret. Of course, stockraisers themselves act as the first line of healers. Based on investigations by the Asela Veterinary Laboratory of Ethiopia, this article describes Ethiopian pastoralists' traditional methods of tick control, toxic plant management, surgery, vaccination and pharmacology. Tick controls take the form of pasture burning, homemade acaricides, salt feedings (or grazing animals on halophytic plants) and hot mineral baths. Plant poisoning may be treated by feeding an antidote plant. Surgical operations span: for demodectic blepharitis, slitting the eyelids of the affected cattle and removing the pustules; bloodletting from the ears of cattle [for unspecified ills]; for blackleg, branding or firing; and midwives' replacement of prolapsed uteri and correction of dystocia in cattle. Boran pastoralists vaccinate against CBPP by placing a piece of lung tissue from an animal dead of the disease under a flap of skin on the forehead of healthy cattle; Afar pastoralists do likewise, but on the tail tip. A rinderpest prophylaxis is to spray corrals and drench healthy cattle with diarrhoeic faeces taken from sick animals and diluted in water. In terms of ethnopharmacology, a Chinese veterinary team working in Ethiopia between 1974 and 1976 identified 22 traditional herbal medicines in the form of powders, tinctures and ointments for treating livestock wounds, gastrointestinal and respiratory problems, skin diseases, pain and pyrexia. In collecting treatment details on 33 384 animals, this team found that 70% were treated using such herbal preparations. Further, the team deemed a number of traditional treatments effective, such as eucalyptus leaf oil as a bacteriostat and *Glinus lotoides* against *Moniezia* and *Thysaniezia* spp. Other remedies studied and found effective by other scientists are also reported here, such as *Phytolacca dodecandra* as a molluscicide that helps control schistosomosis and fasciolosis in humans and animals. Also noted are as-yet-unstudied but promising traditional treatments, such as Boran use of *Commiphora erythraea* to help expel the placenta in both women and livestock or other cattle peoples' feeding of mineral soils. Despite such find-ings, plus similar research in other countries, in Ethiopia 'many veterinarians . . . think of traditional practices as mere superstition . . . [and] the domain of "quacks"' (p. 420). But the authors believe that 'traditional medicine could be useful if applied as an integral part of modern veterinary medicine' (ibid.); and they report that the Chinese veterinary team's promotion of Ethiopians' increased reliance on Ethiopian EVM has been encouraging. At the same time, the authors recommend further evaluation of ethnoveterinary practices by the national veteri-nary service before integrating them into formal healthcare delivery; but 'isolation of the active ingredients should not be a precondition if clinical observation sup-ports the effectiveness of a particular herb . . . claimed to be useful by traditional healers' (p. 421). They also suggest the creation of an association of such healers, plus incentives for them to act as veterinary scouts, in order to save valuable but disappeared ethnomedical knowledge. Other ideas mooted are: importation of veterinary medicinals already improved in other countries, for cultivation in Ethiopia, so as to maintain a continuous supply of herbals; and establishment within the national Veterinary Department of a multidisciplinary unit to coordinate and guide experiments on EVM and to communicate about EVM to veterinary pro-fessionals and students. Such units should incorporate vets, anthropologists, plant taxonomists, pharmacologists and biochemists.

Metailié, G. 1984. Aperçu des principes de la médecine vétérinaire traditionnelle en Chine. *Ethnozootechnie* 34: 43–50.

While the Western world opposes 'folk' to 'official, scientific' veterinary medicine, this is not the case in China. There, a well-accepted and highly formalized system of veterinary medicine apart from either folk or Western scientific practice has existed since the 11th century. This uniquely Chinese approach, which is deductive rather than experimental, rests on the theory of Yin versus Yang, a five-part cosmo-logical classification of elements (wood, fire, earth, metal, water) and correspon-dences posited among these elements, livestock anatomy and certain natural phenomena (seasons, processes of growth and change, colours, taste, physical environment). The author illustrates how application of this complex conceptual system dictates diagnoses and choice of treatment in animal disease.

Miles, Paul. 1997. Letters to the editor: Local remedies. *Draught Animal News* 26: 20–21.

In this letter, a South African rancher writes in to describe his time-tested (since 1958) remedies for injuries to draught animals, based on his own, successful experiences at raising cattle, horses and donkeys, as well as sheep and goats. Applied as soon as possible to burns, eggwhite relieves the pain and heals the damage. For tapeworm in young stock, the following recipe is effective. Boil 100 g of tobacco for 10 minutes in 1 l of water, then strain the liquid and add 2 tea-spoons of salt and 4 of *Aloe ferox* juice. Drench a fasted 3-week-old calf, kid or lamb with 30 ml of this medicament; for older animals, increase the dosage by 15 ml per month of age. For very bad cuts or wounds, boil a good handful of peach leaves in water. Then wash the wound with the cooled peach-leaf water; pack the wound with the boiled leaves; and dress it with a large swab saturated in the peach-water, taking care to keep the wound damp at all times. Change the dressing thrice daily after first washing the wound raw. The rancher recommends this treatment for castration wounds as well as for other, more serious wounds of horses; he finds it gives no rise to proud flesh or white hair. While the remedy may take longer than conventional veterinary treatments, 'the end result is far better and cheaper' he says, most likely due to the prussic and tannic acids in peach leaves. A simpler alternative for healing wounds or abrasions is to apply Stockholm tar, which also repels flies. To stop wounds from bleeding, he applies a wad of spider web. For footrot, the rancher paints a mixture of this tar and powdered copper sulphate onto and between the affected hooves. A pinch of copper sulphate in the eye cures ophthalmia, as does a pinch of chewn tobacco. To draw an abscess, apply a hot paste of laundry detergent and sugar or of the leaf-skin of prickly pear cactus. Some of his horses that are particularly fond of Mexican marigold bushes are always free of ticks and winter lice and in far better condition than their herdmates. So now, the rancher chops up the green bushes, adds salt and, a few days later, bonemeal or dicalcium sulphate and sets this silage out for all stock to lick. Given that many of the ingredients he uses are found worldwide, the rancher-author urges scientific testing of such home remedies. He also notes the value of searching through old books that document traditional tribal remedies – like the 1880 *Materia Medica of South Africa* – as a way of re-discovering useful remedies.

Millour, C. 1984. Les saints guérisseurs du bétail en Bretagne. *Ethnozootechnie* 34: 53–58.

Both historically and currently, popular 'veterinary saints' have been associated with curing and protecting horses, cattle and swine in France. Although typically uncanonized, these saints are prayed to and asked to bless bread for feeding to ailing animals or water for sprinkling over them. In return, they receive pilgrimages and offerings of butter, lard, horsehair, wool, lambs, piglets, money or other items. This article details a long list of these French veterinary saints. The author notes that their cult has diminished in the 20th century. For example, as the number and importance of horses decreased, so did the importance of the saints associated with this species.

Milton, Shaun. 1998. Western veterinary medicine in colonial Africa: A survey, 1902–1963. *Argos: Bulletin van het Veterinair Historisch Genootschap* 18(2): 313–322.

This article overviews colonial veterinary interventions in Africa under four topic headings: invasion, conquest and colonial consolidation; colonial power and veterinary administration; developments in veterinary field administration; and conclusions and post-colonial footnote. The penultimate heading discusses interventions according to major diseases (rinderpest, tick-borne ills, trypanosomosis and FMD). In the process, the author notes one of the paramount reasons and mechanism behind veterinary authorities' consistent denigration of African EVK. This was the need to substitute initial coercive approaches to making Africans adopt Western veterinary tactics with a more 'hegemonic' approach aimed at persuading stock-raisers of the inferiority of their 'primitive and superstitious' ethnoveterinary practices. Substituting such self-policing for direct policing was intended to save on scarce human and financial resources for veterinary services while still maintaining veterinary authorities' position in the colonial power structure. In addition, 'veterinarians were . . . sometimes simply intellectually or ideologically incapable of recognising or utilising, [sic] the depth and experience attached to such local knowledge' (pp. 314–315). Ironically, Africans' initial scepticism about Western techniques was sometimes well-founded. For example, early rinderpest vaccines were unreliable and difficult to apply in the African context. Moreover, they took nearly a week to confer full immunity, which lasted for only a few months thereafter; in the meantime, stock could still be infected and die. As a result, stockraisers saw the authorities as either inept or as wilfully introducing diseases and veterinary regulations as instruments of conquest and control. In one instance, however, authorities did draw upon indigenous practice. This was in their pre-World-War-II adoption of a 'bioeconomic' attack on trypanosomosis via intensive bush clearing. In summary, the author concludes that, backed by racial supremacy and classist notions of the day, veterinary medicine in colonial Africa was by definition interventionist, geared to upholding imperial or settler political-economic interests rather than native stockraisers' well-being. Today, however, 'there is room for optimism . . . In . . . a growing appreciation . . . of the potential of cheap "low input, environmentally sound and sustainable" indigenous practices and the utility of combining Western and African traditions to develop "syncretic options" for the provision [of] a veterinary medicine more appropriate to Africa's ecological, social and economic needs' (p. 320). The author also sees promise in 'sensitively applied' genetic science.

Minja, Mkangare M.J. n.d. Collection of Tanzanian medicinal plants for biological activity studies. Unpublished manuscript. 21 pp.

After warning about the imminent and frightening 'disintegration of the knowledge of medicinal plants in many societies' (p. 2), this paper briefly discusses debates about optimal approaches to medicinal plant exploration. Some natural-products investigators believe that semi-random collection of plants with specific properties is the most rewarding. Others prefer a random selection combined with broad pharmacological screening. Still others argue for ethnobotanical approaches that directly tap the knowledge of local healers. Another method is literature searches. Had ancient Egyptian papyri been searched in greater detail, the world might not have had to wait until the 1940s to discover the antibiotic properties of certain fungi! Also useful are herbarium studies. Opting for the ethnobotanical approach, the author here reports on 65 plant species of veterinary importance that he collected in the Arusha and Kilimanjaro regions of Tanzania based on interviews with herbalists, knowledgeable elderly people and herbal medicine vendors in marketplaces. Samples for later biological screening were taken; and botanical identification was done at the Tropical Pesticides Research Institute and the Animal Diseases Research Institute of Tanzania. The raw results from this ethnobotanical effort are displayed in a table that lists the 65 plants by their Latin and then local names, the plant parts used and their treatment indications in ruminants, poultry, dogs or in general. Occasional mention is made of treatments' use in humans as well, or as fish poisons. Both mono- and polyprescriptions are recorded. Plants that herbalists deemed particularly effective included: a boiled extract of *Adenia volkensii* for expulsion of the placenta; *Adenia gummifera* for FMD; *Fuerstia africana* for skin diseases, including mange; *Zehneria scabra* for wounds; and as powerful anthelmintics, *Cissampelos mucromata* roots, *Senecio lyratipartitus* leaves and *Croton macrostachys* leaves. In conclusion, the author makes a plea for increased inter-institutional cooperation in the study of medicinal plants and, to facilitate this work, the establishment of zonal herbaria.

Minja, M.M.J. 1984. Utilization of medical plants in veterinary practice. In: *Proceedings of the 2nd Tanzania Veterinary Association Scientific Conference. Vol. 2.* Arusha, Tanzania, 4–6 December, 1984. Tanzania Veterinary Association, Sokoine University, Faculty of Veterinary Medicine, Morogoro, Tanzania. Pp. 257–263.

Based on a field survey and 13 publications, this paper mentions seven plants used to treat livestock diseases in Tanzania, plus pharmacological research on some of these plants. The survey showed that traditional remedies were successful in treating cases of generalized debility, helminthosis, loss of milk, infertility, wounds, afterbirth retention, bloat, diarrhoea and snake bite.

Minja, M.M.J. 1994. Medicinal plants used in the promotion of animal health in Tanzania. In: Kakule Kasonia and Michel Ansay (eds). *Métissages en Santé Animale de Madagascar à Haïti: Actes du Séminaire d'Ethnopharmacopée Vétérinaire 'KAGALA', un Partage de Savoirs Burkina-Faso, Ouagadougou, 15–22 Avril 1993.* Presses Universitaires de Namur, Namur, Belgium. Pp. 336–364.

In developing countries like Tanzania, 'herbalists play a crucial role in the healthcare system for both humans and animals. . . . in the rural areas, when an animal falls sick a herbalist is consulted first, and only in case of failure a veterinarian is sought for, who . . . may be miles away' (p. 336). Between 1991 and 1992, renowned herbalists interviewed in three regions of Tanzania (Arusha, Kilimanjaro and Mbeya) cited 103 plant species of 48 botanical families for the cure of 38 animal diseases. Among the livestock diseases that Tanzanian herbalists combat with medicinal plants, the most frequent are gastrointestinal disorders, followed by helminthosis, wounds and urethral infections. The most popular plant part used is leaves (66 out of 117 cases), followed by roots (32), bark (11), seeds (6), whole plants (5) and fruit (1). Doses varied greatly across herbalists. In general, however, herbalists prescribed preparations they knew contained toxic plants in lower doses. For other prescriptions, herbalists took pains to emphasize their safety, even if stockraisers were to overdose with them. In evidence of their confidence in the safety of most of their medicines, herbalists often chew and swallow some themselves to demonstrate. Scores of herbalists' treatments for ruminants and poultry are presented in a 14-page annex to this article, along with the interview guide administered to healer-interviewees. For each treatment the following are noted: plant family and species; the reporting healer's village and district; plant parts used, their preparation and mode of administration; herbalists' mention of human uses of the same remedy; and references to the plant and its properties and uses in published pharmacological literature. One remedy cited in the text consists of spraying powdered *Acacia amythethophylla* Steud and/or *Acacia stulhmannii* Brenan root on the ground near kraals to repel snakes. A treatment for pinkeye is to place *Ocimum gratissimum* seeds in the conjuctival sac until they are washed away by tears. Besides all the usual modes, herbalists often administer medicinal plants via massage, fumigation and smoke inhalation.

Minja, M.M.J. 1998. The Maasai's role in the conservation of eco-systems through widespread practice of ethnoveterinary medicine. Paper presented to the Pastoralists' NGOs Workshop, organized by the Journalists Environmental Association of Tanzania in collaboration with Panos Eastern Africa. Arusha, Tanzania. 10 pp.

Maasai pastoralists of East Africa are famed for their profound ethnomedical knowledge and they enjoy ratios of local healers to human population of between 1:56 and 1:40. Known as *laibons*, the same healers generally treat livestock as well. This paper reports some of the findings from an EVK survey conducted in Tanzania's Simanjiro District by Vetaid teams in collaboration with national research institutes and herbaria plus the Simanjiro Animal Health Learning Centre and local NGOs. While the survey revealed a large number of ethnoveterinary practices, this paper focuses on ethnodiagnoses and ethnomedical action only for the livestock ills that key informants in at least 50% of the survey villages reported as being confidently controlled or cured with EVM. These ills included FMD, ephemeral fever, blackquarter, pyometra [peri-natal and natal difficulties], red-water/babesiosis, tetanus, calf scours, volvulus [twisted bowel], poisoning and infestations of worms, ticks, fleas or leeches. In dealing with these ailments, Maasai have recourse to: numerous botanicals (not yet identified by their Latin names) and other *materia medica* (salt, sodium bicarbonate, honey, ash, urine, muscle) administered in oral, topical and anal prescriptions; surgery, including cautery and phlebotomy; and management interventions. The latter span quarantine, herd dispersal, enforced rest, kraal hygiene, day-long sun baths, manual destruction of ticks, avoidance of places infested with poisonous insects and plants, gradual introduction of stock onto new pastures and prevention of stampedes by keeping a sharp lookout for wild animals and stemming thirsty herds' rush for water. Maasai also prepare homemade vaccines. For blackquarter (for which they have no ethnotherapies), a leg muscle from an animal dead of this disease is boiled in water for 10 hours, along with certain medicinal leaves, buds and fruits. After cooling and straining, the filtrate is administered via intramuscular injection to the whole herd in the amount of 1 cc per animal regardless of liveweight. Other observations of interest are the following. Homemade tick and flea repellents are applied strategically to the anatomical sites most attractive to these pests, such as around the anus, on the dewlap and the tip of the tail and inside the ears. Especially for pyometra, ethnoveterinary treatments mirror those for humans. The author notes that respondents willingly and freely shared their EVK and demonstrated striking diagnostic abilities based on their knowledge of clinical signs.

Mishra, Sunita, Vidyanath Jha and Shaktinath Jha. 1996. Plants in ethno-veterinary practices in Darbhanga (North Bihar). In: S.K. Jain (ed.). *Ethnobiology in Human Welfare.* Deep Publications, New Delhi, India. Pp. 189–193.

A survey of farmers, cattlemen, housewives and veterinarians in 20 villages of one district in India revealed that they all have recourse to a range of plant-based home remedies to treat livestock. The findings reported here span nearly two-score plant species and about two dozen animal ills. The data are organized in a table listing: name or general description of the ailment; where known, Latin plant name; vulgar plant name and parts used; and mode of usage. The authors note that many of the preparations reported here are already well-recognized and utilized in modern (especially human) medicine. Somes examples are: for dysentery in poultry mix wheat flour, garlic pods and mustard oil together and feed to the fowl; for coughs, cold and fever in cattle and buffalo crushed pepper with mustard oil is either fed or put into the animals' ears.

Moktan, D., B.K. Mitchelhill and Y.R. Joshi. 1990. *Village Animal Health Workers in the Koshi Hills (an Evaluation Report).* PAC Working Paper No. 4. Pakhribas Agricultural Centre, Dhankuta District, Koshi Zone, Nepal. 65 pp.

In describing the design and functioning of the above-referenced paravet programme in Nepal, this report notes that farmers' assessments of the diseases most requiring formal veterinary attention in their cattle, buffalo, sheep, goats, pigs and chickens differed in many respects from district veterinary officers' and technicians'. Also, veterinary personnel have difficulty dealing with farmers' locally recognized and defined disease syndromes. Finally, farmers and veterinarians part ways on whether they respectively consider therapeutic or prophylactic measures most needful.

Momha, Catherine, Omer Songwe and Brigitte Sunjo. 1998. HPI: A pace setter in ethnovet medicine. *La Voix du Paysan English* 35: 14–15.

This interview with an HPI/Cameroon Director describes how this PVO first began its EVM work in Bui District with Fulani pastoralists, assuming that local farmers would have little or no EVK. But this assumption proved wrong. In consequence, HPI brought the two groups together to describe the names of plants they use for which symptoms of livestock disease and how long it takes the animals to recover after ethnoveterinary treatment. Veterinarians assisted this process by providing scientific identification of the diseases stockraisers described. As a result of this exercise, nearly 300 medicinal plants were identified and investigation of some prescriptions' effectiveness was begun. An early study found a two-plant dewormer and a coccidiosis treatment that seemed to work well. Also mentioned in this interview are a number of preventive treatments. In 1994 localized Ethnoveterinary Councils were created to apply and disseminate EVK more widely; and participating HPI stockraisers were encouraged to grow 4 × 5 m backyard gardens of medicinal plants and to organize exchange visits amongst themselves. Plans are now underway to establish an ethnoveterinary pharmacy where people can learn about and purchase such botanicals.

Monod, Théodore. 1975. Introduction. In: Théodore Monod (ed.). *Pastoralism in Tropical Africa: Studies Presented and Discussed at the XIIIth International African Seminar, Niamey, December 1972.* Oxford University Press, London, UK. Pp. 8–98.

In the appendix to the introduction of this anthology, the author briefly reviews some of the husbandry measures and related activities, such as weaning methods, that are employed by different pastoral societies in Africa. For example, a thorny liana is attached to the calf's nose. Every time it wants to suckle from its mother, it pricks the dam, who pushes the calf away.

Monreal, Angel. 1989. Uso del catnip (*Nepeta catarea*) en el manejo de los gatos. In: Gerardo López Buendía (ed.). ***Memorias: Segunda Jornada sobre Herbolaria Medicinal en Medicina Veterinaria.*** Universidad Nacional Autónoma de México, Facultad de Medicina Veterinaria y Zootecnia, Coordinación de Educación Continua, México DF, México. Pp. 136–139.

Herbs and other plants provide vital vitamin, mineral and fibre complements to carnivorous diets, like those of cats. However, the use of medicinal plants to modify animal behaviours has been little studied. This paper discusses some of the ways that catnip can be used to produce desirable behaviours in cats.

Monteil, Vincent. n.d. ***Essai sur le Chameau au Sahara Occidental.*** Études Mauritaniennes No. 2. Institut Fondamental d'Afrique Noir (IFAN), St Louis du Sénégal, Mauritania. Project supported by the Centre National de la Recherche Scientifique, Paris, France. 131 pp.

This treatise on the Saharan camel describes camel anatomy, ailments and traditional treatments as used by the herders of Arabia, Syria, Egypt, Sudan, Tunisia, Algeria and Mauritania. Treatments include cauterization, incision, bloodletting, debriding washing, topical applications (including poultices), fumigation, surgery and nasal drenching. This last technique employs a teapot to pour medicinal liquids into camels' nostrils and thus down the oesophagus, also ewe's milk can be squirted directly from the ewe's teat into a sick camel's nostrils.

Morales, Edmundo. 1995. ***The Guinea Pig: Healing, Food and Ritual in the Andes.*** University of Arizona Press, Tucson, Arizona, USA. 177 pp.

Drawing upon the author's firsthand field experiences in Bolivia, Colombia, Ecuador and Peru as well as on numerous secondary sources in anthropology, animal science, archaeology, etc., this book focuses on the myriad practical, social and religious uses of the guinea pig or [hereafter] *cuy* (*Cavia porcellus*) in Andean life, both in past and especially today. The *cuy* was probably domesticated about 5000 B.C. on the Andean Altiplano, where wild guinea pigs are still to be found. Consumption of the *cuy*'s delicious high-protein low-fat meat eventually spread to coastal South America as well, at least by the 1st century B.C. Other parts of Latin America, and now the world, have since taken up *cuy* husbandry; immigrants in the public parks of New York City can be seen barbecuing the animal for picnics! Throughout the Andes today, almost every family – mestizo as well as Indian – keeps at least 20 *cuy*s. Traditionally, women and children own and raise the family *cuy*s, which they can dispose of at their discretion. The animals are kept in the kitchen, where they are warmed by the cookfire, protected from ectoparasites by the smoke and fed on fallen scraps of food, vegetable peelings, a little grain, corn-beer dregs and gathered grasses and other vegetation. Unlike larger animals, *cuy*s and also poultry receive no personal names. Rather, they are identified by physical characteristics. To say that a person has no *cuy*s is to say that she/he lives in the most abysmal poverty imaginable. When a woman lacks a suitable breeding male, however, she may borrow or rent one from a relative or neighbour. Rental is repaid in kind, by a pup from the resulting litter. Traditionally, *cuy*s were raised exclusively as a highly prized festival meat and their manure was used on the kitchen garden. Only recently has the species become a major market commodity. In the 1960s, scientists realized that *cuy*s were shrinking in size because people were selling or consuming their biggest animals in response to the burgeoning demand for meat plus the fact that *cuys* are one of the few agricultural commodities in the region to enjoy a stable market price. Thus, in Peru a breeding programme was begun that produced 2 kg animals by the early 1970s and additional research was undertaken on reproduction and nutrition. Nowadays, backed by such research, large industrial *cuy* operations are found in all the Andean countries except Bolivia and commercial forage-growing operations to support the industry have also appeared. While traditional *cuy* raisers and a new category of mid-sized producers have also benefitted from increased scientific attention to this species, the author expresses profound concern that 'populations that have preserved the *cuy* germ plasm for centuries will most likely lose control of it' (p. xxiii). As he witnessed for a *cuy* project in Ecuador, within the space of only 2 years people had replaced all their original stock with scientifically improved breeds. Moreover, 'the significant cultural traditions that have grown around the *cuy* will be lost to the capitalist economy ... The drive to integrate indigenous peoples into the modern market economy has led Latin American governments to implement development policies that are aggressively changing traditions and values in the Andes' (ibid.). For example, a *cuy* production project for women in Colombia proved so successful that local men tried to take over all the profits while leaving women to do the work. In addition, the widescale commercialization of *cuys* has eroded the species' rich and ancient role in cementing human social relations via gifting and exchange. At the same time, increased commercial marketing can chip away at traditional market-partner relationships, exposing producers to more exploitative terms of trade. And as *cuy* prices to the end-consumer inflate, the many medical treatments, sacrifices and rituals of all ilk in which *cuys* are traditionally employed become more dear and may even have to be foregone by poor people – thus laying them open to all manner of illness and misfortune. Nevertheless, the author sees great potential for improving the lives of the Andean poor via culturally sensitive and popularly led *cuy* development.

Moran, Katy. 1986. ***Traditional Elephant Management in Sri Lanka: The Use of Applied Anthropology.*** MS degree paper, Anthropology, American University, Washington, DC, USA. 103 pp.

This study describes traditional elephant management in Sri Lanka, including its history and associated cultural patterns and economics, plus the technology used in taming and training. Keepers have a special tool, the *ankus*, with which they prod nerve centres near the surface of the elephants' skin. The keepers know and utilize eight different centres in order to control aggressive animals. The pressure exerted with the *ankus* depends on the degree of aggressiveness, but too heavy a pressure can lame the elephant. Keepers use the *ankus* mainly when training an elephant. It is seldom employed on tame animals unless they run amok.

Morgan, George Robert. 1981. 'Sugar bowls' (*Clematis hirsutissima*): A horse restorative of the Nez Perces. ***Journal of Ethnopharmacology*** 4: 117–120.

Nez Percé Indians of the northwestern US traditionally used the roots of *Clematis* spp. as a restorative for horses that had been run or raced to the point of collapse. A root from which the bark has been scraped is briefly inserted into the patient's nostrils. Reportedly, the horse arises almost immediately, albeit with some trembling or convulsions. It is then led into water and bathed, after which it is completely normal and grazes peacefully with the rest of the herd. Similarly, Teton Sioux gave their tired mounts a restoring snuff of dried and powdered *Clematis* root. In essence a sort of smelling salts for exhausted horses, the root clearly seems to have had powerful CNS effects. Also documented in this article are various other plants historically used by North American Indian tribes to improve their horses' speed and/or stamina. To these ends, Omaha and Ponca prepared a horse tonic from *Silphium lacinatum*. Omaha also chewed the corms of *Laciniaria scariosa* L., Hill and then blew them into horses' nostrils. An Omaha horse snuff consisted of dried *Acorus calamus* L. rhizomes. Various preparations of *Clematis* roots, leaves and whole plants also figured in many tribes' ethnomedicine for humans, e.g. as anti-itching treatments, headache cures and stimulants.

Morgan, W.T.W. 1981. Ethnobotany of the Turkana: Use of plants by a pastoral people and their livestock in Kenya. *Economic Botany* 35(1): 96–130.

Plants used by Turkana pastoralists in Kenya can be categorized according to their human-nutritional, medical, pastoral and miscellaneous domestic uses. Some 67 plants of medical value were recorded, including five species for delousing humans and livestock: *Commicarpus plumbagineus, Jasminum fluminense, Celosia schwe-infurthiana, Celosia stuhlmanniana* and *Adenium obesum*. Wounds are dressed with *Caralluma somalica* sap. Placed at either side of the kraal entrance, the sap also protects animals from theft or witchcraft. Camels with coughs are given a *Calotropis procera* drench. *Pseudosopubia hildebrandtii* is tied to the tails of she-camels or cows who refuse their young.

Morna, Colleen Lowe, Grace Gikaru and Femi Ajayi. 1990. Farmers fight pests the natural way. *African Farmer* Nov: 28–33.

Natural pesticides for crops and livestock are discussed in this article. A mixture of boiled tobacco and soap brushed on the hides of tick-infested sheep, cattle and goats once a week for 2 to 3 weeks reportedly serves as an effective acaricide.

Morkramer, Gerd. 1990. Nutzungssyteme der Tierhaltung in Nord-Benin. In: Horst S.H. Seifert, Paul L.G. Vlek and H.-J. Weidelt (eds). *Tierhaltung im Sahel. Symposium 26–27 Oktober 1989.* Göttinger Beiträge zur Land-und Forstwirschaft in den Tropen und Subtropen, Heft 51. Forschungs- und Studienzentrum der Agrar- und Forstwissenschaften der Tropen und Subtropen, Georg-August-Universität Göttingen, Germany. Pp. 141–152.

Animal production systems in northern Benin fall into three categories: extensive pastoralism, agropastoralism and farming systems that incorporate some cattle. But Fulani agropastoralists manage the majority of the region's cattle. About 85% of the Fulani interviewed indicated that they undertake long-distance transhumance. They do so mainly because of dry-season fodder and water shortages rather than because of trypanosomosis, since the tsetse fly is ubiquitous and since most of their animals are trypanotolerant. Because other groups' expanding cultivation has encroached on Fulani's traditional grazing grounds, more and more Fulani house-holds now also transhume during the rainy season, to marginal areas. The increased labour entailed by this added transhumance makes it difficult for agropastoralists to continue their cropping. At the same time, pastoralists' and agropastoralists' stockraising faces fresh challenges: growing scarcity of good forage; restricted

access to water points and salt-cure areas, as more and more fields bisect their
migration routes; and as a result of poorer animal nutrition, lower calving rates and
higher losses to disease. The latter factors influence herd structure, encouraging
Fulani to keep as many female animals as possible in an effort to maximize milk
production and maintain herd size. Studies from other regions indicate that trans-
humants would be willing to adopt other production systems, if they are offered
acceptable alternatives, because their migrations now entail such hard work and
high risks. GTZ has launched an integrated project in Atacora to address these
problems.

Morren Jr., George E.B. 1986. *The Miyanmin: Human Ecology of a Papua New
Guinea Society.* UMI Research Press, Ann Arbor, Michigan, USA.

Pages 88–89 of this ethnography describe Miyanmin pig husbandry. The Miyanmin
castrate male pigs by cauterizing the testes when the pigs are very young. They also
dock [amputate] the tails of all piglets. Sows mate with wild boars in the bush. Piglets
are taken away from the sow soon after birth and are hand-fed with cooked taro. This
practice imprints the piglets on the woman caring for them and prevents them from
becoming feral. The Miyanmin also use this method to domesticate wild piglets.
According to the author, piglet mortality is high.

Morvan, Hervé and Josef Vercruysse. 1978. Vocabulaire des maladies du bétail
en langue Fulfuldé chez les Mbororo de l'Empire Centrafricain. *Journal
d'Agriculture Tropicale et de Botanique Appliquée* 25(2): 111–118.

In the spirit of better informing scientists about pastoralists' veterinary concerns,
this article categorizes the disease definitions and classifications of two groups of
central African Fulani (Mbororo and Fulße) in their native language, Fulfulde. The
authors give the Fulfulde term, the French scientific name where identifiable and
the symptoms cited by stockowners for 47 ailments. The 47 are classed into six
categories: viral; bacterial; parasitic, subdivided by internal and external; fungal;
diverse general terms; and undetermined ills. [Unfortunately, no literal translations
of the indigenous names are provided.] All but the latter category are based on
direct clinical examination of animals with the condition described by the Fulfulde
term. The authors note a general ignorance or disinterest among these pastoralists
as to the aetiology of their animals' ills. Again, however, they emphasize the importance of being able to communicate correctly with stockowners in order to understand and address local veterinary health needs.

Moscoso Castilla, Mariano. 1953 [1942]. *Secretos Medicinales de la Flora
Peruana y Guía de la Maternidad* (2nd edition). Tipografía Americana, Cuzco,
Perú. 262 pp.

Written by a renowned Cuzqueñan herbalist, this volume is designed as a guide to
human, and especially maternal, ethnomedicine of Peru. However, page 261 of the
index conveniently lists ten plants or other substances used in ethnoveterinary
treatments. These include: aloe juice or *capulí*-wood ash with alum and sulphur to
disinfect and cure wounds rapidly and prevent their parasitic infestation; sulphur in
water or pig fat to fatten animals; *barbasco* to treat lice and mange in herd animals;
mocco-mocco, also known as *matico*, to treat saddle sores; *sebadilla*, an alkaloid-
laden plant, to combat ectoparasitism; an infusion of a twig of *accana* with soap

and cooking oil to treat bloat and colics in herd animals; an infusion of pulverized *accana* leaf along with a spoonful of *khechincha* and some *kusmayllu* juice in fermented human urine to combat pulmonary parasites in sheep; and the herb *cicihuataa* to relieve pleurisy.

Mourier-Ballon, M. 1983. *Essai d'Ethnobotanique en Bas-Dauphiné.* Third-cycle doctoral thesis, Université de Lyon II, France.

Unavailable for review.

Mpande, Roger. 1993. Africa case studies. *Appropriate Technology* 20(2): 22.

Tonga of north-western Zimbabwe administer concentrated tamarind liquid for gastrointestinal disorders in humans, but they may also add it to animals' drinking-water as a cure for trypanosomosis.

Mukherjee, Reena and Mahesh Chander. 1997. Women and livestock health: An insight into ethnoveterinary medicine from hills [sic] of Uttar Pradesh. Paper presented to the International Conference on Creativity and Innovation at Grassroots for Sustainable Natural Resource Management, 11–14 January, Ahmedabad, India. 3 pp.

An ethnoveterinary survey in the hill regions of Uttar Pradesh found that livestock are normally treated using traditional methods. Indeed, elders in some communities prefer ethnoveterinary to modern medicines, even when the latter are available cheaply. The study also notes that people do not share their knowledge of traditional methods because they believe that doing so would render the treatments ineffective. But people are more inclined to share their EVK if researchers live with them in their communities and work alongside them for some time. Overall, women in rural areas are less reticent in this regard than men. The authors attribute this last finding in part to the fact that the researchers were also female. But they also feel that women would be the more appropriate participants in EVM R&D in this hill area.

Müller, Julius Otto. 1990. Risiken der Sedentarisierung und Transhumanz-Verhalten 'après-forage' von Peul-Nomaden im Koya (Nord-Senegal). In: Horst S.H. Seifert, Paul L.G. Vlek and H.-J. Weidelt (eds). *Tierhaltung im Sahel. Symposium 26–27 Oktober 1989.* Göttinger Beiträge zur Land-und Forstwirschaft in den Tropen und Subtropen, Heft 51. Forschungs- und Studienzentrum der Agrar- und Forstwissenschaften der Tropen und Subtropen, Georg-August-Universität Göttingen, Germany. Pp. 111–122.

Digging new wells in northern Senegal caused pastoralists to settle near the wells where, at first, their herds increased. But livestock diseases such as *maladie des forages* or 'well disease', caused by the bacterium *Clostridium botulinum*, also then increased. As a result, transhumance may again be on the rise, as herders seek to escape the risks connected with sedentarization. Discussions with herders revealed ten reasons for transhumance. A number of these pertain to animal nutrition and health, i.e.: lack of fodder or of certain forages; avoidance of certain diseases; overutilization of pastures; poor-quality well water; watering problems due to mismanagement of wells; animals' need for salt cures; and fires that destroy large areas of pasture.

Mulvany, Patrick and Francis Njeru. 1993. Makueni's *wasaidizi* – Care in the community. *Appropriate Technology* 19(4): 25.

In describing the start-up of an ITDG paravet programme among WaKamba farmers of Kenya's Makueni District, the authors note that the poorest stockraisers in the service area may be unable to afford even paravets' modest fees and the commercial drugs they sell. The authors suggest that a possible solution to this problem may be to popularize traditional livestock remedies.

Mundy, Paul and Evelyn Mathias. 1999. Participatory workshops to produce information materials on ethnoveterinary medicine. In: E. Mathias, D.V. Rangnekar and C.M. McCorkle, with M. Martin (eds). *Ethnoveterinary Medicine: Alternatives for Livestock Development – Proceedings of an International Conference Held in Pune, India, 4–6 November 1997. Volume 1: Selected Papers.* BAIF Development Research Foundation, Pune, India. Pp. 78–87.

This paper describes a process employed in Africa and Asia to document, validate and publish EVK in the form of a desktop-published manual that field workers can use. The process brings together local livestock healers, scientists, NGO and extension staff in a workshop to present, discuss and revise manuscripts on specific livestock health problems and their EVM solutions, for compilation in a practical field manual. The workshop provides an opportunity for scientists to validate ethnoveterinary practices, since they are able to discuss details of each practice with the local specialists who use it, compare it with standard veterinary methods and judge its applicability and effectiveness based on their own experiences, observations and knowledge of the scientific literature. This approach is also an excellent way to interlink research, extension and the field, in that scientists learn of EVM techniques they may be interested to investigate via clinical trials or other methods; and scientific knowledge is translated into a form that extensionists and stockraisers can use. A team of editors, artists and computer personnel assist the workshop participants in revising, illustrating and desktop-publishing their output. By the end of a two-week workshop, near-camera-ready material for a 200-page manual can be ready. The method can also be adapted for use at the field level. In Kenya, for example, a group of Luo practitioners are developing an ethnoveterinary manual for Luoland. Such manuals have been elaborated for other agricultural topics and then adapted and translated into various languages in Africa, Latin America, Asia and the Pacific simply by disseminating the original computerized disc of the manual *gratis* to NGOs and other development agencies, who then modify it according to their needs and circumstances.

Murdiati, Tri Budhi. 1991. Traditional veterinary medicine for small ruminants in West Java. In: E. Mathias-Mundy and Tri Budhi Murdiati (eds). *Traditional Veterinary Medicine for Small Ruminants in Java.* Indonesian Small Ruminant Network, SR-CRSP, Central Research Institute for Animal Science, Agency for Agricultural Research and Development, Bogor, Indonesia. Pp. 5–11.

A survey of traditional medicine for small ruminants collected 37 prescriptions from 22 farmers in six villages of West Java. The prescriptions are compounded of one to four ingredients comprising local plant parts and juices from, e.g., banana, cassava, coconut, ginger, guava, hibiscus, jackfruit, papaya, potatoes, tamarind, turmeric and more. Other ingredients include everyday items such as salt, sugar, shrimp paste, sweet soy sauce, eggs, honey, human urine, used engine oil and sulphur. The prescriptions are used to treat diarrhoea, scabies, endoparasitism, eye diseases, bloat, inappetence and insect worry. Bloat has four different treatments: drenching with a bamboo-leaf preparation or with coconut oil, covering the belly with a wet black cloth and inserting a stalk of papaya leaf into the anus. A scabicide consisted of ashes from burning an Islamic hat. Farmers reported they seldom seek veterinary help from others, whether local healers or rarely-available veterinarians. The author notes that most of the ethnobotanicals are also used in human ethnomedicine in the region.

Murdiati, Tri Budhi. 1994. Personal communication to C.M. McCorkle at the 11–25 July Workshop to Produce an Ethnoveterinary Information Kit. IIRR, Silang, Cavite, Philippines.

In 1994, a set of on-station trials was mounted in Indonesia to validate a local Javanese treatment for ovine endoparasitism. The treatment consists merely of periodically feeding the sheep whole, immature papaya fruits. Based on prior experiments and review of the pharmacological literature, scientists knew the key parasiticidal constituent resided mainly in the fruit sap. So they collected and administered only the sap itself, instead of following farmers' practice of feeding the whole fruit. The result? In a matter of hours, 80% of the sheep in the high-dosage experimental group and 20% in the medium-dosage group died of acute poisoning.

Murdiati, T.B., Beriajaya and Isbandi. 1994. Penggunaan obat tradisional dalam kaitannya dengan gangguan pencernaan pada domba dan kambing. Paper presented to the Kongres XII dan Konferensi Ilmiah Nasional VI Perhimpunan Dokter Hewan Indonesia, 21–24 November, Surabaya, Indonesia. 12 pp.

Interviews with 68 male and female respondents from one village in West Java, Indonesia revealed that farmers there use 16 different plants to treat small ruminant gastrointestinal conditions such as diarrhoea, worms, inappetence and thinness. The botanical items most frequently mentioned were leaves of *Antidesma bunius*, *Cyclophorus nummularifolius* and *Artocarpus heterophyllus* plus *Zingiber aromaticum* rhizome. [See also Mathias-Mundy et al. 1992 and Wahyuni et al. 1992.]

Murdiati, T.B. and J.S. Manurung. 1991. Uji daun ketepeng (*Cassia alata* L.) untuk pengobatan penyakit kulit (*Psoroptes cuniculi*) pada kelinci. **Penyakit Hewan** 23(41): 50–52.

Based on a traditional Indonesian remedy for scabies in small ruminants, this study tested the efficacy of *ketepeng* (*Cassia alata*) leaves for similarly treating psoroptic mange in rabbits. Ten New Zealand rabbits, naturally infected with *Psoroptes cuniculi* mites in both ears, were randomly divided into a treatment and a control group. The former was treated weekly with a 50% aqueous suspension of *ketepeng* leaves. Scabs collected from both ears were investigated for live mites. After 4 weeks, the number of live mites significantly decreased in the treatment compared to the control group ($P < 0.05$). The number of scabs as well as the area infected also declined. The results suggest that *ketepeng* is effective against psoroptic mange in rabbits.

Murdiati, Tri Budhi and Zakhia Muhajan. 1991. Bibliography on traditional veterinary medicine in Indonesia. In: E. Mathias-Mundy and Tri Budhi Murdiati (eds). *Traditional Veterinary Medicine for Small Ruminants in Java.* Indonesian Small Ruminant Network, SR-CRSP, Central Research Institute for Animal Science, Agency for Agricultural Research and Development, Bogor, Indonesia. Pp. 39–49.

In addition to the products of a large number of *jamu* (traditional medicine) factories, numerous publications demonstrate that the value of traditional medicine has long been recognized in Indonesia. However, the bulk of such products and literature centre on human ethnomedicine. This chapter instead offers 19 abstracts of references of interest for EVM in Indonesia. Seven of the 19 that deal more or less directly with farm animals are reproduced in the present bibliography. The remaining 12 mainly report on pharmacological tests of botanical preparations in laboratory mice.

Murdiati, Tri Budhi and Suhardono. 1990. *Bibliografi Tanaman Obat di Indonesia.* Research Institute for Animal Disease (Balai Penelitian Veteriner), Bogor, Indonesia. 45 pp.

This annotated bibliography summarizes approximately 100 journal articles and conference papers on pharmacological studies of Indonesian medicinal plants plus some 30 books and unpublished manuscripts on different aspects of traditional herbal medicine. A number of the plants discussed are known to be used in Indonesian EVM. Examples are garlic, onion, papaya and *Cassia alata*.

Murdiati, T.B., Sri Wahyuni, H. Sangat-Roemantyo and E. Mathias-Mundy. 1992. Tumbuhan dalam pengobatan etnoveteriner pada ternak ruminansia kecil di Jawa Barat. *Prosiding Seminar dan Lokakarya Nasional Etnobotani, Bogor, Indonesia, 19–20 February 1992.* Pp. 67–70.

Interviews in a village just outside Bogor, Indonesia revealed that smallholders employ some 50 plant species in their ethnomedicines for sheep and goats. *Huni* (*Antidesma bunius*) leaves are the most frequently used, followed by *deduitan* (*Cyclophorus nummularifolius*) leaves and the fruit pulp of *tamarind* (*Tamarindus indicus*). This study demonstrates that EVM is just as important among peri-urban dwellers as it is in remote rural areas. [See also Mathias-Mundy et al. 1992 and Wahyuni et al. 1992.]

Mursof, E.P. 1990. *Pengendalian* Ascaridia galli *Pada Ayam Petelur Dengan Getah Pepaya* (Carica papaya Linn.). MSc thesis, Fakultas Pascasarjana, Bogor Agricultural University, Bogor, Indonesia. 53 pp.

Papaya sap is used in a variety of traditional veterinary medicines in Asia. In this study, the efficacy of sap from immature papaya against *Ascaridia galli* was tested in 15 groups of laying hens. Each group consisted of four 18-week-old birds. Thirteen of the groups were artificially infected with *Ascaridia galli*, while two were left uninfected. Two of the 13 infected groups did not receive any treatment, while the remaining groups were orally treated with different dosages of a 20%

aqueous solution of the sap. Body weight and egg production increased significantly in all treatment groups, but the best results were obtained at a dosage of 1120 mg/animal of sap solution. More than 1500 mg/animal were required for the solution to be lethal.

Mustapha, A.A. and M.T. Fawi. 1966. Control of disease as prerequisite to development. *Sudan Journal of Veterinary Science and Animal Husbandry* 7(2): 46–73.

In discussing the control of trypanosomosis in Sudan, this article notes that cattle-owners have two different names for the disease according to whether it is contracted inside or outside known tsetse-fly-infested areas. The only breed of cattle to survive inside such areas is the Nuba dwarf Koalib, which thus appears to be trypano-tolerant.

Mwangi, E.N. 1996. The role of women in animal husbandry: The Kenyan perspective. In: Karl-Hans Zessin (ed.). *Livestock Production and Diseases in the Tropics: Livestock Production and Human Welfare. Proceedings of the VIII International Conference of Institutions of Tropical Veterinary Medicine held from the 25 to 29 September, 1995 in Berlin, Germany.* Volume II. Deutsche Stiftung für Internationale Entwicklung, Zentralstelle für Ernährung und Landwirtschaft, Feldafing, Germany. Pp. 599–603.

In many Kenyan farming systems, women play a key role in gathering and/or growing fodder and presenting it to livestock. This conference paper further notes that Maasai women have long prepared and applied homemade fly repellents to livestock. These treatments consist of smearing the animals with dung ash or with a concoction of water, milk and tobacco. Maasai women also burn special plants at the homestead to keep flies away from the human and livestock residents. In central Kenya, women manually de-tick animals while milking, or they may apply kerosene to the ticks they discover. They also prepare and apply homemade acaricides made of tobacco leaves boiled with pepper and soap. Kenyan scientists' research has shown a similar preparation involving tobacco and sodium bicarbonate to be effective against ticks. In terms of their traditional roles, women are ideally placed to apply such techno-blended treatments.

Nahar, Zebun. 1986. *A Case Study of Aresa Begum of Bilaspur Village.* OFRD, Joydebpur, Bangladesh.

Six plants used by Bangladeshi villagers to treat colds, coughs and allergies of livestock are noted in this case study. [Abstract based on Gupta et al.'s 1990 annotated bibliography.]

Nair, R. Sabarinathan, S.V.M. Rao and S. Ramkumar. 1999. Perceptions of veterinarians on ethnoveterinary medicine. In: E. Mathias, D.V. Rangnekar and C.M. McCorkle, with M. Martin (eds). *Ethnoveterinary Medicine: Alternatives for Livestock Development – Proceedings of an International Conference Held in Pune, India, 4–6 November 1997. Volume 1: Selected Papers.* BAIF Development Research Foundation, Pune, India. Pp. 243–249.

Since 300 B.C., veterinary medicine has been practised in India, evolving through constant observation of animal ethology and trial-and-error applications of indigenous veterinary treatments. The resulting 'folk findings' have been handed down through the generations, making for a number of practices that are time-tested, environment-friendly, cost-effective, readily available and location-specific. Lately, scientists have become interested in understanding such indigenous technical knowledge and 'farmers' wisdom' in order to utilize it more widely or systematically in animal healthcare. For example, neem leaves, jaggery and areca nut have been found effective in controlling worm infestation. Other promising elements in ethnoveterinary pharmacopoeia include camphor, turmeric, eggwhite, pepper, lemon and ginger, which are widely used for animal ailments ranging from wounds, sprains, fractures, to gastrointestinal disorders. To preserve such knowledge and test, and through R&D expand, its usefulness in present-day systems of animal healthcare, more research is required.

Namada, A.T. 1997. Ethnoveterinary practice among the nomadic pastoralists of northern Kenya. Paper presented to the First International Conference on Ethnoveterinary Medicine: Alternatives for Livestock Development, Pune, India, 4–6 November 1997.

Camels play many vital roles in the life of Gabbra and other pastoralists of northern Kenya, who have a proverb to the effect that 'The camel is second only to God'. Thus it is little surprise that owners pay great attention to their camels' health. They have an extensive vocabulary for camel diseases. And their diagnostic abilities are such that neophyte veterinarians often turn to pastoralists for diagnostic help. Ethnoaetiologies span: for certain diseases, different types of flies or ticks; for orf, bad air; for coughs and pneumonias, contaminated water; in general, contaminated grass and malnutrition; and curses and the evil eye. The author classifies pastoralists' EVK into open versus closed, defined as knowledge that is widely held versus knowledge that is limited to only a few people and/or a specific lineage or clan. The latter is generally kept secret, although non-initiates can sometimes learn it for a price. Understandably, it cannot be found in any books, journal articles, or other publications. However, some 'open' EVK is documented in this conference paper, grouped according to ingredients or techniques. Of course, medicinal herbs of many sorts are used. Old engine oil, brake fluid and tar are employed, mainly for ectoparasitism. Fire or heat is administered with hot irons or stones. Melted sheep fat is applied for dermatomycosis and, mixed with *Commiphora erythraea* gum, for skin lesions. Fat is also administered orally for lameness and, in a sheep's-head soup, for coughs. Milk or ghee figure in wound and ringworm remedies; and plant poisoning is treated by feeding large quantities of camel milk to induce diarrhoea or by drenching with camel milk mixed with laundry detergent, liquid paraffin and castor oil to induce vomiting. Smoke and ash play various roles. Donkeys with strangles are made to inhale the smoke from burning their clipped manes, while also ingesting herbal preparation of onion or garlic. Ash is applied to neonates' navels; and animals with mastitis are positioned over hot ashes sprinkled with water for the steam to bathe the udder. A tick remover consists of kitchen ash mixed with pounded aloe leaves and paraffin or oil. A different tick remover is prepared from a heated paste of camel urine mixed with *C. erythraea* or *C. incisa* gum or resin. Camel urine is also mixed with salty soils to make a general insect repellent. Indeed, salt is a highly prized weapon in camel pastoralists' ethnoveterinary armoury, administered in drenches, washes, baths and topical applications for multiple disorders. Also popular is bleeding, whether from the jugular vein or by incising the skin tissue over swollen or bruised areas. Bleeding is believed to expel 'bad blood'. Some examples of surgical techniques among camel pastoralists of Sudan are: foetotomy; removal of third eyelid carcinoma using an acacia thorn and wooden splints; splinting fractures with bark; and tying the umbilical cord over a calf's back in order to stop bleeding and infection. Pastoralists also take many preventive measures. For instance, they burn accumulated cowdung and any bones lying about. The smoke drives away insects and the fire destroys ticks in the dung and infectious agents, like anthrax spores, in the bones. As a prophylaxis against ectoparasites, camels are taken for dust baths in salty soils. This paper concludes with listings of local disease names and medicinal plants.

NAO. 1998a. Chicks and ticks. *New Agriculturist On-line* 4: unpaginated (www.new-agri.co.uk/98-4/focuson/focuson6.html).

Taking a cue from longstanding and widespread stockraiser practice, researchers at the International Centre for Insect Physiology and Ecology are exploring environmentally safe yet effective methods of tick control. Chickens embody one such control. Scientists have found that within a matter of hours chickens can consume literally hundreds of ticks. Another type of control is the use of neem compounds, pioneered by Indian farmers. Yet a third is organized movement of livestock and poultry according to daily tick activity. Ticks show two diurnal activity peaks (one in the morning and another in the afternoon) and they tend to drop off animals at a specific time of day. As a result, farmers can control [and have done] tick infestations by avoiding grazing at certain times of the day. A blending of local and scientific knowledge could give farmers even greater control over ticks. For example, people could remove stock from pastures at the tick drop-off time and then attack the ticks in the pastures at that moment – whether by the timed release of scavenging chickens onto the pastures or by other means.

NAO. 1998b. Livestock genetic resources. *New Agriculturist On-line* 4: unpaginated (www.new-agri.co.uk/98-4/focuson/focuson10.html).

Farmers have an important role to play in livestock conservation programmes because they know the characteristics of their local breeds. Farmers have long selected or castrated for superior disease resistance, climate adaptation and productivity in their livestock. Around the world, farmers keep over 4500 breeds or strains of domestic animals of more than 40 species. As investigated and documented by organizations like ILRI and FAO, a number of these breeds may carry valuable disease-resistance genes. Examples are: the trypanotolerant N'Dama cattle of West Africa; Ethiopia's Horro and Menz breeds of sheep, which may be resistant to gastrointestinal parasites and which, moreover, are able to survive on very low-quality diets; and the endoparasite-resistant Red Maasai and possibly also Dorper sheep, both of coastal Kenya. Other farmer-developed breeds, like the Shami or 'Damascus' goats of Syria, are noteworthy for their high milk yield and prolificacy under adverse conditions. In Asia, studies are underway on unique breeds like the Taiwan Native Goat and the Chinese Goose. Unfortunately, nearly a third of the world's livestock breeds are currently at risk of disappearing, at an extinction rate of about six breeds per month! There is already far less genetic variation in domestic-animal as compared to plant-crop species. Hence the urgent need to foster scientific and public appreciation of traditional breeds and to support farmers in their stewardship of them via financial, scientific, technical and marketing assistance.

NAO. 1998c. Paravets and plants for animal healthcare. *New Agriculturist On-line* 4: unpaginated (www.new-agri.co.uk/98-4/focuson/focuson5.html).

In its work with paravet programmes in Mozambique and Somaliland, Vetaid has noticed that subsistence farmers in remote communities with little money or access to formal veterinary services of any kind rely on botanical treatments for livestock. In combination with good nutrition and disease prevention, plant-based medicines make for inexpensive animal healthcare. Several such medicines are noted in this short article: a wound poultice of fresh turmeric, guava and artemisia (mugwort) leaves; an anthelmintic drench of fresh betel nuts; and a drench of boiled camphor leaves to relieve cough and fever. While most such plants are found in the wild, Vetaid advises farmers to establish backyard gardens of the species they are most likely to need for livestock healthcare.

Narainswami, B.K. 1998. Ethnoveterinary medicine in India: Status, strategies for integrating it with research and education and methodology for promotion and development. In: E. Mathias, D.V. Rangnekar and C.M. McCorkle, with M. Martin (eds). *Ethnoveterinary Medicine: Alternatives for Livestock Development – Proceedings of an International Conference Held in Pune, India, 4–6 November 1997. Volume 2: Abstracts.* BAIF Development Research Foundation, Pune, India. Pp. 43–44.

India has a rich EVM heritage that sadly is not used properly in development. This is because of EVM's low status in the eyes of veterinarians and stockraisers due to the: lack of standardization of ethnoveterinary medicines, techniques and treatment schedules; inconvenience of preparing and/or administering some types of EVM; seasonal unavailability of certain *materia medica*; paucity of ethnoveterinary treatments against infectious epidemic and systemic diseases; dearth of studies on the economic viability of ethnoveterinary treatments; and general government inattention to EVM. Yet in modern-day India, Western-style veterinary medicine has also been called into question. It has resulted in the resurgence of some diseases; also, there is uncertainty about the components responsible for modern drugs' often-toxic effects; the costs of drugs and other veterinary supplies or infrastructure and of formal training programmes are becoming prohibitive; and veterinary researchers and extensionists are losing credibility with farmers because information from formal research has proved of limited practical relevance to farmers. Taken together, the foregoing factors suggest that there *is* a place for EVM, but that traditional and local practices of animal health and production need to be systematically explored, linking up with formal research. Before designing such an integrated R&D strategy, it is also necessary to determine in which contexts EVM is expected to operate and what may be the real economic gains of livestock farmers from ethnoveterinary as compared to Western treatments. To this end, the author makes the following, stepwise recommendations. Analyse the situation, identify the healthcare problems and possible solutions, decide on objectives and a plan of work, and execute the plan. Standardize ethnoveterinary practices, compare their efficacy with Western equivalents and then advocate only the proven practices. To change the knowledge, attitudes, skills of veterinarians, integrate the standardized and proven practices into college and university veterinary curricula. For extending EVM, also train skilled farmers and veterinary healers in these practices and set them to work as paraveterinarians. To help promote the practices, use individual, group and mass contact educational methods, including audiovisual aids and demonstrations with effective communication (see Narainswami et al.1988). Also back up these methods with management services to would-be farmer-adopters, such as technical advice on the preparation of ethnoveterinary treatments, credit for EVM and other inputs, marketing services, livestock insurance and subsidies for local-level ethnoveterinary programmes.

Narainswami, B.K., C. Resmy and N.K. Kulkarni. 1998. Effective communication for the promotion of ethnoveterinary medicine. In: E. Mathias, D.V. Rangnekar and C.M. McCorkle, with M. Martin (eds). *Ethnoveterinary Medicine: Alternatives for Livestock Development – Proceedings of an International Conference Held in Pune, India, 4–6 November 1997. Volume 2: Abstracts.* BAIF Development Research Foundation, Pune, India. P. 42.

For lack of effective communication, many useful ethnoveterinary practices that could be extended more widely are not reaching the livestock farmers who need them the most, i.e. those for whom Western-style drugs and services are unavailable or prohibitively expensive. Good communicators create shared understandings and impart knowledge in clear ways. To become effective communicators, promoters of EVM alternatives must familiarize themselves with the seven 'Cs' for effective communication: credibility – there must be a climate of belief and earnest desire for information; context – the situation must allow participation and feedback; content – the content must have meaning for the farmer; clarity – the message must be clear and simple and words must mean the same thing to the farmer and the developer/extensionist; channel – established channels of communication respected by farmers must be used; consistency – communication is an unending process that requires repetition to achieve penetration; and capability – this refers to people's availability for and habits of taking in information, their reading ability and their pre-existing knowledge. The promoter of EVM is actually a motivator who must be fully devoted to, identify with and have the confidence of farmers to be successful. Confidence can be won by the careful and gradual introduction of validated ethnoveterinary practices. Also required for effective communication are farmer and promoter cooperation with researchers, so as to convey farmers' real problems from the field to scientists and so as to keep promoters current on EVM findings.

Nass, Klaus Otto. 1990. Tierhaltung als Risikovorsorge und Naturzerstörer – Erfahrungen aus der praktischen Arbeit im Sahel. In: Horst S.H. Seifert, Paul L.G. Vlek and H.-J. Weidelt (eds). *Tierhaltung im Sahel. Symposium 26–27 Oktober 1989.* Göttinger Beiträge zur Land-und Forstwirtschaft in den Tropen und Subtropen, Heft 51. Forschungs- und Studienzentrum der Agrar- und Forstwissenschaften der Tropen und Subtropen, Georg-August-Universität Göttingen, Germany. Pp. 67–82.

Entitled 'Animal Production as Risk Reduction and Environmental Degradation – Experiences from Practical Work in the Sahel', this conference paper argues that Sahelians keep large herds as a form of food security. Especially during droughts, people are thus able to sell animals in order to buy foodgrain without compromising herd composition and future fertility. However, for many reasons, the per-head fodder base is decreasing, leading to increased livestock losses to disease. Under such conditions, animal production can no longer fulfil its food-security role. The author discusses the pros and cons of six alternatives for reducing herd size without prejudicing human well-being. The first is to improve animal health and quality through vaccination and veterinary services; but it is unclear whether such measures would reduce or augment herd size. Theoretically, a second option is bank savings accounts. But this option appears unworkable due to the lack or instability of banking institutions plus on-going inflation in the Sahel. Nor does a third strategy – that of storing millet as a form of wealth – seem viable because grain quality deteriorates over time and community as versus private storage schemes are problematic. A fourth idea is to restrict access to water and forage, as many traditional grazing systems once did. But this is difficult where, as in the Sahel, state controls are limited. For the same reason, a head tax on livestock is difficult; moreover, herders commonly report only 5% to 29% of their animals. A sixth solution might be to provide incentives for herders to plant and protect *Acacia senegalensis* trees, for example through guarantees to buy the gum arabic harvest at a good price. While animal densities in the Sahel need to be adapted to the available fodder, the author warns that stockraisers will keep smaller herds only if they are offered trustworthy alternatives for risk reduction.

National Research Council. 1981. *The Water Buffalo: New Prospects for an Underutilized Animal.* National Academy Press, Washington, DC, USA. 118 pp.

The domesticated water buffalo (*Bubalus bubalis*) hails from Asia and 97% of the species is still found there today. But buffalo have also been an important part of animal husbandry for centuries in Italy and Egypt as well as the Balkan nations, after Arabs brought these animals to the Near East about 600 A.D. Buffalo have since flourished in Brazil and other circum-Caribbean countries; and more recently they have been introduced to the South Pacific. Buffalo come in two basic varieties, Swamp and River, although there is also an identifiable Mediterranean strain. According to the authors, buffalo owners have rarely intervened in breeding. Only in India are there scientifically well-defined breeds. Although it is susceptible to most of the same diseases as cattle in the tropics, the buffalo appears to resist ticks and other ectoparasites, if only due to its wallowing; and healthy buffalo are seldom affected by warble flies or screwworms. Moreover, buffalo rarely suffer from foot diseases despite their affinity for swampy areas. The buffalo gives a rich milk that is higher in butterfat and nonfat solids than that of cattle. In India, buffalo milk is thus prized above all others and fetches a premium price. Its high fat content makes it especially good for processing into a wide variety of products. In much of Asia, the buffalo is prized also for its strength; it can pull not only agricultural equipment but also carts laden with several-ton loads. Besides drayage and field ploughing and harrowing, buffalo are also used for puddling clay for bricks, for racing and in Bulgaria, for clearing snow. Asians generally treat these gentle animals almost as pets; they are typically herded and managed by children and elderly women. Unfortunately, the largest and fastest-growing bulls that would be best for breeding are often castrated as draught animals or sent to slaughter. As a result, in some parts of Asia (notably Thailand and Indonesia) buffalo have been shrinking; they are down from a common maximum weight of 1000 kg to only 750 kg. Moreover, faced with burgeoning demand for meat on both national and international markets, buffalo populations in some countries are actually dwindling. This is the case in Thailand where, contrarily, demand for draught buffalo is on the rise as other sources of power become scarcer and more expensive. In the Philippines, butchers pay such high prices for buffalo meat that farmers sell them even their best breedstock. This volume goes on to extol the buffalo's many virtues and potential uses. A few more examples are: buffalo's tendency to use communal defaecation grounds, such that they are easily trained to avoid contaminating waterways; their ability to fend for themselves for months on end, returning docilely to work thereafter; the female's generosity with her milk, such that she will allow other buffalo calves and even adult animals to suckle. A telling quote is that of an old Taiwanese women, who explains 'To my family the buffalo is more important than I am. When I die, they'll weep for me; but if our buffalo dies, they may starve' (p. 110).

Ndamukong, K.J.N., M.M.H. Sewell and M.F. Asanji. 1987. Productivity of sheep and goats under three management systems at Bamenda, Cameroon. *Tropical Animal Health and Production* 21: 191–196.

This study compared sheep and goat productivity under two modern management regimes and one traditional system of stockraising in Cameroon. Findings revealed that goat growth rates in the traditional system outstripped those in the modern ones. The authors suggest this may be because the modern, paddocked systems did not permit goats to browse very much. Yet browsing reduces the chances of acquiring pasture-transmitted parasites.

Ndamukong, K.J.N., M.M.H. Sewell and M.F. Asanji. 1989a. Disease and mortality in small ruminants in the North West Province of Cameroon. *Tropical Animal Health and Production* 21: 191–196.

This study in Cameroon collected data on mortality, morbidity and the epidemiology of diseases among small ruminants, as well as information on their owners' diagnostic abilities and livestock health controls. Some 18% of stockraisers medicated their animals, whether with modern or traditional remedies. The latter included topical application of spent engine-oil or kerosene mixed with palm oil for the treatment of mange, soremouth (contagious ecthyma), wounds and ticks. Soot mixed with salt was fed for almost any ailment, but especially diarrhoea.

Ndamukong, K.J.N., M.M.H. Sewell and M.F. Asanji. 1989b. Management and productivity of small ruminants in the North West Province of Cameroon. *Tropical Animal Health and Production* 21: 109–119.

A study of sheep and goat management in Cameroon's North West Province found that approximately 20% of farmers wait until after 9:00 a.m. to turn their animals out to graze. Farmers explained that animals are more likely to consume snails and millipedes in still-dew-ridden pastures, which were therefore regarded as a health hazard.

Negron Alonso, Luís. 1966. *La Fiebre Aftosa: Crisis Insólita – El Caso de Vicos.* Thesis, Department of Anthropology, Universidad Nacional de San Antonio Abad del Cuzco, Perú. 89 pp. With English-language annex entitled 'The case of peasant acceptance of livestock immunization', by Luís Negron and H.F. Dobyns, 37 pp.

Conducted as part of the famous Cornell Peru Project in the 1950s and 1960s in the community of Vicos, Callejon de Huaylas, this study documents the socio-economic and cultural impacts of, plus peasants' response to, the first appearance of foot-and-mouth disease in their region. Vicosiños were baffled by the new disease's aetiology and they uncertainly adduced a number of possible causes, including: worms, heat, travellers from afar, a punishment by God, a falling comet or evil winds (both ancient Andean beliefs), airplane exhausts and the vengeance by sorcery of US Peace Corps volunteers who had departed the community. But fully 41% of interviewees were unable to name any cause. Given that this disease produces a fever, the ethnomedicine of Latin America prescribes 'cool' therapies. Peasants' first reaction therefore was to try to treat the epidemic with home remedies such as decoctions of barley, flax and squash; squash poultices; washes of fermented urine or citrus juice and salt; and a number of more idiosyncratic cures. Stockowners also moved their animals to higher, colder pastures in hopes of thus avoiding or assuaging contagion. Vicosiños initially resisted treatment with a Western commercial drug, which did not perform as promised. However, they came to accept preventive vaccination, the effects of which they could rapidly verify firsthand. The authors explore the implications of this case for induced change in the context of 'a practical and convincing demonstration accomplished in terms of a natural experimental design furnished by a serious disaster situation' (Annex p. 27).

Ngwa, A.T. and J. Hardouin. 1989. Traditional weaning practices in the semi-arid zone of Mali. In: R.T. Wilson and M. Azeb (eds). *African Small Ruminant Research and Development. Proceedings of a Conference held at Bamenda, Cameroon, 18th to 25th January 1989.* ILCA, Addis Ababa, Ethiopia. Pp. 77–85.

Under traditional management in Mali, small ruminants of both sexes and all ages are herded together. This means that females can mate while their most recent off-spring is still very young. Pastoralists have developed several weaning methods to prevent the dams from becoming debilitated and bearing weak lambs or kids. Methods include daubing dung on the dam's teats, immobilizing the tongue of the offspring and affixing thorns to the kid or lamb so that suckling pricks the dam. The authors consider such traditional weaning practices effective but crude and suggest that their improvement could contribute to increased livestock output.

Niang, Amadou. 1987. *Contribution a l'Étude de la Pharmacopée Traditionnelle Mauritaniénne.* Thesis, École Nationale de Médecine Vétérinaire, Sidi Thabet, Tunisia. 157 pp.

After describing the geography, climate and vegetation of Mauritania, the author briefly outlines the nation's animal husbandry system, selected economic features of pastoralism and the prevailing livestock diseases. However, the bulk of his thesis deals with medicinal plants traditionally used by Mauritanian pastoralists. In a survey of 53 (mainly Fulani) herders, 58 healing plants were identified. The author details the botanical description, application, preparation, active ingredients and efficacy of 31 of these plants. Based on his survey and an extensive review of the literature, he recommends ten of them for the treatment of eight livestock diseases.

Nimenya, Herman. 1998. La lutte contre l'anémie ferriprive chez les porcelets par un savoir traditionnel. *Le N'Dama: Journal du Sous-Réseau PRELUDE Santé, Productions Animales et Environnement* 11, 12(1&2): 20–21.

With decreased imports of veterinary inputs to Africa thanks to an almost continent-wide economic crisis, stockraisers engaged in non-traditional confinement production of pigs are no longer able to buy key feed supplements and injectible vitamins. As a result, they are experiencing increased piglet losses due to iron-deficient anaemia in sows. Sows kept under traditional, free-range conditions do not have this problem, however, as they will naturally root for iron-rich soil to eat. The author suggests a simple solution for stockraisers formerly dependent on imported iron supplements. Based on traditional healers' longstanding practice of prescribing doses of iron-rich earths to pregnant women, he suggests similarly providing such supplements *ad libitum* to sows in confinement. To ensure that 'clean dirt' is collected, he advises digging to a depth of 20 cm. In general, the author urges African veterinarians to 'draw from their own wells' of 'high-performing' traditional knowledge in order to free African stockraisers from the clutches of what he terms a fictive economic growth imposed by the World Bank.

Nitis, I.M. 1983. Feed analyses: The needs of developing countries. In: G.E. Robards and R.G. Packham (eds). *Feed Information and Animal Production: Proceedings of the Second Symposium of the International Network of Feed Information Centres.* Commonwealth Agricultural Bureaux, UK. Pp. 433–449.

In Bali, farmers traditionally incorporate up to 40% of banana stem in their pig and cattle rations. Originally considered by extension workers as a practice to provide water to the animals, it was discovered that banana stems are also rich in trace minerals. The banana supplement thus helps prevent nutritional diseases.

Njeru, Francis M. 1989. *Results of a Rapid Appraisal of the Traditional Ethnoveterinary Knowledge among the Borana of Garba Tulla Division of Isiolo District.* In-house report (draft). ITDG, Nairobi, Kenya. 25 pp.

Using a simplified ethnoveterinary question list [see publications by Grandin and Young], ITDG staff collected ethnoveterinary information on 24 livestock health problems recognized by Borana pastoralists of Kenya in their cattle, camels, sheep and goats. Between 3 and 5 informants were consulted on each problem. This report presents the resulting raw data. Disorders cited span FMD, CCPP, orf, diarrhoea, bloat, manges and ectoparasites, footrot, ecthyma, eye and ear infections and a number of unidentified conditions. Traditional veterinary *materia medica* mentioned include: grease, spent engine oil and fats (e.g. for orf, lice and ticks, and ecthyma); salty water (for worms); milk (for diarrhoea); tobacco, gum arabic and many other plants [no Latin names given] for a wide variety of ills. These materials are administered topically, orally, intra-nasally and intra-ocularly. Borana's use of commercial drugs is also detailed. Non-pharmacological therapeutic techniques include incising and branding/firing. Borana selectively administer all types of therapies according to animal species, age, sex and reproductive status. For a great many ills, however, informants confessed they knew of no effective traditional or, sometimes, even modern cure. Perhaps because of the paucity of therapeutic responses, Borana take myriad prophylactic measures. These span: vaccinating with modern drugs; branding and firing; controlling ticks; not mixing sick with healthy animals; carefully screening new animals' health before adding them to the herd; moving herds to new grazing areas and to new corrals, ideally on higher, drier ground; avoiding areas infested with certain kinds of ticks, poisonous grasses, soft or wet forage, or contaminants like urine; not grazing near rivers during the rainy season; rotating water points and choosing between well versus river watering according to the disease and the seasons, not watering stock when it is very hot; keeping animals well-fed; not allowing dogs to urinate in corrals; and for certain diseases, immediate sale or slaughter.

Njeru, Francis. 1994. Traditional healers of Ukambani. *Baobab* 14(Jul): 13–14.

While training selected WaKamba farmers in Kenya to become paravets, ITDG staff discovered that local people and healers controlled vast amounts of traditional veterinary knowledge. Livestock healers there are divided into psychics/diviners or herbalists, depending on whether they deal with diseases ascribed to supernatural or natural causes. Herbalists employ animal organs as well as plants in their medicines; and they may specialize in only certain diseases. They are typically paid in kind after a patient recovers. Most herbalists insist that theirs is not a profession but a gift from God, although Kenyan Christians often indiscriminately associate the practice of any form of traditional medicine with evil. Veterinarians, too, look down on all such healers as charlatans. But herbalists confidently treat the more common livestock diseases. Their remedies require analysis; and livestock healers themselves would like help in organizing themselves into groups to receive offical government recognition like that already enjoyed by traditional healers of humans in Kenya.

Noerdjito, M. 1985. Perlu diunkap lebih lanjut: Ramuan dan khasiat obat tradisional bagi ayam. In: Purnomo Ronoharjo et al. (eds). *Proceedings Seminar Peternakan dan Forum Peternakan Unggas dan Aneka Ternak, Ciawi, Bogor, 19–20 Maret, 1985.* Central Research Institute for Animal Science (CRIAS), Jalan Raya Pajajaran, Bogor, Indonesia. Pp. 347–356.

Entitled 'It is Necessary to Intensify the Study of Traditional Remedies for Chickens', this conference paper reports on research into this subject in villages around Malang, East Java, Indonesia. Interviews with 10 chicken farmers revealed that most of the ingredients employed in poultry remedies were the same as those used in traditional human medicines in the area, or as food and spices. The ingredients spanned plants such as *temu ireng (Curcuma aeruginosa), kencur (Kaempferia galanga)* and *temu lawak (Curcuma xanthorrhiza)* and/or condiments such as salt, sugar and chili *(Capsicum frutescens).* The paper lists 25 prescriptions to treat chickens' health problems, including reduced libido in cocks, colds, worms, wounds, stomach problems, inappetence and general unthriftiness. Another list indicates the diseases for which each plant is also used in human ethnomedicine. In some instances, the plants are applied for similar problems in people and animals. *Temu ireng*, for example, is fed to both species as a dewormer. In other cases, the indications differ. For instance, onion is fed to cocks to stimulate their libido, while in humans it is prescribed for coughs, vomiting and an array of other ills.

Noirtin, C. 1975. *Vocabulaire Patois en Pathologie Bovine*. Doctoral thesis, Veterinary Medicine, Ecole Nationale Vétérinaire, Alfort, France. 67 pp.

Unavailable for review.

Nossek, Milan and Carla Verheijden. 1988. *Informe de una Investigación Preliminar de los Cerdos Caseros en la Región de Estelí y Juigalpa* [Nicaragua]. Unpublished manuscript. 21 pp. Union Nacional de Agricultores y Ganaderos (UNAG), Esteli, Nicaragua.

Based on library, laboratory and slaughterhouse research plus field interviews with 96 informants, this manuscript reports on women's farmyard swineraising in Nicaragua. Holdings average two animals per household. The pigs are tethered (15%), penned (22%) or left to run free (63%). Rarely are pens roofed or cleaned; and free-ranging animals often wander into houses, where they transmit zoonotic diseases. (However, people know to palpate the tongue for signs of trichinosis and they destroy any animals with such signs.) Pigs are fed kitchen scraps and dishwater twice daily and occasionally supplemented with maize and whey; pregnant or lactating animals receive no special rations. Drinking water is seldom provided. Aside from castration, breeding is largely uncontrolled. Castration is performed late (between 30 and 90 days of age), using a single or a double incision and timed according to the phase of the moon: waxing for young boars (which is said to diminish bleeding and risk of infection) and waning for older ones. The wound is washed; the scrotum is filled with hot ashes and lime or salt; fig-tree oil or purchased medicaments are applied to the incision; and sometimes an antibiotic is injected. However, castrators' failure to tie off the spermatic cord often results in boars' bleeding to death. To speed fattening, occasionally meat sows are also 'castrated' [i.e. spayed] by cutting the ligaments between the ovaries and the uterus or the abdominal wall, then suturing the incision and applying garlic to it. Sixty percent of informants have ways of detecting pregnancy and imminent parturition; but only 33% and 15% respectively make special preparations for or assist in parturitions. Stockowners perform caesareans when necessary, suturing the incision with nylon thread soaked in pig fat; this procedure saves the farrow, but the sow usually dies within a few days. When weaning fails to occur naturally, people may separate the piglets from the sow, tie a sack over the sow's teats, or, if the sow is not to be bred again, snip off the tips of the teats. While the local *criollo* breed is well-adapted to the climate and diseases of the region, it nevertheless suffers from a variety of health problems. Among live births (92%), neonate mortality averages 15%, mostly from sows' rolling on the farrow (80%) but also from mastitis, metritis, agalactia and attacks by dogs, coyotes and buzzards. These figures are no greater than those for large-scale Nicaraguan hog operations, however. In adult pigs, respiratory ailments are the most common complaint. These are treated with commercial drugs or with a drench of chicken droppings, diesel gasoline and soapy dishwater. Commercial drugs are universally used for the next most-cited health problem: diarrhoeas and digestive disorders. All informants also cited a hoof problem believed to result from a certain spider's urinating on or biting the hoof. Treatments span: washing the hoof with diesel fuel or water and then trimming off the necrotic parts; annointing the hoof with any of a variety of substances (armadillo fat, leaves from the *teposán* tree, hot lemons, the commercial drug *Cascosán*); or bleeding the area and then dressing it with used engine oil, gasoline, creosote or a disinfectant. Prevention consists of tying a string around the hoof. For skin problems like scabies, pig raisers use topical applications of: commercial insecticides; local barks, woods or fruits; or a preparation of engine oil, diesel gasoline, putrefied mud, warm cattle faeces and hot ashes in water. For mastitis, metritis, or agalactia, the belly is vigorously rubbed with hot salt water or *matorral*, or spread with a homemade pomade; a pencillin injection may also be given. People know of no treatments for paralysis of the hindquarters – a common problem due, in some cases, to plant poisoning. Most informants vaccinated once a year against cholera.

Novaretti, Robert and Denis Lemordant. 1990. Plants in the traditional medicine of the Ubaye Valley. *Journal of Ethnopharmacology* 30: 1–34.

In interviews with agrosylvopastoralists in the Ubaye Valley of France's Alpes de Haute Provence, 136 medicinal plants were brought to light. Of these, 32 were employed in ethnoveterinary medicines for sheep and goats. Examples included: thyme, used against FMD; a laxative of *Linum usitatissimum* L.; a withered leek stalk, fed as a digestive; and *Gentiana lutea* L. root, decocted and administered as a digestive, febrifuge, vermifuge or carminative.

NRC. 1992. *Neem: A Tree for Solving Global Problems.* Report of an Ad Hoc Panel of the Board on Science and Technology for International Development. National Academy Press for the National Research Council, Washington DC, USA. 139 pp.

Pages 69 to 70 of this volume on the many virtues of products from the neem tree (*Azadirachta indica* A. Juss.) note some of their ethnoveterinary uses. Traditionally, Indians rubbed crushed neem leaves into open wounds on cattle to eliminate maggots. In Sri Lanka, neem oil is rubbed on cattle as a fly repellent; and research has shown that both the oil and the seed extract deter blowflies from laying their eggs on sheep. The active ingredient in neem, azadirachtin, also exerts an ovicidal effect in eggs of the bloodsucking fly *Stomoxys calcitrans*. Further, trials in Germany have shown that azadirachtin works against intestinal nematodes in animals.

Nur, Hussein M. 1984. Some reproductive aspects and breeding patterns of the Somali camel (*Camelus dromedarius*). In: Mohamed Ali Hussein (ed.). *Camel Pastoralism in Somalia: Proceedings from a Workshop Held in Baydhabo, April 8–13, 1984.* Camel Forum Working Paper No. 7. Somali Camel Research Project, Mogadishu, Somalia and Stockholm, Sweden. Pp. 91–114.

Pages 101 ff. describe Somali camel herders' knowledge of the management of camel breeding and reproductive patterns. Their knowledge spans: age of puberty, sexual maturity, breeding seasons and reproductive life; detailed physiological and ethological signs of heat and pregnancy, the latter including indigenous 'cocked tail' observations that allow detection of pregnancy within 8–15 days after breeding; length of gestation and processes of parturition; twinning rates, abortions and post-natal mortality; suckling behaviour; and castration and culling procedures.

Nuru, Hameed and Denis Fielding. 1993. Traditional knowledge and practices in calf rearing. *Intermediate Technology* 30(3): 33–35.

This article overviews helpful traditional calf-rearing practices among African stockraisers. To make a newborn calf draw its first breath, its nostrils may be tickled with a straw or sprinkled with salt. To induce suckling, salt may also be sprinkled on the calf's tongues, thereby triggering salivation and swallowing. To promote calf survival, Fulani women avoid milking dams for several days post-partum; once milking begins, the women always leave some milk in the udder in order to ensure that newborn and unweaned calves receive sufficient colostrum and nutrition, respectively. Traditionally, Fulani also vaccinated their calves against diseases such as CBPP and FMD, using various homemade vaccines and con-trolled exposure techniques. Among pastoralists in northeastern Africa, cauteriza-tion serves to prevent horn development in calves and to treat hoof problems, chronic wounds and bleeding in animals of all ages. In traditional methods of open castration of calves, herdsmen may tear and sever the spermatic cord by biting it. Especially for calves destined for fattening, however, closed castration may be per-formed by crushing the spermatic cord with a mallet or a stone. This technique wards against the tetanus and secondary bacterial infections that sometimes result from open surgery. Effective weaning strategies are myriad: in Mali, daubing dung on the dam's teats; among Somali, tying off the teats; elsewhere, placing a rope bit on the calf; alternatively, affixing thorns to the calf's mouth or the dam's udder; among Maasai, covering the udder and/or distracting the calf with salt; and among Borana pastoralists of East Africa, incising the calf's muzzle so that suckling pains the calf. Somali herders may likewise slice the calf's tongue or insert a stick in its nose or tongue. Alternatively, they may simply separate the calf from its dam. The authors note some caveats about certain of these practices. For example, cauteriza-tion can be dangerous in cases of infectious disease because it may depress anti-body production through the release of histamines. And of course, any kind of open surgery increases the risk of infection. However, they conclude that 'there is a lot for modern veterinary science to learn by studying' Africans' calf-rearing practices.

Nuwanyakpa, Mopoi Y. 1992. *Partnership with Heifer Project International for Integrated Rural Agricultural Development and Environmental Sustainability: A Concept Paper and an Unsolicited Proposal.* HPI, Bamenda, Cameroon. 79 pp.

HPI has been promoting livestock development in Cameroon since the 1970s. This concept paper overviews HPI/Cameroon activities at the time of writing, within the framework of this PVO's overarching philosophy and goals. Pages 40 ff. discuss the creation of HPI/Cameroon's EVM project. A highlight of this effort was the establishment of a Council of Experts on Ethnoveterinary Medicine, drawn from exceptionally experienced stockraiser-healers throughout the Northwest Province. The 12 experts on the council were selected as the oldest and most experienced from among 60 volunteers who responded to HPI letters of invitation; the 60 names were originally generated in project consultations with HPI extensionists. As a result of these experts' input, plus other factors, HPI livestock work has shifted to the use of EVM wherever feasible. Since 1989, only herbal medicines have been promoted for the control of helminths in both beef and dairy cattle. As of 1990, the use of modern medicines in HPI rabbit projects was discontinued. And in 1992, HPI began to promulgate herbal and other traditional treatments for poultry. HPI trains selected local stockraisers in ethnoveterinary treatments at the stockraisers' own expense and the project then helps establish trainees as barefoot veterinarians. HPI also holds 'ethnovet field days' which have proved popular occasions for Fulani herders to exchange EVK. Since 1990, Western-trained vets from the provincial veterinary school, the national zoological research institute (IRZ) and the government livestock agency have joined in these efforts. Other outcomes of HPI's emphasis on EVM have been that the Chief of the IRZ Veterinary Department has embarked on the study of several ethnoveterinary medicines and government veterinary officers have begun independently to seek out the specialized assistance of HPI-trained 'ethnoveterinarians'. Meanwhile, training in EVM has been extended to native farmers as well as Fulani herders. At present, HPI is disseminating traditional remedies for 33 economically important ailments of cattle, small ruminants, poultry and rabbits. To support this work, a herbarium has been established and scientific identification of the approximately 300 veterinary medicinal plants so far identified is underway. In addition, backyard gardens for these plants are being promoted; and HPI is assisting provincial forest reserves in adding land for *in situ* conservation of the plants.

Nuwanyakpa, Mopoi, James Devries, Cristopher Ndi and Sali Django. 1990. *Traditional Veterinary Medicine in Cameroon: A Renaissance in an Ancient Indigenous Technology* (draft). HPI, Bamenda, Cameroon. 66 pp.

While also introducing conventional veterinary training topics, this draft manual lays out the compelling arguments for and highlights specific examples of ethnoveterinary alternatives based on HPI/Cameroon's EVM and Fulani Livestock Development Project. The authors also detail project start-up methods. Initially, HPI/Cameroon worked with a cadre of 12 expert Fulani 'ethnoveterinarians' selected for their long EVM experience from among 60 volunteers in all five divisions of Cameroon's Northwest Province. Across 4 months in 1989, these 12 men, aged 47 to 93, were interviewed individually and also brought together to share their vast EVK on 36 cattle ailments they considered important, plus ethnopharmacological and -surgical treatments for these ills. The men also described the pros and cons of traditional and modern veterinary and husbandry practices based on their personal experiences. While these experts agreed on cattle disease terms and symptoms, they differed somewhat in their range of treatments. It was found that a single plant species may be used to treat different diseases and, conversely, one disease can be treated with different plants. This means that, at any given time, at least one botanical should be available to address a given health problem; and at other times, multiple complementary botanicals can be brought to bear on the problem, thus enhancing treatment effect. About 5% of the experts' treatments centred on magico-religious procedures. However, this manual includes only ethno-prophylactic and -therapeutic measures grounded in active biological principles. The manual lists 14 emically defined cattle ills and experts' varied plant prescriptions for them. Further, it presents preliminary comparisons between the cash costs of selected EVM versus conventional treatments. Needless to say, EVM won out in this regard. For example, a local remedy that proved 92% effective against worms in calves was also more than 31 times cheaper than its Western equivalent. Even a home remedy for tick control that was compounded of a commercial insecticide powder and burnt engine oil (also purchased) proved nine times cheaper than the most common acaricide available commercially in Cameroon. A concluding section of the manual offers tips 'to other Third World' R&D workers who hope to initiate EVM projects or other local-knowledge initiatives in their countries, based on the Cameroonian authors' firsthand experiences with the HPI effort.

NVV. 1995. From nasal blocks to broken legs: Tamil way of health. ***Honey Bee*** 6(4): 9–10.

Thirteen local health and husbandry treatments plus two food-product techniques used on livestock by Tamil-speaking groups in India are reported here, taken from the NVV Network's newsletter. Five of these were contributed by an elderly herbal veterinarian: for discharge from the ears, apply ash of burnt *Helicteres isora* pods in coconut oil; for 'frog disease' in cattle – diagnosed by a squatting position, flexed fetlocks and hair standing on end – feed two doses for one day of *Clerodendron phlomoides* leaves soaked in water; for nasal obstructions, give nose drops made from one *Solanum xanthocarpum* fruit in goat urine that has been buried in a clay pot for a week; for eye diseases, a non-smoker chews black pepper and spits it into the patient's eyes; finally, for ephemeral fever – signalled by inappetence and erection of hair over the entire body – feed boiled horse gram and have three girls of the same name and age-group winnow kitchen ash over the animal's whole body. Other treatments noted include the following. For several days after castration, bulls will not take food; so, to sustain post-operative animals nutritionally, just before castration farmers give them a maceration of 2 leaves of *Cardiospermum halicacabum*, one bottle gourd, 200 ml of neem oil and a farm egg. To facilitate expulsion of the placenta, certain vines are tied around the cow's neck and she is fed several pounded *Abrus precatorius* seeds. Casts for broken legs are made from a paste of powdered *Acacia leucophloea* bark in water, bandaged over by a cloth kept moist for about 10 days. *Euphorbia tortilis* latex is applied to swollen knee joints. Myiasis is treated with *Leucas aspera* extract. A common treatment for FMD is to fumigate the cattle yard and the affected animals by burning a mixture of neem leaves, dry fish wastes and turmeric powder. Both animals and humans are given *Solanum indicum* fruits to suck on in order to reduce toothache pain and kill germs in the sufferer's mouth. Regularly feeding goats the pods of *Acacia leucophloea*, *Cynodon dactylon* and *Prosopis juliflora* greatly improves the taste and quality of their meat. To curdle fresh goat milk quickly, add *Wrightia tinctoria* latex.

NVV. 1996a. Transgenic marriage, cough balls and organic jaggery: *Nam Vazhi Velanmai*. ***Honey Bee*** 7(1): 8.

This article describes two veterinary treatments recommended by a traditional healer plus one indigenous haymaking technique, as reported in the Tamil-language version of *Honey Bee*. For bites from snakes and other poisonous creatures, feed livestock pounded *Aristolochia bracteolata* leaves mixed with an equal quantity of fresh butter. To relieve coughing and asthmatic wheezing, give boluses of pounded garlic, cumin and *Ficus tinctoria* every morning for 3 days. To store sorghum and maize stalks for prolonged periods, sprinkle common salt over every layer of straw as it is stacked up, using approximately 10 kg of salt per acre of straw.

NVV. 1996b. Beer for bullocks and appetizers for animals! ***Honey Bee*** 7(2): 9.

Various Indian cures for cattle are noted here, as described by readers of the *Nam Vazhi Velanmai* Network newsletter in Tamil Nadu State. A kilogramme of macerated, pounded *Wrightia tinctoria* leaves are fed to cure diarrhoea. A tonic drench for over-worked bullocks consists of neem and *Pterocarpus marsupium* bark fermented in water, to which black cumin and palm jaggery are added. For heart trouble, bullocks are drenched with a hot aqueous mixture of human urine, *W. tinctoria* leaves and chilli powder, accompanied by three blows to the chest in the region of the heart. Rectal prolapse is cured with a drench of macerated *Mimosa pudica* or tortoise-shell ash. For ephemeral fever, a drench of pounded leaves and seeds of *Abrus precatorius* and *Pergularia daemia* in cow urine is given; an alternative is drenching with cannabis plants macerated with jaggery and diluted in hot water. At the same time, a supplement of ground, soaked rice, field beans, black gram and horse gram is fed. For inappetence, a cloth filled with crushed tamarind pods, green chillies and salt is tied over the tongue for 2 hours.

NVV. 1996c. Crab cares and castor cures! *Honey Bee* 7(3): 9.

In this regular *Honey Bee* column, farmers and developers alike report on various local livestock treatments in Tamil-speaking areas of India. For retained placenta, macerated *Grewia flavescens* root is fed. A paste prepared from 1 handful each of the pounded leaves of *Polygala grinerisis, Andrographis alata, Acalypha indica, Cynodon dactylon* in 100 ml of neem oil and 200 ml of warm water is administered [in an unspecified way] for poisonous bites; for the remainder of the day, the patient is fed only dry paddy straw for 1 day and the animal is not allowed to bathe for 15 days thereafter. Cattle poisoned by eating *Aloe vera* are drenched thrice daily with crushed *Pedalium murex* and *Bauhinia racemosa* in water, administered through a hollow bamboo funnel. Acute external swellings are plastered with a paste of curd mixed with the pounded outer rind of *Datura metel* pods or pounded *Solanum indicum*. Drenches for constipation include: 200 ml of castor oil; 200 g of powdered castor seeds in water; or crushed *Terminalia arjuna* bark in water. Feverish cattle should be denied green grass, given only hot water to drink and made to inhale smoke from burning a cloth dipped in pig blood, poultry manure, turmeric powder and human hair. Cattle with pharyngitis are fed bamboo and *Dodonaea viscosa* leaves. If the throat is obstructed by some foreign material, a sort of metal cup is inserted into the cattle's mouth, a folded-up gunny sack is placed on its head between the horns and then the animal is given a blow on the sack. This should cause the foreign item to be expelled into the cup [a sort of modified Heimlich manoeuvre]. A multiplex treatment for animals with FMD is to: isolate them by penning in a separate shed; feed bananas soaked in castor oil overnight, as well as pork cooked in *Panicum miliare* water; wash the hooves in water in which dried fish have been soaked; and apply kerosene to the cleft of the hooves. For poor lactation, feed either 100 to 200 g of tapioca tubers or 2 kg of powdered bajra grain with 1 kg of brinjal. In foot injuries from ploughs, feed the animal a live field crab with grass and keep it working.

NVV. 1996d. Butter-milk, honey bees and tamarind: Tamil farmers show the way. *Honey Bee* 7(4): 11–12.

In this compilation of farmer practices and scientist commentary from the Tamil version of *Honey Bee*, one man recommends establishing bee colonies to enhance pollination of the difficult yellow variety of coconut palm. Mud pots hung upside down on trees or poles reportedly will attract natural colonies of bees within a couple of months. For increased energy and milk production in cattle, another man suggests daily feeding 1 to 2 kg of tamarind seeds that have been baked, pounded to remove the husk and then soaked overnight. Drenching with 3 cloves of garlic, 10 pepper seeds and an unstipulated quantity of *Stephania japonica* root, all ground together and diluted in hot water, cures inappetence. A febrifuge drink for livestock consists of a handful of *Wrightia tinctoria* leaves, a palm-sized piece of bark of *W. tinctoria*, 1 chilli pod and 3 or 4 garlic rhizomes all ground together and diluted in 0.5 l of water; if this is administered in the morning, the fever is down by evening. A drench for kidney stones consists of filtering 500 g of crushed *Bryophyllum* spp. leaves in 500 ml of water; 250 ml of the filtrate is given twice daily for 8 to 10 days. A one-day drench of 100 g of salt, 2 turmeric rhizomes and the extract of a handful of young *Cassia senna* leaves in 0.25 l of raw cow's milk, topped up with water to make 1 l, induces heat in livestock. To promote conception, give cows 1 *Semecarpus anacardium* seed per day for 3 days and leave off deworming with *Aloe vera*; then feed 250 g of sprouted wheat seed for 15 days. An alternative to these last two treatments is to feed the extract of 1 leaf of *Aloe vera* for 3 days, followed by daily feedings of 200 g of sprouted Bengal gram for 2 weeks. Ten problem cows (2 cattle, 8 buffalo) given this treatment conceived and a plan is now in place to test it on 100 animals.

NVV. 1997a. Irrigation through melons, moth control through marigold. ***Honey Bee*** 8(1): 15.

In Tamil-speaking parts of India, a wound and myiasis treatment that can be stored for up to 3 years is made from 2 l of *Datura metel* leaf extract, 100 g of copper sulphate and 1 l of coconut oil boiled together until dry. Casts for fractures are fashioned of a paste of *Mucuna pruriens* or *Ormocarpum sennoides* leaves bandaged over the broken bone. To prevent corneal opacity in cattle, an extract of ground *Barberea cuspidata* leaves, 6 ground *Piper nigrum* seeds and chewn tobacco and betelnut is squeezed through a cloth into the eyes. An antacid drench for cattle is made by pounding together 2 fruits and 4 leaves of *Strychnos nux-vomica* and then diluting the mass with water.

NVV. 1997b. 'Tulsi' cures poultry too. ***Honey Bee*** 8(3): 7.

This article reports the results of a workshop held in India's Tamil Nadu State for men and women farmers to document innovative practices for sustainable natural resource management. Several such practices deal with respiratory disorders of poultry, which are a chronic problem in the region. One treatment is oral administration daily for 3 days of pounded *Ocimum* sp. leaves in an amount of about 100 g per 1000 birds. To reduce head and facial swelling of birds with respiratory disorders, 0.5 kg of dried and powdered *Tragia involucrata* root is put in their feed for 2 days. This amount is also sufficient for a flock of 1000. A complete cure reportedly can be effected by adding 1 kg of palm sugar or palm jaggery to their drinking water for the next 2 days.

NVV and SIRPI. 1994. Lateral learning among animal healers: A workshop on indigenous veterinary practices. ***Honey Bee*** 5(3): 16.

This article describes the outcome of a one-day workshop on indigenous veterinary practices hosted by the *Num Vazhi Velanmai* Network (a *Honey Bee* affiliate) and the local NGO SIRPI. Held in a village of Tamil Nadu State, India, the workshop was attended by 30 farmers (12 of them women) from four adjacent villages. Participants prepared a list of common practices for cattle. These included: a *veeli*-leaf (?) drench for coughs; also to control coughs, fumigation by burning incense along with a cloth soaked in pig blood or, alternatively, burning the skin of a pangolin (an anteater-like creature); as a dressing for leg wounds, a lukewarm solution of boiled sheep droppings, water-soaked tamarind seeds and termite-mound soil; for blackquarter, pork soup mixed with *Panicum miliare*; *Aloe barbadensis* juice and, a week later, sprouted Bengal gram, fed to anoestrus cows; for neck swellings, topical application of any of the following – wax and coconut oil, *Madhuca longifolia* kern oil, crushed *Muyal kathazhai* leaves or crushed steamed onion. For plough wounds to the sole, a heated plough rod is held just above the wound while fermented rice water is poured down the rod. Feverish or shiver-legged cattle are adorned with a necklace of *Abrus precatorius* plus a three-time sprinkling of ash from the animal's head to its tail, ideally performed simultaneously by three different women with the same name. Another practice is stock-buyers' feeding crushed tamarind leaves and twigs to small ruminants put up for sale; the tamarind acts as a diuretic, causing the animals to expel extra water fed them by the seller, thus allowing the buyer to judge their real weight.

Nwude, N. and M.A. Ibrahim. 1980. Plants used in traditional veterinary medical practice in Nigeria. *Journal of Veterinary Pharmacology and Therapeutics* 3: 261–273.

This article draws upon library research and inquiries among herders and other local people about medicinal plants employed in traditional veterinary medicine in Nigeria. It lists 92 such plants; their vernacular names in English, Hausa, Igbo, Yoruba and Fulani; the animal species for which the plants are used; their indications; and aspects of the plants' preparation and administration. The authors give several examples of plants with proven pharmacological effectiveness. They strongly recommend the integration of traditional with modern veterinary medicine.

Oakeley, Roger. 1998. *Experiences with Community-based Livestock Worker (CLW) Programmes, Methodologies and Impact: A Literature Review.* Veterinary Epidemiology and Economics Research Unit, Department of Agriculture, University of Reading, Reading, UK. 32 pp.

This review of paravet programmes worldwide notes a growing consensus with respect to the place of EVK in such initiatives. 'Appropriate training' is emphasized; that is, training that uses local terminology and attempts to meet producers' expressed needs. This approach necessitates careful background study of EVK, of existing production systems, of livestock species and health problems in the specific local context and so forth. Increasingly, paravet programmes are actively incorporating traditional remedies and ethnoveterinary skills into training, not only as a means of harnessing valuable local knowledge but also as a way to reduce dependence on expensive and sometimes-inaccessible Western drugs. However, as a number of authorities in the field of EVK caution, the technical soundness of many traditional treatments is still unknown. Thus, such treatments should be investigated before they are incorporated into paravet curricula. That said, there is growing agreement that Western veterinary technologies should not be advanced to the exclusion of local ones. Because Western drugs may be harder to come by locally than traditional remedies, however, demands on paravet programmes to offer them may be great. As at least one author has noted, ironically sometimes proponents of 'participative' approaches and local technology are reluctant to acquiesce to stockraisers' demand for powerful Western drugs and chemicals.

Oba, Gufu. 1994. *The Role of Indigenous Range Management Knowledge for Desertification Control in Northern Kenya.* Research Report No. 4. Environmental Policy and Society (EPOS) Programme, Uppsala and Linköping Universities, Sweden. 40 pp.

Pastoralists of Northern Kenya base their assessment of range quality on vegetation, along with other factors. In a normal year, pastoral livestock distributions correlate closely with the abundance of preferred range-plant species. A browse plant favoured by goats is *Cadaba glandulosa* which, say pastoralists, also 'cleans up' the rumen.

Obel-Lawson, Elizabeth. 1992. *The Paravets of Loumbol.* Arid Lands Information Network (ALIN), Dakar, Senegal. 14 pp.

In an ALIN paravet effort among Fulani agropastoralists of Senegal's Ferlo Reserve, as trainees, communities selected 'mostly young, wealthy herders who did not know much about traditional treatments. Most of this knowledge is jealously guarded by the old practitioners, who do not teach it to just anybody' (p. 11). No women were chosen for training, even though women are often the first to detect sick animals. Few details of ethnoveterinary treatments were noted during paravet project design – only 'burning specific parts of the body, draining blood from the tongue, bone splinting, bone setting, use of herbs . . . mixed with water or buried as a fetish' (p. 13). The author further comments that, although Fulani's traditional veterinary treatments worked well in the past, some are no longer effective because of their animals' feeble health.

Ohta, Itaru. 1984. Symptoms are classified into diagnostic categories: Turkana's view of livestock diseases. *African Study Monographs* 3 (supplementary issue): 71–93.

This article examines how the Turkana, an East African pastoralist group, recognize, classify and cope with livestock diseases. The author describes the etymology, aetiology and treatment of 37 such ills as classified by the Turkana and eight words used to describe symptoms. Disease names mostly derive from typical clinical signs or from post-mortem observations. The Turkana are aware of the contagiousness of many diseases. The author concludes that the Turkana disease classification system is highly complex, but that pathogenic explanations and curative measures are not very advanced. Ethnoveterinary treatments and procedures include medicines, bleeding, cauterization, castration and other surgical techniques.

Ohta, Itaru. 1987. Livestock individual identification among the Turkana: The animal classification and naming in the pastoral livestock management. *African Study Monographs* 8(1): 1–69.

In the notes on pages 63 through 66, this article offers some insights into the perinatal care of livestock among Turkana pastoralists in northwestern Kenya. Turkana have three different castration methods for their livestock: beating (the scrotum is beaten with a wooden hammer), cutting (the scrotum is cut open and the testicles and seminal ducts removed) and biting (the seminal duct is bitten off). They classify parturitions into four categories: two types of abortion, premature births and normal parturition. The herders know when their animals are about to give birth and they help the dams as much as possible during the expulsion stage. Turkana pay great attention to the dam–offspring bond because of their concern with milk production and the calf's health. They take several countermeasures when the dam refuses or loses her offspring. In the latter case, they make a dummy of its skin, give the dam an orphan to adopt, or allow the previous offspring, if it is still young, to suckle again.

Oluyemi, J.A., D.F. Adene and G.O. Ladoye. 1979. A comparison of the Nigerian indigenous fowl with White Rock under conditions of disease and nutritional stress. ***Tropical Animal Health and Production*** 11: 199–202.

This comparative study of Newcastle disease in indigenous Nigerian chicks versus White Rock chicks suggests that the former have some natural resistance to the disease. Upon exposure of unvaccinated chicks, the White Rocks suffered 100% mortality; but mortality among the unvaccinated indigenous birds was significantly less ($P < 0.05$). 960 chicks were used for this trial (equal numbers of White Rock and indigenous Nigerian chicks). The chicks were fed either balanced or deficient diets and were either vaccinated or not against Newcastle disease. The deficiency in the diet was largely in respect of crude protein. In previous studies, indigenous chicks were shown also to have greater resistance to *Salmonella gallinarum* than exotic breeds.

Omondi, N.F. 1996. ***T.M.W.G. Efforts in Ethnoveterinary Medicine and Miot Traditional Healers of Transmara and Bomet Districts, Kenya.*** In-house report. Kilgoris, Kenya. 4 pp.

The Transmara Western Group (TMWG) is a small association of traditional healers and voluntary researchers in Kenya. The group has identified and documented the names of plants of ethnoveterinary importance in their region. It has also drawn up a list of local, *miot* herbalists who now meet regularly to exchange ideas on ethno- and Western-scientific veterinary medicine. On the ethnoveterinary side, the group mounted a project to combat ecto- and endoparasites using neem, which has decreased mortality among participants' livestock. Conversely, on the Western-scientific side, thanks to researchers' sharing their knowledge, *Leucaena* and *Calliandra* spp. have become more widely accepted as useful fodders among the region's Kipsigis and Maasai peoples.

Omondi, Naftally Felix. 1998. Mapping animal diseases. ***Footsteps*** 34: 10.

The Transmara Western Group (TMWG) is a small team of volunteer researchers in Kenya who promote sustainable development by building upon local knowledge. Based on TMWG experiences, this brief article describes how to do simple on-farm and community maps to locate occurrences of livestock disease vis-à-vis significant natural, social and other features in a given area. Whether one-by-one or in workshops, such maps can then be combined to embrace larger areas in order to facilitate discussion and problem-solving for questions like the following. Are certain diseases more common in some areas than others? If so, why? What could be done to combat them? How far are people from the nearest veterinary help? Where are critical medicinal plants to be found? TMWG application of this mapping + discussion technique across 4 years in Kipsigi and Maasai communities of Transmara District revealed many important issues. For example, farmers there rank ECF as the most serious disease, but they cannot afford the commercial treatments for it. For the same reason, farmers are no longer able to dip large cattle herds regularly. Home spraying of animals is done mainly by women, but they lack the proper training and equipment. Most tick-borne diseases are treated by local herbalists. Lack of water for livestock is a serious problem that forces herds to range farther, thus increasing the spread of ticks. And much more. Such findings have fed directly into TMWG livestock development planning. In the veterinary arena, they have led TMWG to focus on producing low-cost remedies locally in conjunction with traditional livestock healers.

Ondieki, P.G. and N.F. Omondi. 1997. Linking ethnoveterinary medicine and modern medicine. ***Indigenous Knowledge and Development Monitor*** 5(1): 18.

The Transmara Western Group (TMWG) is a small, private, volunteer self-help team of livestock experts, social scientists and traditional healers in Kenya. It is searching for local solutions to animal health problems, since modern medicines are either unavailable or too expensive. At the moment, TMWG is working to identify plants yielding extracts that can combat ECF.

Ontañón Moreno, Victor. 1989. Fitoterapía veterinaria. In: Gerardo López Buendía (ed.). ***Memorias: Segunda Jornada sobre Herbolaria Medicinal en Medicina Veterinaria.*** Universidad Nacional Autónoma de México, Facultad de Medicina Veterinaria y Zootecnia, Coordinación de Educación Continua, México DF, México. Pp. 141–155.

'Often, valuable understandings of the medicinal actions of plants have been obtained by observing animal behaviour. Cats and dogs, for example, cure their stomach disorders by eating bitter herbs, while sick sheep seek out yarrow. A wild bear suffering from henbane poisoning has recourse to fresh Carlina Angelica roots to cure itself. Rats store mint for the winter. In the first days of spring, hungry bears search for bear garlic (*Allium ursinum*). Ants sow thyme throughout their anthills. Wounded deer roll in alpine plantain. Swallows use celandine ("swallow herb") juice to open their hatchlings' eyes. With tomato juice, crows chase fleas from their nests. Rheumatic cattle lie down in fields of buttercups. And snakebitten iguana find an antidote in camomile.' (Thomson, cited in Ontañón)

The foregoing citation opens this article, which lists dozens of bibliographic items on veterinary phytotherapy. Beginning with 18th-century French books and journals, items span Asian, Australian, European, North and Latin American sources that describe home remedies for animals or veterinary-pharmacological studies based on plant and other materials on all these continents plus Africa. The author then groups several scores of plants named in these sources into 42 categories by pharmacological function (analgesics, anthelmintics, etc.).

Opasina, B.A., O.O. Dipeolu and B.O. Fagbemi. 1983. Some ectoparasites of veterinary importance on dwarf sheep and goats under traditional system [sic] of management in the humid forest and derived savanna zones of Nigeria. *Revue d'Élevage et de Médecine Vétérinaire des Pays Tropicaux* 36(4): 387–391.

Among other things, this article notes that greater attention is being paid to Africa's dwarf sheep and goat breeds because of their probable genetic tolerance of the intense heat and the many tropical diseases of the forest and forest-border zones of West Africa.

Orprecio, J.L. and D.L. Catcnero [sic]. 1992. A community animal health volunteer training programme in the Philippines. In: P.W. Daniels, S. Holden, E. Lewin and S. Dadi (eds). *Livestock Services for Smallholders: A Critical Evaluation of the Delivery of Animal Health and Production Services to the Small-scale Farmer in the Developing World.* Proceedings of an International Seminar held in Yogyakarta, Indonesia, 15–21 November 1992. INIANSRE-DEF, Bogor, Indonesia. Pp. 235–237.

The observations of Catchero and Orprecio n.d. concerning the place of EVM in an HPI paravet programme in the Philippines are reiterated in this conference-paper abstract.

Orskov, Bob. 1992. Global communications: Pastoral innovation from Mongolia. *Honey Bee* 3(3&4): 7.

Mongolian herdsmen have been making what the author considers 'excellent' mineral blocks for centuries. The ingredients are condensed milk, sodium carbonate, wheat bran, onion leaves and other unspecified items. The blocks are set out to dry on top of herders' tents, where they become so rockhard that they cannot be attacked by fungi. Among other things, hypothesizes the author, the blocks provide selenium, which is an essential trace mineral that is probably limiting to livestock raised on the poor soils in Mongolia.

Oseguera, M.D. 1998. Heridas de piel en équidos de trabajo de México curados con métodos alternativos. In: Magdalena Escamilla Guerrero, Rosa María Parra Hernández and Angélica María Vargas (eds). *3er. Coloquio Internacional sobre Équidos de Trabajo.* División de Educación Contínua, Facultad de Medicina Veterinaria y Zootecnia, Universidad Nacional Autónoma de México, México DF, México. Pp. 125–127.

This conference paper addresses skin wounds of pack horses and donkeys in Mexico. Among other things, it notes that poor people there cannot afford formal veterinary care or commercial drugs for wound care. Based on experiences of the mobile veterinary clinic of the national university, the author recommends a successful alternative treatment based on EVM. It consists of simply washing the wound with soap and water, removing any foreign matter, allowing the area to air dry for a bit and then generously dressing it with honey and, if available, a little gauze. This procedure should be repeated daily until the wound heals. The author notes that animal owners themselves can easily afford and apply this treatment.

Oyedipe, F.P.A. 1977. Institutionalization of semi-sedentarism: The Hausaji Fulani nomads at Kainji revisited. Paper presented to the Conference on the Aftermath of the Drought. Kano, Nigeria. Pp. 10 and 11.

Among many other things, this paper describes how Fulani quickly became frustrated with proffered, post-drought veterinary and other services that never materialized – such as promises to help herders with their animal-health and predator-control problems. But whenever Fulani complied with government requirements to report disease outbreaks or predator attacks to veterinary or game-reserve authorities, the promised help was not forthcoming. Thus herders soon quit making such reports or seeking assistance in the form of veterinary drugs. Instead, 'They want to rely on their own resources as much as possible; if they fail, they leave all to "Allah"' (p. 11).

Pachegaonkar, M.R. 1998. Homoeopathy in ethnoveterinary medicine. In: E. Mathias, D.V. Rangnekar and C.M. McCorkle, with M. Martin (eds). *Ethnoveterinary Medicine: Alternatives for Livestock Development – Proceedings of an International Conference Held in Pune, India, 4–6 November 1997. Volume 2: Abstracts.* BAIF Development Research Foundation, Pune, India. P. 44.

Conventional drugs are costly; many have undesirable side effects; and chemoresistance due to the frequent and often indiscriminate use of such drugs in livestock poses a danger to people, animals and the environment. Homeopathic medicine offers a possible alternative. Veterinary homeopathy was introduced in 1833 when the German veterinarian Johan Wilhelm Lux published a pamphlet entitled *Isopathik der Contagionen*, based on the principle that all diseases carry within themselves the means of their cure. Lux also started a periodical on veterinary homeopathy entitled *Zooaiasis*. Nearly two decades ago, the Sheep Breeding Farm of India's Maharashtra Sheep & Goat Development Corporation Ltd conducted a series of homeopathic trials, the results of which have been published elsewhere. This paper reviews the application of Lux's theories to livestock in general, but especially small ruminants. Homeopathy has been successfully employed for both prevention and treatment. Examples are the prevention of anthrax in small ruminants and of pox in cattle, sheep and goats. With regard to treatment, homeopathic approaches have proven most effective in diseases commonly encountered in clinical practice such as mastitis, summer diarrhoea, three-day fever, bloat, contagious ecthyma, burns, injuries and fractures.

Padmakumar, Varijakshapanicker. 1996. *Traditional Knowledge and its Application in Veterinary Medicine by Livestock Farmers in Kerala (South India).* MSc thesis, CTVM, University of Edinburgh, Edinburgh, UK. 72 pp.

A survey among 150 farmers and 18 traditional healers in Kerala, India found that 75% of the farmers use traditional methods to treat their animals' diseases, especially bloat, diarrhoea, fevers, FMD, helminthosis and mastitis. Treatments were mostly plant-based and included such ingredients as garlic, ginger, neem, pepper, tamarind and turmeric.

Padmakumar, V. 1998. Farmers' reliance on ethnoveterinary practices to cope with common cattle ailments. *Indigenous Knowledge and Development Monitor* 6(2): 14–15.

Now an assistant manager at the Malabar Regional Co-op Milk Producers Union in Kerala, India, the author describes findings from his University of Edinburgh post-graduate researches on EVK in two traditional cattle-raising districts of Kerala. There, he interviewed 150 farmers (32 of them women) selected at random from those supplying milk to local cooperatives plus 18 livestock healers, also chosen at random. Findings revealed that about 75% of the farmers used ethno-veterinary medicines, with 70% administering them themselves. The main reason farmers gave for employing EVM were its lack of side effects, its low cost and the absence of modern veterinary services. EVM is used mainly for FMD, mastitis, fever, bloat, diarrhoea and helminthosis, most commonly employing pepper, ginger, turmeric, garlic, neem and tamarind. Farmers say these treatments are generally effective for these diseases, depending upon the stage and severity of the problem. People usually have recourse first to home remedies, then to local livestock healers and only lastly to modern veterinary medicine if it is available. In Kerala, EVM is intimately linked with Ayurvedic medicine. Indeed, healers buy some of their *materia medica* from Ayurvedic pharmacies to supplement those they gather on their own. The majority of healers treat only 5 to 10 cases a month, in return for token earnings. They operate by vending their medicaments along with their expert advice to the worried stockowner, who then administers the treatment at home. However, exceptionally successful healers may see more than 50 patients a month. Such individuals support themselves from EVM, often making up their own herbal pills and hiring tribal people from the forest areas to collect plant materials for them.

Padmakumar, V. 1999. Ethnoveterinary medicine in Kerala (south India). In: E. Mathias, D.V. Rangnekar and C.M. McCorkle, with M. Martin (eds). *Ethnoveterinary Medicine: Alternatives for Livestock Development – Proceedings of an International Conference Held in Pune, India, 4–6 November 1997. Volume 1: Selected Papers.* BAIF Development Research Foundation, Pune, India. Pp. 30–31.

Under the hegemony of Western science, traditional/indigenous knowledge has been accorded little importance in the past. Especially in the tropics, however, vast numbers of stockraisers still depend on such knowledge and its associated treatments for most of their animal healthcare. Indigenous methods are often cheap, sustainable and free of negative side effects. A survey conducted among 150 farmers and 18 traditional healers in Kerala, India to ascertain the level of use of ethnoveterinary practices showed that nearly 75% of farmers and all healers use traditional methods to treat their animals, especially in cases of mastitis, fever, bloat, diarrhoea, helminthosis and FMD. *Materia medica* include spices such as pepper (*Piper nigrum*), ginger (*Zingiber officinale*), turmeric (*Curcuma longa*) and garlic (*Allium sativum*), plus preparations from neem (*Azadirachta indica*) and tamarind (*Tamarindus indica*). Although local knowledge has its limitations, there is tremendous scope for its application, especially in a suitable blending with Western techniques.

Padua, Ludivina S. de. 1989. Medicinal plants in animal health care. Paper presented to the Sixth Asian Symposium on Medicinal Plants and Spices, 23–28 January, Bandung, Indonesia. 9 pp.

This conference paper reports on a study in the Philippines that revealed 116 plant species employed in Filipino treatments for animals. The most widely used plants are also the most widely available ones. These include mainly fruits and vegetables such as bananas, coconuts, papayas and red peppers but also inedibles like betelnut and tobacco. Most of these materials are applied to multiple diseases. Banana, for example, is employed in prescriptions for diarrhoea, digestive disorders, urinary tract infection, wounds, skin problems, mites, ticks and fleas. Other plants have more specific applications, such as feeding betelnut to expel intestinal parasites. In total, some 56 livestock diseases were found to be treated or managed with medicinal plants.

Padua, Ludivina S. de. 1991. Plants for animal health care. *Sustainable Agriculture* 3(1): 24.

In the Philippines, medicinal plants play an important role in the healthcare of both farm animals and pets, especially given the country's worsening economic situation. Animal species treated with plant medicines include cattle, horses, swine, goats, poultry and dogs. A wide variety of common ailments in these species are treated with plants, as are production problems such as decreased milk and egg yields, and inappetence and weight loss. Both mono- and polyprescriptions are prepared and administered in a wide variety of ways. Through experience and continued use, farmers have established dosages for certain prescriptions and diseases. In all, 116 plant species from more than 50 families are employed in the Philippines today. Some formulations that practitioners have found particularly effective are: for lice, a wash of decocted or pounded-together plant parts of *Vitex negundo* and *Strychnos nux-vomica* leaves with *Curcuma longa* rhizomes; for respiratory infections, a paste or bolus of *V. negundo* and *Ocimum basilicum* leaves, *Ricinus communis* root, ginger rhizome and powdered *Piper nigrum* fruits; and for increasing milk secretion in cows, a concentrated aqueous extract of *Citrus aurantium* roots, *Achyranthes aspera* leaves and *Acorus calamus* rhizome applied to the udder. The author emphasizes that attention to developing veterinary products from plants would go far in solving many of the Philippines' problems in animal production and healthcare while reducing the nation's dependence on expensive imported medicines.

Paine, R. 1964. Herding and husbandry: Two basic concepts in the analysis of reindeer management. *Folk* 6: 83–88.

Unavailable for review.

Pal, D.C. 1980. Observations on folklore about plants used in veterinary medicine in Bengal, Orissa and Bihar. *Bulletin of the Botanical Survey of India* 22(1–4): 96–99.

This article reports on 20 plant species of 19 genera from 16 families as used by Kondh, Monda, Lodha, Oraon and Santal tribes in India to treat their cattle, buffalo, sheep, goats and poultry. Details of prescriptions are also given. For example, an antidote for plant-poisoning in cattle consists of a drench of 100 grams of *Canna indica* L., 21 black peppers and 25 grams of ginger boiled together in rice water. To ensure proper foetal development and enhance milk production, cows are given a decoction of *Daedalacanthus roseus* T. roots with 50 ml of country liquor.

Palacios Ríos, Félix. 1985. Tecnología del pastoreo. In: Heather Lechtman and Ana Maria Soldi (eds). *La Tecnología en el Mundo Andino: Runakunap Kawsayninkupaq Rurasqankunaqa. Tomo I: Subsistencia y Mensuración.* Imprenta Universitaria de la Universidad Nacional Autónoma de México, México DF. Pp. 217–232.

Much of the same material found in Palacios Ríos 1988 is included in this book chapter. However, the chapter contains a brief section devoted to Aymara ethnoscientific categories of llama and alpaca disease. One of the most feared such diseases is *wila wichhu* (bloody diarrhoea), which decimates the camelid young. Producers attribute this to drinking 'hot' standing water and they treat the condition with lemon water or vinegar. Ectoparasitism is endemic. Lice are treated with soot, ash and alpaca lard. Mange produced by biting and burrowing mites is combated with applications of a volcanic sulphur mixed with melted lard. Other camelid diseases recognized by these Aymara stockowners include: *tongo tongo*, described as sores that form in the throat; *chiqollo*, an intestinal parasite that is treated with infusions of bitter herbs; and *chawlla lago*, a liver fluke. The author emphasizes how producers daily examine their animals, one by one, for any signs of disease or for unusual behaviour such as loss of appetite, excessive thirst and irascibility, so that they can then form accurate diagnoses and take prompt therapeutic action.

Palacios Ríos, Félix. 1988. Tecnología del pastoreo. In: Jorge Flores Ochoa (ed.). *Llamichos y Paqocheros: Pastores de Llamas y Alpacas.* Editorial Universitaria UNSAAC for the Centro de Estudios Andinos Cuzco, Cuzco, Perú. Pp. 87–100.

In describing the range management and animal husbandry system of alpaca raising in an Aymara community of the high punas of southern Peru, this chapter touches upon a number of indigenous practices and beliefs that directly or indirectly impact upon animal health. For example, to prevent diarrhoea, animals are not grazed in icy or dewy pastures or near stagnant water, where moist conditions promote parasitic infestation. When diarrhoeal disease strikes nevertheless, producers administer lemon and vinegar, although they ruefully note that these remedies are rarely effective. The greatly dreaded *sarna* (mange) of alpaca is evaluated during an annual ceremony when newborns are counted; all infected animals receive a topical application of alpaca fat plus sulphur or ash, depending on the type of parasite. Endoparasitism is treated with herbal infusions. Careful genetic selection is practised in an annual breeding ceremony and the alpacas are mated with human assistance. Neonates and pregnant and lactating females are given special care and feeding and herds are divided and ranged by sex and age. The author notes that disease is a critical limiting factor in native alpaca production and that stockraisers are always alert to idiosyncratic behaviour in each of their animals so as to detect any early signs of illness.

Palacpac-Alo, Anna Marie. 1990. Save your animals! Try medicinal herbs. *The PCARRD Monitor* 18(2): 3,8.

'Keeping animals in good shape is not . . . easy, what with the spiralling cost of feedstuffs and livestock medicines' and the 'lack of veterinarians in the barrios' (p. 3). Part of the solution to these problems may lie in medicinal herbs. This article reports findings from a project in the Philippines entitled 'Assessment, Identification and Utilization of Medicinal Plants for Animals'. Based on the EVK of backyard and smallholder stockraisers, the project has found a number of local herbs that offer immediate relief of common ailments like parasitism, wounds and diarrhoea in buffalo, cattle and goats. Parasitism is the major problem for rural stockraisers. A few examples of their herbal responses to endoparasitism are drenches of: pounded *Vitex negundo* L. leaves in water; half a glass of dried and powdered *Leucaena glauca* L. seeds in water (but not for pregnant animals); the juice of 0.5 to 1 kg of washed and pounded *Cajanus cajan* L. leaves or of the same amount of *Momordica charantia* L. leaves; or 8 to 10 powdered seeds of *Areca catechu* L. in water. These and other preliminary findings are based on a benchmark survey that has established preliminary indications of efficacy. The survey will be followed by: bioassay toxicity studies of promising plants for livestock; field trials on the 'best bets' among the plants thus screened; and finally mass propagation and multiplication of the most effective plants.

Palanivelu, A.P. 1997. Jeevakarunya: Use of gentle methods in veterinary practice. In: Anil Gupta (ed.). *International Conference on Creativity and Innovation at Grassroots for Sustainable Natural Resource Management, January 11–14, 1997: Abstracts.* Indian Institute of Management, Ahmedabad, India. P. 150.

As a follower of a certain Tamil saint, the author eschews the use of toxic or painful medicines, rough handling and for herbivores, animal-based products in livestock healthcare. A specialist in treating poisonous bites, injuries and fevers, he describes his own, more 'gentle' veterinary remedies [not detailed in the abstract].

Pande, C.B. 1999. Zeetress – a promising anti-stress and immuno-modulator: A review. In: E. Mathias, D.V. Rangnekar and C.M. McCorkle, with M. Martin (eds). *Ethnoveterinary Medicine: Alternatives for Livestock Development – Proceedings of an International Conference Held in Pune, India, 4–6 November 1997. Volume 1: Selected Papers.* BAIF Development Research Foundation, Pune, India. Pp. 126–132.

Stress is a very common but often unnoticed health problem in the livestock industry. With the high animal densities and constant push for ever-higher product yields of intensive management systems, however, stress is unavoidable. Stressors significantly increase the plasma corticosteroid level, resulting in excess protein catabolism, which in turn causes diminished production, poor feed conversion and immunosuppression. The commercial polyherbal formulation Zeetress is based on familiar traditional botanicals *Emblica officinalis*, *Ocimum sanctum* and *Withania somnifera*. Zeetress regularizes the plasma corticosteroid level and thus prevents excessive protein catabolism and its sequelae. It also minimizes stress-induced depletion of Vitamin C (ascorbic acid) and stimulates humoral as well as cell-mediated immune responses.

Pandey, S.N., M. Sabir and A.K. Srivastava. 1998. Pharmacological actions of some medicinal plants having uterotonic activity. In: E. Mathias, D.V. Rangnekar and C.M. McCorkle, with M. Martin (eds). *Ethnoveterinary Medicine: Alternatives for Livestock Development – Proceedings of an International Conference Held in Pune, India, 4–6 November 1997. Volume 2: Abstracts.* BAIF Development Research Foundation, Pune, India. Pp. 45–46.

In India, a number of medicinal plants have traditionally been used to treat reproductive disorders in domestic animals. Due to the adoption of Western-style veterinary medicine, however, knowledge and use of such ethnobotanicals has declined dramatically. This paper reports on evaluations of various pharmacological parameters of five such plants that are all applied as uterotonics: *Adhatoda vasica, Gardenia gumnifera, Leptadenia reticulata, Plumbago zeylanica* and *Viburnum stellulatum.* On chemical examination, *A. vasica* was found to contain alkaloids, glycosides, phenolic components and sterols; *G. gumnifera* contained glycosides, phenolic compounds and amines; *L. reticulata* contained alkaloids, glycosides, phenolic compounds and sterols; and *V. stellulatum* contained alkaloids, glycosides, amines and sterols. The five plants produced varying degrees of analgesic, hypnotic and hypotensive effects in dogs and rats. *Adhatoda vasica* increased both the rate and amplitude of respiration, while the other plants mildly inhibited respiration. None of the five had any effect on the nictitating membrane. On the isolated uterus of rat, collected during the metoestrus phase of the oestrous cycle, *A. vasica* had a mild stimulatory effect; and on the uterus collected during the oestrus phase, it induced marked rhythmicity. On the isolated full-term gravid uterus of rats, *A. vasica, P. zeylanica* and *L. reticulata* markedly increased the tone of spontaneously motile tissue, while *G. gumnifera* and *V. stellulatum* did not. Still other important pharmacological and therapeutic actions of these plants were investigated.

Parasuraman, Aroor. 1994. Practices from Tamil version, 'Num Vazhi Velanmai' 1 (3&4). *Honey Bee* 5(2): 19.

In Tamil-speaking India, to reduce mortality rates in rabbits, newborns are given 3 ml of honey in warm water (human infants, too) and 21-day-olds receive a deworming drench of several ground papaya seeds in about 10 ml of water.

Parent, R. 1994. *A Few Alternative Treatments in Rural Veterinary Medicine.* In-house report of Project SCLD. Extension Service West, Provincial Delegation MINEPIA, Bafoussam, Cameroon. 40 pp.

Written by a veterinarian, this booklet is designed to inform African veterinary technicians of valid alternatives to conventional veterinary treatments that they can themselves prepare and administer using locally available plant and other materials such as palm oil, engine grease, bleach and vinegar. Livestock species mentioned include large and small ruminants, monogastrics and rabbits. Remedies draw upon both traditional and modern, plant and non-plant ideas and ingredients. Examples of some of the 17 preparations described are an antifungal lotion, a laxative, a disinfectant for animal quarters and a treatment for coccidiosis in rabbits. A warming ointment compounded of strong red and yellow peppers soaked in table oil for 10 days and then mixed with engine grease is recommended for massaging stock with tendonitis, pulmonary congestion, or intestinal disorders.

Parida, Nisith R. 1997. Punyakoti the truthful test. *Undhyoo* 12: 79.

This press release article highlights several presentations on EVM made by Indian scientists and farmers at the International Conference on Creativity and Innovation at Grassroots, held in India in 1997. A Dr Veena outlined a simple yet reliable pregnancy test for cattle, which she drew from an ancient Egyptian method employing the subject cow's urine and wheat seed. Veena has since standardized this test and named it *punyakot* after a cow in Kannada legend who risked her life to uphold the truth. In response to Dr A.M. Thakar's description of the use of custard apple seeds to control various livestock parasites, some attendees commented on the seeds' possible neurotoxicity. A farmer discussed some traditional livestock treatments from his native state of Uttar Pradesh and pled for mechanisms to keep this knowledge alive in farm youth.

Parodi C., Bruno Giovanni, Eugenio Martínez Bravo and Dora Martínez Olivares. 1989. Investigación etnobotánica medicinal veterinaria en Zacatecas: Comunicación preliminar. In: Gerardo López Buendía (ed.). *Memorias: Segunda Jornada sobre Herbolaria Medicinal en Medicina Veterinaria.* Universidad Nacional Autónoma de México, Facultad de Medicina Veterinaria y Zootecnia, Coordinación de Educación Continua, México DF, México. Pp. 162–171.

In 1981, the Medicinal Plant Project of Mexico's Zacatecas State University designed three questionnaires to explore rural people's knowledge of and success with medicinal plants in animal and human ethno-medicine and -dentistry. The questionnaires were distributed in 28 rural secondary schools in 17 of the state's 56 municipalities for students to take home and complete along with their elders. For each plant, the questionnaires asked about 13 variables, which were later encoded in a conventional DBIII database. From the questionnaire on EVM, 248 out of 380 informants' responses were statistically analysed, based on a criterion of at least five animals treated for a specific disease with a given plant. A total of 82 plant species used on cattle, equines, swine, poultry, dogs and cats were thus identified. Of the 82, 47 also appeared among the 202 plants mentioned for human ethnomedicine. Based on consistent reports of their therapeutic success in livestock, 14 ethnoveterinary treatments were tagged for future, in-depth clinical trials, to be conducted for and with farmers themselves. This paper presents statistical and treatment details for 12 of these 14: *Agave* sp., *Allium cepa, Ambrosia artemisiifolia, Andropogon citratus, Artemisia mexicana, Citrus limonus, Eysenhardtia polystachy, Fraxinus uhdei, Jatropha dioica, Physalis* sp., *Verbesina* sp. and *Yucca zacatecana.* Meanwhile, comparative information is being sought in literature on Zacatecan ethnomedicine dating from the 16th century forward, in order to detect to what extent such phytotherapeutic knowledge is being retained or lost. The overarching goal of this ongoing project is to characterize clinical ethnomedical knowledge and practice, rather than to validate them phytochemically or pharmacologically. Even though the latter such studies suggest that, 'in more than 90% of cases, popular references to the use of medicinal plants are essentially correct as to their described effects, ultimately pharmacological studies . . . are divorced from the application . . . of the . . . plants in their traditional form . . . and are limited . . . to a select public of researchers, with almost no possibility of getting the eventual benefits [of this research] out to the [farming] population' (p. 163). Indeed, in developing countries such phytochemical and pharmacological research often serves as little more than a 'Third World sweatshop for transnational pharmaceutical companies' (ibid.).

Parra C., Alejandro. 1989. Aplicaciones prácticas de la herbolaria a la medicina curativa en rumiantes. In: Gerardo López Buendía (ed.). *Memorias: Segunda Jornada sobre Herbolaria Medicinal en Medicina Veterinaria.* Universidad Nacional Autónoma de México, Facultad de Medicina Veterinaria y Zootecnia, Coordinación de Educación Continua, México DF, México. Pp. 88–91.

The author recounts his personal experiences as a veterinarian using herbal remedies, alone or in combination with commercial ones, on cattle in the tropics and high plains of Mexico. Eleven plants are cited [without Latin names] as effective cures for diarrhoeas, constipation, colics, conjunctivitis, mange, wounds, bites, sores, myiasis, abscesses and tumours, rheumatism, phlebitis, inflamed nerves and sunburn. Non-botanical items such as bran, flour, vinegar, salt, olive oil and vaseline also figure in many of these remedies. The author makes a plea for systematic scientific and clinical study of all such cures in order to bolster practical experiences like his own. He argues that professionals have an ethical duty to investigate such remedies, since stockraisers appear to be using them more and more.

Patel, Bhikhubhai G. 1994. A farmer's report from south Gujarat. *Honey Bee* 5(2): 8.

Farmers in south Gujarat, India give 100 to 150 ml of dilute lime water mixed with feed to cows that have just calved. Continued for 3 months, this treatment reportedly prevents milk fever. For the same reason but as another way of administering the lime, some farmers paint their water tanks with lime twice weekly.

Patel, K.K., J.H. Suthar, D. Koradia, A. Raval, A. Pastakia, C. Srinivas, S. Muralikrishna, H. Patel, R. Sinha and A.K. Gupta. 1997. Survey of Grassroots Innovations Part XIX. *Honey Bee* 8(2): 13–15.

Rajasthani camel herders give overheated camels 5 kg each of curd and barley flour. Elsewhere, livestock diarrhoea is cured by a warm infusion of 200 g each of *Butea monosperma*, *Madhuca latifolia* and *Acacia catechu* bark; after cooling overnight, 2 bowls of the filtered liquid are given the patient twice daily for 2 days. Extract of green *Syzygium cuminii* bark given morning and evening for three days cures kidney stones in bullocks. Using a similar treatment regime, swollen and painful joints due to overwork or excessive loads of bullocks can be soothed with a balm of 100 g each of *Moringa* spp. bark and *ghodakhundi* (?) plant. Animals that stop ruminating can be given 200 to 300 g of crushed *Moringa* spp. and 500 g of jaggery in water, followed by crushed *Balanites* spp. bark in 200 ml of water. To expel the placenta, give the cow a cooled decoction of 300 to 400 g of *Rivea hypocrateriformis* leaves, 250 g of jaggery, 50 g of *suva* (?) and 25 g of ash from burnt *Sesamum indicum* stalks.

Patel, Kirit K., Jitendra H. Suthar, Dilip Koradia et al. 1997a. Survey of grassroots innovations part XX. *Honey Bee* 8(3): 11–13.

One Indian stockraiser treats hair loss on the tail of his animals by applying boiled and then cooled sesame oil to the bald areas thrice daily for a month. A woman ensures placental expulsion by feeding dams 1 kg of rice smeared with groundnut oil 3 or 4 hours afer calving; if the placenta is not dropped within 8 hours, she feeds 7 to 8 *Abrus precatorius* seeds. For problems of repeat breeding, Indian treatments are to feed livestock fine sand and a few crushed *Lawsonia inermis* leaves that have been soaked in water overnight in an earthen vessel, or 200 g of ghee and 500 ml of sugar solution. To increase buffalo's milk yield, 250 g of cooked rice is fed twice a day for a week. To set fractured bones, a cast is made of powdered charcoal from burnt *Capparis decidua* stems mixed with ghee. Wounds are dressed daily for a week with a paste of several goat droppings and 1 or 2 leaves of *Cassia auriculata* pounded together. A paste of butter with ashes from burning 200 g of onion relieves yoke gall.

Patel, K.K., D. Koradia, P. Rohit, C.H. Parmar, C. Srinivas, S. Muralikrishna, H. Patel, R. Sinha, A.K. Gupta and P. Shah. 1997b. Survey of Grassroots Innovations Part XXI. *Honey Bee* 8(4): 15–17.

Indian cattle raisers use different methods to increase milk production. One is to feed the boiled mixture of a cotton ball, *Acacia nilotica* beans and pearl millet at milking time. Another is to add the inner kernel of mango pits to cattle feed. To cure swollen udders and teats, stockraisers apply the juice of *Salvadora persica* leaves twice daily for 2 days. For common colds in cattle, they feed 150 g of groundnut oil daily, add onions to the feed and give an evening drench of decocted leaves of *Ocimum sanctum, Trachyspermum ammi*, mint and tea or tea powder for 3 to 4 days. Bullocks with kidney stones are drenched with juice of *jamun* (?) fruit skin twice daily. An Indian scientist notes that this and related diuretic treatments can help stone expulsion; but if the urine is completely blocked, they should not be used.

Patel, K.K., D. Koradia, P.H. Rohit, C.H. Parmar, C. Srinivas, S. Muralikrishna, H. Patel, R. Sinha, A.K. Gupta and P. Shah. 1998a. Survey of Grassroots Innovations Part XXII. *Honey Bee* 9(1): 15–17.

Indian ethnoveterinary practices reported here include: feeding 1 or 2 basketfuls of fresh *Bambusa bambos* leaves to promote rapid explusion of placenta; to cure urinary problems, drenching with 100 ml per day for several days of 1 kg of *Boerhavia diffusa* roots decocted in 2.5 l of water until the water is reduced to 1 l; and for myiasis, washing the wound, pouring buffalo milk on it to draw out the maggots for manual removal, then cleaning and dressing the wound with a paste of crushed *Momordica charantia* (known to have antibacterial, antifungal, insecticidal and styptic properties). To control fleas on cattle, one woman cleans out her cattleshed using a broom made of dry *Madhuca indica* and spreads about 100 g of the leaves of this strong-smelling plant around the shed. In addition, she rubs 10 to 15 *Moschosma polystachym* plants on the bodies of the flea-bitten animals. For ticks, she does likewise with a mixture of 50 g of turmeric powder in 100 g of castor oil.

Patel, K.K., D. Koradia, P.H. Rohit, C.H. Parmar, C. Srinivas, S. Muralikrishna, H. Patel, R. Sinha, A.K. Gupta and P. Shah. 1998b. Survey of Grassroots Innovations Part XXIII. *Honey Bee* 9(2): 14–16.

Various ethnoveterinary treatments from around India are reported here. The arthritic limbs of cattle are massaged with a decoction of 1 kg of the inner bark of the *Moringa pterygosperma* tree, boiled in 4 l of water until the liquid is reduced by half. Cattle with diarrhoea are drenched with 500 g of powdered *Tamarindus indica* seeds in 250 g of water every day for a week or so. A general poultry tonic consists of 100 g of Indian laburnum (*Lassia fistula*) pods ground with water and mixed with the essence of 1 garlic knot and 2 onions in 100 ml of water.

Patel, P.R., F.S. Kavani and M.P. Pande. 1992a. Farmers' practices in animal husbandry. *Honey Bee* 3(3&4): 7.

Post-partum cows suffer from low calcium, leading to shivering. Indian farmers remedy this by feeding an appetite-stimulating mixture of fenugreek, sesame and other seeds with black pepper. Pre-partum cows are denied mustard straw in the belief that this fodder can cause abortions. Therapeutic cautery or firing, using an iron rod, is applied to animals with chronic joint pain and acute inflammation: farmers say this technique increases blood circulation.

Patel , P.R., F.S. Kavani and M.B. Pande (commentators). 1992b. Animal husbandary [sic]. *Honey Bee* 3(3&4): 18–21.

This article details 13 categories of disorders in cattle, camels and poultry that are treated with a variety of locally available *materia medica* in India, as reported by *Honey Bee* readers and evaluated by this newsletter's Technical Committee of Livestock and Veterinary Sciences. Cattle disorders and their corresponding treatments span: urinary blockages – various bark, millet-pollen, barley and other plant drenches; female infertility – castor-oil or banana-extract or -leaf feedings; postpartum care – sugar drenches; endoparasites – castor- or mustard-oil laxatives followed by prompt removal of the resulting dung from the cattle-shed, to prevent further infestation; yoke gall – topical applications of root extracts, of dry-cell battery powder and oil, or of a certain leaf first chewed by the farmer; fractures – a plaster of fenugreek seed-flour with bamboo splints; an unspecified ailment, possibly muscle inflammation – stand or float the animal in deep water or startle it with a noise or black cloth and drench it with tea; ingrown horns – a moist dressing of millet flour and human hair; loose teeth – feeding a crushed bark-and-root mixture; flatulence – a drench of *Cucumis sativus* seeds; udder inflammation – sprinkling on the udder a solution of salt or white-alum or a suspension of *Aegle marmelos* and *Cenchrus* sp. leaves, crushed together; food poisoning – repeated rubs of termite-mound soil inside the mouth or of newspaper ash with jaggery. Examples of general poultry remedies include pounded-up garlic, onion and *Cuscuta reflexa* in the birds' drinking water, or rabbit faeces mixed with *C. reflexa* vines.

Patel, P.R., F.S. Kavani, K.M. Jadhav and R.M. Patel. 1993. Control of milk fever in cattle. *Honey Bee* 4 (2&3): 13.

In this article, Indian scientists report on helpful farmer practices to prevent or control milk fever in cattle and buffalo cows. Milk fever is characterized by chills, weakness, anorexia and recumbency, all linked to a colostrum-related calcium deficiency. To prevent milk fever in the first place, for several days after calving, cows should be milked only partially so as to leave the udder half full of colostrum. If milk fever strikes nevertheless, farmers take immediate action to warm the cow by building a fire near it, covering it with gunny/grain sacks and/or covering the sides of its shed to block chill winds. Light exercise, in the form of slowly walking the cow, forces the animal to get up and increases blood flow to the legs. During and/or before the calving period, cows are fed laxative but energy-giving foods such as boiled *bajra* (?), jaggery, edible oils, ghee and eggs, plus appetite-inducing seeds like those of fenugreek or *Anethum graveolens*. A mixture of salt, turmeric, ginger, cumin, asafoetida and black pepper also helps stimulate appetite and expel rumen gases. For very severe cases of milk fever, however, a veterinarian should give an intravenous injection of calcium.

Patel, P.R., C.B. Prajapati, M.T. Panchal and J.J. Hasnani. 1998. Sarcoptic mange in rural camels (*Camelus dromedarius*) and its treatment – A useful ethno-medical practice. In: E. Mathias, D.V. Rangnekar and C.M. McCorkle, with M. Martin (eds). *Ethnoveterinary Medicine: Alternatives for Livestock Development – Proceedings of an International Conference Held in Pune, India, 4–6 November 1997. Volume 2: Abstracts.* BAIF Development Research Foundation, Pune, India. P. 46.

Mange is the second most important health problem of rural camels. Predisposing factors are poor husbandry, overcrowding, malnutrition, fatigue, long hair coat, lack of green fodder in the diet and worm infestation. A total of 702 skin scrapings from 269 camels in rural India showed that about 27% of the animals were infected with *Sarcoptes scabiei*. As remedies, camel owners commonly apply castor oil, *karanja* (*Pongamia glabra*) oil, or burnt engine oil on the skin lesions once or twice a week for several months, after which improvement is usually observed. These remedies' efficacy is probably due to the fact that such viscous oils prevent *Sarcoptes* larvae from migrating, thus interrupting the parasite's life cycle.

Peacock, Christie. 1996. *Improving Goat Production in the Tropics: A Manual for Development Workers.* Oxfam, Oxford, UK. 386 pp.

This thorough-going manual on goat production in the tropics recommends a number of useful practices that are characteristic of many traditional EVM systems around the world. To treat the bloat, diarrhoea and pain of acidosis, common materials such as oil, charcoal and sodium bicarbonate can be introduced into the rumen using a tube. Charcoal can also be helpful in absorbing the toxins produced by enterotoxaemia. Good hygiene and separation of infected animals are keys to battling contagious agalactia. Broken bones can usually be repaired by simple splinting techniques and rest, especially for kids. To combat the burrowing mites of sarcoptic mange, a proven treatment is a castor-bean (*Ricinus communis*) wash, which is rich in the insecticidal chemical ricin. The chopped castor-bean leaves and stems are heated in water just to boiling, at a ratio of 1:50 by weight. Citing Matzigkeit (1990), the author notes seven common plants from which natural medicines can be prepared to repel or control ectoparasites. For small herds of goats with only minor tick challenge, manually killing ticks by piercing them with a needle or thorn is often sufficient to control these pests; moreover, children can perform this task. Pen feeding greatly reduces goats' exposure to ticks and other ecto- and endo-parasites. Commercial acaricides may not be a viable option in smallholder production systems unless all livestock owners act together. So 'It may be better to try to keep a balance between the disease challenge from the ticks and the goats' resistance to the challenge' (p. 193). In the latter regard, as a result of both natural selection and owners' selective breeding, '. . . tropical goats are well adapted to surviving in tropical environments with . . . high disease challenge' as well as high temperatures, poor-quality feeds and limited water (p. 262). So far, there has been little threat to genetic maintenance of indigenous races of tropical goats from crossing with alien breeds. Besides castration, goat raisers have a number of traditional methods for controlling breeding. Separation of the sexes is used mainly where goats are penned most of the year. For rangestock, aprons made of leather or canvas can be tied around bucks' midriffs until mating time, when the aprons are then removed or twisted 'round. A penis string may be employed in the same fashion. Looped at one end around the testicles and at the other around the prepuce, the string deviates the extended penis to left or right. When it comes to castration, a common traditional method consists of crushing the spermatic cord between two pieces of wood using a hammer or stone. However, this method can result in only partial castration. In addition to controlling breeding, castration speeds animal growth rate and increases carcass fat content by reducing the energy spent on fighting and mating; it also lessens the odour of buck meat. Finally, the author notes that 'Psychological support and encouragement' are important in treating and nursing sick goats because otherwise 'They tend to sink into a depression from which it is often difficult for them to recover' (p. 217).

Peillen, D. 1972. Recueil de recettes vétérinaires de Joréguiberry. **Bulletin du Musée Basque** 57(3): 113–144.

Unavailable for review.

Pelant, Robert K. 1991. Health care programs for small ruminants. In: Harvey D. Blackburn (ed.). **Small Ruminant Production: Systems for Sustainability. Proceedings from a Workshop for the PVO and University Communities, June 20–21, 1991.** University of Maryland, College Park, Maryland, USA. Pp. 111–128.

A few ethnoveterinary practices from India are described in this conference paper. Leaves from the custard apple tree are fed to expel roundworms in buffalo calves. Neem leaves are used to discourage fly strike and myiasis. Both of these trees' leaves are used and recommended by the veterinary departments of Madras' Christian College and the Tamil Nadu Veterinary University of India [as part of the Ayurvedic system].

Pélissier, Paul. 1966. **Les Paysans du Sénégal. Les Civilisations Agraires du Cayor à la Casamance.** Imprimerie Fabrègue, Saint-Yrieix, France.

When an epidemic strikes, Diola pastoralists of Senegal send their animals away to friends and family because, according to the author, they are incapable of treating the animals themselves (p. 763).

Peña Bellido, Luís Beltran. 1975. **La Agropecuaria Tradicional en la Provincia de Chumbivilcas – Cusco.** Thesis, Department of Agronomy, Universidad San Antonio Abad del Cusco, Perú. 163 pp.

This thesis constitutes a wide-ranging social, economic, technological and ideological description of agropastoralism in the southern Peruvian department of Chumbivilcas. Chapter IV, 'Traditional Stock Raising in Chumbivilcas' not only outlines basic husbandry techniques, but also details many aspects of folk veterinary therapies to combat both internal and external parasites, diarrhoeas, bloat, haemorrhages, infections, fractures, saddle sores, lameness, placenta retention, abortion and poisoning in livestock (pp. 139–148). Ethnotherapies involve: different salts, clays, sulfur, lime and other minerals; drenches, unguents and plasters using a great variety of plant preparations (e.g. banana leaves, latex, indigo, in addition to sylvan and domesticated plants of the sierra), often along with other items like the ubiquitous llama fat as well as lard from other species, and poultry droppings, urine, blood, sugar, ash, soap and 'fresh snakes' (the latter used to bind fractures); sun baths and smoke cures; bleeding, lancing and cauterization. Many of the treatments are reportedly effective.

Peña Haaz, Nelly, Estela Ana Auró Angulo and Héctor Sumano López. 1988. Evaluación comparativa del efecto nematodicida del ajo (*Allium sativum*), sus extractos liposoluble e hidrosoluble y el tartrato de amonio y potasio en carpa (*Cyprinus carpio*). In: Luz Lozano Nathal and Gerardo López Buendía (coordinators). ***Memorias: Primera Jornada sobre Herbolaria Medicinal en Veterinaria.*** Universidad Nacional Autónoma de México, Facultad de Medicina Veterinaria y Zootecnia, Coordinación de Educación Continua, México DF. Pp. 124–129.

Mexican aquaculture is plagued by internal parasites which often go untreated because commercial products are too expensive, give unsatisfactory results, are not always available, often leave harmful chemical residues and their dosages are difficult to determine. From time immemorial, garlic has served as an excellent anthelmintic in both humans and domesticated mammals. This preliminary study sought to determine whether it might also be effective for fish. Both egg counts and necropsies showed that ground garlic is a more effective nematocide than various garlic extracts or than standard chemical treatments. The authors suggest that garlic can be very profitably and easily used by small fish farmers in Mexico, with the only drawback being its strong odour.

Percy, Fiona. 1995. Existing local knowledge: Does it help participatory development? *Baobab* 20 (Jul): page number unknown. [Article taken from the Arid Lands Information Network website, http://alin.utando.com/percy.html.]

In working with Samburu pastoralists and their extensive knowledge of animal health, ITDG/Kenya noted that herders were worried that this existing knowledge (which allows them to keep their herds healthy without recourse to veterinarians) was being lost. Part of the reason for its disappearance was that when Samburu children attend school, they lose confidence in their parents' knowledge. This concern on the part of Samburu has led ITDG/Kenya to produce booklets for use in local schools, based on its work in participatory research and validation of effective traditional treatments for livestock. At a broader level, an ITDG/Kenya multinational workshop on existing local knowledge such as EVM concluded that such knowledge is vital in promoting sustainable development by enabling communities to take the initiative. Workshop participants thus strongly recommended its validation and application, its use in building local people's confidence and in widening technology options and better transfer of findings on local knowledge from research to extension.

Perevolotsky, Avi. 1985. *Los Pobladores de los Despoblados: Goat Herders in Piura, Peru.* Technical Report No. 33. SR-CRSP, Department of Rural Sociology, University of Missouri-Columbia, Columbia, Missouri 65211, USA. 174 pp.

Based on participant observation, slaughterhouse records and a survey of more than 200 pastoral households, this report analyses the ecological, social, economic and political context of goat husbandry in Piura, Peru. Chapter 3 on goat raising (pp. 22–47) includes descriptions of breeding, genetic selection, housing, watering and feeding. Septicaemia, pneumonia, mastitis, parasitism, plant poisoning and *coquera* are the most common ailments among goats in Piura. *Coquera* is a disease affecting the muscles of the digestive system. According to local herders, it is related to a poor diet consisting mostly of *algarrobo* pods. The author reports that plant materials are only rarely used to treat sick goats and that there is no evidence of a well-developed ethnoveterinary system among these herders. The last chapter of this report investigates whether goats overgraze the *Despoblado* region.

Perezgrovas Garza, Raúl. 1988a. Les bergères Tzotziles et leurs brebis: Une bienveillance de longue date. *Habbanae* 49: 15.

In addition to the information noted in other articles by this author, here three native Mayan animal domesticates are mentioned: dogs, ducks and turkeys. Once again, the unique and sacred position of sheep among Tzotzil Maya Indians of Mexico's Chiapas highlands is noted. That is, in contrast to cattle, pigs and chickens, sheep are never sacrificed and eaten, whether for ritual or nutritional purposes. Rather, sheep are treated more like members of the family.

Pérezgrovas Garza, Raúl. 1988b. Ovicultura indígena en los altos de Chiapas: Aportación Tzotzil a las costumbres pastoriles Españolas. In: Rodolfo Uribe Iniesta (ed.). *Medio Ambiente y Comunidades Indígenas del Sureste: Prácticas Tradicionales de Producción, Rituales y Manejo de Recursos.* Comisión Nacional de los Estados Unidos Mexicanos para la UNESCO, IV Comité Regional, Gobierno del Estado and Secretaria de Educación, Cultura y Recreación del Gobierno de Tabasco. Tabasco, Mexico. Pp. 140–151.

Sheepraising as practised by Tzotzil Maya of Mexico's Chiapas highlands represents a uniquely 'autochthonous' system, built up from a marriage of Spanish and Maya religious and husbandry traditions. Sheep first reached Mexico in 1493, travelling as ship's food-animals on Columbus' second voyage. From that time forward, Amerinds have been elaborating their own blend of management and healthcare methods, as suited to their particular social, economic, ecological, ideological and historical circumstances. This article describes Tzotzil shepherdesses' practices for pasturing, housing, watering, docking, treating and naming their animals – all in the context of ancient Maya cosmology and ethnomedicine, but as syncretized with Spanish Catholicism. For example, prayers, votive candles and offerings to the patron saint of sheep or other 'animal saints' figure in local veterinary medicine, alongside ritual practices based on Mayan notions of animal souls. Herbal medicines are also used, whether for such supernatural conditions as evil or 'hot' eye or for natural ones such as general unthriftiness (locally termed *aire* or 'air'). Particular medicinal plants mentioned include *Adiantum andicola*, *Allium sativum* and *Nicotiana tabacum*. Shepherdesses are especially knowledgeable about pasture plants that produce, or 'are associated with, ovine health problems like poisoning, bloat and fasciolosis. For example, they link the last to plants that grow in the same moist habitat as that of the liverfluke's snail host.

Pérezgrovas Garza, Raúl. 1989–1990. La apropriación de la ovinocultura por los Tzotziles de los altos de Chiapas: Un pasaje de la historia desde la perspectiva etnoveterinaria. *Anuario CEI* 3: 185–198.

Taking an ethnoveterinary perspective, this article from the Centro de Estudios Indígenas of UNACH's *Anuario* journal traces the history of the adoption of sheep-raising by Tzotzil Maya Indians of Mexico's Chiapas highlands. It first addresses the fascinating question of how a Spanish tradition of large-scale transhumant pastoralism managed by men mainly for meat production was transformed into a system of settled small-scale stockraising managed by native Indian women for wool production within a culture that had never known herding. The remainder of the article describes contemporary Tzotzil sheep husbandry: housing, corralling and grazing patterns; muzzling and watering practices; knowledge of toxic plants; and herbal medicines. Illustrating from the most important sheep disease of the region (fasciolosis), discussion emphasizes how husbandry of this introduced livestock species has been functionally folded into and guided by ancient Maya cosmological and ethnomedical beliefs, as well as astute ethnoecological understandings – even though the latter, too, are cast in an ideological idiom. [For greater detail, see the annotations of other Pérezgrovas publications.]

Perezgrovas, Raul. 1992a. Animal health care by Indian shepherdesses in southern Mexico. In: John Young (ed.). *A Report on a Village Animal Health Care Workshop – Volume II: The Case Studies.* ITDG, Rugby, UK. Pp. 76–80.

Extensive research is being conducted into the animal healthcare and husbandry system of Tzotzil Maya shepherdesses in Mexico's Chiapas State. As part of this research, three herbal remedies recommended by the shepherdesses to combat gastrointestinal parasites were clinically evaluated. Two of these consist of feeding sprigs of *Teloxys ambrosioides* or the mashed seeds of the giant pumpkin *Cucurbita maxima*. [The third remedy is not mentioned here.] Initial trials have shown a significant reduction in faecal egg counts of gastrointestinal nematodes and oocysts of *Eimeria* spp. within a week of treatment. While parasites are never totally eliminated, such folk remedies are virtually 'costless'. Moreover, unlike commercial medicaments, they are culturally acceptable to shepherdesses, who reject any drug in the form of pills, tablets or injectable liquids. The author expects that, perhaps with further research on dosing regimes, these traditional treatments can be very efficient in parasite control. Participatory on-farm trials on the treatments are now underway. The trials are managed by shepherdesses themselves, using their own sheep. At first, the women objected to researchers' collecting faeces directly from sheep; but eventually the shepherdesses agreed that this procedure did not harm their animals. Now, more and more women are asking to participate. This is the best indication of appropriate research. The long-term goal is to elaborate a calendar for the regular administration of botanicals, in adequate frequency and combinations, in order to keep parasite burdens as low as possible in lieu of commercial products.

Perezgrovas, Raul. 1992b. Collecting and using ethnoveterinary information. In: John Young (ed.). ***A Report on a Village Animal Health Care Workshop – Kenya, February 1992.*** ITDG, Rugby, UK. Pp. 6–11 of Appendix 5.

Drawing on the author's work with Tzotzil Maya shepherdesses of Mexico, this pictorial presentation of how to collect and apply EVM data encapsulates the ideal ER&D attitude and approach. The first rule of ER&D is 'Be nice to people'. The second rule is 'Repeat rule 1'. After that, there are no rules in the sense that researchers must 'leave all preconceived ideas behind' (p. 9). In terms of scientific inputs, the importance of an interdisciplinary approach cannot be overemphasized. Beyond the veterinary and animal sciences, inputs from agronomy and ecology are usually needed. The social and related sciences should also always be involved: social anthropology, sociology, linguistics and certainly economics. Depending on the role of animals in the farming system, additional expertise is also required. For the work with Tzotil, for example, experts in fibre analysis and processing and in textile production were needed for the project because the goal of Tzotzil sheep-raising is wool production and weaving. Based on the author's own research experiences, the paper gives examples of methodologies for gathering ethnoveterinary data from all these perspectives with the ultimate goal of producing a 'package' approach to people's animal health problems that builds on local knowledge and resources as much as possible.

Perezgrovas, Raúl. 1996. Sheep husbandry and healthcare among Tzotzil Maya shepherdesses. In: Constance M. McCorkle, Evelyn Mathias and Tjaart W. Schillhorn van Veen (eds). ***Ethnoveterinary Research & Development.*** Intermediate Technology Publications, London, UK. Pp. 167–178.

In Mexico, where the ovine population has been declining over the last 20 years, the small municipality of Chamula, in the highlands of Chiapas State, has the highest sheep density in the country. The area is inhabited by different groups of Maya Indians, including the Tzotzil. Tzotzil derive up to 40% of their income from raising sheep for wool, which is performed entirely by women under a traditional management system. More than 400 years have passed since sheep were first introduced to the region by Spanish priests and landlords. During that time, Tzotzil women have developed a unique relationship with, and husbandry system for, their animals. For example, they believe that every sheep has a soul; therefore eating mutton (but not beef) is taboo. [This belief is not surprising given that the Tzotzil goal of sheep production is wool, not meat.] Based on interviews in 30 Chamula hamlets, this chapter overviews Tzotzil sheep management and describes how Indian shepherdesses perceive, prevent and cure the most common sheep diseases. Grazing is rotated seasonally: during the June to November rains, sheep graze communally owned pastures; during the subsequent dry season, they enjoy the rich stubble of the harvested maize fields; thereafter, the flock is moved to the forest where they can browse until the rains return. A unique management technique is muzzling sheep on their way to grazing grounds in the early morning so that the hungry animals cannot eat ripening crops, poisonous plants, or the still-dew-ridden grasses that harbour infective parasites or their hosts. Another astute and environmentally friendly husbandry technique is bucket-watering so that sheep cannot ingest aquaphilic vegetation that shelters the snail host and infectious larvae of liver fluke. Furthermore, this practice protects streams, their banks and the often-unique flora and fauna of riparian habitats from degradation or disturbance by trampling and grazing; and it has the added benefit of keeping stock from fouling water supplies also used by people. Shepherdesses also take care to keep animal quarters clean. The women who use temporary corrals to manure their fields move the structures every 6 weeks; women with permanent and often roofed structures muck them out every 8 to 10 weeks. With regard to livestock (and human) diseases, these are defined in terms of syncretic Mayan/Catholic concepts wherein good and evil forces struggle over the soul of an animal and where an owner's emotional state can affect the health of her flock, making the animals 'sad' and thus prone to disease. Sadness can be triggered by situations such as: someone other than the shepherdess-owner's tending the flock; the owner's talking or even thinking about selling her animals, which women say the sheep can sense; arguments and fights between husband and wife that transmit their anger to the flock; and the shepherdess' laziness and inattention to her animals. The ethnoaetiology, physiopathology and treatment of fasciolosis are illustrative of shepherdesses' disease concepts and responses. They term this disease 'water necklace' or 'water bag' after its characteristic sub-mandibular oedema. Most often, they attribute it to animals' ingesting various aquaphilic plants [see above], which they say produce the 'little leaf animals' (i.e. flukes) that can be seen upon practical necropsy of the liver. Homemade drenches of *Eupatorium ligustrinum* sprigs, with known anti-inflammatory properties, are a popular water-bag therapy; the same drench is used for ovine diarrhoea. An alternative is a drench of fresh-ground garlic in homemade rum; this remedy also treats bloat. Still other herbal preparations are prescribed for fasciolosis. However, if its cause is diagnosed as sadness, then a complicated ritual cure is instead indicated. A clear understanding of a people's management and ethnoveterinary concepts and practices has immediate implications for new approaches to the development of livestock health and productivity. It reveals what practices may be effective and should be reinforced – like many Tzotzil husbandry techniques and the view that lazy and inattentive shepherdesses may indeed sadden their animals by allowing them to graze in unhealthy places. It also points up concepts and practices that may be less helpful – like the *E. ligustrinum* drench, which may reduce the jaw swelling but not attack the root cause of fasciolosis – where inputs from modern science can be beneficial. Finally, it can teach developers the importance of being more emotionally sensitive and culturally informed. For instance, Tzotzil would be profoundly shocked if some over-enthusiastic developer were to suggest they raise a dual-purpose wool/meat sheep for consumption (just as would Muslims or Jews if it were suggested they raise and eat pigs). From stockraisers like Maya shepherdesses, Western scientists and developers may well learn some new lessons about how to keep more livestock 'souls' happy and thus healthy and productive.

Perezgrovas, Raul. 1997. Ethnoveterinary research & development in Latin America. Paper presented to the First International Conference on Ethnoveterinary Medicine: Alternatives for Livestock Development, Pune, India, 4–6 November 1997.

Major initial contributions to ER&D in Latin America came from Peru, where the work of Dr Constance McCorkle on an international and multi-university livestock development project in the early 1980s later led her to propose ER&D as a new field of study. The other major site of ER&D was Mexico, where various university groups conducted research and held a number of academic meetings beginning in the 1980s on the historical, social and cultural importance and the biomedical efficacy of traditional veterinary and husbandry techniques for Mexican stockraisers. Such work as was carried out elsewhere in Latin America was also mainly based in universities, notably of Bolivia, Brazil, Chile and Venezuela. In general, ER&D in Latin America has followed a trajectory of: collecting and recording EVK; testing plant remedies; investigating husbandry and breeding practices; and at least in Peru and Mexico, conducting participatory research involving communities in on-farm trials on local treatments and breeds. Some noteworthy features of ER&D in Latin America are: its close attention to spiritual, supernatural or magical components in ER&D; and its inclusion of species such as guinea pigs and the South American camelids. Looking across the ER&D scene in Latin America as of 1997, some important shifts have been: the addition of more countries to the EVK map, as it were, such as Costa Rica, Ecuador and Guatemala; the increasing involvement of NGOs; and as a result, an overall growth in ER&D studies and development efforts of all sorts. But much remains to be done. More projects, R&D funding and consciousness-raising are required across the board.

Perezgrovas, Raul. 1999. Ethnoveterinary studies among Tzotzil shepherdesses as the basis of a genetic improvement programme for Chiapas sheep. In: E. Mathias, D.V. Rangnekar and C.M. McCorkle, with M. Martin (eds). *Ethnoveterinary Medicine: Alternatives for Livestock Development – Proceedings of an International Conference Held in Pune, India, 4–6 November 1997. Volume 1: Selected Papers.* BAIF Development Research Foundation, Pune, India. Pp. 32–35.

In Mexico's Chiapas Highlands, sheep are considered so sacred that they are never killed or eaten. This is not surprising in view of the fact that sheepraising is a mainstay of Tzotzil Maya Indians' livelihoods. Women's wool processing alone generates up to 36% of their households' annual income. The women are responsible for all aspects of sheep husbandry. Their management system is a simple but efficient one, designed to keep the animals healthy and productive. Medicinal plants are used to treat certain sheep diseases, but others are prevented through flock management strategies. Worldwide, most ER&D has focused on veterinary (and especially botanical) treatments for livestock. But a large body of traditional knowledge exists about other aspects of local animal husbandry and production, which likewise deserves to be documented and validated. An example is Tzotzil shepherdesses' traditional knowledge of wool production and of breeding to improve fleece quality. This paper reports on participatory research, aimed at blending such knowledge into appropriate programmes of formal genetic improvement, in which shepherdesses ranked their criteria for desirable breeding animals primarily by characteristics of their wool (e.g. combination of short and long fibres, shape and length of locks, absence of kemp) and secondarily by overall fleece quality (softness, colour, lustre, appropriate growth for shearing). Women's criteria result from their daily handling of wool and their centuries-long observation of flocks. In Chiapas sheep, the combination of a primary coat of long coarse fibres plus an undercoat of short, finer ones makes the fleece especially appropriate for manual spinning and weaving on the native backstrap loom. Research is now under way to: quantify emic characteristics of 'good' fleeces by the proportion of long to short fibres (range 1:2 to 1:5); translate emic measures of fibre length into etic ones, to establish objective selection criteria; and characterize fleece softness by fibre diameter and amount of kemp. Presently, shepherdesses' fleece gradings are assigned a gross score between 1 (poor) and 4 (excellent) for input into a genetic improvement programme. Statistical analysis will establish which objective parameters derived from local expertise can be best used to develop appropriate selection indices for better-quality wool and fleece in Chiapas sheep.

Pérezgrovas, Raúl, Hilda Castro, Althea Parry, Marisela Peralta, Lourdes Zaragoza, Pastor Pedraza and Gudalupe Rodríguez. 1995. El borrego Chiapas: Concepto actual e indicadores productivos de un importante recurso genético. *Anuario IEI* 5: 307–339.

While this article covers much of the same ground as other publications by Pérezgrovas and colleagues, it constitutes one of the more comprehensive technical summaries of the UNACH group's genetic research on the Chiapas sheep. Among other things, the article notes that the shepherdesses who steward this breed practise an active programme of genetic selection based on fleece colour. Also, on-station experiments confirm that shepherdesses' shearing schedules make for the maximum possible wool harvest. Given UNACH's now-extensive database on Tzotzil sheepraising, the authors conclude without reservation that 'under the particular conditions of the mountain regions of Chiapas, both the indigenous management system as well as the Chiapas breed itself have characteristics that make them superior to the methods of modern animal science and to specialised ovine races, respectively' (p. 308). Known as *batsi chij* or 'true sheep' in Tzotzil, the Chiapas landrace represents a unique, antique and invaluable source of ovine biodiversity, carefully husbanded for half a millennium.

Perezgrovas, Raul and Norma Farrera. 1999. Sustainable options for sheep extension and development derived from ethnoveterinary research in highland Chiapas, Mexico. In: E. Mathias, D.V. Rangnekar and C.M. McCorkle, with M. Martin (eds). *Ethnoveterinary Medicine: Alternatives for Livestock Development – Proceedings of an International Conference Held in Pune, India, 4–6 November 1997. Volume 1: Selected Papers.* BAIF Development Research Foundation, Pune, India. Pp. 202–205.

ER&D among Tzotzil Maya shepherdesses of Mexico has helped launch a research programme on genetic improvement of their local sheep, in which the women's knowledge provides the framework for breeding animals that produce heavier fleeces with higher quality wool. An important part of this effort will be the introduction of superior individuals of the local, Chiapas breed of sheep into village flocks. Previous such endeavours on the part of government extensionists lacked any understanding of Tzotzil culture and sheep husbandry systems, relying instead on male-oriented Western extension schemes for alien breeds. These schemes proved useless among Tzotzil, where sheep are sacred animals cared for exclusively by women within a unique, non-Western cultural context. This paper reports on participatory research conducted to gather, register and validate Tzotzil shepherdesses' traditional practices of sheep lending and acquisition as input into the design of a sustainable programme for introducing superior animals from the experimental farm of the University of Chiapas. Individual and group interviews revealed that: most shepherdesses (41%) prefer to lend out stud rams for short periods (2 to 45 days); others (31%) deal with breeding needs by direct purchase of animals, mainly young ewes; a third mechanism (16%) is to exchange sheep for clothes or agricultural products like maize and beans. Only 12% of respondents were inclined to use a government-recommended system of long-term animal loans combined with shareherding of lambs. These findings were shared with a small group of respected Tzotzil shepherdesses, to design with them an 'ideal' extension programme. In brief, the women opted for a programme in which superior rams selected by shepherdesses would be lent to or purchased by the women during their sheep's oestrous season, while all other rams would be separated from the flock. Animals defined as superior according to womens' own choice of sexes, ages and phenotypes would also be sold from the experimental farm, under a monthly payment plan. Another option would allow a shepherdess to acquire these superior farm-raised animals by exchanging poultry or pigs as well as sheep from her own flock, or even clothes or agricultural products. Women interested in long-term animal loans could receive several ewes and a ram during three years of shareherding lambs. The foregoing options add up to a framework for a truly appropriate breeding extension programme for Tzotzil sheepraisers. In a preliminary experiment, superior Chiapas rams were lent out for three months to ten villages. The rams adapted well to local conditions; and shepherdesses and their neighbours responded positively to the programme. In sum, extension programmes based on indigenous knowledge and practice and designed along with the beneficiaries themselves promise greater success than conventional, top-down, gender-biased and alien interventions.

Pérezgrovas, Raúl, Pastor Pedraza and Marisela Peralta. 1991–1993. Cría de ovejas por los indígenas de los altos de Chiapas. Algo más que lana para el telar. *Anuario IEI* 4: 73–91.

Winner of the 1991 national Solidarity Prize for groups working to improve the lot of Mexico's poor, this article, subtitled 'More Than Just Wool to Weave', overviews the philosophical framework and general findings from a decade of UNACH research on the semi-sacred sheepraising of Tzotzil Maya Indians in the Chiapas highlands. UNACH began this work because, in Chiapas, a nationwide programme to replace nativized *criollo* sheep with Rambouillets, that would supposedly produce four times as much wool, proved a disaster. The Rambouillets all died within weeks of being distributed. Government workers' response was to accuse indigenous recipients of eating the animals, despite Tzotzil's taboo against mutton. In contrast, UNACH scientists saw this effort to replace the local Chiapas breed, wrongly despised as inferior, as reductionist, at best. At worst, they liken it to trying to solve livestock production problems and the associated poverty among oppressed and stigmatized stockraisers by bringing in Aryan men as studs to Amerind women! To correct the ignorance and arrogance of such top-down livestock development programmes as the Rambouillet fiasco, UNACH instituted a participatory, bottom-up and largely field-based R&D agenda that considers every aspect of local stockraising systems – not only standard technical topics but also historical, religious, cultural and ecological factors plus a focus on women, who often have important stockraising roles or, as among Tzotzil, may even be the main stockraisers. A highlight of the present article is a comprehensive, 1982–1991 bibliography of relevant publications by UNACH scientists and collaborators. Some of the research findings mentioned include the following. Tzotzil weaving technology draws on ancient indigenous methods of native cotton processing. At least once a year, on the day of the saint said to have given sheep to Tzotzil, shep-herdesses carry salt, coloured ribbons and a token lamb to church to be blessed. Throughout the year, they also implore this saint to protect their flock, intoning the names of all the animals' grazing grounds, watering spots, trails and each sheep's personal name. Not only do Tzotzil consider sheep to be family members; they also believe that, along with certain other animal species, sheep are often literally the 'soulmates' of people. Thus, if a sheep falls sick or dies, so will its human soul-mate. Hence the taboo on killing or eating sheep, as well as Tzotzil resistance to culling (as the Rambouillet programme required). Tzotzil ethnoaetiologies centre on Maya notions of disease as the result of underworld gods winning temporary ascendancy over heavenly gods. Thus ritual as well as herbal and husbandry methods figure heavily in Tzotzil EVM.

Perezgrovas, Raul, Pastor Pedraza and Marisela Peralta. 1992. Animal healthcare by Indian shepherdesses: Plants and prayers. *ILEIA Newsletter* 8(3): 22–23.

This article covers the same information as Perezgrovas, Peralta and Pedraza 1993.

Pérezgrovas, Raúl, Marisela Peralta and Althea Parry. 1995. Más y mejor lana en el borrego-Chiapas. Un proceso de investigación interactiva con pastoras indígenas. *Anuario 1995 – Centro de Estudios Superiores de México y Centroamérica, Universidad de Ciencias y Artes del Estado de Chiapas.* Pp. 190–206.

To date, studies of sheepraising among the Maya mountain-women of Mexico's Chiapas State have centred on traditional management systems, ethnoveterinary knowledge and genetics. These studies have been characterized by a participatory-rural-appraisal (PRA) approach coupled with an interdisciplinarity that integrates animal science, reproduction and genetics, veterinary medicine and anthropology. However, the University of Chiapas scientists who pioneered this approach have now expanded their work to include wool production and processing, which are the paramount reasons for Maya sheepraising, plus an even more interactive research strategy. The latter embraces not only academics but also extensionists and arte-sanal wool processors and weavers as well as shepherdesses, with the latter three groups playing a greater decisioning role in research. Current research focuses on establishing correspondences between subjective local criteria versus quantitative scientific assessments of wool output and quality, with an eye to improving selec-tive breeding accordingly. A sophisticated conceptual model of genetics drives this effort: that of an 'open nucleus flock' of breeding animals. This flock is built up from an elite nucleus, later combined with genetic inputs from ordinary commu-nity flocks. All animals are selected according to criteria that locals and scientists together agree capture the 'best' wool-producing rams and ewes from among the hardy Chiapas landrace. Initial criteria for the elite nucleus were: a simple pheno-typic distinction according to colour (for which the genotypic correlates had already been scientifically established); an age of 2 to 4 years; a verifiable pedi-gree; and good health. Interestingly, because of Mayan ideological proscriptions on selling 'animal souls' [see other Pérezgrovas abstracts] – and especially those rep-resenting prime breedstock – it took considerable time and money to constitute this elite nucleus. Shepherdesses would sell a prize animal only if they were in acute economic distress; and even then, they would not accept less than three to four times the national market price. Under management conditions closely paralleling those of villages, the elite nucleus was established on-station, where it underwent further objective assessments (for body and fleece weight, fibre length and milk production). Then, expert native processors/weavers and shepherdesses came to the station to make their own assessments, using a variety of PRA scaling, ranking and matrix exercises to codify and evaluate the variables they deemed most important for wool output and quality. Based on these local experts' criteria (cf. p. 195), a further cut was made in the elite nucleus. Meanwhile, standard community-level criteria for genetic selection within family flocks were also identified. In 1995, community animals chosen on the latter bases were added to the elite nucleus to form the open nucleus, from which improved breedstock will eventually be returned to the participating communities under an animal-dissemination and extension programme to be designed by shepherdesses themselves. Meanwhile, in their co-researcher role, weavers and shepherdesses regularly re-evaluate fleece development in the open nucleus flock during biannual shearings and decide upon animals to withdraw. Researchers do likewise, using a numeric ranking scale and statistical analysis and then comparing it with the local experts' findings. The authors make the important point that, for certain kinds of information, more honest, accurate and detailed ethno-assessments can be obtained on-station, where people are not pressured to sell or rank their own or neighbours' animals. Another finding was that, in deciding on sheep purchases and sales, shepherdesses took into account animal temperament, age and reproductive status as much as or even more so than variables directly related to wool quantity or quality. Of course, all such considerations have implications for wool production and/or overall flock management and pastoral labour. But a concern for temperament also reflects shepherdesses' beliefs about proper relationships with the 'animal souls' in their charge. Processors/weavers and shepherdesses all evaluated wool quality in relation to local processing technology. This perspective generated variables to breed for that were quite different from those of large-scale industrial processors. The essential point is that an interactive research approach captures every type of beneficiary input, not only economic and technological but also sociocultural and religious.

Perezgrovas, Raul, Marisela Peralta and Pastor Pedraza. 1993. The woollen souls of Chiapas. *Appropriate Technology* 19(4): 21–23.

Tzotzil Indians of Mexico have been raising their sacred breed of highland sheep for 400 years. The shepherdesses use phytotherapies, say prayers to St John the Baptist (a patron saint of sheep) and hold curing ceremonies for their flocks. A project in Chiapas, Mexico is conducting clinical evaluations of three Tzotzil herbal treatments in an effort to determine the most appropriate dosing regime. Findings are now available on two of the treatments. Specifically, feeding sprigs of *Teloxys ambrosioides* or the mashed seeds of *Cucurbita maxima* – traditional cures for ovine stomachache and diarrhoea, respectively – significantly reduces the number of eggs of gastrointestinal nematodes and oocysts of *Eimeria* spp. within one week.

Perezgrovas, Raul, Marisela Peralta and Pastor Pedraza. 1994. Sheep husbandry among Tzotzil Indians: Who learns what from whom? In: Kate Kirsopp-Reed and Fiona Hinchliffe (eds). *RRA Notes Number 20: Special Issue on Livestock.* IIED, London, UK. Pp. 69–70.

As the title of this article hints, 'Local people may lack formal education but they have plenty of experience and empirical knowledge that technicians should look into and learn from' (p. 69). The authors suggest that an ethnoveterinary approach to understanding stockraising systems is more productive and informative than arrogant 'developmentalist' stances. '. . . we can learn a great deal about animal management and health when (and if) we listen carefully and respectfully to those who, educated or not, know better' (ibid.). This point is illustrated by the authors' participatory approach to EVK fieldwork among Tzotzil Maya shepherdesses of Mexico's Chiapas state as compared to government extensionists' dictatorial approaches to livestock development in the area. In addition to findings reported in other Perezgrovas and colleagues' publications, some astute local husbandry practices noted here include Tzotzil's supplementation of sheep with mountain salt and their management of reproduction by exchanging rams and isolating post-parturient ewes.

Peries, Leonard. 1989. A herbal recipe to chase away the insects. *ILEIA Newsletter for Low External Input and Sustainable Agriculture* 4(3): 27.

In describing the many uses of neem (*Azadirachta indica*) in pest control in Sri Lanka, the author notes the use of crushed fresh turmeric cooked in *neem* oil to dress festered wounds of livestock. The application causes any maggots to quickly drop off, keeps away flies and other insects and greatly speeds healing of the wound.

Perre, D. 1983. *Médecine Vétérinaire Populaire en Haute-Loire.* Doctoral thesis, Ecole Nationale Vétérinaire, Lyon, France. 80 pp.

Unavailable for review.

Perry, B.D., B. Mwanaumo, H.F. Schels, E. Eicher and M.R. Zaman. 1984. A study of health and productivity of traditionally managed cattle in Zambia. *Preventive Medicine* 2: 633–653.

This study in four Zambian provinces is based on a questionnaire survey, a serological survey and a sentinel herd scheme for disease surveillance among 27 cattle herds. It reports on herd size and composition, calving percentage, offtake, mortality rates and herders' own assessment of the relative importance of different diseases. Interviewees considered ticks, unthriftiness, cutaneous oedema and sudden death the most important animal health problems. Other ailments discussed include mastitis, lameness, diarrhoea, blackleg, tick wounds and nervous symptoms that in many cases may be caused by heartwater.

Peters, Henk. 1992a. Chad's Ishtirak paravets. *Appropriate Technology* 19(4): 33.

The same EVK information is offered here as in Peters 1992b.

Peters, Henk. 1992b. Paravet programme of the Ishtirak project, Chad. In: John Young (ed.). *A Report on a Village Animal Health Care Workshop – Volume II: The Case Studies.* ITDG, Rugby, UK. Pp. 32–38.

In the process of setting up the Oxfam-funded Ishtirak (Arabic 'association') paravet programme in central Chad, project personnel found ethnoveterinary treatment options very limited. They noted only four remedies: cautery with hot irons on painful or injured sites and for diarrhoea; the use of cattle urine and *Balanites aegyptica* leaves to dress wounds; *Acacia nilotica* seeds used [in unspecified fashion] against trypanosomosis; and recourse to rituals by Islamic priests [also for unspecified conditions].

Philipot, J.M. 1978. *Le Practicien 'Salarie': Étude d'un Nouveau Mode de Relation Éleveurs Vétérinaires.* Thesis, Veterinary Medicine, Toulouse, France.

Unavailable for review.

Phillips, Roger. 1987. *Herbs and Medicinal Plants.* Elm Tree Books, London, UK. 160 pp.

The plants described and depicted in this book are mostly from human ethnomedicine. However, the author notes that in Sweden, necklaces of garlic cloves are hung around the necks of animals to protect them from trolls or to prevent goblins from stealing milk from cows.

Phin, Pham Cong. 1997a. Integrated rice-duck cultivation in Vietnam. *ILEIA Newsletter* 13(4): 17.

Duck raising is an ancient profession in Vietnam. There, farmers have long supplemented their birds' feed by releasing ducklings into harvested paddy fields to glean fallen rice grains. In 1994, an added variant on this age-old post-harvest practice was borrowed from Japan and tested in Vietnam by the Sustainable Agriculture Promotion Centre of Haiphong in conjunction with the Haiphong Garden Association. The technique consists of releasing 10-day-old ducks into recently transplanted rice fields at a density of about 190 birds per hectare. The ducklings' feeding helps control insects, snails, weeds and even mice. So that the birds will not damage the crops, however, they are removed from the fields before the rice ears form. By this time, the ducklings are big enough for slaughter. This technique promotes not only rapid and healthy duckling development but also chemical-free cropping. Participating Vietnamese farmers are enthusiastic about the modified practice, as are Chinese, Koreans and Taiwanese. Recently, Tanzanians have also begun to experiment with this money-saving and rapid-fattening organic alternative.

Phin, Pham Cong. 1997b. Rice–duck integrated cultivation in Vietnam. Unpublished paper.

An earlier and longer version of the above-referenced 1997 article by the same author, this paper offers some additional observations on integrated rice+duck raising. In Vietnam, traditionally farmers carefully controlled hatching such that ducklings grew big enough to forage on their own just as rice paddies were harvested. Originally, ducks were forbidden to enter paddy fields until after harvest. But in an innovative system created some 10 years ago by a number of Japanese farmers, 10-day-old birds are released into 10-day-long transplanted fields, where they provide various pest- and weed-control and tilth benefits at the same time that the ducklings grow healthier and fatten faster. As a result, farmers reaped bumper harvests with little or no agrochemical inputs. This system has been shown to reduce the cost of rice production by about US $200 per hectare as compared with normal paddy cultivation, due to savings on both agrochemical inputs and human labour. In addition, human and environmental health benefitted from the reduced use of chemicals. Indeed, in Japan's 1993 crop failure, only adherents to this innovative duck+rice system reaped much rice. In short order, this farmer-designed system spread to more than 10 000 families in Japan and thence to other Southeast Asian and even African nations. The original inventors are now experimenting with more complex crop–livestock integrations, in the form of a rice+duck+fish+azolla farming system.

Pierre, Brigitte. 1994. La médecine vétérinaire traditionnelle en Haïti: Actes du Séminaire d'Ethnopharmacopée Vétérinaire 'KAGALA', un Partage de Savoirs Burkina-Faso, Ouagadougou, 15–22 Avril 1993. In: Kakule Kasonia and Michel Ansay (eds). *Métissages en Santé Animal de Madagascar à Haïti: Actes du Séminaire d'Ethnopharmacopée Vétérinaire 'KAGALA', un Partage de Savoirs Burkina-Faso, Ouagadougou, 15–22 Avril 1993.* Presses Universitaires de Namur, Namur, Belgium. Pp. 309–332.

Stockraising in Haiti is mainly a traditional family enterprise. Indeed, 95% of the nation's households keep livestock. But few families can afford to spend much on animal healthcare. In any case, formal veterinary services and medicines are limited. This article argues for studies to sort magico-religious veterinary practices from 'those that are really effective and beneficial for the animal as based on scientific research' (p. 310), so as to place a wider and more credible range of treatments in the hands of smallholder stockraisers and rural veterinary agents. To this end, based on a 1984 study in one area of Haiti, the author presents Haitians' naturalistic remedies for 12 categories of ailments in pigs, along with the ailments' vernacular names in Haitian Creole, their clinical signs as described by local swineherds and their presumed scientific aetiologies. For each treatment, the plant parts used, their form of preparation (including any additive ingredients) and mode of administration are noted in tabular form. Additives include blood, chemicals for seed preservation, DDT, lamp oil, milk, salt, sugar and urine. Also described for each ailment is the frequency with which interviewees cited a given traditional treatment plus the percentage of interviewees who choose to: apply a traditional treatment themselves; buy and administer a commercial medicine themselves; go to a local veterinary practitioner; slaughter the ailing animal; or simply do nothing. For example, for diarrhoea in pigs, the corresponding percentages are 76%, 0%, 11%, 4% and 9%. Local diarrhoea remedies are based on drenching with varied preparations of one of three plants (used by 96% of interviewees) or with salt water (4%). For one of the three plant remedies (based on *Psidium guajava*), seven different prescriptions were found, according to the plant parts people used. For the other two (*Citrus aurantifolia* or *Pavonia spinifex*), there was 100% agreement on the parts and form of preparation. The other 10 pig ailments addressed are: intestinal problems, eye disorders, paralysis of the hindquarters, itching skin diseases, cysticercosis, fevers (probably due to septicaemia or viral infections), malnutrition, fractures, coughs, general unthriftiness (probably due to endoparasites and vitamin and mineral deficiencies) and vomits. Haitian remedies span both mono- and polyprescriptions, although the former seem to predominate. Forms of plant-part preparation run the gamut from raw to smoked or oxidized; and modes of administration include oral, topical (including compresses, plasters, friction and baths), inhalation, and eye and ear drops. Examples of non-plant treatments are: for CNS problems, administering an inhalation of burning rubber (6%) or drenching with Kola, the national carbonated drink (25% of interviewees); and for coughs, holding the patient's head under water (8%). Also noted are prayers and rituals, used alone or in company with naturalistic interventions.

Pillai, Nelliah. 1989. *Periya Mattu Vagadam.* B. Rathina Nayajar & Sons Publishing, Madras, India. 203 pp.

A compilation of the traditional veterinary practices first described in ancient Tamil palm-leaf manuscripts, this volume documents more than 250 cattle maladies and their plant-based treatments. Among the health problems noted are infertility, poor milk yield, snakebite, diarrhoea, rinderpest and FMD. Some examples of FMD treatments are: applying pulverized *Acorus calamus* and *Sesbania grandiflora* to the mouth, nostrils and feet; washing the hooves with water in which dried fish has been soaked and/or spraying the fish-water over cattle yards; spreading burnt fish scales in cattle yards; drenching plus externally applying *sukku naripal* (?) grass, *Madhuca indica* cakes, sandalwood and leaves of *Pergularia daemia, Calotropis gigantea* and neem, all crushed together. For constipation – diagnosed by excessive water intake and bloody urine – cattle were fed ground-up *Acorus calamus*, mustard, *Sida acuta* leaves and Moringa.

Piyadasa, H.D. Wasantha. 1994a. Personal communication to C.M. McCorkle at the 11–25 July Workshop to Produce an Ethnoveterinary Information Kit. IIRR, Silang, Cavite, Philippines.

In Asia, poultry are often kept in buffalo's night-time quarters, where the fowl gobble up any ectoparasites that survive wallowing. The buffalo lie down and obligingly lift their legs so the birds can reach the parasites still clinging to difficult sites like the britch and axilla.

Piyadasa, H.D. Wasantha. 1994b. Traditional systems for preventing and treating animal diseases in Sri Lanka. *Revue Scientifique et Technique de l'Office International des Épizooties* 13(2): 471–486.

Traditional veterinary medicine in Sri Lanka is mainly based on the Indian Ayurvedic system, which attributes diseases to an imbalance in the bodily humours of wind, bile and phlegm. Approximately 2000 traditional veterinarians practice in Sri Lanka today, most on a part-time basis. They use over 250 species of medicinal plants plus 28 mineral and animal products in their prescriptions for cattle, buffalo, horses and elephants. Oral remedies can be prepared as decoctions, fresh mixtures of plant juices, fermented plant materials and boluses. Herbal medicines can also be instilled into the eyes, ears or nostrils. Both mono- and polyprescriptions are prepared. An example of the latter is an anthelmintic bolus for calves, which is prepared from the young leaves of nine plant species plus copper sulphate. Another example is a general medicinal inhalation made of 21 ingredients, including powdered antler and ivory, bat faeces and moulted snakeskin. Dry (smoke) and wet (steam) inhalations of strong-smelling substances are given both therapeutically and prophylactically, usually accompanied by incantations. Smoke is administered by burning the *materia medica* over red-hot charcoal in a clay brazier that is held under the patient's nostrils; at the same time, the patient may be covered with sacking or mats to concentrate the smoke. The brazier may also be walked 'round the animal so as to expose its skin to the smoke. Medicinal steam is generated by placing a heated stone into the medicinal plant juices inside a clay vessel. To treat indigestion, constipation, emaciation and colic in ruminants and as a general precaution against epidemics, symbols may be branded on various parts of the body. When an epidemic strikes, some practitioners may diagnose 'anger of the gods' and treat accordingly, e.g. by prescribing a small pouch of medicine or an 'enchanted thread' (p. 481) to be tied around the neck of each animal in the herd. A highlight of this article is its description of EVM and husbandry practices for elephants. To take a few examples: impaction and constipation are treated by a smoke inhalation of cinnamon and neem; castration is performed by rapidly rubbing together two sticks placed cross-wise above the testes; and elephant handlers know how to locate 97 nerve centres on their animals and to stimulate these centres by goad or heel in order to control these mighty beasts. Based on animal conformation, behaviour and purpose, native veterinary practitioners classify elephants and cattle into 10 and seven families, respectively; and they recognize different disease susceptibilities across families within each species [perhaps akin to disease-tolerant strains or breeds?]. Also, practitioners draw diagnostic and ethnopharmacological information from animal feeding behaviour. For instance, if they see an elephant eating *Erythrina variegata* leaves or *Capsicum* spp. plants in preference to other forages, they diagnose worms or indigestion, respectively. Other diagnostic methods include taking the patient's pulse (usually in the jugular vein), examining the eyes and interviewing the owner. Traditional practitioners generally keep their EVK secret. Their knowledge passed only from father to son, via oral instruction, practical assistanceship and sometimes also centuries-old ola-leaf manuscripts.

Pollak-Eltz, Angelina. 1987. Veterinärmedizinische Kenntnisse der venezolanischen Volksheiler. *Curare* 10: 246–248.

In nearly all Venezuelan villages, there are *curanderos* 'curers' who often treat both animals and people. This article describes these healers' ethnoveterinary practices in two locations: the peninsula of Paria in Sucre Province, where farmers keep only a few goats, chickens and pigs; and the plains of Apure, where cattle raising predominates. Many *curanderos* use both local and commercial drugs. The article briefly names local plants and practices for treating livestock fevers, coughs, udder infections, diarrhoeas and other gastrointestinal problems, *hormigon* (footrot?) and several other conditions. Often, *curanderos* are expert bonesetters of fractures in ruminants, dogs and cats. They push the broken bones back into place, splint them and apply *preparados* (plasters?) made from soaking certain materials in herbs and alcohol. For a horse with broken bones, healers generally advise slaughter because they know there is little chance the animal will recover. Some curers also perform conjurings and prayers on behalf of distant livestock patients afflicted by, e.g., worms or snakebite. The sick animal often receives some herbal remedy in addition to the spiritual one, however. In snakebite cases, for instance, garlic and tobacco are rubbed into the bite. Although the author does not comment on the efficacy of all the treatments described in the article, she opines that the results of this and similar studies could be useful to veterinarians and pharmacologists.

Pompa, Gerónimo. 1984. *Medicamentos Indígenas: Colección Extraída de los Reinos Vegetal, Animal y Mineral – Indice para sus Aplicaciones* (51st edition). Corporación Marca, Caracas, Venezuela, for Editorial América. 341 pp.

This volume details 456 plant, animal and mineral substances used in the human ethnomedicine of Venezuela. Veterinary applications are also occasionally mentioned, e.g.: the shade of the *achiote* tree and/or a solution of powdered *achiote* on the animal's forehead and behind its ears, to treat sunstroke; a paste of *auyama* leaves and salt to combat ectoparasitism and *arestín*, an ailment of the heel; and a bath of squash-leaf juice to repel flies. Further, the volume includes a lengthy annex entitled 'Ailments of Horses and their Manner of Cure' wherein nearly 50 local definitions of equine afflictions and their ethnotherapies are described, often with compelling firsthand evidence of their effectiveness. With an acumen too extensive to detail here, it is clear that the horsemen and women of the Venezuelan savannas have a highly refined, empirical appreciation of their mounts' ills and needs.

Porter, Barbara A., Tjaart Schillhorn van Veen and J.B. Kaneene. 1988. The future of traditional veterinary medicine in Africa. Unpublished paper. College of Veterinary Medicine, Michigan State University, East Lansing, Michigan, USA.

This paper describes the evolution of veterinary medicine since the first domestication of animals and briefly reviews the state of the art among contemporary African pastoralists. In addition to a magico-religious component, traditional veterinary medicine includes surgical and obstetrical techniques, prophylactic management practices, knowledge of epidemiological features of some diseases and a broad spectrum of traditional drugs. An example from WoDaaße herders demonstrates the complexity of traditional views of animal healthcare. Modern veterinary interventions should consider traditional practices as practical alternatives to Western medicine.

Porter, Mimi. 1998. Physical therapy. In: Allen M. Schoen and Susan G. Wynn (eds). *Complementary and Alternative Veterinary Medicine: Principles and Practice.* Mosby, Inc., St Louis, Missouri, USA. Pp. 201–212.

Physical therapy involves the use of noninvasive physical measures in the treatment and, more rarely, the diagnosis of disease and injury. Typically, its goals are pain reduction and/or the patient's return to full motor function and strength. Illustrating from the author's own experience with horses, this chapter describes some of the tools and techniques used by the veterinary physcial therapist. Electrical stimulation is used for pain relief, absorption in oedema, wound healing and amelioration of muscle atrophy and spasm. Iontophoresis, defined as the introduction of drugs via electrically stimulated ion transfer, is applied for, e.g., tendonitis, epicondylitis, bursitis, acute arthritic flare-ups and musculoskeletal inflammations. Ultrasound offers a means of heating deep-tissue structures – for instance, so as to temporarily increase their extensibility before exercise. Superficial cold or heat treatments, given via ice packs or hot packs, warm-water baths, infrared lamps and electric heating pads, respectively stimulate or restrict blood flow, thereby producing analgesic effects or halting inflammation. Finally, stretching exercises are commonly prescribed for, e.g., relieving trigger-point pain, stimulating tissue remodelling and enhancing balanced movement and thus reducing the likelihood of injuries. Also briefly mentioned are low-level laser, magnetic-field and massage therapies.

Porter, Mimi and Mary Bromiley. 1998. Massage therapy. In: Allen M. Schoen and Susan G. Wynn (eds). *Complementary and Alternative Veterinary Medicine: Principles and Practice.* Mosby, Inc., St Louis, Missouri, USA. Pp. 213–216.

Whether applied pre- or post-performance, massage can increase circulation, release scar tissue, balance muscle function and calm and relax the patient. This chapter discusses different massage techniques and their veterinary applications. Techniques include: trigger-point, acupressure and ice massages; craniosacral therapy or 'energy work'; effleurage (firm strokes); tapotement or cupping (gentle, rhythmic blows); friction; and passive range-of-motion exercises. The authors caution against conditions or sites in which massage should not be used, such as infected lesions, torn muscles and acute haematomas.

PPEA-PRATEC. 1989. *Manejo Campesino de Semillas en los Andes.* Serie Eventos de Técnicos. No publisher given, Lima, Perú. 554 pp.

This volume is one in a series of publications on indigenous technologies in the Andes. [See also CEDECUM 1988, PRATEC 1988a&b, PRATEC 1989 and PRATEC-CEPIA 1988.] Despite its misleading title, 'Farmer Seed Management in the Andes', it describes a number of ethnoveterinary and animal husbandry techniques. Technology No. 193 details an effective method for controlling the snail hosts of the liver fluke that infest Andean pastures. No. 203 deals with ethnotherapies for a wide variety of diseases of dogs, pigs, poultry, horses, cattle, sheep and guinea pigs. Prescriptions involving differing combinations of wild plants, garden vegetables, grains, seeds, fruits, spices, eggs, milk, oils, fats, alcoholic beverages, human urine, animal dung, salts, minerals, soaps, ashes, kerosene, diesel oil, used motor oil, insects, snakes and purchased medicaments such as Alka-Seltzer, glycerin and iodine, sometimes along with whippings, amputations, smoke inhalations and religious gesticulations are given for treating diseases as varied as bloat, endo- and ectoparasites of many types, wounds, infections, rabies, plant poisoning and the evil eye. Preventive measures for some diseases are also described, such as burning old tyres in animal quarters or sprinkling corrals with lime or creosote to cleanse them of parasites. No. 206 offers similar information for curing colics in both animals and human beings. Other animal-related technologies include castration of guinea pigs (No. 192), traditional cheese-making techniques (No. 190), wool dyeing methods (No. 207) and native pasturing patterns and flora (No. 197).

Pradhan, S.K. 1998. Can fish scare water cat? Insights from Tripura. *Honey Bee* 9(1): 6.

In India's Tripura region, where multi-species fish farming [akin to mixed grazing] is commonly practised, farmers have elaborated some unique pisciculture strategies. For one thing, contrary to scientists' recommendations, they raise *Labio kalbose* fish in with the other six to eight species they grow. They say the brightly shining eyes of *L. kalbose* frighten off a troublesome nocturnal otter that preys on fish, thereby helping to protect the other, more desirable species. Moreover, they note that the fast-moving kalbose compels the other fish also to move frequently, which increases their growth. Some Tripura fish farmers further disagree with scientists that only exotics like *Catla catla* and silver carp (*Hypophthalmichthys moltrix*) make for high production and returns. Rather, they find that indigenous fish like *Amblypharyngodon mola* and *Esomus danricus* give better yields year-round and fetch higher market prices. In contrast, scientists consider such species as good only for feeding the exotics. Yet the indigenous species fetch higher market prices: e.g. Rs 80 to 100 per kg versus silver carp's Rs 20 to 25. By not growing the carp, farmers realize much better overall returns since it is not necessary to purchase much artificial feed. This is because Catla eat some of the indigenous species and the remainder are harvested and sold. Besides fish, Tripura farmers also raise poultry and pigs. Diarrhoea is one of the most common diseases of their poultry. To combat it, farmers feed: onion or citrus juice; turmeric with salt; or a teaspoonful of country liquor. A traditional anthelmintic and all-round prophylaxis and tonic for swine is *Thysanolaena maxima* seeds in *Pterospermum acerifolia* bark extract, fed four times a year. Throughout India, crosses of exotic with local pigs are very popular, but few people can afford to own an exotic breeding boar. The boar can be hired out to co-villagers in exchange for a stud fee of one piglet from each litter sired.

Prajapati, R.B. and L.S. Hiregoudar. 1976. Treatment of psoroptic mange of buffaloes with mineral and plant oil. *Indian Veterinary Journal* 53: 150–151.

A clinical trial was carried out to test the efficacy of three local treatments for mange in India. Fifty 5–8-year-old buffaloes with mange were divided into five equal groups one of which was left untreated as control. The four other groups were treated with either unused engine oil, burnt engine oil, *karangi* (?) oil, or the commercial drug Lazin. Applications were made every 3rd day, altogether seven times. The most effective treatment against psoroptic mange in buffalo was the unused engine oil. However, from an economic point of view, the burnt engine oil proved cheaper and nearly as effective as the unused oil.

Prakash, Jai. 1998. Modern methods in formulation and evaluation of herbal medicine. In: E. Mathias, D.V. Rangnekar and C.M. McCorkle, with M. Martin (eds). *Ethnoveterinary Medicine: Alternatives for Livestock Development – Proceedings of an International Conference Held in Pune, India, 4–6 November 1997. Volume 2: Abstracts.* BAIF Development Research Foundation, Pune, India. P. 49.

Over centuries, the human race has acquired tremendous medical/veterinary knowledge and technologies from the exploration of the medicinal properties of plants. This has created a treasure trove of pharmacognostic knowledge in different cultures and civilizations. In India, for instance, the history of herbal veterinary medicines dates back to the Mahabharata of 5000 B.C., recorded in the form of Nakul Samhitas. Herbal medicines have been and still are used in animal healthcare throughout the world. Besides being effective and economical, such medicines have a long record of safety. Plant-based compounds such as digoxin, morphine, atropine, taxol, vincristine and colchicine, to name just a few, present a broad range of pharmacological activity. Yet the importance of botanicals in modern medicine is often underestimated. This need not be the case, however, because today, herbal medicines developed on the basis of traditional knowledge can be subjected to extensive scientific research, the better to establish their safety and clinical efficacy and to standardize their formulation. Also, applying good manufacturing practices and total quality management guidelines can ensure more predictable and dependable preparations, thus restoring the historical status of plant-based medicines.

Prasad, Durga. 1995. Hatching eggs: Batulu Narsayya's way. *Honey Bee* 6 (2): 8.

This article recounts the visit to an indigenous duck-hatchery operation in India's Andhra Pradesh State by a branch manager of the State Bank of India, who was seeking creditworthy agricultural activities to fund. The hatchery was conceived, constructed and operated by a Mr Batulu ('Ducks' in the local language) Narsayya and his wife. They sell 1-to-2-day-old ducklings from batches of 5000 to 7000 eggs that they incubate in a homemade system of temperature- and humidity-controlled pits. Their system employs one sub-pit for water, a fireplace in another sub-pit for heating the larger pit and ordinary thermometers to indicate when to adjust the fireplace flame. Incubation lasted the normal 28-day cycle for ducks. Depending on the quality of the eggs, the hatching rate ranges from 40% to 80%, which is considerably higher than that of mechanized incubators. The system is also more energy-efficient than mechanized ones. In economic terms, it has an extremely low break-even point; and the market for ducklings appears to be unlimited, as the Narsayyas had approximately half a year's orders pending. The system's only drawback is its labour-intensiveness, as the eggs must be moved every 4 hours. However, the bank manager worked out a way to semi-mechanize the operation so as to reduce such drudgery while still keeping costs far below those of commercially-made incubators.

Prasad, G., V.D. Sharma and A. Kumar. 1982. Efficacy of garlic (*Allium sativum* L.) therapy against experimental dermatophytosis in rabbits. *Indian Journal of Medical Research* 75(Mar): 465–467.

Topical application of a crude extract of garlic in a concentration of 1:10 in distilled water was shown to combat dermatophytosis in rabbits without causing any side effects.

PRATEC. 1988a. *Rondas Campesinas y Tecnología Andina: Taller Regional Norandino de Tecnologías Campesinas.* Editorial Adolfo Arteta, Lima, Perú. 86 pp.

Like PPEA-PRATEC 1989, PRATEC 1988a&b and 1989, CEDECUM 1988 and PRATEC-CEPIA 1988, this booklet documents and contributes to a methodology for recovering indigenous knowledge in the Andes. Page 31 briefly describes several ethnoveterinary practices on the Peruvian altiplano. To prevent bloat in ruminants, producers dose their animals with a preparation of two native plants, *paico* and *haycha*. To relieve swelling of the udder in lactating cows, they apply a decoction of another plant, *hinojo*. For ovine diarrhoeas, they drench with powdered mustard flowers in whey (Spanish *suero de vaca*).

PRATEC. 1988b. *Saber Campesino Andino: I Taller Regional Sur-andino de Tecnologías Campesinas.* G. y G. Impresores, Lima, Perú. 61 pp. plus 13 pamphlets totalling 149 pp.

The aim of this publication is the same as that of PRATEC-CEPIA 1988. The attached pamphlets are in fact a continuation of the technology numbers presented there, but with a focus here on the Peruvian altiplano. Page 23 of the booklet mentions the effectiveness of *tarwi* water against ectoparasites of alpaca. [See also Avila Cazorla et al. 1985a&b, Jiménez et al. 1983, Sánchez n.d. and Tillman 1983.] Technology No. 26 outlines an indigenous treatment for broken bones among herd animals. No. 68 prescribes drenching with a decoction of the *ajana ajana* plant to combat endoparasites in both ruminants and humans. No. 77 describes a topical application of ashes, urine and commercial herbicides to combat bovine ectoparasitism. It also gives a recipe for fattening cattle, based on aquatic forages from Lake Titicaca combined with barley and salt. Several other animal or range management techniques are also described.

PRATEC. 1989. *Sorochuco: Chacra Campesina y Saber Andino – II Taller Regional Nor-andino de Tecnologías Campesinas.* PPEA-PRATEC, Lima, Perú. 385 pp.

This volume represents a continuation of PRATEC 1988a. It lists 30 rural Andean technologies (Nos. 130–160) from Peru's Cajamarca Department. No. 153 describes a prophylaxis for bovine ectoparasites in which cattle are washed with a mixture of powdered dish detergent and fresh-ground *chirimoya* fruit. No. 154 details two home remedies for ovine footrot. The first consists of cleaning the hoof with a decoction of a native plant called *matico*, then cutting away the rotted parts and rubbing the raw areas with a heated lemon and salt. An alternative cure is to rub hot sheep fat into the trimmed areas; apply a poultice of burnt, ground *matico*; and then bind the hoof with a clean rag or a piece of plastic for 2 days, meanwhile keeping the animal out of damp or muddy places. Other animal-related technologies described in this volume include cheese and butter making, natural dyes for wool and on-farm plough manufacturing.

PRATEC-CEPIA. 1988. *Tecnologías Campesinas de los Andes.* Editorial Horizonte, Lima, Perú. 621 pp.

This volume is the result of a 6-day meeting in 1987 in Cajamarca, Peru of 34 institutions concerned to 'rescue traditional knowledge among Andean producers' (1988: 9). The volume provides detailed instructions and drawings for 60 Andean technologies, two of which concern ethnoveterinary practices. Technology No. 26 describes how stockowners of the Peruvian altiplano treat fractured leg bones of sheep with a hot poultice compounded of a local locoweed (*Astragalus* sp.), human urine, dried snake flesh and coarse brown sugar. The poultice is applied to the realigned bones, the leg is then tightly bandaged and splinted and the animal is kept close to home. When properly done, the animal reportedly recovers within a month or so. Technology No. 27 reports indigenous Andean cures for liver fluke and gastrointestinal parasites in sheep and cattle by drenching with an infusion of *amaro* (*Webebaueri* sp., Asteraceae family). Faecal egg counts taken at 4, 7, 15 and 21 days after treatment showed a decrease in the eggs of various endoparasites. Technologies Nos. 29, 42, 43 and 44 respectively describe supplemental feeding techniques for guinea pigs, indigenous pasture rotation systems, local methods of cattle identification and marking and home preparation of high-energy rations for plough oxen.

PRELUDE. 1993a. Rapport de commission du groupe II. *Lettre du Sous-Réseau PRELUDE: 'Santé, Productions Animales et Environnement'* Supplément du Bulletin PRELUDE 22–24: unpaginated (5 pp.).

One outcome of PRELUDE's first inter-regional seminar on traditional African veterinary pharmacopoeia was the formation of subregional workgroups. This article gives an example of Group II (Burkina Faso, Chad, Ivory Coast, Niger) efforts to identify common veterinary uses of specific medicinal plants across countries in the group, using a standardized information-collection and reporting form. The form is organized in five parts: pathology – disease description/perception, country, local-language and probable veterinary-scientific names for the disease, livestock species affected and season(s) of occurrence; plant – the vernacular name, Latin name (family and genus), synonyms and milieu of the principal plant used in remedies for the disease; preparation – season and developmental stage for harvesting the plant, parts used, their mode of conservation and preparation and associated plants; administration – route and quantity of remedy; and 'other information' – human medical uses and other remarks. The example given is for snakebite and snake spittle in the eyes. While various plants are used to treat these problems across Group II, comparison of findings revealed that one plant was mentioned in all countries responding (no data were available from Chad): *Securidaca longipedunculata*. Details of its use are reported according to the standardized format. In addition, findings from the phytochemical and pharmacological literature on this plant are referenced, in indication of properties that support its antivenin action. Part of the function of the PRELUDE newsletter is to disseminate such comparative findings, since botanicals that are widely used for the same livestock ailment across several countries are more likely to be effective and to be 'good bets' for further research.

PRELUDE. 1993b. Séminaire africain inter-régional sur la pharmacopée vétérinaire Avril 15–22, 1993, Ouagadougou, Burkina-Faso: Synthèse des travaux du groupe I. *Lettre du Sous-Réseau PRELUDE: 'Santé, Productions Animales et Environnement'* 3: 2–4 plus 4 pages of tables.

This synthesis of findings from the PRELUDE subregional Group I (Guinea Bissau, Mali, Mauritania, Senegal) highlights ethnoveterinary botanicals for gastrointestinal parasites and trypanosomosis. Comparison across countries revealed a commonality in the respective use of *Cordyla pinnata* and *Khaya senegalensis* in remedies for these two ills. The report also notes other plants used in Group I countries for these and other animal health problems. Some examples are: in Guinea Bissau, a decocted or macerated drench of *Afromomum melegueta* rhizome or seeds for dysentery, wounds and other ailments; also in Guinea Bissau, a decoction of *Solanum incanum* roots, fruits or leaves as a drench for vomiting or neuralgia and as eyedrops for conjunctivitis; in Mauritania, the use of fresh, pounded *Datura metel* leaves as a poultice for inflammations; and in Senegal, a drench of the macerated green leaves or stalks of Euphorbiaceae for strangles in horses.

Primov, George. 1984. *Goat Production within the Farming System of Smallholders of Northern Bahia, Brazil.* Technical Report No. 35. SR-CRSP, Department of Rural Sociology, University of Missouri-Columbia, Columbia, Missouri 65211, USA. 160 pp.

This report is based on interviews with 50 goat smallholders in northeastern Brazil's Bahia State. It describes production strategies in the context of crop and livestock sectors of the farm production system, plus goat production, consumption and marketing patterns. Most people recognize the relationship of their goats' poor health to malnutrition. But goats receive supplementary feeding only when producers fear the animals may die. However, 72% of the interviewees provided their goats with salt. Pages 118–123 discuss goat diseases as classified, diagnosed and traditionally treated by producers. Diseases include caseous lymphadenitis (perhaps the most serious ailment in that region), intestinal worms, rabies and footrot.

Priyanto, Dwi, Agus Suparyanto, Isbandi, Sri Wahyuni, Tri Budhi Murdiati and Evelyn Mathias-Mundy. 1991. *Pengetahuan Veteriner Tradisional Peternak Domba/Kambing dan Appliaksinya (Studi Kasus Dua Desa di Kapubaten Bogor).* SR-CRSP Report, Balai Penelitian Ternak, Ciawi, Bogor, Indonesia. 48 pp.

A multidisciplinary team assessed healthcare practices of smallholders for sheep and goats in Nagrak and Pasir Gaok Villages of West Java, Indonesia. Study methods included transects, observation, inspection of animal condition, analysis of secondary data and key-informant interviews. This report details: small ruminant management, breeding, feeding and diseases as described by farmers and observed by the research team; farmers' choice of treatment approach, whether rest, medication, slaughter or sale; and remedies for each health problem, ranked by whether key informants regarded their efficacy as low, medium or high. The two villages' different management systems made for different diseases and treatments. In Nagrak, most animals were in excellent condition. They were kept in raised barns with slatted floors, where they were fed under a cut-and-carry system supplemented daily with cassava peels. Farmers knew the peels could be toxic and occasionally an animal might die from their cyanide content. But farmers observed that animals could grow fat on it. In Pasir Gaok, animals were grazed on a rubber plantation and their condition was much poorer. They probably had higher worm burdens than Nagrak stock due to Pasir Goak's extensive management system. These findings demonstrate that even villages in the same general region may have very different husbandry and healthcare systems and consequently may require different livestock development approaches. [See also Mathias-Mundy et al. 1992.]

Puffet, H. 1985. Pharmacopée vétérinaire traditionelle des éleveurs du sud-Niger. *Tropicultura* 3(1): 14–15.

Stockraisers of Niger continue to use mainly their own, traditional veterinary medicines, which are greatly appreciated and well-mastered. A 1983–1984 survey among sedentary stockraisers and healers in 40 villages of southern Niger sought to compile this EVK in a form that livestock field agents could understand and use. A total of 773 people were interviewed singly or in groups. Together, they mentioned 42 livestock ailments and 94 local plants used in their treatment. Treatment information was systematically collected for the following parameters: name of the ailment or of its principal symptom; species treated – cattle, sheep, goats, horses, camels or 'all species'; plant parts used – leaves, bark, roots or whole plant; mode of preparation – powder for external application, fumigation, decoction, infusion, plaster or bath; and treatment outcome – very good, good, medium, passable or very mediocre. Illustrative findings are presented here in tabular form, organized according to 19 medicinal plants used. A fuller report of 55 pages is available for field agents' use. Here, the author makes the following, additional observations: pastoral and transhumant stockraisers of Niger probably have a 'richer and more complete' (p. 15) EVK than the sedentary people interviewed; livestock healers prefer to keep certain aspects of EVK secret, which makes research difficult; the identification in Western terms of local disease and plant names posed some problems; and future studies should pay more attention to details of dosage amounts and frequencies.

Pullan, N.B. 1980. Productivity of white Fulani cattle on the Jos Plateau, Nigeria. III. Disease and management factors. *Tropical Animal Health and Production* 12: 77–84.

This article describes the importance of disease and management factors for the productivity of traditionally managed herds of white Fulani cattle on Nigeria's Jos Plateau. Researchers found that epizootic diseases were not a major limiting factor in productivity, given the decline of the two major such diseases – rinderpest and CBPP. Rather, productivity was compromised more by management-related ills, including streptothricosis, liver fluke, coccidiosis and parasitic gastroenteritis. The only traditional treatment mentioned in the article is manual removal of ticks from cattle.

Purba, Anny Victor. 1986. Phytochemical investigation of *Leucas lavandulifolia* J.E. Smith. *Medika* 8(12): 718–722.

A phytochemical investigation of *Leucas lavandulifolia* was carried out in Java, Indonesia, where this plant is commonly applied to stinking wounds of livestock, in order to cleanse them of larvae. The plant is also used for eye sores, a gargle and in veterinary surgery for inflamed callosity. A phytochemical analysis of the plant led to the isolation of vanilin and a crystalline mixture of the glycosides of three common plant sterols: sitosterol, stigmasterol and campesterol.

Puyvelde, Luc van. 1994. Importance sur le plan biomédical des produits naturels en matière de santé: Le CURPHAMETRA à Butare. In: Kakule Kasonia and Michel Ansay (eds). *Métissages en Santé Animale de Madagascar à Haïti: Actes du Séminaire d'Ethnopharmacopée Vétérinaire 'KAGALA', un Partage de Savoirs Burkina-Faso, Ouagadougou, 15–22 Avril 1993*. Presses Universitaires de Namur, Namur, Belgium. Pp. 101–110.

In Rwanda, CURPHAMETRA (Centre Universitaire de Recherche sur la Pharmacopée Traditionelle) has been conducting ethnomedical and ethnoveterinary drug trials, based on ethnobotanical information collected from traditional practitioners and local people. To take one example, Rwandan peasants have long used the powdered roots of *Neorautanenia mitis* mixed with butter to cure mange in calves. Bioassays showed that *N. mitis* did indeed have an acaricidal ingredient, specifically 12a-hydroxyrotenone. A solution and an ointment of *N. mitis* were prepared and tested on mange-infected rabbits and then on 500 human patients with scabies in a double-blind trial that included a commercial scabies treatment as a control. Every person given the *N. mitis* treatment was cured, with no side effects. The solution and ointment were then commercialized, thus providing a national alternative to expensive imported scabicides that few rural Rwandans could afford. This study also illustrates the value for human health of ER&D.

Puyvelde, Luc van. 1996. Ontwikkeling van plantaardige geneesmiddelen in Rwanda. *Rainforest Medical Bulletin* 3(2): 5–7.

This article describes the development and industrial production in Rwanda of low-cost, safe and effective plant medicines based mainly on existing ethnomedical and -veterinary knowledge in the country. Work began with the establishment in 1971 of a centre for research on traditional medicine (CURPHAMETRA) that involved the University of Rwanda, government and foreign funding, both foreign and Western-trained Rwandan physicians and scientists of various disciplines, plus the enthusiastic participation of traditional healers. As of 1980, 11 well-established remedies prepared from cultivated Rwandan and a few imported plants were successfully tested, put into local production and brought to the national market in attractively packaged and culturally acceptable formulations. These 11 were followed by a scabicide [see Puyvelde 1994], a fungicide and a previously unknown pesticide, all developed from indications garnered from indigenous Rwandan plant medicine. The CURPHAMETRA case stands as a model for how interdisciplinary and transcultural cooperation can build upon ethnomedical knowledge to create new industries and bring to market improved but still inexpensive traditional remedies and/or new medicaments based on them

Rabari, Unaji Chelaji (and other Maldharis of Sembalpani). 1995. Traditional episodic institutions for dealing with FMD. *Honey Bee* 6(4): 17.

Maldhari or Charvah pastoralists are landless villagers who raise cattle and buffalo in the forests of a remote part of India's Gujarat State. There, FMD is an economically serious disease that can spread rapidly unless strict quarantine measures are promptly instituted. Stock with FMD lose weight, give less milk and abort within 2 months of conception. Based on informal interviews in one Maldhari village, this article describes traditional social institutions that these pastoralists have elaborated to control FMD. When only one or two animals are discovered to be infected, their owner must immediately alert his neighbours and confine the patients to their cattle-shed, where they are stall-fed until their [unspecified] treatment is completed. Under no circumstances are infected animals allowed to use communal grazing grounds or water points. When more than two animals are infected, confinement and stall-feeding become impractical; so villagers meet to assign a particular area of the forest and one water point for the patients' exclusive use, plus a single route (usually the shortest) for the animals to take to the forest. If a majority of a community's stock are stricken, the elders inform all neighbouring villages and keep the infected animals out of the other villages' grazing areas. Because these rules have been elaborated by the pastoralists themselves, they are rarely broken. Transgressors are roundly socially ostracized; upon acknowledging the error of their ways, the offenders must pay a fine of 15 kg of foodgrain to the community and must invite the whole community to tea, there to ask forgiveness with folded hands from every inhabitant. Informants said that these rules are largely effective in containing FMD and thus preventing major economic losses, but that they do not completely eradicate the disease because it is difficult to keep strays out of other communities' quarantined areas.

Rahman, Abdur, Muzahid Uddin Ahmed and Abdus Salam Mia. 1976. Studies on the diseases of goats in Bangladesh: Mortality of goats under farm and rural conditions. *Tropical Animal Health and Production* 8: 90.

This study of goat management systems in Bangladesh revealed that goat mortality was higher on farms than under extensive rural conditions. This discrepancy may be explained by the facts that village goats are kept in small numbers; belong to women and children, who give the animals individualized care and attention; and have larger areas in which to forage. This short communication does not state whether this is due to forage, disease or other factors.

Rahmann, G. 1996. Acceptance of vaccination campaigns in nomadic societies – The case of nomads in the Butana/eastern Sudan. In: Karl-Hans Zessin (ed.). *Livestock Production and Diseases in the Tropics: Livestock Production and Human Welfare. Proceedings of the VIII International Conference of Institutions of Tropical Veterinary Medicine held from the 25 to 29 September, 1995 in Berlin, Germany.* Volume II. Deutsche Stiftung für Internationale Entwicklung, Zentralstelle für Ernährung und Landwirtschaft, Feldafing, Germany. Pp. 559–564.

This conference paper suggests that one of the reasons some Sudanese nomads cling to ethnoveterinary treatments is their misunderstanding of Western ones. A case in point is vaccinations, which some nomadic tribes mistakenly believe should have an immediate therapeutic effect on already-sick animals. When such effects do not materialize, nomads may reject the vaccines. Rejection of other kinds of Western drugs also results from negative outcomes attendant upon nomads' own misapplication of them. The author opines that, in general, nomads place little faith in government-directed measures and campaigns. Moreover, he says, they do not worry about diseases until these have actually struck.

Rai, Samuel. 1997. Kuntz, a multipurpose plant. *ILEIA Newsletter* 13(1): 31.

Kuntz (*Thysanolaena maxima* R.) is a multipurpose plant cultivated in India. Farmers rate it as one of the best fodders for milk production and it is used in both human and animal ethnomedicine. Feeding kuntz to cows with retained placenta reportedly stimulates immediate expulsion of the placenta.

Rajan, S. and M. Sethuraman. 1997. Traditional veterinary practices in rural areas of Dindigul District, Tamilnadu, India. *Indigenous Knowledge and Development Monitor* 5(3): 7–9.

This article records 16 plants employed in (mostly internal) EVM in India's Tamil Nadu State: *Aegle marmelos, Allium cepa, Ceiba pentandra, Calotropis gigantea, Cissus quadrangularis, Datura metel, Erythrina suberosa, Lablab purpureus, Leucas aspera, Luffa acutangula, Musa paradisiaca, Piper betle, Solanum surat-tense, Tamarindus indica, Tribulus terrestris* and *Zingiber officinale*. Other items found in the ethnoveterinary medicine chest of the region are sugar, which is sprinkled into the eyes of cattle with cataracts, and bamboo splints, which are used along with a paste of powdered black gram seeds and eggwhite to treat broken bones of cattle. Instead of the paste, gingelly oil may be applied to the fracture site twice a day. Cattle, buffalo, goats, pigs, chickens and dogs are the main species treated.

Stockraisers themselves perform a majority of the treatments. But sometimes a specialist in plant-based remedies for animals is required. This is the *tharakar*, who also works as a livestock broker. These men all belong to a single family of hereditary indigenous practitioners, who are very secretive about their knowledge. The authors draw a distinction between 'day-to-day' treatments, which centre on externally visible signs, versus other treatments that require greater herbal knowledge and skills and centre on internal disease.

Ralalarisoa. 1985. *Les Plantes Médicinales Commercialisées sur les Hauts-plateaux – Possibilités d'Emploi en Médecine Vétérinaire.* Memoire de Fin d'Etudes, Departement Elevage, Université de Madagascar, Antananarivo, Madagascar. 106 pp.

Madagascar has long been known for its wealth of medicinal plants and they continue to be widely used throughout the nation in daily healthcare for humans and animals. Indeed, plant use is increasing due to Madagascar's lack of foreign exchange for importing commercial drugs. The most popular medicinal plants are sold in marketplaces. This student study had three aims: to census commonly sold plants that can be of veterinary use; to collect and review literature on the pharmaceutical properties of such plants; and to conduct a limited number of simple, informal tests of some of the plant medicines' effects on cattle and swine diseases, following prescriptions provided by stockraisers and other interviewees. For the first aim, buyers and sellers of 81 medicinal plants in markets and around Antananarivo were interviewed as to the plants' uses. As might be expected in a town environment, the vast majority of uses turned out to be for humans. Tests of three different plant solutions for treating scrapes on pigs were inconclusive, as were those for another three plants supposed to enhance growth when fed to unthrifty piglets. Likewise for three other concoctions for porcine mange. However, various preparations of three plants for treating bovine dermatophilosis proved promising (*Tetradenia fructicosa* Benth, *Ricinus communis* and *Centella asiatica*). The author concludes with a plea for more rigorous studies on plant medicines for both humans and animals in Madagascar. With these and with proper plant conservation measures, he sees potential for a local herbal industry to contribute to reliable yet inexpensive healthcare in the nation. There is also the possibility of attracting pharmaceutical firms to Madagascar – instead of the nation's exporting crude botanicals and then re-importing extracts and drugs made from them, as it presently does.

Ramdas, Sagari R. and Nitya S. Ghotge. 1996. Ethnoveterinary Research in India: An Annotated Bibliography. Unpublished manuscript. ANTHRA, Hyderabad, India. 60 pp.

This bibliography offers 214 abstracts of publications dealing with EVK in India. Forty-five abstracts concern ancient texts on Indian veterinary medicine for different species (horses, elephants, cattle) as well as research on such texts. Another 134 abstracts cover: selected books on indigenous medicines plus clinical studies to validate the medicines; veterinarians' practical field experiences; and methods for recording EVK in rural communities. Also included are annotations of 35 EVK references from countries other than India. The annotations are preceded by an introductory discussion that traces the history of EVM in India from ancient times and Ayurvedic texts through the 20th century, outlining local practices prevalent among different Indian stockraising communities today. The introduction also explores policy efforts across time to integrate traditional animal healthcare systems with the dominant, Western-allopathic model.

Ramírez Valenzuela, M. 1994. Los antiguos métodos de profilaxis de las enfermedades animales. *Revue Scientifique et Technique de l'Office International des Epizooties* 13(2): 343–360.

Beginning with hunters of the Neolithic, this article overviews ancient methods of preventing animal disease as 'an important part of the historic development of veterinary medicine' (p. 343). Neolithic cave paintings in France attest to the early use of magic to protect preferred species, along with fences used both to corral captured herd animals and protect them from predators. The practice of hanging up protective items dates from antiquity. In early Mesopotamia, for instance, clay tablets with prayers to beneficient gods were hung up to ward against the seven demons believed to cause livestock and human ills. Also in Mesopotamia, in addition to hexes, exorcisms, sacrifices and divinations to ward against diseases, priests were called upon to purify stables as a way of preventing livestock ailments. As reported in various studies, certain Egyptian priests also practised semi-empirical veterinary arts, mainly for sacred cattle. Besides magico-religious rites, they administered cold and hot baths, massages, fumigations, cauterizations, bleeding, castration and various plant-based and other medicines to livestock. High-level officials also existed to oversee the care of horses and geese. Many Egyptian methods of disease prevention and treatment were taken up by Greeks, Romans and Moslems. Greeks were the first to develop the doctrines of the four elements and of humoral balances, applied equally to animal and human health. Aristotle wrote about clinical signs of disease in oxen, horses, donkeys, pigs, birds, bees and elephants, along with prophylactic and therapeutic treatments. Early Greek veterinarians also advised of the greater importance of prevention over curing. An early Roman prophylaxis for sheep mange consisted of washing the animals with water or wine in which *Lupinus albus* seeds had been soaked, followed 3 days later by washing with sea or salt water. For epidemic diseases, Romans had recourse to hygienic controls on faeces and diseased carcasses, quarantine, avoidance strategies such as dispersal of healthy animals to new or distant environments – although most of their methods for preventing rabies were misguided. An early Roman medical/veterinary text lists 540, 180 and 100 treatments of plant, animal and mineral origins, respectively. Similar observations to those for the Roman empire apply to the ancient Indian, Chinese and Islamic worlds. An early Indian king ordered construction of veterinary hospitals and the cultivation of medicinal herbs. Arabs established the first pharmacies and developed phytochemistry. In Europe of the Middle Ages, veterinary medicine was more oriented to supernatural causes and prophylaxes. But empirical specialists in horse medicine arose; and some 10th and 11th century scholars emphasized the importance of analysing clinical signs in arriving at treatments, along with the importance of 'affection and good management' (p. 353) in maintaining equine health. Meanwhile, stockraisers themselves employed many plant-based treatments. With the advent of continent-wide epidemics of livestock disease in post-Renaissance Europe, modern Western veterinary medicine began to evolve, along with laws for controlling such epidemics.

Ranaivoson, Andrianasolo, Jean Rajaonarison, Rosa Ranaivoson, Désiré Rambelomanana and Arsène Andrianavalona. 1982. *Effet du* **Cannabis sativa** *ou* **Rongony** *sur la Maladie de Teschen.* In-house report. Département de Recherches Zootechniques et Vétérinaires, no place of publication given, Madagascar. 9 pp.

A clinical trial was conducted in Madagascar to validate the traditional use there of *Cannabis sativa* as a prophylaxy for the viral encephalomyelitis of swine known as Teschen. However, pigs administered *C. sativa* and subsequently inoculated with the virus all died. In evaluating this finding, the researchers point up several possible flaws in the trial's design: inoculation is not equivalent to natural infection on-farm; the test pigs were of a different breed from those raised in traditional areas; and the conditions in which the test animals were kept on-station differed greatly from those for livestock in village farms.

Ranaivoson, Andrianasolo, Rosa Ranaivoson and Désiré Rambelomanana. 1984. *La Dermatophilose a Madagascar: Epidemiologie et Lutte.* Centre National de la Recherche Appliquée au Développement Rural, Département de Recherches Zootechniques et Vétérinaires, Antananarivo, Madagascar. 58 pp.

In passing, this study of dermatophilosis (also known as cutaneous streptothricosis or mycotic dermatitis) in livestock of Madagascar notes the results of an experiment on a [traditional?] plant-based remedy. The treatment consisted of weekly applying a decoction of equal parts of the *tanatanamanga* and *borona* plants [no Latin names or preparation details given] to the affected parts of 111 cattle after scraping away the scabs that are characteristic of the disease. With two or more applications, more than half the cattle were fully cured; and all but seven of the remainder experienced slight to considerable improvement. *In vitro* studies of *tanatanamanga* extracts were then planned, in order to discover the active ingredient(s).

Rangel, Rosa and José Luis Felipe Ortiz. 1985. Medicina tradicional para animales en dos comunidades de la Meseta P'urhépecha. Unpublished manuscript. URM/Dirección General de Culturas Populares/SEP, Uruapan, México. 60 pp.

This study reports on more than 30 ailments of cattle, horses, pigs, sheep, donkeys and poultry in two P'urhé communities of Mexico, along with 38 medicinal plants and seven other curative materials used to treat these ills. The P'urhé people distinguish between two types of animal ills: those that can be cured locally and those that require the attention of a veterinarian. Nevertheless, before calling in a veterinarian, stockowners always try to treat their animals themselves using indigenous therapies, patent medicines, or both. Many of the same medicinal plants are used for both human beings and animals. Also, plants that ailing animals are observed to consume are often thereafter incorporated into the human ethnopharmacopoeia. [Annotation based on information in Argueta Villamar 1988.]

Rangnekar, D.V. 1992a. BAIF's experience in developing delivery systems to provide services on the door-step of smallholders. In: P.W. Daniels, S. Holden, E. Lewin and S. Dadi (eds). *Livestock Services for Smallholders: A Critical Evaluation of the Delivery of Animal Health and Production Services to the Small-scale Farmer in the Developing World – Proceedings of an International Seminar, Yogyakarta, Indonesia 15–21 November 1992.* INIAN-SREDEF, Bogor, Indonesia. Pp. 360–363.

The BAIF Development Research Foundation is an Indian NGO that promotes integrated rural development nationwide. Among its many operational principles are doorstep delivery of services to farmers and, in the case of research, an on-farm emphasis coupled with a respect for indigenous knowledge. BAIF's largest development thrust is its dairy cattle programme, initiated in 1969. This seminar paper notes the recent addition to the programme of studies on indigenous treatments for livestock in order to gain more information about herbal remedies.

Rangnekar, D.V. 1992b. Study of traditional livestock production systems of the pastoralist and their [sic] perceptions about the production system and attitude to change. Paper presented to the Workshop on Transhumant Pastoralism in Gujarat. Indian Institute of Rural Management, Anand, Gujarat, India. 10 pp.

Based on the work of the Indian NGO BAIF in 11 districts of Gujarat State, this workshop paper reports on traditional husbandry practices in two communities of pastoralists there. Pastoralists in India are widely characterized as 'a menace to the rural society . . . so stubborn and resistant to change that they do not desire even to consider possibility [sic] of accepting new technologies or more productive and profitable production systems' (p. 1). The author argues that, in fact, over time and also recently pastoralists have themselves undertaken changes in their stockraising strategies in response to shifts around them. Some examples are found in the realm of herd composition and breeding. Due to uncertain rainfall and thus diminished feed resources, during the past decade Gujarat pastoralists have added more goats and buffalo to their herds. Also, they have instituted controls on bucks such that there will be only one kidding per year, corresponding to the time of greatest forage abundance. For cattle as well as goats, pastoralists have used a time-tested system of breeding that involves careful selection and rotational use of male animals. This system has resulted in a particularly hardy and strong cattle breed (the Kankereg) prized by neighbouring farmers as draught animals. But pastoralists also vary their selection criteria in order to respond to farmer demand for varying coat colours, horn shapes and body conformations in different parts of Gujarat State. Also noted is pastoralists' astute knowledge of feed resources and their practice of mixing their own rations from locally available feedstuffs that research has shown to be good sources of nondegradable protein. Indeed, both their breeding and feeding practices mirror many of the most 'modern' recommendations from, respectively, animal nutritionists as to feed supplementation and rumen manipulation, and geneticists and reproduction specialists as to avoidance of inbreeding. In sum, the author reiterates that, on the one hand, pastoral traditions are not static; but on the other hand, sometimes pastoralists' 'resistance to change . . . is a blessing in disguise' (p. 2).

Rangnekar, D.V. 1997. BAIF's experience in developing delivery systems to provide services at the door steps of smallholders. *FAO Electronic Conference on Principles for Rational Delivery of Public and Private Veterinary Services. January–March 1997.* 2 pp.

Studies of traditional livestock feeding systems by the Indian NGO BAIF show that, where diets are slim in proteins and minerals, Indian stockraisers feed supplements of protein-rich local plants, including various bushes, creepers, flowers, leaves and pods. BAIF is working to improve and extend feeding systems based on these traditional practices, recommending increased quantities of tree products in animal diets.

Rangnekar, D.V. 1999. Developing livestock health management systems. Paper presented to the International Seminar on Integrated Approach for Animal Health Care, 4–6 February 1999, Calicut, Kerala, India.

Livestock are not only a part of the human food chain, but also an important source of income for small farmers. Current animal healthcare services, however, do not meet the needs of the clientele. They have limited coverage and the adoption of preventive disease control and other measures is low. To become more effective and efficient for small farmers, health services should become a tool for development. Besides treating sick animals, services should cover breeding and feeding and help animals to produce at their full potential. They should recognize the value of local knowledge and combine both allopathic and alternative types of veterinary medicine such as Ayurveda, folk medicine and homeopathy. But in addition to treating sick animals, services should include breeding, feeding and other husbandry aspects in order to help animals reach their full productive potential.

Rangnekar, Sangeeta. n.d. *Traditionally Used Fruits and Flowering Plants for Animal Treatment. A [sic] Initial Report Based on Extensive Observations in Some Districts of Maharashtra, Gujarat, Rajasthan.* Women [sic] Organisation for Rural Development, Ahmedabad, India. 11 pp.

Based on extensive discussions in the mid-1990s with men and women farmers, this report documents flowering and fruit plants commonly used in several underdeveloped areas of India to treat everyday livestock ills (species unspecified). A total of 48 treatments involving 37 plants are described under the following headings: tick control, wounds and maggots, worms, poisoning, chicken diseases, bleeding, repeat breeding, footrot, milkstone, cough and pneumonia, diarrhoea, liver disorders and skin diseases. Colour photos are included for 16 of the plants. A few examples of treatments are: a wound paste of burnt mango-tree bark and coconut oil; for myiasis, a daily dressing of one crushed wild onion; to stop bleeding in cuts and wounds, *Jatropha curcas* latex; an anthelmintic feed of *Cucurbita pepo* seeds; for coughs and pneumonia, a twice daily chest-wrap of heated *Carica papaya* leaves; for diarrhoea in large animals, a 3-day, thrice-daily drench of 10 teaspoons of *Lawsonia alba* seeds soaked in water; for liver disorders, a drench of *Achyranthes aspera* roots crushed in buttermilk; a paste of jasmine flowers to reduce itching in skin diseases. The author underscores the flexibility, multivalence and availability of such local remedies, in that a choice of treatments involving different plants usually exists for any one animal disease and, conversely, a given plant is often employed in treatments for different diseases.

Rangnekar, Sangeeta. 1992a. Role of women in livestock production and health management. In: John Young (ed.). *A Report on a Village Animal Health Care Workshop – Volume II: The Case Studies.* ITDG, Rugby, UK. Pp. 138–144.

Research on women's roles in stockraising in India revealed that women are knowledgeable about major animal diseases. They spot the onset of disease quickly since they are keen observers and know each individual animal's behaviour. Women also know many traditional veterinary treatments and medicinal plants for livestock. Further, women are especially knowledgeable about nutritious fodders for different species (buffalo, cattle, goats) and sexes (cows, bullocks) of animals. For mastitis, women recommend feeding a mixture of oil and turmeric and applying turmeric or certain tree leaves to the udder. Remedies for FMD lesions include: walking animals through hot sand; and applying linseed oil and turmeric to the lesions or, if there is myiasis, kerosene. Women treat tympany by drenching with a mixture of linseed oil, ginger, turmeric and asafoetida, and by tying the animal's mouth open with a piece of wood. Retained placenta is cured by feeding bamboo leaves or a mixture of oil, bran and grain. For anoestrus, stock are fed the seeds of a certain forest tree. Neem leaves are fed to deworm goats. Special fodders consist of: cotton seed and cottonseed cake, to increase the yield and fat content of milk; *Acacia* and *Prosopis* spp. pods and seeds, for the same purposes plus inducing heat; the creeper *Tinosperma cordifolia* and leaves of *Alangium* spp., *Bassia latifolia* and *Butea monosperma* to improve milk production; neem leaves, to do likewise in goats; and *B. latifolia* flowers, to improve bullock condition. Not surprisingly, women stockraisers have proved apt students in training on how to deliver other kinds of animal health and extension services to women.

Rangenekar, Sangeeta D. 1992b. Women farmers' views on animal health and production services in India. In: P.W. Daniels, S. Holden, E. Lewin and S. Dadi (eds). *Livestock Services for Smallholders: A Critical Evaluation of the Delivery of Animal Health and Production Services to the Small-scale Farmer in the Developing World – Proceedings of an International Seminar, Yogyakarta, Indonesia 15–21 November 1992.* INIANSREDEF, Bogor, Indonesia. Pp. 223–226.

Tribal and pastoral women in India carry out many critical management tasks such as cleaning animals and their quarters, feeding and milking stock, and harvesting, processing and marketing dairy products. While women's range of livestock tasks varies according to household socioeconomic status, most know the behaviour and temperament of every animal in their family herds. Thus women are often the first to observe signs of sickness or other changes in animal condition. Women also control considerable knowledge of local feed resources and veterinary plants. They may administer home remedies themselves or they may consult a local livestock healer. In the 1200 families of diverse socioeconomic status interviewed by the author, 70% to 80% of women respondents said they turn to such healers before going to a veterinarian because 'he [the healer] is easily available and uses locally available cheap medicines effectively against some ailments'. In contrast, 'veterinarians . . . administer drugs as they feel and farmers incur heavy expenditure [sic]' (p. 226). The same percentage of women said they believe in evil spirits as causes of livestock disease and that they 'make special worship for the sick animal' (ibid.).

Rangnekar, S.D. 1996. Study on role of women in animal husbandry in rural parts of western India. In: Karl-Hans Zessin (ed.). *Livestock Production and Diseases in the Tropics: Livestock Production and Human Welfare. Proceedings of the VIII International Conference of Institutions of Tropical Veterinary Medicine held from the 25 to 29 September, 1995 in Berlin, Germany.* Volume II. Deutsche Stiftung für Internationale Entwicklung, Zentralstelle für Ernährung und Landwirtschaft, Feldafing, Germany. Pp. 608–611.

Conducted in rural parts of India's Gujarat and Rajasthan States, this study found that women there have a profound knowledge of livestock ethology and production characteristics and are able to describe each individual animal under their care accordingly. Women in arid and semi-arid areas are also expert at selecting and storing protein- and energy-rich feeds like acacia pods, *Ziziphus* leaves, groundnut hay and *mahuva* flowers. Women then later process and present these feeds according to individualized animal performance. Furthermore, women know effective traditional medicines for disorders like tympany, inflammations and swellings, foot problems, skin diseases and certain types of anoestrus.

Rangnekar, Sangeeta. 1997. Rural women: The hidden innovators as experienced while studying livestock production. Paper presented to the International Conference on Creativitiy and Innovation at Grassroots, January, Ahmedabad, India. 5 pp.

Discussions with rural women in India's Maharashtra, Gujarat, Rajasthan and Madhya Pradesh States about their roles in ruminant and poultry production revealed that women control considerable knowledge of bovine nutrition and of traditional veterinary practices. Discussants identified a variety of local tree and shrub fodders that are fed to cows to improve the quantity and quality of their milk. To improve the fat content of buffalo milk, women also wash and feed a certain weed (*Cassia critica*) that they gather in their grain fields. Women also prepare a special cattle feed made up of tree pods, cotton seed, grain, salt and tamarind; they cook the mixture before feeding to make it more digestible. Several treatments in particular were found to be widely and effectively used by women. FMD foot ulcers are dealt with by walking the animal through hot sand or by applying hot sand to the lesions. An alternative is to apply linseed oil and turmeric powder, along with kerosene if there is myiasis. Women treat tympanitis by drenching with a mixture of linseed oil, ginger and turmeric and asafoetida powder or by tying a piece of wood into the patient's mouth so as to keep its mouth open. Poultry receive important feed supplements in the form of daily kitchen wastes. At night, the birds' basket-coops are hung along the eaves of the home or are installed on top of a long bamboo, where nocturnal predators cannot reach.

Rangnekar, Sangeeta. 1999a. Participatory studies with women on ethno-veterinary practices for livestock health management. In: E. Mathias, D.V. Rangnekar and C.M. McCorkle, with M. Martin (eds). *Ethnoveterinary Medicine: Alternatives for Livestock Development – Proceedings of an International Conference Held in Pune, India, 4–6 November 1997. Volume 1: Selected Papers.* BAIF Development Research Foundation, Pune, India. Pp. 36–40.

This paper reports on studies of women's ethnoveterinary knowledge, aptitude and practices (KAP) in stockraising groups of pastoralists, tribals and farmers of the western Indian states of Gujarat, Madhya Pradesh and Rajasthan. Regional and social KAP variations were determined and indirectly validated. For example, it was found that tribal women knew more about medicinal plants than did women in the other two groups. Women living near a city or a veterinary dispensary were the only ones to turn first to veterinarians when they felt they needed professional help with livestock health problems. Other women consulted local healers (who are mostly men) before approaching veterinarians. The reasons they cited for this pref-erence ranged from cost factors to long-term association or personal relationships with healers, greater credibility of and confidence in such traditional practitioners and greater ease of access to local healers than to veterinarians. Regardless of region, social organization or production system, however, nearly all women had some knowledge of, and used, traditional veterinary treatments. This paper lists treatments for mastitis, foot and mouth ulcers, tympany, retention of placenta, anoestrus, diarrhoea, bleeding, ecto- and endoparasites and footrot. The author concludes by noting that women play an important role in the health management of their livestock. She recommends that women should be included in the valida-tion of traditional remedies as well as the training and orientation programmes for paravets.

Rangnekar, Sangeeta. 1999b. Farmer perceptions of livestock health services. Paper presented to the International Seminar on Integrated Approach for Animal Health Care, 4–6 February 1999, Calicut, Kerala, India.

This paper gathers together the results of various studies conducted across the last 10 years on livestock production and health in western India's Rajasthan, Gujarat and Madhya Pradesh States. The studies sought to understand farmers' perceptions and priorities as affected by socioeconomic status, area and gender. The goal was to appreciate better the health systems in existence and farmers' needs so as to plan services more effectively. Topics studied spanned: livestock in rural systems, stockraising objectives, farmer perceptions, women's roles in animal healthcare and veterinary services.

Rao, G.S., Jawahar Lal, S. Chandra and J.K. Malik. 1998. Studies on the effects of ethnobotanicals on the goat trachea. In: E. Mathias, D.V. Rangnekar and C.M. McCorkle, with M. Martin (eds). *Ethnoveterinary Medicine: Alternatives for Livestock Development – Proceedings of an International Conference Held in Pune, India, 4–6 November 1997. Volume 2: Abstracts.* BAIF Development Research Foundation, Pune, India. P. 51.

Stockraisers treat their animals' respiratory diseases with a number of medicinal plants, yet little is known about these ethnobotanicals' effects on the smooth muscles of the ruminant airway. The *in vitro* study reported here investigated five different plant extracts in this regard: alcoholic extracts of *Piper nigrum* fruits, *Allium sativum* bulbs and *Syzygium aromaticum* buds, and essential oils of *Eucalyptus* sp. leaves and *Cedrus deodara* wood. Tracheae were collected from freshly slaughtered goats at the local abattoir and the specimens were then chilled in Kreb's-Henseleit solution. Next, smooth muscle strips of 3 to 4 cm were dissected from the mid part of the trachea and mounted in an organ bath (20 ml) containing Kreb's-Henseleit solution ($37 \pm 0.5°C$) continuously bubbled with air. The tissues were allowed to equilibrate for 1 hour under a constant tension of 1 g. Responses were recorded by a force displacement transducer, connected to an ink-writing oscillograph. The relaxant effect of various extracts was seen on the pre-contracted tissues with histamine (10–5M) and carbachol (10–8M) [sic]. The *S. aromaticum* extract (1 mg/ml) completely relaxed both histamine and carbachol-induced contractile responses, whereas the other extracts and the essential oils did not alter either response. To further confirm *S. aromaticum*'s effect, the tissues were pre-treated with the extract (1 mg/ml) for 15 minutes before exposing them to histamine and carbachol. The extract completely blocked the contractile responses to both agonists; and this effect was reversible.

Rao, S.V.N., A.W. Den Ban, D.V. Rangnekar and K. Ranganathan. 1995. Indigenous technical knowledge and livestock. In: Kiran Singh and J.B. Schiere (eds). **Handbook for Straw Feeding Systems.** ICAR, New Delhi, India. Pp. 119–128.

In discussing the importance of studying indigenous technical knowledge and comparing it with modern equivalents, this chapter mentions the Indian practice of applying turmeric and mustard or coconut oil to livestock wounds as an example of an indigenous technique that is easier and cheaper to apply than turning to modern, external inputs such as antibiotics or formal-sector veterinary services.

Rao, V.N., H.C. Joshi and Abhay Kumar. 1983. Therapeutic efficacy of garlic (*Allium sativum*) against *E. coli* infections in chickens. **Avian Research** 67(1): 26–27.

Garlic was tested *in vivo* for its efficacy in combating *E. coli*, taking advantage of a poultry flock known to be infected. Across 4 days, 35 out of the 900 birds in the flock had died from the infection. After the flock was fed a ration of 4% garlic chips, only three birds died the following day; thereafter, there was no further mortality. The therapeutic effect of garlic was further confirmed by the *in vitro* sensitivity of an *E. coli* isolate to an aqueous extract of garlic in the ratio of 10:1.

Rappaport, Roy A. 1968. **Pigs for the Ancestors: Ritual in the Ecology of a New Guinea People.** Yale University Press, New Haven, Connecticut, USA. 311 pp.

This cultural-ecological ethnography focuses upon the complex relations among the Maring Tsembaga of New Guinea, their plant crops, pigs and their broader physical, human and spiritual environment. Pages 69–70 note that the Maring frequently explain illnesses in both people and animals by reference to the contamination of the ground by supernatural *tukump*, corruption disseminated by a spirit, or by *kum*, an infection of the earth sent by sorcery. The appropriate therapy consists of relocating one's homestead.

Rath, Sabyasachi. 1994. Madhuchakra. *Honey Bee* 6(2): 9–10.

In India's Tamil Nadu State, livestock enteritis is controlled with an aqueous drench of 100 g of dried ground ginger and 2 ground pepper seeds or with a bolus of cold *ragi* (a family food?) and pig fat. Indigestion or anorexia is remedied by a single feeding of 100 ml of gingelly oil and a bunch of *Calotropis* leaves. Ingestion of a hen's egg, red soil and 0.5 kg of tomatoes helps cows to conceive. To increase milk production, bottle gourd, fenugreek, coconut, black gram and palmyra jaggery are pounded together and fed to the cow for 3 days. To get rid of lice, goats and cattle are washed with water in which tobacco has been soaked. For cattle with FMD, neem oil is applied between the toes thrice daily. For asphyxia, water or castor oil is poured into one nostril so that any material blocking it will be ejected through the other nostril.

Rathore, Hanwant Singh, Shravan Singh Rathore and Ilse Köhler-Rollefson. 1999. Traditional animal health services: A case study from the Godwar area of Rajasthan. In: E. Mathias, D.V. Rangnekar and C.M. McCorkle, with M. Martin (eds). *Ethnoveterinary Medicine: Alternatives for Livestock Development – Proceedings of an International Conference Held in Pune, India, 4–6 November 1997. Volume 1: Selected Papers.* BAIF Development Research Foundation, Pune, India. Pp. 162–170.

Godwara, located in south-central Rajasthan, is an area rich in livestock. There, nomadic Raika pastoralists herd sheep, goats and camels; land-owning castes of Rajput and Jat raise cows and buffalo; and donkeys are kept by scheduled castes and backward classes like Kumhars, Kalbelia and Bhat. This paper reports on a study conducted by the NGO Lokhit Pashu-Palak Sansthan on local disease concepts and treatments in Godwara. Treatments spanned herbal and non-herbal preparations, surgical techniques and firing. The authors endeavour to give some general assessments of the efficacy of a few treatments. But ultimately, they point out that without prolonged comparative studies, one can only speculate about efficacy. Still, they found that certain camel diseases (notably rheumatism, bronchopneumonia and wry-neck syndrome) that resist conventional therapies seemingly responded to firing with a hot iron. The study also provided insights into stockraisers' choice of animal healthcare provider. Although Godwara boasts an extensive network of government animal hospitals, rural people rarely access it. Instead, they prefer self-treatment or consultations with a traditional healer or a spirit medium (*bhopa*). Not surprisingly, nomadic pastoralists are most likely to resort to self-treatment. In contrast, settled groups usually turn to a local healer and, if the healer fails them, to a *bhopa*.

Raval, S.K., R.G. Jani and P.R. Patel. 1998. Value of camphor for the treatment of blood in milk. In: E. Mathias, D.V. Rangnekar and C.M. McCorkle, with M. Martin (eds). *Ethnoveterinary Medicine: Alternatives for Livestock Development – Proceedings of an International Conference Held in Pune, India, 4–6 November 1997. Volume 2: Abstracts.* BAIF Development Research Foundation, Pune, India. P. 52.

In the dairy industry, mastitis and milk abnormalities can sharply curb profits. This study discusses the efficacy of camphor (*Camphora officinarum*) for treating stock with blood-tinged milk. Camphor contains a volatile acid that has a styptic action. In villages near Anand, India 21 buffalo clinically observed to have blood in their milk were given 2 camphor-in-banana tablets twice a day. Before and after the camphor therapy, milk samples of these animals were tested for both clinical and occult blood using a strip cup and benzidine tests in the laboratory. Affected animals recovered within 3 to 5 days. Treatment costs per animal were calculated and the cost:benefit ratio for camphor was compared with that of other drugs. Findings indicated that camphor is effective and cheap; moreover, it is widely and easily available in India.

Ravindra, D. and K.R. Rao. 1999. Ethnoveterinary medicine – a boon for improving the productivity of livestock in rural India. In: E. Mathias, D.V. Rangnekar and C.M. McCorkle, with M. Martin (eds). *Ethnoveterinary Medicine: Alternatives for Livestock Development – Proceedings of an International Conference Held in Pune, India, 4–6 November 1997. Volume 1: Selected Papers.* BAIF Development Research Foundation, Pune, India. Pp. 144–154.

Despite relentless government efforts across the last 50 years, India's formal veterinary system is far from satisfactory by world standards. Yet the nation's vast livestock resources are pivotal in providing employment for small and marginal farmers. And largely thanks to such farmers, India ranks first in world milk production and 19th in broiler production. In the modern veterinary sector, 45 670 veterinary institutions cater to the healthcare needs of 322 085 million adult units (data estimated for 1996). This makes for only one veterinary institution for every 7052 adult units. Yet the National Commission on Agriculture's goal is a ratio of 1:5000 by the year 2000. The lack of veterinary institutions is especially acute in states like Bihar, Gujarat, Madhya Pradesh, Maharashtra, Rajasthan, Uttar Pradesh and West Bengal, where the gap is more than 50%. When it comes to veterinary personpower, there is a gap between the supply of and demand for veterinarians to the tune of 27 459. Finally, the supply/demand gap for veterinary products in 1996 is estimated at US $180 to $250 million, assuming an expenditure of 2% to 2.5% of the value of livestock products on veterinary medicines. The foregoing figures need to be considered realistically in the light of the financial implications of trying to bridge such gaps with conventional veterinary medicine, i.e. the costs of establishing a veterinary institution, training a veterinarian, or building the infrastructure for manufacturing veterinary products. When all such costs are taken into account, the advantages of valid ethnoveterinary solutions as a way of bridging these gaps in animal healthcare institutions, practitioners, products and infrastructure become evident. Ethnoveterinary solutions seem particularly attractive in a country like India, where traditional treatments have been used and documented for centuries; where there is a clear market demand for practitioners, which demand could well be filled by traditional healers who have been given some formal training; and where an industry in ethnoveterinary pharmaceuticals already exists. To exploit the potentials of EVM, what is needed are: creation of an organizational structure, like regional work stations linked to a central policy body; measures to exploit existing resources in order to standardize EVM treatments and practices; and development of a national database on livestock populations, veterinary infrastructure and so forth, so as to identify where best or first to target EVM support.

Raviprakash, V. and M. Sabir. 1983. Scope of herbal medicines in veterinary practice. ***Veterinary Research Journal*** 6(1): 1–9.

This article reviews the role of Ayurvedic veterinary medicine in India and then discusses several traditionally-based commercial preparations. An example is the drug Wopell[TM], which is compounded of *Mallotus philippensis, Butea frondosa, Embelia ribes, Areca catechu* and *Dryopteris filix.* In one form or another, this compound has been used as an anthelmintic for more than 3000 years.

Ravis-Giordani, G. 1981. ***Les Communautés Pastorales du Niolu.*** Doctoral thesis, Université René Descartes, Paris, France.

Unavailable for review. However, based on Brisebarre 1985a, see especially Chapter 14, Part 6, 'Les Soins Au Troupeau', pp. 436–447.

Raychaudhri, S.P. (ed.). 1964. ***Agriculture in Ancient India.*** ICAR, New Delhi, India.

Reportedly, pages 144 to 151 of this publication describe some 86 ethnoveterinary practices used in ancient India, with disease treatments divided into nasal, oral and ocular. [Abstract based on Gupta et al.'s 1990 annotated bibliography.]

Razafindrakoto, Ch. n.d. ***Contribution à l'étude de l'efficacité d'une Cucurbitacée (Voatovon-Dolo) contre certains parasites internes des ruminants.*** In-house report. Département de Recherches Zootechniques et Vétérinaires, no place of publication given, Madagascar. 12 pp.

A trial was carried out in Madagascar to evaluate the effect of a certain *Cucurbitae* species traditionally used in treating cestode infestations of livestock. The plant trial made use of three sheep and three bovids. One sheep was given one spoonful of powdered dried *Cucurbitae* seeds, the second sheep received two spoonfuls and the third none. A similar design was used for the bovids. The plant appeared to have significant positive results on sheep and cattle, but further work is needed to confirm this.

Reddy, K. Raja and G. Sudarsanam. 1987. Plants used as veterinary medicine in Chittoor District of Andhra Pradesh, India. ***International Journal of Crude Drug Research*** 25(3): 145–152.

In the forests of Chittoor District in India's Andhra Pradesh State, between 1980 and 1985 the authors consulted reputed traditional healers (*pasuvaidyulu*) from a wide variety of tribal and non-tribal groups on their knowledge of ethnoveterinary plants. Consultations lasted from a few hours to several weeks, depending upon an interviewee's knowledge and/or his willingness to reveal it. Some healers (especially the sacred elders) were reluctant to expose the depth of their knowledge in the belief that doing so would render their drugs ineffective. Nevertheless, together healers described 57 plant prescriptions for cattle disorders, along with the dosage and duration of treatment. A few examples follow. Emaciated cattle are administered a decoction of *Acacia sundra* stem bark mixed with cumin seed and ginger paste for 4 days. *Solanum nigrum* L. leaf juice is applied to castration wounds of oxen. *Tylophora indica* leaves, garlic cloves and pepper fruits are ground into a paste and given as an antidote for cyanide poisoning. Non-plant materials figuring in some prescriptions include salt, jaggery, buttermilk, eggwhite and pig fat. The majority of remedies are monoprescriptions, however. In concluding, the authors note that modern medicine is gradually eroding the use of crude herbal drugs.

Reddy, V.N. Viswanatha. 1999. Holistic approach of treating animals. Paper presented to the International Seminar on Integrated Approach for Animal Health Care, 4–6 February 1999, Calicut, Kerala, India.

The author advocates a holistic approach to treating livestock. A list of nine pathologies is provided with a choice of allopathic, herbal and homeopathic treatments. For example, the mouth lesions of FMD can be treated with allopathic antihistamines and antibiotics, with bananas dipped in sesame seed oil as a herbal topical application, or with homeopathic pills of zinc. The author also stresses the importance of good feeding and management in reducing the incidence of disease.

Reddy, V.N. Viswanatha, B.K. Narainswami and N. Nomesh Kumar. 1998. Holistic approach of treating animals. In: E. Mathias, D.V. Rangnekar and C.M. McCorkle, with M. Martin (eds). ***Ethnoveterinary Medicine: Alternatives for Livestock Development – Proceedings of an International Conference Held in Pune, India, 4–6 November 1997. Volume 2: Abstracts.*** BAIF Development Research Foundation, Pune, India. Pp. 58–59.

One way of moving toward more sustainable systems of animal production is to take a holistic healthcare approach that integrates homeopathic (Ho), Ayurvedic (Ay) and allopathic (Al) medicines. The choice of methods and their combination depends on the disease and the availability of drugs. Holistic approaches are gaining favour because of increasing awareness of problems with allopathic drugs, such as toxicity, inappropriateness and non-availability. This paper suggests holistic treatments for five bovine health problems. A holistic treatment for active FMD consists of: rinsing with a mouthwash of *Hydrastis* and *Semper Vivum Tectotrum* combined with feeding pills of Zincum Metallicum 200, Nitric Acid 200, Variolium 200 and Mercksol 200 (Ho); feeding ripened banana dipped in pig fat or gingelly (*Sesamum indicum*) oil (Ay); and washing the mouth lesions with 4% washing soda (Al). To combat FMD's after-effects in female animals (i.e. anoestrus and reduced milk yields), an integrative treatment is: feeding pills of Ipecac 30, Thyroidinum 30 and Aurum Iodum 200 (Ho) along with germinated *Trigonella* spp. seeds and fried gingelly seeds in jaggery (Ay); and injecting compounds having iodine or giving potassium iodide or Thyroxine tablets (Al). Recommended for eversion of the uterus are: feeding Opium 200 pills with or without Carboveg (Ho); applying an extract of *Mimosa pudica* to the everted uterus and also giving the extract orally (Ay); and injecting epidurally amyl alcohol (Al). For repeat breeders, pills of Aurum Iodum 200 and Thyroidinum 30 (Ho) can be fed along with Aloes Compound tablets (Ay) and prostaglandin or GnRH or hCG injections (Al) can be given. Mastitis may be treated by: feeding Bryonia 200, Belladonna 200 and Echinesiae 30 (Ho); applying a paste of turmeric, millet and butter, and also feeding *Abrus precatorious* (Ay); injecting antibiotics, antihistamines and liver extract parenterally (Al); and infusing antibiotics intramammarily (Al). For any of these diseases, homeopathic, Ayurvedic or standard allopathic treatments can be employed individually; or different combinations of the three can be employed depending upon considerations of cost and efficacy. However, when used properly, holistic approaches have a definite advantage over individual methods.

Reed, J.B.H., D.L. Doxey, A.B. Forbes, R.S. Finlay, I.W. Geering, S.D. Smith and J.D. Wright. 1974. Productive performance of cattle in Botswana. *Tropical Animal Health and Production* 6: 1–21.

A field investigation was undertaken in six areas of Botswana to determine how management, environment and possibly aphosphorosis affected the body condition and reproductive performance of range cattle there. The authors found that in areas where cattle raisers were wealthy men who owned or controlled better grazing areas and who held 'enlightened ideas' (p. 6), cattle performance was much better due to these men's use of up-to-date preventive veterinary inputs such as acaricides, anthelmintics, vitamin injections and dietary supplements. In other areas, however, use of such inputs was limited and performance was thus lower, due to 'the ignorance, apathy or financially embarrassed state of the owners' (ibid.).

Rege, J.E.O. 1998. African domestic ruminant genetic resources: What are they worth and can value be added? *Currents* 17/18: 24–30.

Whether in terms of species, breeds or strains, down through the ages Africans have developed a great diversity of farm-animal genetic resources. For ruminants, these span some 100 to 150, 50 to 60, and 45 to 50 breeds or strains of cattle, sheep and goats, respectively. There is also a large but undetermined number of indigenous breeds or strains of chickens and other poultry species. Africa further boasts substantial genetic diversity in pigs, mules, horses, donkeys and dromedary camels. With regard to the comparative productivity of ruminants, ample research indicates that under the conditions in which indigenous African livestock are typically raised, specialized imported breeds are simply no match. Moreover, most studies have shown that indigenous breeds can be as, if not more, productive than European ones. This is especially true when viability and maintenance requirements as measured by liveweight are taken into account, along with the lower risk factors of husbanding animals specifically adapted to the high environmental stresses of Africa. In addition, stockraising based on indigenous breeds 'is more environmentally friendly as it is invariably associated with little or no input of chemicals, e.g. veterinary therapeutic and curative drugs' (p. 26).

Reid, J.A. 1930. Some notes on the tribes of the White Nile Province. *Sudan Notes and Records* 8(2): 149–209.

Among nomadic Arab pastoralists of Sudan, the camel alone provides the transport, milk and fibre that in other cultures come from horses, cows and sheep. These camel pastoralists migrate in parallel lines so as to avoid cutting across, and so fouling, each other's grazing grounds. The herds are 'salted' at a water hole or lake that is naturally salty. Camels are categorized by age according to the number of teeth they have. The most common camel diseases are trypanosomosis, internal haemorrhaging and mange. The herdsman diagnoses trypanosomosis by smelling the camel's urine. A diseased animal is isolated and may be given a complex 3-year-long treatment to 'immunise' it against trypanosomosis. Camels that survive this treatment become extremely valuable because they can travel farther south, where heavy rains make for high tsetse fly populations.

Rekha, S.T., Jagdish S. Matti and B.K. Narainswami. 1998. Ethnoveterinary medicine for ruminants. In: E. Mathias, D.V. Rangnekar and C.M. McCorkle, with M. Martin (eds). *Ethnoveterinary Medicine: Alternatives for Livestock Development – Proceedings of an International Conference Held in Pune, India, 4–6 November 1997. Volume 2: Abstracts.* BAIF Development Research Foundation, Pune, India. Pp. 53–54.

Herbal medicines that can be prepared from locally available resources are often effective, less expensive and more eco-friendly than commercial veterinary drugs. This paper reports findings from a 1997 study of farmers' traditional herbal medicines for ruminants in Shimoga District, Karnataka State, India. For example, *Tagetes erecta* (African marigold) leaves and camphor are ground together, heated and applied to the foot ulcers of FMD. The buccal ulcers of FMD are likewise treated with ground-together jaggery (50 g), salt (15 g) and *Swertia chirata* roots (15 g); also, a portion of this preparation is fed to the sick animal. To treat rabies, people drench with crushed-together *S. chirata*, *Piper longum*, *Brassica juncea* (mustard), dry ginger, onion, *Tylophora indica*, *Vitex negundo* and *Andrographis paniculata* and mango leaves in buttermilk and hot water. Blackquarter is treated with a twice daily drench, for 3 days, of *Trianthema decandra* juice mixed with 5 g of *Capsicum frutescens* (chilli) powder and 5 g of crushed garlic. Mastitic stock are given a 3- to 4-day hot-water drench of the following ingredients ground together: the leaves and bark of *Albizia amara*, *Vitex negundo*, *Adhatoda vasica*, the leaves of *Tinospora cordifolia*, *P. longum* and 0.25 kg of garlic. Also, a paste of *T. cordifolia* leaves is smeared on the udder. To control external parasites, 10 tablespoons of powdered *Butea monosperma* bark mixed with buttermilk are applied all over the body; an alternative application is a fine paste of *Leucas aspera*, *Clerodendrum inerme* and *Azadirachta indica* leaves mixed with *Curcuma longa* L. (turmeric) powder. Internal parasites are controlled by a drench of turmeric powder in *Agave americana* (century plant) leaf juice. For severe diarrhoea, animals are drenched with onion in buttermilk. Even from these few examples, it is evident that the spectrum of local treatments is wide. Veterinary science should take a closer look at them.

Rennie, T., D. Light, A. Rutherford, M. Miller, I. Fisher, D. Pratchett, B. Capper, N. Buck and J. Trail. 1997. Beef cattle productivity under traditional and improved management in Botswana. *Tropical Animal Health and Production* 9: 1–6.

In Botswana, 92% of cattle are raised under a traditional 'cattle post' management system in which the animals are maintained on unenclosed grazing land. The animals are not accompanied by a herder during the day; and they are corralled at night only if they are near cultivated areas or if there is danger from predators. Under this system, controlled use of bulls and oversight of calf weaning are difficult and calf mortality is higher than on ranches. Yet these herds of indigenous Tswana cattle produce 85% of all beef for export. The research reported here investigated to what extent the Tswana breed would respond, without any genetic modification, to more intensive and 'modern' management as represented by '"reasonably acceptable" fenced ranch conditions' (p. 5). In brief, results revealed a substantial decrease in calf mortality and significant increases in calving percentages, 7-month calf weight and post-weaning growth among ranched cattle as compared to controls.

Ridder, N. de and K.T. Wagenaar. 1986. A comparison between the productivity of traditional livestock systems and ranching in eastern Botswana. In: P.J. Joss, P. W. Lynch and O.B. Williams (eds). *Rangelands: A Resource Under Siege. Proceedings of the Second International Rangeland Congress.* Cambridge University Press, Cambirdge, London, New York, New Rochelle, Melbourne, Sydney. Pp. 404–405.

In comparing traditionally raised versus ranched cattle in Botswana in the 1970s, the authors found that productivity of the former was significantly lower when expressed as weight of weaner calf per cow per year. However, this relationship was reversed when productivity was calculated on a per hectare basis, even when the negative impacts on beef production of draught power and milk offtake for human consumption from traditional herds were factored in. Overall, on a per-hectare basis, Botswana's traditionally raised, multi-purpose herds can be considered as 95% more productive than the single-purpose beef cattle on ranches.

Riley, Bernard W. and David Brokensha. 1988. *The Mbeere in Kenya Volume II: Botanical Identities and Uses.* University Press of America, Lanham, Maryland, USA. 348 pp.

This volume lists the numerous uses that Kenya's Mbeere tribe makes of plants in their environment as, e.g. living hedges, hive timber, corks and medicines. Plants employed in Mbeere veterinary treatments include: *Sarcophyte piriei* H. for anthrax or for expulsion of the placenta in cattle; *Ficus* sp. leaves for diseased or barren heifers or cows; *Euphorbia candelabrum* T. latex for myiasis; *Cissus cactiformis* G. for cleaning and dressing wounds; and the oily sap of *Commiphora madagascarensis* J., which is rubbed on chickens and other livestock to rid them of lice and fleas.

Ritter, Hans. 1990. Soziokulturelle Aspekte der Tiere bei den Twareg. In: Horst S.H. Seifert, Paul L.G. Vlek and H.-J. Weidelt (eds). *Tierhaltung im Sahel. Symposium 26–27 Oktober 1989.* Göttinger Beiträge zur Land-und Forstwirschaft in den Tropen und Subtropen, Heft 51. Forschungs- und Studienzentrum der Agrar- und Forstwissenschaften der Tropen und Subtropen, Georg-August-Universität Göttingen, Germany. Pp. 39–66.

This conference paper on Sahelian stockraising discusses the origin of Twareg animal names as well as myths and rites relating to animals and how these influence Twareg's use of animals and their products. For example, eating meat from camels that have received a name and thus have become individualized – such as riding or racing mounts – is taboo. But slaughtering and eating 'anonymous' animals such as transport camels is not.

Rivers, W.H.R. 1906. *The Todas.* Macmillan and Co. Ltd, London, UK and New York, New York, USA. *Ca.* 749 pp.

This ethnography explores the social and especially religious lifeways of the Toda of India's Nilgiri hills as these relate to the heart of all things Toda: their semi-wild buffalo. In particular, numerous ideological beliefs and practices surround the management of, and the processing of products from, the sacred herds of the Toda dairy-temple system. The clarified butter and soured whey that the temples produce are distributed amongst each temple's associated villages. From the anthropologist-author's description, many such ideological elements are suggestive of practical husbandry, veterinary and public-health measures. For example, the temples are maintained apart and distant from household herds and are staffed by dairymen/priests in a ratio of perhaps one priest per every seven animals. These men, who may serve for as long as 15 years, are subject to a wealth of regulations on personal hygiene, behaviour and product handling. Depending upon their office, priests must: constantly wash their hands and use mainly the right hand for their husbandry duties; wear a certain garment, which never leaves the dairy; avoid being touched by any ordinary person and not touch many areas and things both inside and outside the dairy; never prepare any food-stuffs other than the temple dairy products; periodically or after a night away from the dairy, wash themselves from head to foot; never visit markets or attend a funeral; remain celibate; and much more. A minimum of five times per year, dairymen regale their charges with salt mixed with soured buttermilk, water and a certain tree bark (*tudr*). Served up in a hole in the ground, some of these feed-ings coincide with seasonal events, such as the first spring grass or first frost, that have implications for animal health. Very young calves are penned separately; and for their first 2 weeks of life, they are allowed to suckle all their dams' milk. Before milking, the teats are smeared with butter. The vessels used to harvest, churn and boil the milk are kept scrupulously clean. Moreover, they are never used for any other purposes and they never leave the dairy-temple, where they can be handled only by the dairymen/priests. If new earthen vessels are pur-chased in the marketplace, before they can be used they are scrubbed inside and out with a *tudr* bark, washed three times and then filled with water and set to boil over the dairy fireplace for some time. Wherever possible, sacred dairies have their own, untainted water supply for all their washing, cooking and product-processing needs. Ideally this is a spring, a separate stream, or at the very least an upstream site different from those used for ordinary herds and household needs. Although disease is largely viewed as a punishment from the gods, if a livestock epidemic breaks out in an area, the sacred herd is promptly moved to one of the other dairy-temples on its annual transhumant route. Clan temples exchange animals as needed for breeding or re-stocking. When a calf (usually male) is to be sacrificed, the priests have tricks to induce its dam to suckle a foster female calf. All three animals are penned together for several days on a bedding of certain grasses and leaves; after trampling, these materials are rubbed on the calves' backs along with some milk, so the dam will lick and nurse them both. The object is to confuse the cow into continuing to nourish the foster calf after her own is removed. If this trick fails, the skin of the slaughtered male calf is placed on the foster female. Taken together, all the foregoing practices imply expert maintenance of strong, genetically vigorous pools of disease-free and productive stock that consistently furnish their worshipful public with safe and healthy dairy foods – the mainstay of the Toda diet. [See also Walker 1986 and 1989.]

Roa R., María de los Angeles. 1989. Uso de la acacia para el tratamiento de diarrea en un grupo de antilopes y un dromedario. In: Gerardo López Buendía (ed.). *Memorias: Segunda Jornada sobre Herbolaria Medicinal en Medicina Veterinaria.* Universidad Nacional Autónoma de México, Facultad de Medicina Veterinaria y Zootecnia, Coordinación de Educación Continua, México DF, México. Pp. 133–135.

Dazzled by commercial pharmaceuticals, clinical veterinarians have forgotten that many plant medicines can give just as good results when employed correctly. Vets may quickly recall this fact, however, when they have no commercial drugs at hand or when such products have failed to solve the health problem they are treating. This conference paper recounts zoo managers' and veterinarians' successful experiences, under just such circumstances, in treating diarrhoea in a camel and, later, a herd of antelope by feeding them leaves of the leguminous mimosa tree, *Acacia cyanophila*.

Robin, B. 1994. Les parasites en Europe et leurs traitements décrits dans la seconde moitié du XVIIIe siècle. *Revue Scientifique et Technique de l'Office International des Épizooties* 13(2): 559–580.

This article discusses the study and practice of parasitology in 18th-century Europe. Contemporary scientific diagnosis, control and treatment of the following parasitoses are noted: liver flukes, bots and other myiases, lice, ticks, roundworms, flatworms and sarcoptic mange. Liver fluke disease was prevented by avoiding low-lying swampy pastures, turning animals out to graze only after dew or rain has dried and keeping animals on large, airy pastures. Treatments centred on feeding oats into which various ingredients had been mixed (e.g. salt, antimony, saltpetre, absinth buds, human urine) and giving water high in minerals such as copper sulphate. Bots were sometimes treated surgically as well as medically, by trepanation and curettage of the sinus cavities. For lice and ticks, separation of infested animals was recommended, along with washes made variously of salt, tobacco, mercury, brandy and corrosive materials. Vermicidal drenches were also many and varied. Of all the diseases discussed, however, treatments for mange were the most diverse. They usually consisted of topical unguents made from ingredients such as mercury, sulphur, tobacco, tar and turpentine. Shepherds were encouraged to scrape mange lesions with a specially manufactured pincer and then apply the unguents to the open sores. To ensure that the medicine would adhere to the sores, in the winter and summer, respectively, unguents were made oilier or drier by the addition of lard or soot. Not until WWII did chemical insecticides like organochlorines and piperazine gain wide use in European veterinary parasitology. And the first anti-parasitic vaccine did not appear until the 1960s.

Robinson, Patrick. 1992. Indigenous knowledge in yak/cattle cross-breeding and management in high altitude Nepal. In: Devika Taman, Gerard J. Gill and Ganesh B. Thapa (eds). *Proceedings of the Workshop on Indigenous Management of Natural Resources, Dhulikhel, June 8–9, 1992.* Winrock International, Kathmandu, Nepal. Pp. 139–148.

Yak/cattle cross-breeding is actively promoted throughout the Himalaya-Karakorum region of Nepal and in many other mid- and high-altitude zones of central Asia. Cross-breeding reaps the benefits of hybrid vigour and genetic adaptation to a wider range of altitudes and environmental conditions than that enjoyed by either parent of the cross.

Roe, Frank Gilbert. 1955. *The Indian and the Horse.* University of Oklahoma Press, Norman, Oklahoma, USA.

The Hidatsa believed that castrated horses did not tire so easily in soft and swampy ground. Only experts could perform castrations. With the Cree, on the other hand, castration was a job anybody could do and there were no ritual correlates involved in the procedure (pp. 258–259).

Roepke, Dean. 1989. Indigenous practices warranting the interest of the veterinary medical community. Personal communication (letter) to E. Mathias of 22 January 1989. 3 pp.

Many modern veterinary practices have arisen from traditional ones. In North America, drenching animals with corn syrup for ketosis has evolved into drenching with glucose solution. In central Europe, mastitis was treated with pure distilled alcohol to alter vascular pH. This practice has now been replaced by antibiotics. In Africa, colonists adapted traditional peoples' use of *Tephrosia vogelii* leaves against cattle ticks by preparing the leaves as a wash, which the colonists then applied successfully to their dogs as well as cattle.

Roepke, Dean A. 1996. Traditional and re-applied veterinary medicine in East Africa. In: Constance M. McCorkle, Evelyn Mathias and Tjaart W. Schillhorn van Veen (eds). *Ethnoveterinary Research & Development.* Intermediate Technology Publications, London, UK. Pp. 256–264.

Drawing upon the author's 5 years' experiences as an HPI veterinarian in East Africa, plus a rich historical literature, this chapter focuses on traditional preparations of local plants as antifungals, antivirals, anthelmintics, ectoparasiticides, styptics, cathartics, laxatives, diuretics and antidiuretics, antivenoms and still more. Information is provided on the chemical action and *in vitro* efficacy of many of these traditional medicines. The author summarizes four particular lessons learned from his work in East Africa. First, traditional veterinary practices often parallel Western techniques – as when he first observed smallholders injecting the milk of unripe coconuts subcutaneously as a fluid- and electrolyte-replacement therapy for young stock with scours, much as humans are given a drip to offset the dehydration of acute diarrhoea. Second, some ethnoveterinary practices appear to be just as effective as, and far more sustainable than, their Western commercial counterparts. An example is WaSwahili's equal, if indeed not greater, success in treating dermatophilosis in cattle using seed oil of the tree *Hydnocarpus wightiana* Blume, as compared to the author's HPI-prescribed antibiotics, which were locally available only from the project and would likely disappear with the project. The third lesson is that such EVK is in danger of being lost or suppressed. For example, early 20th-century Europeans in the tropics used to cultivate *H. wightiana* in order to use the seed oil as a topical treatment for leprosy; but it has since been forgotten in Western medicine, along with many other therapies and prophylaxes recorded in a wealth of colonial literature. The fourth lesson is that, given all these considerations, EVM can offer a much-needed alternative or complement to Western-style medicine; conversely, past and present Western medicine can in turn inform and refine local techniques. For example, in one district of Tanzania, the author introduced a group of 35 dairy farmers to an old Western-world anthelmintic, made of the pulped root of the male shield fern (*Dryopteris filix-mas* Schott) at a dosage adapted from early Western pharmacopoeias; faecal samples indicated the treatment was effective with no side effects. The larger point is that, from whatever sources, traditional botanicals and other treatments can be rescued, 're-applied', and, perhaps after some modest field trials, more broadly extended. As the cost of modern medicines spirals and as traditional ones are forgotten, stockraisers may otherwise be left with no weapons to combat their animals' ailments.

Roersch, Carlos and Liesbeth van der Hoogte. 1988. *Plantas Medicinales del Surandino del Perú.* Visual Service S.R.L. for the Centro de Medicina Andina, Cuzco, Perú. 297 pp.

This book lists 55 of the plants most commonly used in human ethnomedicine in the southern Andes of Peru. It identifies each by its Latin and local names, describes the species' habitat, gives its classification in the Latin American hot/cold medical system, notes the parts of the plant most often employed and then details its mode of application to numerous diseases. No mention is made of ethnoveterinary applications aside from the discussion on page 168 of *muña* (*Minthostachys andina*), a plant of extremely widespread use whose pharmacological action was first demonstrated in veterinary research on its effectiveness against ectoparasites in a variety of animal domesticates. [See also Caballero Osorio 1984a&b.] The primary value of this volume for ethnoveterinary research lies in its thoroughly professional treatment of the Andean plants listed, most of which also figure in the management of animal health in the region.

Röeth [sic], Gitta. 1997. Blending human and plant based knowledge systems: Dominican pest management practices – Part I. *Honey Bee* 8(3): 16–17.

Smallholders in the highlands of the Dominican Republic have long used *Citrus aurantium* and *Piper aduncum* against fleas and mites in livestock (and humans), *Ocimum gratissimum* for myiasis and *Allium sativum* and *Carica papaya* against intestinal parasites. [Details of treatments are not given.] Stimulated by biodynamic and organic agriculture ideas introduced by a development project, young farmer-students in one village are now experimenting with their traditional ethnomedical *materia medica* to see if they can be adapted to generate herbal pesticides for their plant crops, as they cannot afford commercial ones. However, farmers who have tried the new herbal preparations note that, while they work, they are practical only for small plots like kitchen gardens because of the work entailed in gathering and preparing the plants. The author suggests that with more support from extension and development services, ways to scale up the technology could be found.

Rohrbach, J.A. 1986. Herbal medicine, its application in veterinary medicine. *The Veterinary Annual* 24: 208–214.

This article provides a brief introduction to the veterinary applications of herbal medicine and overviews their history beginning with ancient Ayurvedic writings up to Amerindian practices. The raw materials, growth, harvesting and preparation of medicinal plants are discussed; and in some cases, specific veterinary applications are recommended. An example is the use of *Valeriana officinalis* for nervous disorders. Administered orally in large quantities, it excites the nervous system. In small doses, it exerts a calming effect on animals aroused by external factors, but not by inherent defects in temperament.

Romero Ramírez, Carlos, Arcelia R. del Castillo R., Adriana C. Martínez M. and Carlos J. Calderón F. 1988. Estudios preliminares de los efectos antibacterianos, antiparasitarios y toxicológicos de la raíz del chilcúan. In: Luz Lozano Nathal and Gerardo López Buendía (coordinators). *Memorias: Primera Jornada sobre Herbolaria Medicinal en Veterinaria*. Universidad Nacional Autónoma de México, Facultad de Medicina Veterinaria y Zootecnia, Coordinación de Educación Continua, México DF. Pp. 134–143.

Since pre-Colombian times, the root of *chilcúan* (*Helosis longipes*) has played a prominent role in Mesoamerican ethnomedicine. Rural Mexicans today employ it as a local anaesthetic in humans and an insecticide in livestock. The studies presented here demonstrate its potential effectiveness in an alcohol extract for combating *E. coli* and *Staphylococcus aureus* and the larva of two fly species that parasitize sheep and horses.

Ruhanga, Jean Damascène. 1998. Integration-valorisation de la médecine vétérinaire traditionnelle: Les initiatives de la société Rwandaise. *Le N'Dama: Journal du Sous-Réseau PRELUDE Santé, Productions Animales et Environnement* 11, 12(1&2): 8–13.

With impetus from its Ministry of Scientific Research, Rwanda has created a University Centre for Research on Traditional Pharmacology and Medicine (CURPHAMETRA), including veterinary medicine. CURPHAMETRA activities span: (1) study and understanding of traditional Rwandan medicine, including phytochemical and pharmacological research on medicinal plants found in the nation; (2) in-country production of medicines and other economically useful products, based on findings from (1); and (3) likewise, incorporation of ethnomedical training into Rwandan university curricula. In 1982 CURPHAMETRA established a dispensary of traditional medicine with six healers who had received some training in modern medicine. This mechanism was designed to stimulate dialogue between traditional and modern practitioners, dispel negative attitudes among the latter about the former and help healers to begin formally organizing. A somewhat similar initiative was a Catholic priest's 1978 establishment of the Bare Center of Traditional Medicine (CMTB), which has since won the support of Rwanda's Ministry of Public Health. However, both the dispensary and the CMTB work mainly only with herbalist-healers, to the exclusion of other Rwandan practitioner-types like midwives, diviners, sorcerers and poisoners. But these groups also often employ botanicals. (However, the CMTB later added traditional psychiatrists, for human patients.) The author asks: is not the exclusion of other kinds of practitioners perhaps a perversion of traditional medicine, a stripping away of some of its essential elements and cultural meanings? Is a synthesis somehow possible, he wonders? Otherwise, he fears an 'absorption of traditional by modern medicine' that will 'do more harm than good to the population [of Rwanda]' (p. 11). The remainder of the article discusses the many problems encountered in both centres in bringing traditional and modern medical practitioners together. The author advises that 'Since the sociocultural context of health and illness cannot be universalised . . . Each country should find a health system appropriate to its society' and ' . . . one cannot pretend to assure . . . collaboration with traditional medicine without first seeking to understand the logic that underlies its practice' (p. 12).

Sackmann, W. 1994. Anthrax in Switzerland during the early 19th century. *Revue Scientifique et Technique de l'Office International des Épizooties* 13(2): 537–543.

Based on records from a farm in Switzerland that suffered a devastating attack of enzootic anthrax in the 1800s, this article describes prophylactic and therapeutic measures taken at the time, albeit with limited success. These included: fumigating stables with vinegar and juniper berries; providing clean, fresh drinking water frequently; quartering stock in cool, shaded places; and bathing them in cold water. A 17th-century anthrax remedy consisted of saltpetre, saffron, alum, egg white and the urine of a young boy administered in an unspecified fashion. Likewise for several kinds of oil, including turpentine, walnut, juniper and oil from church lamps. For acute cases, a special variant of seton application or 'pegging' was used, in which a dried hellebore root (*Helleborus niger, H. viridis*, or *H. pupurascens*) was inserted under the skin. As a foreign body, the root produced pus; but it was also expected to exert specific pharmacological effects. In Switzerland, root pegging dates back at least to the 1500s and the practice survived into serious European veterinary textbooks of the 1950s [see also Marusi and Bochhi 1983 and Blancou 1994a]. Additional observations of note in this account include the following. As a last resort in combatting recurrent anthrax on his farm, the farmer in question turned to magic and religion. He purchased a black billy goat to expel the evil; but the goat, too, succumbed to anthrax. In addition, although himself a Protestant, the farmer asked Catholic monks to perform an exorcism; but ultimately the government forbade any religious intervention. Although the aetiology and epidemiology of anthrax was poorly understood, stockraisers of the time knew to quarantine sick animals and to bury the carcasses of animals with anthrax in deep graves, taking into account soil humidity and underground watercourses. And a Swiss veterinarian of the period made the astute observation that outbreaks of anthrax in some areas were linked to fertilizing pastures with gypsum mined from deposits that, in retrospect, must have been infected with anthrax spores.

Salcedo, Mario B. 1986. *Un Herbolario de Ch'ajaya Revela sus Secretos.* Artes Gráficas El Buitre for SOBOMETRA and SENPAS, La Paz, Bolivia. 165 pp.

Written by a well-known Bolivian herbalist, this book lists 238 disease symptoms in human beings and 108 plants, fruits, vegetables, spices and other items used in their treatment. In only one case is mention made of ethnoveterinary applications. This is the plant *Psoralea glandulosa*, known in the Spanish of Bolivia, Mexico, Peru and Chile as *culén* (Quechua *williya*, Aymara *wallwa*, Kallawaya *llallirikicho*). The author details the species' habitat, geographic distribution, morphology, history of discovery, use and exploitation, and notes that an infusion of *culén* is an antidote to locoweed poisoning in herd animals.

Salih, M.A. Mohamed. 1992. *Pastoralists and Planners: Local Knowledge and Resource Management in Gidan Magajia Grazing Reserve, Northern Nigeria.* IIED Dryland Networks Programme, IIED, London, UK. 37 pp.

Among Fulani pastoralists interviewed in northern Nigeria, many responded that local veterinary knowledge was being lost as healers who could accurately diagnose and treat animal diseases were becoming fewer and fewer. Respondents also mentioned six plants used in Fulani cattle treatments: for brucellosis, powdered *Terminalia avicennioides* bark fed with salt; for delivery delays and birthing pains in cows, the same preparation but with *Cucumis pustulatus*; for haemonchosis in calves, a drench of *Dichrostachys cinerea* seeds, *Aristolochia albida* bark and *Parkia clappertoniana* soaked in water; and for poisoning, *Bridelia ferruginea* bark. This article also notes Fulani's conscious breeding for cattle that can thrive under a wider range of drought and disease challenge.

Sánchez V., Clemente. n.d. Avances sobre el Proyecto Alpaca Convenio UNTA-NUFFIC, 'Control de la sarna de alpacas con alcaloides del tarwi'. In: *II Anales del Conversatorio Nacional Multisectorial sobre Desarrollo de Camélidos Sudamericanos.* Instituto Nacional de Investigacion y Promocion Agropecuaria. Pp. 153–154.

This abstract reports the results of experiments with *tarwi* (*Lupinus mutabilis*) water [see Tillman 1983], an ancient Andean treatment for camelid ectoparasitism, to validate its effectiveness scientifically. As of 1 month after topical treatment with *tarwi* water, all of the experimental alpaca recovered fully. The author mentions that similar trials have been conducted with lice in alpaca, *Melophagus* in sheep and demodectic mange in dogs.

Sandford, Dick. 1981. Pastoralists as animal health workers: The Range Development Project in Ethiopia. *Pastoral Network Paper* No. 12c. Agricultural Administration Unit, ODI, London, UK. 8 pp.

This paper summarizes the experiences of the Rangeland Development Project in Ethiopia with the installation of pastoralists as 'veterinary scouts', i.e. animal health workers. The author discusses the scouts' role, remuneration, selection, supervision and training. He concludes that the employment of scouts resulted in the pastoralists' support for the project. But veterinary scouts' potential can be tapped only if the veterinary service as a whole is effective. Disease surveillance is necessary.

Sangat-Roemantyo, Harini and Soedarsono Riswan. 1991. Ethnobotanical aspects of medicinal plants for ruminants in Java. In: E. Mathias-Mundy and Tri Budhi Murdiati (eds). *Traditional Veterinary Medicine for Small Ruminants in Java.* Indonesian Small Ruminant Network, SR-CRSP, Central Research Institute for Animal Science, Agency for Agricultural Research and Development, Bogor, Indonesia. Pp. 1–4.

To treat their ruminants, farmers in Java exploit at least 23 plant species belonging to 15 families. Of these, ginger is the most frequently used. Also included are cash crops such as shallots, garlic, tobacco, pineapple, papaya and guava. Traditional phytotherapies were most often administered for diseases of the digestive tract (worms, diarrhoea, bloat), but also for wounds, anaemia, colds, anorexia, skin problems and inappetence. Popular plant preparation techniques are direct feeding, grinding, or boiling. Botanical *materia medica* are often mixed with other ingredients such as eggs and honey. Farmers grow most of the plants themselves, in home gardens or plots near the home.

Santra, Ajit Kumar. 1992. The role of AFPRO in animal husbandry projects in Manipur State, India. In: John Young (ed.). *A Report on a Village Animal Health Care Workshop – Volume II: The Case Studies.* ITDG, Rugby, UK. Pp. 117–122.

The Indian NGO AFPRO has long experience in implementing animal husbandry programmes throughout the nation with every type of farm animal. As part of its livestock development efforts, it encourages the use and dissemination of helpful traditional husbandry practices.

Sapre, V.A. 1999a. Scope of homeopathy in veterinary practice. In: E. Mathias, D.V. Rangnekar and C.M. McCorkle, with M. Martin (eds). *Ethnoveterinary Medicine: Alternatives for Livestock Development – Proceedings of an International Conference Held in Pune, India, 4–6 November 1997. Volume 1: Selected Papers.* BAIF Development Research Foundation, Pune, India. Pp. 211–222.

Homeopathic remedies have long been used for veterinary applications. Although texts on this subject are available, the curricula of veterinary colleges and universities in India do not mention it. Also, published reports on this subject are rare in India, although veterinary practitioners have had encouraging experiences with it. Thus, for Indian veterinarians who do use homeopathic remedies, their main source of information is books and practitioners of homeopathy for humans. The author has been a teacher of medicine at Nagpur Veterinary College since 1968, where he also treats and supervises the healthcare of animals at the college's Cattle Breeding Farm. There, he began experimenting with homeopathic treatments for livestock. For example, when seven cows with obstinate *Corynebacterium* infections of the mammary glands refused to respond to the routine intramammary and systemic application of antibiotics, he gave the homeopathic drug Phytolacca 200 X tincture to the cows for 10 days. All the animals showed remarkable improvement and five were cured completely. In a comparative study on subclinical mastitis, as confirmed by bacterial isolation, 87% of 45 affected quarters treated homeopathically recovered whereas the recovery rate was only 27% for another group given antibiotics. Thereafter, research was extended to homeopathic treatments for FMD, with very encouraging results. Subsequently the college conducted research on the use of homeopathic drugs for various ills in some 500 animals at three different locations, where findings have also been very encouraging. As a result, the college has come out with homeopathic remedies for about ten common animal health problems and the drugs are being applied in clinical practice with good results. Overall, there appears to be no harm in using homeopathy in cases for which there is no specific therapy in allopathy. Viral diseases, antibiotic-resistant infections and conditions of unknown aetiology are some examples. But homeopathic cures specifically for veterinary application need to be authenticated for use in clinical practice.

Sapre, V.A. 1999b. Use of homeopathic drugs in the treatment of animal diseases. Paper presented to the International Seminar on Integrated Approach for Animal Health Care, 4–6 February 1999, Calicut, Kerala, India.

A comparison is reported between the homeopathic drug phytolacca and oxytetracycline intramammary infusion in the treatment of mastitis. Sixty six percent of the 15 quarters treated with phytolacca recovered while in the 15 quarters treated with oxytetracycline the recovery rate was 20% as determined using the California Mastitis Test (CMT). In a multilocational study over 5 years, 566 cases of FMD that failed to respond to allopathic treatment after 3 days showed a 66% recovery rate when treated homeopathically. The recovery rates following homeopathic treatment of 15 other common diseases are reported. Recommendations are made for the homeopathic treatment of prolapse of the vagina, wounds, indigestion and diarrhoea. It is concluded that homeopathy has potential for the treatment of animal diseases and that its monitored use should be encouraged.

Sastry, M.S. 1986. Indigenous drugs in veterinary practice. *Indian Veterinary Medical Journal* 10: 88–92.

This historical overview of indigenous drugs used in Indian veterinary medicine describes many plant-based medicines and remarks on the resurgence of interest in them. Some of the plants cited include *Aristolochia bracteata*, *Embelia ribes* and *Butea frondosa* as anthelmintics, and *Leptadenia reticulata*, *Asparagus racemosus* and *Euphorbia* spp. as galactagogues. *Withania somnifera* and *Mucuna prurita* reportedly stimulate the libido and male sexual behaviour of goats.

Satrija, F., P. Nansen, S. Murtini and S. He. 1995. Anthelmintic activity of papaya latex against patent *Heligmosomoides polygyrus* infections in mice. *Journal of Ethnopharmacology* 48: 161–164.

Several tests to validate traditional remedies utilizing pawpaw (*Carica papaya*) in anthelmintic preparations for livestock proved positive [cited in Fielding 1998].

Sautier, Denis and Heraldo Amaral. 1989. Integrated pest management or integrated system management? *ILEIA Newsletter for Low External Input and Sustainable Agriculture* 4(3): 6–8.

This article describes the great variety of wild plants employed in central Brazil to combat pests and diseases of food crops, livestock and humans. Page 6 briefly mentions the use of banana leaves and an extract of garlic against ectoparasites of swine.

Saxena, M.J. 1998. Present status of ethnoveterinary research and development. In: E. Mathias, D.V. Rangnekar and C.M. McCorkle, with M. Martin (eds). *Ethnoveterinary Medicine: Alternatives for Livestock Development – Proceedings of an International Conference Held in Pune, India, 4–6 November 1997. Volume 2: Abstracts.* BAIF Development Research Foundation, Pune, India. P. 55.

A large proportion of the world's livestock still depend on EVM for their healthcare. Many EVM practices offer viable alternatives to conventional veterinary medicine and are especially relevant for developing countries with limited financial resources.

Because of this, ER&D has become a fertile area for technology development. An interdisciplinary approach is essential because of the multiplicity of factors and insights involved. EVM includes a wide spectrum of techniques that can be improved through techno-blending. Conversely, modern science also benefits by drawing upon local knowledge of animal healthcare and husbandry. ER&D covers topics in enterprise development, environment, healthcare delivery, public health, education, socioeconomics, planning and policies, as well as more strictly veterinary and husbandry subjects. These aspects are discussed in relation to present and future veterinary needs in India.

Schillhorn van Veen, T.W. 1979. Influence of animal husbandry on the occurrence of tropical fascioliasis (*F. gigantica*). ***Proceedings of the American Association of Veterinary Parasitologists.*** P. 11.

In West Africa, fasciolosis occurs mainly in the savanna area, where climatic conditions are favourable to the intermediate snail host *Lymnaea natalensis*. The incidence of fasciolosis depends on seasonal variations in snail populations and in livestock movements. Young snails are present mainly during the rainy season and at the beginning of the dry season. During the rainy season, however, most nomadic herds traditionally were moved out of areas with high densities of young snails to other areas less favourable to *Lymnaea* survival and development. Removal of the herds also made fewer host animals available to *F. gigantica* in snails reaching maturity. This traditional epidemiological model of limiting grazing in snail-infested areas during the wet season was applied on a smaller scale to a farm with fluke problems, where it reduced outbreaks of acute fasciolosis in sheep. This on-farm experience served as a sort of 'mini test' of an indigenous management technique, while at the same time illustrating how valuable traditional husbandry practices can be adapted and applied to current stockraising situations.

Schillhorn van Veen, Tjaart W. 1984. Observations on animal health, especially approaches to identify and overcome constraints in the subhumid zone of West Africa. In: J.R. Simpson and Phylo Evangelou (eds). ***Livestock Development in Subsaharan Africa: Constraints, Prospects, Policy.*** Westview Press, Boulder, Colorado, USA. Pp. 303–317.

This chapter discusses constraints to livestock production, the history of veterinary services and developments in animal health delivery in West Africa. The author criticizes the fact that until recently disease control measures in Africa concentrated on eradication of major epidemic diseases such as rinderpest and CBPP, while the day-to-day problems of stockowners were largely ignored. He recommends the introduction of animal health packages and stresses the importance of epidemiological surveys and of an integrated approach to disease control.

Schillhorn van Veen, T.W. 1985. General aspects of small ruminant health: Management, technology and extension. In: R.T. Wilson and D. Bourzat (eds). ***Small Ruminants in African Agriculture.*** ILCA, Addis Ababa, Ethiopia. Pp. 94–106.

In addition to presenting examples of management practices, new technologies and infrastructural changes that can improve the production and marketing of sheep and goats, this chapter notes that the literature offers few controlled studies of the differential effects and impacts at farm and village level of instituting many kinds of simple husbandry practices [often found in traditional management systems]. These neglected practices include: enclosing animals at night, separating the sexes, fencing off pastures, feeding salt, controlling breeding and introducing legumes into the diet.

Schillhorn van Veen, Tjaart W. 1986. Some considerations in the approach to measure and prevent animal health problems in traditionally raised livestock. Adapted English version of a paper presented to the workshop 'Les méthodes de la recherche sur les systèmes d'élevage en Afrique intertropicale', Dakar-Mbour, Senegal, February 1986. 21 pp.

This paper reviews basic epidemiological principles, methods for disease control and prevention and their possible applications to livestock raised under traditional management systems. Examples refer to the USA and Africa. Livestock producers and associations should be involved in planning disease surveillance and veterinary improvement programmes. Because owners everywhere are concerned about their animals' health, they are generally receptive to veterinary interventions; but the acceptance rate also depends on the value of the animals. Interventions should combine treatment with instructions about hygiene and health maintenance.

Schillhorn van Veen, T.W. 1993. The present and future veterinary practitioners in the tropics. *The Veterinary Quarterly* 15(2): 43–47.

The present and future role of ethno- as well as conventional medicine in the work of veterinarians in the tropics is mentioned in this article. Ethno- and alternative veterinary medicine is today increasingly recognized by orthodox veterinarians and international drug companies. Similarly, local perceptions of the patterns and economic importance of different diseases are now often seen as useful for understanding the limitations of introducing Northern veterinary technologies to the South. In the future, traditional medicine and paraveterinary support may provide the most cost-effective approach to animal healthcare in the tropics.

Schillhorn van Veen, Tjaart W. 1996a. Personal communication to C.M. McCorkle of unspecified date. Washington, DC, USA.

Based on his decade of experience as a veterinary professor and practitioner in Nigeria, the author recounts how Fulani pastoralists have 'genetically engineered' the Keteku breed of cattle by crossing their Bunaji breed – which is mainly geared to milk production in the West African savannas – with N'Dama cattle – which are a trypanotolerant rainforest breed. As a result, Keteku cattle can thrive under a wider range of drought and disease challenge.

Schillhorn van Veen, Tjaart W. 1996b. Sense or nonsense? Traditonal methods of animal disease prevention and control in the African savannah. In: Constance M. McCorkle, Evelyn Mathias and Tjaart W. Schillhorn van Veen (eds). *Ethnoveterinary Research & Development.* Intermediate Technology Publications, London, UK. Pp. 25–36.

As documented as far back as ancient Egyptian papyri and the Bible, African herders have long exercised many useful strategies to reduce the risk of livestock disease. Strategies can be broadly classified as either ecological or physiological. The former is commonly used to forestall exposure to non-fatal and especially fatal diseases when the disease pressure is intermittent, localized and to some extent avoidable, as with fasciolosis (see Schillhorn 1979), trypanosomosis, CBPP, rinderpest, anthrax and blackleg. Examples of ecological methods of disease prevention based on avoidance of disease vectors or infected locales and maximization of access to good forage and minerals are: migration and other seasonal herd movements; shorter-term 'tactical' movements; isolation and quarantine; herd dispersal; timing of diurnal and nocturnal grazing and watering regimes; and mixed grazing. The ecological category also embraces numerous mechanical means to control flies, ticks, mosquitoes and maggots. Such techniques include: fly repellents in the form of homemade washes and powders, leather blinkers and protective hedges and smudge fires of insecticidal plants; deliberate overgrazing, clearing, or burning of rangelands to destroy pest habitat; manual removal of ticks, followed by burning them or feeding them to poultry; nowadays commercial insecticidal dips, sprays, washes and powders; and various methods of wound care to forestall myiasis. Physiological methods aim to prevent or control (usually enzootic) disease by modifying endogenous processes so that when disease does strike, major losses can be averted. The classic example is astute traditional methods of immunization – both directly via crude vaccines and indirectly via controlled exposure to diseased animals. A related technique is to ensure that newborns gain immunities by suckling colostrum. Another physiological method is controlled breeding and/or selective stud-animal acquisitions to improve herd resistance or tolerance to pests and diseases as well as other environmental stresses. For example, Fulani who migrate into a new area always buy local bulls (even if they are of a different breed) with the express purpose of enhancing their stock's adaptation to local conditions. Such practices have endowed Africa with breeds and strains of livestock that resist such diseases as trypanosomosis, heartwater and in some cases ovine intestinal parasites. Examples of such breeds are N'Dama, Muturu and Baoulé cattle, and Djallonké and Maasai sheep. In sum, to answer the question posed in the title of this article, from the perspective of Western veterinary medicine, many of the disease control and prevention strategies invented and employed by African herders are anything but nonsense.

Schillhorn van Veen, Tjaart W. 1997a. Sense or nonsense? Traditional methods of animal parasitic disease control. *Veterinary Parasitology* 71: 177–194.

In addition to overviewing traditional movement, management, breeding, housing and vaccination strategies for preventing or controlling parasitic livestock diseases [also see Schillhorn van Veen 1996b], this article addresses ethno-diagnostic and -semantic aspects of traditional animal healthcare and husbandry systems worldwide – all in cultural-historical and modern-development contexts. Drawing upon his own and others' research, the author catalogues an impressive array of accurate ethnodiagnostic techniques based on sensory appreciation of faeces, urine, milk and lymph nodes. For example, Fulani diagnose chronic fasciolosis by observing consistently dry and hard faeces. Samburu detect ECF by palpating the parotid lymph nodes. And Bedouin and/or Twareg diagnose trypanosomosis or intestinal diseases by respectively tasting the milk or smelling the breath of suspect animals. This last technique has only recently received wider attention in conventional medicine. Local disease names may also signal sensitive herder knowledge of disease processes and linkages. An example is coastal Kenyans' varying words for ECF in exotic cattle as versus in native calves or adults, as per the different clinical incidences and outcomes of ECF in these three classes of cattle. In like vein, Nigerian herders distinguish lexically, and correctly, between more and less dangerous ticks epidemiologically. But ethnodiagnostic and related understandings of pathophysiology often falter when it comes to diseases with multiple underlying causes that vary according to time and place, diseases with complex parasitic life cycles or invisible modes of transmission and diseases never before encountered in an area. An example of the first is unthriftiness. In Africa, where herders consider it a major problem, this syndrome goes by many names: *nagana* in East Africa, *sammore* among Hausa and *joola* or *wilsere* for Fulani of Nigeria or Niger; and the syndrome may have nearly as many underlying parasitic, nutritional, or other causes. An example of the second case is Ecuadorean highlanders' failure to distinguish lungworm infections from other pneumonias and to distinguish their different modes of transmission; not until an earthquake in the 1980s destroyed the tightly closed barns in which highlanders kept their animals did they discover the benefits of staking stock outside. To take another example, sometimes stockraising peoples are ignorant of fasciolosis' association with aquatic snails. Nevertheless, they may recognize a proximate linkage, such as the hydrophilic plants that harbour the snail and take appropriate action – like central Yemeni shepherds' removal of such plants or Tzotzil Maya's muzzling and bucket-watering of their sheep so as to prevent contact with the plants (and thus the snail host). With or without a conscious understanding of the biological mechanisms involved, stockraisers around the world have long practised mixed and alternate grazing. Especially when unrelated species are mixed (e.g. ruminants with non-ruminants), this is an effective way to control many gastrointestinal helminths. In parts of Russia, for instance, floodplain pastures are shared by ruminants and geese; Kirghiz herders graze sheep and horses together; and Africans mix cattle, sheep, goats and camels together or, on the eastern steppes, domestic ruminants and wildlife like zebra. Meanwhile, many folk remedies have been demonstrated to alleviate the symptoms, if not always the causes, of parasitic diseases. In sum, from a scientific viewpoint, some traditional practices have great value for control of parasitic disease, some have complementary value, others may have limited or no value and some may even be harmful. Nevertheless, a consensus is emerging about the useful application of all but this last category, at least under specific conditions. Significantly, at its 1996 convention, the American Veterinary Medical Association recognized botanical, nutraceutical, chiropractic, physical therapy, massage, acupuncture and related 'acu' techniques and holistic medicine as 'modalities . . . to be offered in the context of a valid veterinarian/client/patient relationship' (p. 178). Today, schools of veterinary medicine in places as far-flung as China, Ethiopia, India, Mexico, Eastern Europe and the USA offer training in traditional, alternative and complementary animal healthcare. Acceptance of non-conventional medical practices has been facilitated by advances in scientific understandings of population medicine and the benefits of integrated disease management. More sophisticated epidemiological and physiologial knowledge has also elucidated traditional practices previously dismissed as irrational. Outside the veterinary profession, however, there is disagreement about the need to validate such practices. Efforts in this regard are sometimes blurred by debates over intellectual property rights. And insofar as traditional disease-control methods form part of a 'package' of management and other [even spiritual] interventions or are highly site-specific, their validation and subsequent transfer to other contexts is problematic. In the Middle East, for instance, the tradition of grazing native Awassi sheep on pastures with good stands of *Artemisia* spp. seems to produce a natural anthelmintic effect. But it is unclear whether this effect could be duplicated by introducing *Artemisia* to the heavily fertilized and degraded pastures and the different sheep breeds of, say, the Netherlands. The trick perhaps is to transfer the principles of traditional methods, modified according to the target agroecological and socioeconomic system and blended as-needed with conventional epidemiological or veterinary interventions.

Schillhorn van Veen, Tjaart W. 1997b. Untitled contribution. *FAO Electronic Conference on Principles for Rational Delivery of Public and Private Veterinary Services, January–March 1997.* 2 pp.

In his response to the above-cited conference, the author comments on the need for greater access to animal health products on the part of veterinarians and farmers in remote rural areas. In some areas, traditional medicines and practices are also difficult to obtain. Moreover, they may be discouraged or forbidden by veterinary officials, even in the absence of any orthodox solutions.

Schillhorn van Veen, Tjaart W. 1998. One medicine: The dynamic relationship between animal and human medicine in history and at present. *Agriculture and Human Values* 15(2): 115–120.

Drawing upon both historical and up-to-the-minute examples, this journal article explores the dynamic interface between human and animal medicine. In many traditional agrarian and pastoral societies, human and livestock healthcare techniques and practitioners evolved side by side – often with veterinary observations informing human medical knowledge and practice – and were substantially one and the same. As Western biomedical science came to the fore after the Renaissance, this 'one medicine' began to differentiate into two, although they continued to be intertwined. For example, in European veterinary schools, the earliest teachers were often physicians with rural experience and thus some knowledge of animal as well as human diseases. Today, veterinary and human medicine seem to be re-converging, at least in the domains of pathophysiology and epidemiology. There, via more sophisticated biomedical concepts and tools, each informs the other to the benefit of both people and livestock. For example, the one-medicine concept is exploited in the study of zoonosis and zoo-prophylaxis, comparable human and animal diseases (e.g. AIDS in humans and monkeys), animal models for human diseases and the human–animal bond (as in the mutual benefits of pet-keeping). At the same time, both medicines are increasingly harking back to their early roots in herbal and other treatment traditions in a search for 'new' healthcare ideas and approaches in response to people's growing dissatisfaction with current clinical care for themselves and their animals. Indeed, a return to a revised 'one medicine' would yield greater benefits for all species via a more pluralistic approach to healthcare.

Schinkel, Hans-Georg. 1970. *Haltung, Zucht und Pflege des Viehs bei den Nomaden Ost- und Nordostafrikas: Ein Beitrag zur traditionellen Ökonomie der Wanderhirten in semiariden Gebieten.* Veröffentlichungen des Museums für Völkerkunde zu Leipzig, Heft 21. Akademie-Verlag, Berlin, Germany.

This monograph on livestock breeding and management among pastoralists of east and northeast Africa is based on an extensive review of the literature. The author describes four ways that pastoralists provide their animals with salt. In breeding, selection is restricted to male animals. Somali herders fit their rams with leather aprons to prevent uncontrolled mating; the Maasai do likewise with sheep and cattle. For the same reason, Baggara tie up the penises of their rams. Pastoralists have developed several methods to stimulate the milk flow in mothers whose offspring have died (p. 250). Chapter 6 deals with treatment and prevention of livestock diseases. The author summarizes pastoralists' measures in these regards as: fleeing and avoiding areas where epidemics occur; preventing disease through indigenous vaccination and other means; cauterization; applying herbal remedies and other treatments to wounds; removing external parasites; magic; drenching with infusions; feeding herbal tonics; lighting smudge fires; and bleeding. Schinkel illustrates each measure with numerous examples from the literature.

Schoen, Allen M. 1994. *Veterinary Acupuncture: Ancient Art to Modern Medicine.* American Veterinary Publications, Goleta, California. 699 pp.

This volume introduces veterinarians to a vast storehouse of information on the current status of veterinary acupuncture, based on research from the Western world as well as from China. Wherever possible the scientific basis of acupuncture is discussed, in addition to traditional Chinese medical theories. Chapter titles include: efficacy of acupuncture, history and concepts, anatomy and classification of acupoints, neurophysiologic basis of acupuncture, oriental concepts, techniques and instrumentation, acupuncture in small animals, acupuncture in large animals, failures in veterinary acupuncture, veterinary chiropractic care and Chinese herbology in veterinary medicine.

Schram, Louis M.J. 1954. *The Monguors of the Kansu-Tibetan Frontier: Their Origin, History and Social Organization.* American Philosophical Society, Philadelphia, Pennsylvania, USA.

The Monguors geld their horses by cutting the scrotum with the sharp edge of a freshly broken cup. They treat the wound with wine and salt and then suture it with thread from a woman's needle box. After the operation, the horse is prevented from lying down for several days (p. 112b).

Schwabe, Calvin W. 1978. *Cattle, Priests and Progress in Medicine.* The Wesley W. Spink Lectures on Comparative Medicine Vol. 4. University of Minnesota Press, Minneapolis, Minnesota, USA. 274 pp.

Among many other topics, this text describes healers of both people and cattle among northeast African pastoralists and their medical knowledge (pp. 40–49). Besides using magic to treat diseases they don't understand, the Nuer, Maasai and other cattle-herders have developed medical skills such as surgery, bonesetting, bleeding, cauterization, castration and obstetrical procedures. Pastoralists know of many ethnoveterinary drugs and their languages contain rich vocabularies for pathological changes in cattle. Herders are familiar with the idea of contagion and try to avoid the impact of infectious diseases through management practices such as keeping some of their cattle in another person's pasture; thus some animals will probably survive an epidemic. Maasai vaccinate their cattle against CBPP. [According to the author, a new 1984 edition of this volume is available].

Schwabe, Calvin W. 1980. Animal disease control. Part II. Newer methods, with possibility for their application in the Sudan. *Sudan Journal of Veterinary Science and Animal Husbandry* 21(2): 55–65.

Dinka pastoralists of southern Sudan enjoy the services of a certain type of traditional healer of both humans and livestock: the medical *atet*. The author suggests that these specialists could be enlisted in the aid of more comprehensive and cost-effective disease surveillance and other veterinary programmes. In the past, veterinarians and other development workers have tended 'to dismiss traditional healers . . . as magicians and witch doctors and to regard all of them as liabilities rather than potential assets' (p. 62). But this view is 'completely unjustified' in the case of *atet*, who are knowledgeable in anatomy, physiology, disease pathology/diagnosis and wound and abscess surgery, bonesetting and obstetrics [see Schwabe 1996 and Schwabe and Kuojok 1981]. This prestigious and widely consulted cadre of healers could become what the author terms 'accredited *atet*' via some basic education in the form of healthcare demonstrations in their own language. Training could usefully include, e.g. concepts of asepsis, use of basic Western drugs and diagnostic skills, the latter so as to enable *atet* to report diseases appearing in the cattle camps promptly. In addition, they could be trained to collect blood, stool and other specimens, prepare blood films and so forth. 'Such a . . . "grassroots" basis for a disease intelligence network . . . could not only increase immensely the potential for useful work by . . . existing . . . veterinary personnel but could provide an extent and quality of information-for-action about diseases unmatched elsewhere in the "developing world"' (p. 63). The author sees little likelihood of competition and jealousy between accredited *atet* and government vets or veterinary assistants because the former would not be educated outside his local language and cattle-camp environment; he would merely continue to occupy his already demonstrably useful community niche, but fulfilling it more effectively. Indeed, the author believes that *atet* acting as 'shoeleather epidemiologists' would make for a better and more fully and professionally utilized official veterinary service with higher morale.

Schwabe, C.W. 1981. Animal diseases and primary health care: Intersectoral challenges. *WHO Chronicle* 35: 227–232.

This article makes the point that, especially (but not exclusively) where medical practitioners for livestock and humans are traditionally one and the same, it seems only sensible to coordinate across health sectors as many aspects as possible of health-worker training, medical infrastructure, service delivery and national epidemiological intelligence systems.

Schwabe, Calvin W. 1984. A unique surgical operation on the horns of African bulls in ancient and modern times. ***Agricultural History*** 58(2): 138–156.

Medical knowledge in ancient Egypt appears to have evolved along rational rather than purely magical lines because of linkages among agricultural, religious and medical practices. Cattle played an important role in the life and religion of the early Egyptians and priests became involved in cattle husbandry and healing. Knowledge of human medicine may have derived in large part from comparisons with animals. With this hypothesis in mind, the author investigates the meaning of a surgical horn operation for the culture of contemporary Dinka in southern Sudan and presents evidence that this operation has been performed for at least 4500 years.

Schwabe, Calvin. 1987a. ***Traditional Veterinary Medicine of the Nilotic Dinka and Ancient Egyptians Compared.*** Working Paper No. 40. Agricultural History Center, University of California, Davis, California, USA. 21 pp.

This paper compares some practices and beliefs of the *atet* – Dinka healers in southern Sudan who perform wound and abscess surgery, bonesetting, horn surgery, castration and obstetrical procedures – with those of ancient Egyptian priests. As evident from ancient Egyptian illustrations, a unique form of horn surgery in selected bulls carried out by present-day *atet* was also performed in the Nile Valley at least 4500 years ago. Both *atet* and Egyptian priests acquire(d) anatomical knowledge from dissecting sacrificial animals. Other similarities exist in their physiological theories concerning animating forces and the source of semen. Findings suggest that Egyptian healers did not separate human from veterinary medical practice; neither do contemporary *atet*.

Schwabe, Calvin W. 1987b. Traditional veterinary medicine of the Nilotic Dinka and the ancient Egyptians compared. ***Abstracts from the 23rd World Veterinary Congress, 16–21st August 1987, Montreal, Canada.*** P. 372.

Several practices of modern-day Dinka animal healers or *atet* resemble those of ancient Egyptians. One is a complex cosmetic operation on cattle whereby one horn is surgically trained upwards and backwards and the other downwards and forwards. Other parallels are found in Dinka and Egyptian ethnomedical beliefs – probably based on their empirical observations during the slaughtering and butchering of animals – that semen originates in the spine and that fresh muscle contains the animating principle of life.

Schwabe, Calvin. 1996. Ancient and modern veterinary beliefs, practices and practitioners among Nile Valley peoples. In: Constance M. McCorkle, Evelyn Mathias and Tjaart W. Schillhorn van Veen (eds). ***Ethnoveterinary Research & Development.*** Intermediate Technology Publications, London, UK. Pp. 37–45.

In delivering healthcare services of any sort, most poor countries confront a basic quandary. Money for costly conventional interventions such as mass vaccinations is scarce, but so is money for the disease intelligence that would permit more tightly targeted interventions. In the absence of such intelligence, strategies such as mass vaccination are tremendously expensive because they must reach and inoculate all animals and humans, many of whom may not actually be at risk. A possible solution is to link up certain sorts of traditional healers in stockraising societies with official veterinary/medical services so as to enhance primary health-care delivery and disease surveillance. This chapter describes several types of such healers among the Dinka of the upper Nile, along with some of the healers' often-very-sophisticated veterinary/medical acumen and skills, as in surgery and obstetrics. Ethno-physiological theories, ethnoanatomy, disease beliefs and taxonomies, and the origins of some of the foregoing in bull sacrifices are also discussed, along with parallels in Maasai veterinary medicine. Traditional veterinary/medical beliefs, practices and practitioners among these Nilotic peoples are compared with ancient Egyptian antecedents to illustrate their durability across millennia, which in turn suggests their possible empirical validity.

Schwabe, Calvin W. 1998. Integrated delivery of primary health care for humans and animals. *Agriculture and Human Values* 15(2): 121–125.

Illustrating from the case of a pilot children–cattle immunization scheme in southern Sudan, this article emphasizes the cost-effectiveness and other benefits of piggy-backing human healthcare onto veterinary services, especially for remote, poor or nomadic peoples.

Schwabe, Calvin W. and Isaac Makuet Kuojok. 1981. Practices and beliefs of the traditional Dinka healer in relation to provision of modern medical and veterinary services for the southern Sudan. *Human Organization* 40(3): 231–238.

For communication and cooperation between indigenous healers and Western practitioners to be possible, the beliefs and techniques of the former must be well understood by the latter. The authors used field interviews and observations to collect information on ethnoveterinary and ethnomedical knowledge and practices of the Agar Dinka in southern Sudan. There are four more-or-less distinct classes of Dinka healers, each of which practises on both people and animals. This article mainly deals with the *atet*, who have many practical skills such as wound and abscess surgery, bonesetting, obstetrics and castration, all of which are described in detail. The Dinka control considerable anatomical knowledge as a result of dissecting cattle and goats. Their knowledge of human anatomy entirely derives from comparison with animals'. Their physiological knowledge, too, seems to be based on examination of dissected animals. The *atet* and some cattle owners recognize several infectious diseases, including anthrax, CBPP, rinderpest, foot-and-mouth disease, tuberculosis and fasciolosis. Many of their observations on these diseases are at least partially correct scientifically, although the reasoning behind the Dinka idea of contagion may differ from that of Western science. Because of their skills and knowledge, *atet* could undergo specialized training and be integrated into healthcare delivery systems for livestock and also for people. *Atet* could also serve as an epidemiological intelligence network to assist government livestock services.

Schwartz, Cheryl. 1998. Chinese herbal medicine in small animal practice. In: Allen M. Schoen and Susan G. Wynn (eds). *Complementary and Alternative Veterinary Medicine: Principles and Practice*. Mosby, Inc., St Louis, Missouri, USA. Pp. 437–449.

Based on the author's 14 years of clinical experience in the USA, this chapter gives examples of the successful application of some 15 common Chinese herbal formulae to digestive, musculoskeletal and renal disorders in small animals. Also discussed are the general theory, treatment principles, herb classifications, formulae, dosages and time of administration involved in traditional Chinese herbal medicine (TCM). Although TCM can be used according to Western diagnoses, in the author's opinion it is most effective when deployed according to its own canons because these allow formulae to be specifically designed for the individual patient. Nevertheless, TCM can profitably complement Western veterinary treatments. Herbs are particularly helpful for chronic conditions requiring long-term therapy, because they can be given for more extended periods than Western drugs before producing deleterious effects and they work to restore and improve organ function. Herbs are also helpful for vague, unrecognizable ills such as digestive disturbances, for which Western diagnostic tests may be inconclusive. Further, they provide an alternative for animals that are sensitive or allergic to standard Western drugs. The author briefly discusses several Western controversies surrounding TCM. One is the lack of scientific studies and, relatedly, of quality controls on herbals. However, these *materia medica* have been used and evaluated for at least a thousand years on huge numbers of patients in what essentially constitutes an early form of meta-analysis, in which a large number of cross-sectional studies are interpreted for their general principles and conclusions. And at least in China, there are strict controls on the manufacture and use of patent herbs. A corollary issue is that Western practitioners look for specific amounts of active constituent in a herb, whereas herbologists believe it is the whole plant or mineral that gives treatment quality by acting synergistically on a greater range of health conditions. Indeed, disease and its treatment are perceived in an entirely different and much more holistic, way in TCM. For one thing, TCM encompasses multiple cause and effect variables, whereas Western medicine tends to recognize and treat only single cause-effect relations. For another, TCM endeavours to treat imbalances *before* they manifest clinically as full-blown diseases. These concepts are sometimes difficult for Western practitioners to accept.

Schwartz, Horst J. 1990. Produktionsleistung und Produktivität von Dromedaren. In: Horst S.H. Seifert, Paul L.G. Vlek and H.-J. Weidelt (eds). ***Tierhaltung im Sahel. Symposium 26–27 Oktober 1989.*** Göttinger Beiträge zur Land-und Forstwirtschaft in den Tropen und Subtropen, Heft 51. Forschungs- und Studienzentrum der Agrar- und Forstwissenschaften der Tropen und Subtropen, Georg-August-Universität Göttingen, Germany. Pp. 171–186.

This paper reviews the distribution, performance, breeds, reproduction, calf mortality, feeding and nutrition, and diseases of the dromedary camel. It also discusses the results of two studies. The first compared the performance of three camel herds: two kept on commercial ranches for meat and transport; and one kept by nomadic pastoralists for milk production under traditional management, which splits she-camels into subherds according to whether they have male or female offspring. Based on indices for several production parameters, the ranch herds appeared to perform better; but they were partially subsidized by income from cattle and sheep fattening. If these subsidies were factored out, then returns to labour, capital and possibly per-head land use for nomadic herds would probably prove to be as high, or even higher, than for ranch herds. The second study compared performance indicators of dromedaries, cattle, goats and sheep kept under traditional versus improved management systems. In the former system, goats performed best, followed in rank order by dromedaries, sheep and cattle; in the latter, the order was goats, sheep, cattle and lastly dromedaries. Although production values for all species increased under improved management, the magnitude of the increases differed greatly: cattle improved their performance by 93%, sheep by 77%, goats by 35% and the dromedary by only 13%. These results suggest that dromedaries are already so well-adapted to their arid ecological niche that management improvements can enhance this species' production performance only slightly.

Schwartz, H.J. and M. Dioli. 1992. *The One-Humped Camel* (C. dromedarius) *in Eastern Africa: A Pictorial Guide to Diseases, Health Care and Management.* Verlag Josef Margraf Scientific Books, Weikersheim, Germany. 282 pp.

This volume describes and provides a number of colour photos of ethnoveterinary treatments (pp. 110–132) and traditional management practices (pp. 111–142) in eastern Africa. There, camel castration is routinely performed by making two longitudinal incisions in the scrotum, pulling out the testes and then slicing them off with straight cuts. Other livestock, however, are castrated using a bloodless method that entails crushing the spermatic cord between two sticks. Camel disorders are treated with oral and topical herbal preparations (e.g. ointments and rinses). Branding, which enhances localized blood flow, is used in treating wounds, abscesses and fractures. Suckling is controlled by tying soft bark to dams' teats or covering the udder with a basket. A basket may also be affixed over the anus of a she-camel that refuses to accept her own or a foster calf. The basket blocks defaecation until it is removed, at which time the explosive expulsion of faeces simulates pre-parturition pains, making the female more receptive to a calf that may or may not be her own [also see Bernus 1981].

Scoones, Ian. 1994. Browse ranking in Zimbabwe. In: Kate Kirsopp-Reed and Fiona Hinchliffe (eds). *RRA Notes Number 20: Special Issue on Livestock.* IIED, London, UK. Pp. 91–94.

A group of male farmer-stockraisers in Zimbabwe ranked 120 local tree and browse species according to their value for cattle, goats and donkeys. The 32 species rated as the most highly favoured for cattle were then compared with researcher recommendations according to such factors as crude protein content, digestibility, etc. A follow-on ranking of selected browse species for cattle probed the criteria behind farmers' ratings. Some of the criteria that emerged were early shooting of leaves, good taste/saltiness, high water content and palatability of dry leaves. Overall, results revealed that stockowners' rankings tally closely with quality assessments based on chemical analysis, as other such studies have likewise found (e.g. Bayer 1990). Taken together, such findings suggest that farmer rankings can be a reliable yet cost-effective alternative to massive laboratory screenings as a way of informing fodder improvement programmes. For the successful conduct of such rankings, however, the author offers an insightful set of guidelines, as follows. Do not confound preference with availability. Differentiate among livestock species and between plant parts. Take note of seasonal plant phenology and of the fact that drought years are often different. And investigate with different informants.

SEARCA. 1989. Rural folk use medicinal herbs in curing sick animals. *The SEARCA Diary* 18(4): 6–7, 10.

A survey of Filipino farmers found they use 116 different plant species belonging to 50 botanical families in animal healthcare. These plants treat 56 health problems such as: respiratory infections, diarrhoea, fever, skin diseases, eye infections, wounds, parasites, decreased lactation, loss of appetite and weight, sprains and muscular fatigue. Plants are used singly or in polyprescriptions. The treatments are administered in the feed or water, as a drench, bath, wound irrigation or poultice. Examples of the plants include: banana, betel, cashew, coconut, garlic, ginger, guava, onion, pepper and sweet potato.

Sebastian, Matthew K. 1984. Plants used as veterinary medicines, galactagogues and fodder in the forest areas of Rajasthan. *Journal of Economic and Taxonomic Botany* 5(4): 785–788.

This article reviews further plants [also see Sebastian and Shandari 1984] used by forest people of Rajasthan, India to promote livestock health, productivity, nutrition and safety. The leaves of *Abrus precatorius* L. and *Calotropis procera* are burnt together and the ash given to post-partum does to cleanse their stomachs. *Pedalium murex* L. leaves thicken milk that has been diluted with water. Leaves of *Nyctanthus arbor-tristis* L. placed under goats' tongues at night silence the animals, making them harder for thieves to locate.

Sebastian, M.K. and M.M. Shandari. 1984. Some plants used as veterinary medicines by Bhils. *International Journal of Tropical Agriculture* 2(4): 307–310.

An ethnobotanical survey among Bhils of Rajasthan, India recorded 16 plants of local veterinary importance. To take several examples, *Abelmoschus moschatus* is used as a tonic for cattle and buffalo that stop ruminating. *Dichrostachys cinerea* L. is administered for colic, followed by *Tinospora cordifolia*. The Bhil ethnoveterinary pharmacopoeia also includes items such as eggs, which are given to animals with broken bones, and jaggery, which serves as an antidote for poisoning.

Sedoeka, Masaga Shushuda. n.d. Veterinary practice in Barbaig [sic] Area, Hanang District, Arusha, Tanzania. Unpublished manuscript. Livestock Field Office, Katesh, Arusha, Tanzania. 4 pp.

Among Barabaig pastoralists of Tanzania, traditional botanical treatments were identified for the following ten livestock diseases: anthrax, cancer, ECF, helminthosis, mange, meningitis, pneumonia, retained placenta, salmonellosis and trypanosomosis. However, only the local names of the plants were noted. Plant parts used included leaves, pods, roots, bark, milk from shoots and fruit. Stored human urine was also employed as a wash for mange and fleas.

Seguin, Jean. 1980 [1941]. *L'Art de Soigner Gens et Bêtes en Basse-Normandie.* Guénégaud, Paris, France. Pp. 91–101.

Treatments for some 17 livestock ailments are described in this book chapter for pre-WWII from Normandy, France. For colic in horses, 'pseudo-veterinarians' [farmers] recommend giving water to the animal to drink in which a shirt soiled with menstrual blood has been soaked. For bloody diarrhoea, *médécins de bêtes* or 'animal doctors' smear pepper under the tail. FMD is treated using oil, vinegar, or pepper to disinfect the mouth; preventive measures are also taken, such as isolating infected animals and running stock through antiseptic footbaths. Some farmers treat haemoglobinurea (bloody urine) with oral auto-vaccination, by giving the ailing animal the bloody urine it has just expelled. For a pig suffering from 'bad blood', the strategy is to draw the disease to a single part of the anatomy (say, the ear) by sewing a piece of *Helleborus foetidus* root to that part.

Seifert, S.H. 1990. Humanhygienische und wirtschaftliche Bedeutung der Brucellose in der Tierhaltung des Sahel. In: Horst S.H. Seifert, Paul L.G. Vlek and H.-J. Weidelt (eds). *Tierhaltung im Sahel. Symposium 26–27 Oktober 1989.* Göttinger Beiträge zur Land-und Forstwirschaft in den Tropen und Subtropen, Heft 51. Forschungs- und Studienzentrum der Agrar- und Forstwissenschaften der Tropen und Subtropen, Georg-August-Universität Göttingen, Germany. Pp. 187–200.

This paper discusses the aetiology and epidemiology of brucellosis and its hygienic and economic consequences for animal production in the Sahel. There, nomads are aware that this disease causes livestock abortions. They therefore maintain a minimum herd size and they especially keep many cows in order to ensure herd survival and sufficient milk production. While most Sahelian pastoralists boil milk and milk products before consuming them, nomads of Sudan do not. Consequently, the incidence of human brucellosis among these Sudanese groups is higher, paralleling that found in their herds.

Sejuro Nanetti, Olivia. 1988. *Plantas Medicinales Utilizadas por los Curanderos de Nasca: Registro Gráfico Botánico.* Boletín de Investigaciones en Tecnologías Nativas No. 5. Gráficos de Editorial e Imprenta DESA for CONCYTEC (Consejo Nacional de Ciencia y Tecnología), Lima, Perú. 59 pp.

A compilation of interviews with native healers of Peru's Nazca Valley, this slim volume seeks to document fast-disappearing knowledge of ethnopharmacology in the region, along with complete details of its application in medical, social and ceremonial terms. Only one interview mentions an ethnoveterinary treatment (p. 41). A complex cure for injuries, it involves a church-like ritual in miniature plus some 13 ingredients, including a human skull, lamp oil, salt, a fetish bundle of red ribbons, as well as numerous plants. The author's concluding recommendations are equally valid for veterinary, as well as human, ethnomedicine: that traditional medicine be recognized and made available as a useful alternative to Western medicine, especially in rural areas; that a seed bank of medicinal plants be established; and that pharmacies sell traditional as well as modern pharmaceuticals.

Serres, H. 1969. L'engraissement des zébus dans la région de Tananarive selon la technique du 'boeuf de fosse'. *Revue d'Élevage et Médecine Vétérinaire dans les Pays Tropicaux* 22(4): 529–539.

In the town of Tananarive, Madagascar, there is a demand for fatty and even very fat beef, unlike much of the rest of Africa. To meet this demand, men in the rice-growing villages near the town make cheap purchases of old (up to 12 years), thin, but large-bodied cattle – preferably from the south of the island – at the dry season's end (October) and then place them in a pit, where they are fattened for sale to Tananarive slaughterhouses. The selection of such aged animals from the south favours fattening in at least two ways: their phosphoro-calcium needs have already largely been met; and as proven survivors of the extra-long dry season in the south, they are apt to put on weight quickly. When first bought, the animals are put to work threshing the local rice harvest. This task slims and fatigues them further, making them hungrier and more apt to accept confinement. The pit is dug on the side of a hill so as to facilitate the animal's ingress and, just before slaughter, egress; and it is furnished with a stone manger constructed in such a way that feed cannot fall or be tossed out. Pits are roughly rectangular constructions averaging about 20 m². They are oriented to the trade winds in such a way as to protect the animal from rainfall but also to rinse out its bedding. A maximum of two animals may be quartered in a pit, but they are physically separated within it so that neither can appropriate feed from the other. For the first month (November), the cattle are fed rice straw mixed with gathered green plants, mainly *Cynodon dactylon*, *Digitaria horizontalis* and *Setaria pallidefusca*. Once accustomed to this intensive feeding, the animals receive only the green fodder, at a rate of 60 kg per day, throughout January, February and March. If an animal fails to eat all its ration regularly, it is removed from the pit and re-sold. After early rice and groundnut harvesting begins in February–March, the 'pit beef' also receive re-sprouted rice plants and groundnut tops. Sweet potato leaves and vines are added to the rations in April and, especially in May–July, cassava leaves and tubers. By July's end, all forage has been exhausted and, happily, the cattle have reached their maximum weight of 380 to 430 kg for 'fat' animals and 430 to 480 kg for 'very fat' ones, with some weighing as much as 500 kg. Their meat is well marbled and fetches a premium consumer price. Fatteners may as much as double their original cash investment in the purchase price of an animal. They also reap an excellent manure for use on the sweet potato plots. However, it should be noted that such fattening operations require on average 2 hours' work daily, which is done by the man who owns the animal(s). Also required is a certain minimum hectarage of ricelands. But this traditional 'pit beef' system is a classic example of astute crop/livestock integration. It also demonstrates a keen local appreciation of animal nutrition.

Servai, T.M. 1997. Stemming erosion of knowledge: Who will follow in the steps of Thiru Mutthu Servai? *Honey Bee* 8(4): 9.

Thiru Mutthu Servai is a 90-year-old farmer renowned for his ethnoveterinary skills, although 'nobody from the younger generation is willing to learn his store of knowledge'. Thus this short article documents two of his remedies before they become completely lost. He treats hypothermic or shivering cattle by covering them with a gunny/grain sack soaked in fermented rice water and then warmed over a rice-husk fire; he then pours *Clerodendrum phlomidis* extract over the sack. He treats fractures with a combination of internal and external measures: the patient is fed a mixture of crushed *Acorus calamus*, *Helicteres isora*, 6 peppers, a few *Foeniculum vulgare* seeds, three handfuls of *vatha madakki* (?), a pinch of *kasturi* [castor?] and some water; then the fractured bone is covered with ground *C. phlomidis* leaves and bandaged over after splinting with bamboo sticks.

Shanklin, Eugenia. 1985. *Donegal's Changing Traditions: An Ethnographic Study.* Gordon and Breach Science, New York, New York, USA. *Ca.* 229 pp.

Appendix C of this ethnography deals with animal husbandry and health in north-west Ireland. There, cattle are wintered in byres and fed on hay. If a bovine becomes sick, farmers will call a veterinarian. In contrast, sheep are pastured virtually year-round and seldom receive supplementary feed. The author describes common nutritional deficiencies and infections in both species and farmers' response to these problems. Sheep farmers rarely consult a veterinarian, while cattle owners do so whenever they cannot immediately identify and solve a problem. Sheep are bred for 'hardiness' i.e. the ability to survive on poor pasture and in adverse weather. Disease resistance is an important, but secondary, selection criterion.

Shanklin, Eugenia. 1996. Care of cattle versus sheep in Ireland: South-west Donegal in the early 1970s. In: Constance M. McCorkle, Evelyn Mathias and Tjaart W. Schillhorn van Veen (eds). *Ethnoveterinary Research & Development.* Intermediate Technology Publications, London, UK. Pp. 179–192.

Whether they are English-Protestant or Gaelic-Catholic, farmers of the harsh far-north County Donegal in Ireland operate a dual livestock production system: one a highly controlled and intensive regime of cattle raising, the other an extensive, rangestock system of sheepraising. These Irish farmers draw many distinctions between, and hold very different attitudes towards, the two species. The result is that calf and lamb mortality rates in Donegal were, respectively, the lowest and nearly the highest in all of Ireland. Based on 14 months' anthropological field research with a sample of 30 Donegal farmers during 1970–1971, this chapter seeks to explain these differences. Cattle were generally kept year-round near the house and byre, where they received mineral blocks, hay and commercial meals or concentrates; in addition, they were grazed in lush, lowland paddocks. In contrast, sheep receive no feed supplements; and they are left unattended for most of the year on rough, unfenced mountain pastures, where a number may starve or freeze to death, especially lambs. For both species, the major health problems are parasitism and infectious diseases; Donegal farmers also cited several supernaturally-linked ills. Fasciolosis is the paramount parasitic problem. Across the year, farmers regularly drenched cattle with a commercial flukicide, but drenchings for sheep were more irregular even though this species is exposed to greater fluke challenge. Concerning other endoparasitoses, Donegal farmers recognized the existence of roundworms in both species, but did not accept that these can cause significant economic losses. Few recognized lungworm infections and those who did thought that their flukicides controlled lungworm – when in fact, the only lungworm treatment available in Donegal at the time was an injection. All knew about gid, or ovine tapeworms; and this was the only sheep disease that all agreed should be referred to a veterinarian. The major ectoparasite was warble flies (*Hypoderma* spp.), which lay their eggs in cattle's hides, causing thousands of pounds of damage to hides each year and – unknown to many Donegal cattle – depressing milk and meat production. Strangely, however, few farmers treated against warbles. In cattle, calf scours (diarrhoea) was a common infectious disease that most people treated with home remedies. Although it can also occur in sheep, no one in the sample mentioned it, probably because there is less opportunity to observe the health problems of these unattended animals. Redwater (babesiosis or piroplasmosis) was another, much-feared but little understood disease of cattle. For sheep, braxy (malignant oedema) was the most common infectious disease. A virulent *Clostridium* that kills sheep almost overnight, braxy is sometimes linked with predisposing injuries such as wounds from fighting among rams or lacerations of the vulva from parturition. While Donegal farmers took great pains to avoid cattle injuries, which are linked to another species-specific clostridial disease (blackleg or blackquarter), they did not do so for sheep. However, all vaccinated against braxy, as there was no known cure. A minor but ancient ovine disease was contagious conjunctivitis. Although Donegal farmers confessed their ignorance of its aetiology, they accurately diagnosed it by the characteristic white film over the eye. Some people were skilled at snipping out a piece of the film and then pulling away the rest with a needle and thread, a delicate but effective operation. Other home remedies were to put ground glass, household bleach, or acid in the eyes. Two tick-borne diseases were common among Donegal sheep: pains, or tick pyaemia; and louping ill, or ovine encephalomyelitis. Dipping was the only 'solution' to these ailments at the time, given that the only vaccine for louping ill was withdrawn from the market due to production and quality-control problems. Farmers were incensed by this move, because they greatly preferred vaccinations to dipping. They said vaccines are less fallible in that they come in ready-made doses whereas dips have to be 'mixed up'. Also, vaccines last longer, whereas dips must be repeatedly administered. They also complained that government had outlawed the best dips, such as those with DDT, and used sub-standard compounds in the county dipping pits. Contrarily, farmers mixed their dips weaker than was prescribed and often left the sheep in for shorter periods, for fear of side effects. Finally, farmers noted that evil eye can befall cattle, but not sheep. So they took precautions like identifying others' cattle as their own if a person believed to have the evil eye inquires after an owner's herd; and some Catholic farmers sprinkled holy water on newly acquired animals. Overall, much greater husbandry and healthcare attention clearly was extended to Donegal's more valuable cattle. Yet economics alone do not fully explain farmers' attitudes and behaviours. For example, people who treated cattle inhumanely were punished by law; but not so for sheep. And when at one point, the market price of cattle fell to nearly zero, veterinarians received no fewer calls to treat this species, whereas they were rarely called upon to treat sheep no matter what the market price. Finally, both archaeological and ideological evidence points to cattle as highly prestigious and semi-sacred animals for Donegal farmers. The result is a simple but shrewd and centuries-old model of stockraising in Donegal: maximize production from cattle and minimize losses in sheep. Put another way, sheep are deployed so as to take maximum advantage of annual agroecological opportunities with minimal risk to the stockraising enterprise as a whole. In some years, extra money will be made on the sheep; in others, they may fetch little or nothing. But in any event, with nothing much invested in them, nothing much will be lost. Meanwhile, there will always be cattle to provide the family with milk, meat and some longer-term economic security. Ideological considerations help protect against mishandling or squandering this long-term investment. Such findings have obvious implications for what new husbandry and healthcare techniques stock-raisers may, or may not, be willing to accept.

Shannon, David. 1996. Personal communication to M. Martin of 1997. 3 pp.

In Scotland, the Edinburgh Zoo has established a herb garden to grow *materia medica* for the zoo animals. An experienced veterinarian recommended 14 plants to be cultivated and applied as follows. Feeding rosehips (*Rosa rugosa*) provides B vitamins that promote healthy growth and maintenance of hooves, horns and hair. Rosehips are especially good for preventing cracked hooves in equines. Comfrey (*Symphytum officinale*) leaves serve as a soothing dressing for skin wounds. The powerful effects on the heart and circulatory system of extracts of foxglove (*Digitalis purpurea*) have been known for hundreds of years; they increase the force and at the same time slow the frequency of the heartbeat. Inhalations of the aromatic leaf-oil of eucalyptus are useful in treating bronchitis and other respiratory problems. Mint acts against spasms of the stomach wall and aids expulsion of intestinal gas; it is helpful for bloat in bovines and some forms of equine colics. Dandelion (*Taraxacum officinale*) extract increases bile production in the liver. An infusion of holly (*Ilex aquifolium*) leaves combats rheumatisms and helps keep muscles and skeletons strong. Cleavers or 'sticky willie' (*Galium aparine*) relieves bladder and kidney infections and urinary stones. Chloroform mixed with morphine derived from the poppy plant (*Papaver somniferum*) controls diarrhoea in canines, bovines and equines. Used with discretion, poppy also serves as a mild narcotic to ease pain. Coltsfoot (*Tussilago farfara*) is used in herbal cough mixtures. The marshmallow *Althaea* possesses soothing qualities and is useful for treating bowel inflammations.

Sharland, Roger. 1992. 'Barefoot vets' for sheep and goats. *Footsteps* 10(Mar): 2–3.

In the late 1970s and early 1980s, the ACROSS Project in Mundri District, southern Sudan, instituted a sort of paravet programme to combat one of the biggest animal health problems there: parasitism. ACROSS paid attention to local/traditional treatments as well as modern, commercial ones. For instance, besides chemical sprays and dips for ectoparasites, it recommended applications of sheanut butter or used engine oil. For controlling ticks, animals could be brushed with a mixture made from soaking 1 l of fresh pounded leaves of the fish-poison bean plant (*Tephrosia vogelii*) in 1 l of water. For endoparasites, if commercial drugs were unavailable or too expensive, the project suggested asking local healers how they treated worms in livestock and/or people. Some plants reported to ACROSS as being effective for controlling endoparasites of livestock were: a decoction of *Treculia africana* var. *africana* roots or of *Morinda morindoides* leaves and fruits; *Chenopodium ambrosioides* leaf juice; and young neem leaves, mixed in with the feed at regular intervals.

Sharma, Kumar and [no initials] Sridhar. 1987. Historical background and analysis of scientific content of ancient Indian literature on practices for the treatment of diseases in domestic animals. *Indian Journal of History of Science* 22(2): 158–163.

Traditional Indian veterinary prescriptions are cited in this article. One example is a drench for tympanitis made of the juice extracted from pounding together ginger, pepper, salt, asafoetida and a few shavings of the bark of the drumstick tree and then mixing in a little country liquor. Another example is the use of aloe as a purgative for equines. [Abstract based on Gupta et al.'s 1990 annotated bibliography.]

Sharma, L. 1993. Innovations from the hills of Bhutan. *Honey Bee* 4(2&3): 6.

In the hills of Bhutan, castration of livestock is performed with a hammer. Castration wounds are dressed with a turmeric-powder and mustard-oil mix as an antiseptic. To induce heat in sterile cows, powdered pigeon droppings are fed once monthly for 3 to 4 months. To enhance heat, stock are given salt during ovulation; once an animal has been inseminated, salt is restricted for about 3 weeks to prevent abortion. Worms in calves are diagnosed by the animals' foul-smelling breath. A dewormer of curds and buttermilk that has been kept overnight in a copper container and then diluted in water is said to expel the worms in the space of a day.

Sharma, L.D., H.S. Bahga and B.K. Soni. 1967. Anthelmintic screening of three indigenous medicinal plants against *Ascaridia galli* in poultry. *The Indian Veterinary Journal* 44: 665–668.

A clinical trial was carried out in India to test for anthelmintic activity in poultry of three plants generally believed to have vermicidal properties: *Cordia dichotoma, Terminalia chebula* and *Vernonia anthelmintica*. Alcoholic extracts of all three plants were trialled on 65 three week old chicks. The chicks were divided into five groups. Group 1 was the control, group 2 was given 150 mg of piperazine, and groups 3, 4 and 5 were given the three plant extracts respectively. *Terminalia chebula* and *V. anthelmintica* showed the best results *in vivo* as anthelmintics.

Sharma, P.K and V. Singh. 1989. Ethnobotanical studies in Northwest and Trans-Himalaya. V. Ethno-veterinary medicinal plants used in Jammu and Kashmir, India. *Journal of Ethnopharmacology* 27: 63–70.

An ethnoveterinary survey in India's Jammu and Kashmir States collected 18 plant-based recipes for livestock, all of them administered with buttermilk or bread. A prescription for diarrhoea in water buffalo and cattle is compounded of *Aesculus indica, Gentiana phyllocalyx, Rumex acetosa* and *Verbascum thapsus*. For tonsilitis, crushed *Gerbera gossypina* root is given after first scouring the patient's tongue with a comb. This root is also said to be a good health tonic.

Sharma, Satish Kumar. 1997. Nest strainers and tuber-indicators: Grassroots wisdom from Rajasthan. *Honey Bee* 8(4): 13.

To sieve their ghee and buttermilk, many Rajasthani villagers use the half-built, funnel-like nests of *Ploceus philippinus* birds. People seek out nests before the birds have lined them with mud or cattle dung. Before use, a nest is washed several times with clean water to remove any dirt.

Sharma, Satyavan. 1987. *Treatment of Helminth Diseases – Challenges and Achievements.* Communication No. 3816. Central Drug Research Institute, Lucknow, India. 100 pp.

This report reviews drugs available for helminthoses, including a few natural products. Arecoline, isolated from the seeds of the betelnut palm (*Areca catechu*), is an old anthelmintic possessing high activity against tapeworms in dogs, especially

Taenia solium and *Taenia saginata*. Pumpkin seeds, containing cucurbitine, are also active against *T. saginata*.

Sharma, Sureshwar N. 1967. Scope of extension education in veterinary science. *Punjab Veterinarian* 7: 30–32.

Extension work should take into account veterinary services, animal feeding, animal breeding, and animal management and hygiene. Above all, it should study and make use of existing practices through discussion with villagers as well as experts.

Shata, Mohammed M. 1976. A review of anthelmintic treatment in the northern states of Nigeria. *Student Veterinarian* 7: 27–32. Association of Veterinary Medical Students, Ahmadu Bello University, Zaria, Nigeria.

This review spans both traditional and modern methods of treating gastrointestinal parasites and flukes in livestock of northern Nigeria. Traditional anthelmintics primarily consist of herbal drugs and, more recently, oils, copper sulphate mixed with soda-arsenate and nicotine infusions. During the last 20 years stockowners have also adopted some commercial drugs. Many new anthelmintics are now on the market. Before recommending any of them for use in Nigeria, however, the author argues that the local spectrum of helminths and their epidemiology should be studied to determine which drugs are most suitable for and effective under Nigerian conditions.

Sheaffer, C. Edgar. 1998. Homeopathy in food animal practice. In: Allen M. Schoen and Susan G. Wynn (eds). *Complementary and Alternative Veterinary Medicine: Principles and Practice.* Mosby, Inc., St Louis, Missouri, USA. Pp. 515–519.

In contrast to much of conventional veterinary medicine and even crude drugs, homeopathic treatments for livestock are safe, economical, easy to store and implement, able to accommodate idiosyncratic ills and require no withdrawal period before consumption of treated animals' milk, meat, or eggs. This short chapter lists a number of common homeopathic treatments that are suitable for use with ruminants, horses and camelids of different ages and reproductive statuses. In addition to botanical *materia medica*, the use of 'nosodes' is discussed. Nosodes are homeopathic remedies prepared from usually-autogenous disease products such as body fluids and secretions, for example mastitic milk. Supportive therapies for homeopathic treatments generally involve supplementing and controlling patients' diets, adding electrolytes to their drinking water, maintaining ambient hygiene, and massaging. Some examples of health problems for which the chapter names treatments are: neonate birth shock and dystocia injuries; anaemia, colic, worms and diarrhoea; anoestrus, male infertility and other reproductive problems; retained placenta; mastitis; and a variety of metabolic disorders. The chapter concludes with a thumbnail overview of recent research on homeopathic treatments for farm animals.

Shirlaw, Leslie Hamilton. 1940. A short history of Ayurvedic veterinary literature. *Indian Journal of Veterinary Science* 10: 1–39.

A brief but concise history of Ayurvedic veterinary literature, this article touches on Ayurveda's mythological origins, the beginnings of veterinary medicine in India, Indian cattle doctors, early studies in veterinary anatomy and early veterinary authorities. Ancient treatments for horses, elephants and cattle are described. For example, for elephants' wounds, the animal is made to swallow butter to 'draw out the iron'. The sores are then fomented with swine's flesh. According to the literature, the *materia medica* of Ayurvedic veterinary and human medicine largely overlap. The most frequently used plants were: *Phyllanthus emblica, Terminalia balerica* and *T. chebula*; ginger, garlic, mustard, neem; long, round, red and black pepper; salt, sesame oil and betel. Animal excreta, urine, bones, burnt feathers, milk, ghee and honey were also employed.

Shirokorogoff, Sergiei M. 1924. *Social Organization of the Manchus: A Study of the Manchu Clan Organization.* Royal Asiatic Society, Shanghai, China.

Manchus widely practice artificial incubation of chicken eggs. In a tall pottery tube, layers of 30–40 eggs are alternated with layers of bran. The tube is placed on a heated divan or *nahan*, a common furnishing in Manchu houses, for 23–24 days until the chicks hatch (p. 134).

Sikana, Patrick, Peter Bazeley, Dadson Kariuki and Zeremariam Fre. 1992. The Kenya Livestock and Pastoral Programme: Some Observations and Recommendations. Unpublished in-house report. ITDG, Nairobi, Kenya. 71 pp.

This extensive external review of the KLPP fully endorses the programme's growing focus on EVK, especially in light of concerns about the cost-effectiveness of some of the relatively expensive Western therapies in which programme paravets are trained. The price of such treatments may be such that only richer stockraisers can afford paravet services. The report makes several observations and recommendations with regard to future ER&D on the KLPP which are of wider applicability. First, the authors feel that ethnoveterinary treatments should be critically evaluated in the same way as any modern veterinary techniques employed by paravets. Second, while local people's propensity to experiment with EVK should be encouraged where appropriate, possible negative effects of 'certain contingent coping strategies' should be examined. Third, the confusion between stockraisers' disease categories and those of clinical veterinary medicine needs to be clarified during paravet training. Fourth and finally, the authors note that the incorporation of traditional medicine into paravet programmes may help combat EVK's negative associations with backwardness and witchcraft in many people's minds.

Sikarwar, R.L.S. 1996. Ethno-veterinary herbal medicines in Morena District of Madhya Pradesh, India. In: S.K. Jain (ed.). *Ethnobiology in Human Welfare.* Deep Publications, New Delhi, India. Pp. 194–196.

In remote areas of India, no formal veterinary services are available. Farmers therefore depend mainly on local herbal medicines to treat their livestock. Based on first-hand interviews with farmers in one such area, this article enumerates and gives general prescriptions for 35 plant species belonging to 33 genera and 27 families that are employed to treat 15 types of health problems in cattle, buffalo, sheep, goats and horses. Problems span: wounds, cuts, abrasions and dislocated bones; anoestrus and poor lactation; worms, colics, constipation and diarrhoea; lice; conjunctivitis; bronchitis, anthrax and FMD. In addition to plant materials, ingredients such as whey, alum, liquor, coal powder and jaggery figure in various of the prescriptions.

Sikarwar, R.L.S. 1999. Less-known ethnoveterinary uses of plants in India. In: E. Mathias, D.V. Rangnekar and C.M. McCorkle, with M. Martin (eds). *Ethnoveterinary Medicine: Alternatives for Livestock Development – Proceedings of an International Conference Held in Pune, India, 4–6 November 1997. Volume 1: Selected Papers.* BAIF Development Research Foundation, Pune, India. Pp. 103–107.

Comparative studies on the ethnobotany of different regions within or between countries and continents can provide valuable insights into the uses and properties of plants plus the breadth and depth of indigenous knowledge. For the last 4 years, the Institute of Ethnobiology at India's National Botanical Research Institute has been conducting such a study on India and Latin America. Findings reveal that both regions make the same ethnomedicinal uses of a number of plants. Such discoveries lend credence to the medical-veterinary claims that local people make for these plants. Naturally, the study also found that, for some plants, their medical applications were little known and used or unknown in India as compared to Latin America and vice versa. Such information can be very useful, in that ethnobotanical knowledge from one region can be shared with other regions where the same plant species are found. This point is illustrated for the ethnoveterinary uses in Latin America of 17 such plants that, with some further analysis, could potentially be likewise exploited in India. An example is Latin Americans' use of an infusion of *Ceiba pentandra* bark to help post-parturient cows expel the placenta.

Sikarwar, R.L.S., A.K. Bajpai and R.M. Painulli. 1994. Plants used as veterinary medicines by aboriginals of Madhya Pradesh, India. *International Journal of Pharmacognosy* 32(3): 251–255.

This article lists 31 species of plants, under 28 genera and 26 families, that native forest-dwelling peoples in ten districts of the central Indian State of Madhya Pradesh use to treat ailments of their cattle, buffalo, sheep and goats. The health problems thus treated span coughs, wounds, swellings, diarrhoea, stomach pain, intestinal worms, lice, dislocated joints and bones, retained placenta, eye disorders, paralysis and hoof and skin diseases. Bread, buttermilk, whey, salt and jaggery also figure in the ethnopharmacopoeia.

Silver, Robert J. 1998. Ayurvedic veterinary medicine. In: Allen M. Schoen and Susan G. Wynn (eds). *Complementary and Alternative Veterinary Medicine: Principles and Practice.* Mosby, Inc., St Louis, Missouri, USA. Pp. 451–466.

Ayurveda (lit. 'the science of life') is the ancient holistic healing system of India. It involves the integration of herbal medicines with diet, massage, exercise, purification and (for humans) meditation in order to balance natural elements as they relate to patient constitution. This chapter summarizes the background, history and principles of Ayurvedic medicine and presents practical applications of Ayurvedic herbal therapies to animals. Historically, Ayurvedic thought served as the basis for traditional Chinese medicine. Ayurveda's Purusha and Prakruti correspond to the latter's Yin and Yang and to male and female energies. The medical goal is to keep this duality in balance by manipulating and/or applying the three prime attributes of Prakruti (the *tridosha* of wind, bile and phlegm) in relation to the five Ayurvedic elements (ether, fire, earth, air, water) as derived from these attributes and translated into ethereal, radiant, solid, gaseous and liquid matter, respectively. The five parts of plants parallel these elements, although herbs are also categorized according to seven tissue elements: plasma – leaf juice, blood – resin and sap, muscle – softwood, fat – gum and hard sap, bone – bark, marrow and nerve tissue – leaf, reproductive tissue – flowers and fruit. Plant parts are chosen for medicinal use according to their characteristics with respect to the *tridosha* and its three corresponding seasons of the year along with the five elements, plus classification according to taste (sweet, sour, salty, pungent, bitter, astringent) and temperature/moisture (hot/cold, wet/dry and all the permutations thereof). Clearly, Ayurveda theory is very complex. Likewise for Ayurvedic diagnostic techniques, which span pulse palpation, urine examination, visual observation of numerous body parts, interrogation (of human patients) and finally a six-step disease analysis. Treatment is divided into two categories. The first is prophylaxis, which involves diet, lifestyle, herbal medicines and regular purification exercises. The second is therapy, which is further divided into three types: purification, alleviation and a combination of the two. The author presents examples of the veterinary use of nine common Ayurvedic plant medicines, with information on the botany, pharmacology, actions, energetics, target organs, dosages and research publications for each. The plants are: *Withania somnifera, Boswellia serrata, Coleus forskohli, Commiphora mukul, Gymnema sylvestre, Phyllantus amarus, Picrorrhiza kurroa,* neem and turmeric. Also noted are three special Ayurvedic tonics, one of which is mineral-based.

Sindhu, S., B.K. Narainswami and K. Amitha. 1998. Role of women in ethnoveterinary medicine research, development, and promotion. In: E. Mathias, D.V. Rangnekar and C.M. McCorkle, with M. Martin (eds). *Ethnoveterinary Medicine: Alternatives for Livestock Development – Proceedings of an International Conference Held in Pune, India, 4–6 November 1997. Volume 2: Abstracts.* BAIF Development Research Foundation, Pune, India. P. 56.

In most of the rural developing world, livestock production is a family enterprise in which men, women and children all take part, yet all typically control different kinds of knowledge regarding the rearing and healthcare of livestock. In many societies, women have more practical such knowledge as they are the ones who actually take care of animals when men leave the farm or family, e.g. in search of jobs, for military service or trade and so forth. Yet women's EVK is seldom recognized or recorded and livestock development projects generally work only with men. An invisible barrier often blocks women's access to the benefits of such projects and to other kinds of development information and activities. A good example is paraveterinary projects worldwide, where trainees are overwhelmingly male – as are the majority of veterinary professionals and trainers. For instance, research by international working groups on science and technology have found that India ranks third in the world in terms of highly trained scientists and technicians; but only 28% of such professionals are female and the number of women in the veterinary field in India is negligible. Likewise for research, in which women stockraisers are seldom consulted about their EVK, their opinion of the relative efficacy of local and Western treatments and so forth. To be successful, however, any development programme must involve all relevant actors. This means that ethnoveterinary research, development and promotion must be based on a clear understanding of gender roles in stockraising. For instance, it is important to know about gendered decision-making roles regarding livestock management and about how women's knowledge and opinion may affect men's decisions and vice versa. To improve women's participation in ethnoveterinary medicine and meet the challenge of sustainable animal production, researchers and developers need to identify and understand women's role in ethnoveterinary medicine, design and disseminate ethnoveterinary technologies that are appropriate for female as well as male stockraisers, and select research and extension strategies that involve women in every aspect of ER&D.

Singh, Ajit and J.D. Kohli. 1956. A plea for research into indigenous drugs employed in veterinary practice. *The Indian Veterinary Journal* 32(4): 271–280.

This article briefly reviews Indian ethnoveterinary literature and then presents some 30 plants culled from this literature that the authors feel merit closer attention. Examples of such plants are *Cucumis pseudo-colocynthis*, given to horses as a purgative, and *Leea robusta*, administered to cattle with diarrhoea or dysentery.

Singh, M.P. 1987. Tribal medicinal plants used in animals [sic] diseases of Chhotanagpur. *The Indian Forester* 113(11): 758–759.

The preparation and use of 15 ethnoveterinary prescriptions collected from tribal medicinemen in Chhotanappur, India are described in this article. For draught bulls injured by the plough blade, *Annona squamosa* Linn. leaves are bandaged on the wound. Cattle with dysentery are given a decoction of *Atylosia scarabaeoides* Benth. seeds and aerial parts. Heated *Calotropis gigantea* R. Br. leaves are applied to the swollen legs of cattle. A paste of 2 to 3 *Cassia fistula* Linn. roots and black pepper mixed into *Artocarpus heterophyllus* leaf juice is applied to cattle's swollen throats. Myiasis is treated with *Crotalaria linifolia* L. pounded with common salt. The tuber juice of *Curculigo orchioides* Gaerin serves as drops for eye ailments. For fevers, *Cyanotis tuberosa* tubers pounded with common salt is given. An antiseptic for ulcers and wounds is made from pounded *Eclipta alba* Hassak roots in *Carthamus tinctorius* oil. For serious diarrhoea as well as throat swellings, a paste of *Entada pursaetha* Benth. seed cotyledon mixed with ashes of *Polyporus fungus* from *Shorea robusta* trees is applied. Animals that cease to masticate are fed a paste of *Euphorbia thymifolia* Linn. plants and *Scoparia duleis* leaves. Sprains are dressed with a thick decoction of *Erycibe paniculata* Roxb. leaves and stems and neck wounds with a paste of *Jatropha gossypifolia* Linn. The fibrous dry mesocarp *Luffa cylindrica* R. is used as a fumigant for cattle suffering from 'dyspersia' [sic].

Singh, N., Ramesh Kumari, R.S. Yadav, M.A. Akbar and B.P. Sengupta. 1994. Effect of some commonly used galactagogues on milk production and biogenic amines in buffaloes. *Pashudhan* Mar: 4–5.

To cope with milk-yield problems, veterinarians prescribe various drugs, hormones, chemical stimulants and minerals. But most of these treatments are expensive; and some have hazardous side effects. Thus the present study was undertaken to test several herbal galactagogues traditionally used in India and now marketed commercially. Although these herbals' positive effects on milk yield are well-known, they have never been formally evaluated. This study investigated their influence on feed intake and ruminal and circulatory biogenic amines, as well as on milk yields. One non-treatment control group and three experimental groups of four Murrah buffaloes each were established. The three galactagogues tested were: India Herbs' 'Galog', Vet Pharma's 'Hi-Milk' and Haryana Vet Health Product's 'Milkup'. These were fed daily for 20 days at evening milking times in the amount of 50 g, 50 g and 30 g, respectively. In brief, all treatment groups significantly increased milk yields compared to controls across the 90-day trial period. Also, these groups consumed significantly lower quantities of dry matter per kilogram of milk produced, indicating that the herbals make for better utilization of nutrients. Further, significantly higher levels of volatile fatty acids in the treatment groups indicated better energy supply for milk production. Protozoal populations, species and size were remarkably higher as well, signalling good ruminant health. Varied and complex, but beneficial, effects of the herbals on biogenic amines were also observed. Of the three galactagogues, Galog was the most effective overall.

Singh, Rakesh. 1992. Farmers' innovations in eastern Uttar Pradesh. *Honey Bee* 3(3&4): 12.

This short communication notes two indigenous livestock treatments among farmers of India's Uttar Pradesh state. Animals suffering from digestive orders or flatulence are fed pure, clarified butter oil (*ghee*) as a laxative. The hooves and mouths of stock with FMD are washed with an alum solution and the animals are made to walk in mud twice a day.

Singh, Sukhdov. 1987. Where the neem tastes sweet. *Folklore* 28(11): 259–265.

The neem tree has many uses in India, including ethnoveterinary ones. In the case of cowpox, keeping cattle under neem trees, putting neem extract in the drinking water and applying neem oil on the pox sores, all help animals recover from the disease. Neem is also used in a medico-religious ceremony as an FMD prophylaxy. Neem does in fact have antibiotic properties.

Slaybaugh-Mitchell, Tracy. 1995. *Indigenous Livestock Production: An Annotated Bibliography of Husbandry Practices.* Bibliographies in Technology and Social Change, No. 8. Technology and Social Change Program, Iowa State University, Ames, Iowa, USA. 87 pp.

This annotated bibliography deals with traditional animal husbandry practices worldwide, including animal breeding, feeding, healthcare, housing and harvesting of animal products (including drawing off blood for human consumption). General management is also discussed, including herding practices and range management.

A few animal health practice examples are given: hand removal of ticks by Fulani herders, annual bathing of sheep by Bedouin and Fellahin shepherds in Asia to clean the wool and avoid ectoparasitism, management strategies such as herd movement, selective grazing and watering.

Snow, W.F. 1996. Information sources and participatory appraisal for the assessment of African animal trypanosomiasis in the Gambia. In: Karl-Hans Zessin (ed.). *Livestock Production and Diseases in the Tropics: Livestock Production and Human Welfare. Proceedings of the VIII International Conference of Institutions of Tropical Veterinary Medicine held from the 25 to 29 September, 1995 in Berlin, Germany.* Volume I. Deutsche Stiftung für Internationale Entwicklung, Zentralstelle für Ernährung und Landwirtschaft, Feldafing, Germany. Pp. 308–314.

In assessing disease constraints to livestock production, many sources of complementary information can and should be tapped. One that is often overlooked, however, is affected stockraisers' own awareness and assessment of the diseases at issue. This conference paper reports on how PRA data from stockraisers significantly and cost-effectively complemented other sources in gauging the significance of trypanosomosis for agropastoralists in the Gambia. Cattle keepers there recognized and had local names for, both the disease and its tsetse-fly vector, although they did not always causally link the two. Also, via interviews, transects and mapping of grazing movements and site types (e.g. fields and fallows, woodlands and village, riverine sites, places swept by bush fires), stockraisers gave valuable information on varying patterns of cattle-tsetse contact by time of year and locale. Indeed, these PRA exercises revealed a 'remarkable similarity' (p. 313) between stockraisers' and scientific monitoring programmes' assessment of the seasonal prevalence of trypanosome infections and tsetse abundance. Thus, emic inputs can reduce the need for costly and time-consuming technical personpower and provide a shortcut to understanding epidemiological problems. However, the author cautions that, while rural people are often well-aware of animal health problems, environmental changes and their interrelationship, PRA participants may still require technical assistance in describing these factors and in then formulating appropriate village-level solutions.

Soegiharti, S., Jociswati and A. Sardjiman. 1968. *Ekstraksi dan Daya Anthelmintica Beserta Pengaruh* Cucurbita moschata *Duchesne Semen Terhadap Gastrointestinalis.* Final Report. Faculty of Pharmacology, Gadjahmada University, Yogjakarta, Indonesia. [pp. nos. unknown.]

Cucurbita moschata seeds have long been used in homemade Indonesian anthelmintics for ruminants. This study isolated cucurbitin, the active compound in the seeds. Then, cucurbitin's efficacy against *Fasciola* from buffalo and *Haemonchus* from goats was tested *in vitro* and compared to the anthelmintic efficacy of *C. moschata* emulsion. The isolated compound showed higher activity than the emulsion.

Solanki, Rehmatbhai PeerKhan. 1997. Indigenous veterinary surgeon. In: Anil Gupta (ed.). *International Conference on Creativity and Innovation at Grassroots for Sustainable Natural Resource Management, January 11–14, 1997: Abstracts.* Indian Institute of Management, Ahmedabad, India. P. 150.

Mr Solanki is a shepherd-healer from one Indian community, where he provides surgical as well as medical care to farm animals. He acquired his craft from his father and from his own observations and learnings. He serves both rich and poor, those who can pay and those who can't, although he himself remains poor. However, his community helps out his family when unusual expenses arise. And recently, his community acknowledged his services through an award.

Sollod, Albert. 1981. *Patterns of Disease in Sylvopastoral Herds of Central Niger. An Epidemiological Study of Herd Health in the Niger Range and Livestock Project Zone.* The Niger Ministry of Rural Development and USAID, Niamey, Niger. 116 pp.

This technical report on the nature and importance of diseases in pastoral herds of Niger is based on interviews, examinations of herds and individual animals, trials with vaccinations and medications, necropsies, and discussions with members of the livestock service. The prevalence and epidemiological features of approximately 25 diseases are described. Recommendations for combating and preventing these ills take into account cultural traits, the production system, herder attitudes, available infrastructure and environmental factors. An extension system within the livestock service could provide herders with animal health commodities and information. This service should focus on *herd* health rather than on individual animals. If the healthcare delivery system addressed problems that pastoralists themselves consider important, they would then be willing to pay for the service, thus making it self-financing. Limited amounts of mobile research equipment would be useful for further monitoring the prevalence and importance of diseases under field conditions. Annexes to this report include, among other things, proposals for developing disease survey and control capabilities, studying herding dynamics, and mounting training programmes for extension agents and livestock personnel.

Sollod, Albert E. 1983. The influence of trypanosomiasis on the animal disease taxonomies of the Fulße. Paper presented to the 26th Annual ASS Meeting, Boston, Massachusetts, USA, December 7–10, 1983.

This paper compares livestock disease concepts among two Fulani groups (Fulße in Burkina Faso and WoDaaße in Niger), investigates the influence of trypanosomosis on their disease classifications and suggests implications for livestock development efforts. Trypanosomosis, a tsetse-borne protozoan disease, occurs in the Fulße region but not in the arid habitat of the WoDaaße. *Wilsere* is an important disease concept among the Fulße. While it refers to various clinical signs caused by trypanosomosis, it also glosses symptoms of non-trypanosomal diseases such as mastitis, blindness and retained placenta. Veterinary services in the Fulße region should therefore take care to accurately translate stockowners' diagnosis of *wilsere* and should be equipped with a simple microscope in areas where trypanosomosis is present. In contrast to the unifying disease concept of the Fulße, which is probably influenced by the varying manifestations of trypanosomosis, the WoDaaße regard different disease syndromes as single entities. Moreover, they distinguish acute from chronic diseases. Hence, for working with the WoDaaße, a precise glossary of WoDaaße and scientific animal health terms could prove most useful for veterinary projects.

Sollod, Albert E. and James A. Knight. 1983. Veterinary anthropology: A herd health study in central Niger. In: ***Third International Symposium on Veterinary Epidemiology and Economics.*** Arlington, Virginia, 6–10 September 1982. Veterinary Medicine Publishing Company, Edwardsville, Kansas. Pp. 482–486.

The authors see veterinary anthropology as a fusion between epidemiology and the anthropology of pastoralism. Insight into a people's culture helps epidemiologists understand livestock disease patterns, which are often culturally determined. Veterinary anthropology also enables epidemiologists to tap pastoralists' knowledge of animal health and production. It uses anthropological research techniques such as participant observation and interviews. A detailed description of a herd health study in Niger performed in 1981 illustrates the concrete applications of veterinary anthropology. This study used the following methods: interviewing herders about current or past herd health problems; examining health status and general condition of herds on a group basis; assessing natural and artificial components of the environment; conducting trials with vaccines and medications and recording the herders' perceptions about these; keeping detailed records of observations and interviews and analysing the day's findings each evening; performing necropsies of 16 sheep and goats and sending specimens to laboratories for analysis; clinically examining and treating individual animals; soliciting opinions about local diseases from Niger Livestock Service personnel; and analysing samples of local soil and salt. During the study period, the authors – a veterinarian and an anthropologist – observed at least 24 diseases. They were able to associate some of them to management practices and ownership by specific ethnic groups and to determine cultural and socioeconomic influences leading to the expression of some diseases. The socioeconomic assessment of disease importance reflects the herders' rather than the outsider's point of view. The authors propose a veterinary extension system utilizing pastoralists as extension agents.

Sollod, A.E. and C. Stem. 1991. Appropriate animal health information systems for nomadic and transhumant livestock populations in Africa. ***Revue Scientifique et Technique de l'Office Internationale des Épizooties*** 19(1): 89–101.

Developed under relatively simple, sedentary production conditions, Western veterinary models have proved powerless to address herd health problems in African pastoral regimes, which are managerially complex, mobile and thus subject to high environmental variability. To design a truly appropriate animal health information system for pastoral systems, a 'veterinary anthropology' approach is needed that takes EVK into account. This article offers a number of methodological tips on the conduct of ER&D with respect to, e.g. survey or interview instruments and timelines, geographical and informant sampling frames, and interpreters [see also Stem 1996]. It also discusses the importance of clarifying culturally-bound disease complexes, both for pastoralists and for personnel involved in epidemiological monitoring or care delivery. Particularly problematical in this regard are highly inclusive disease syndromes that are named and recognized among pastoralists but that do not correspond to any Western nomenclature. An example is the concept of *wilsere* among Fulße pastoralists of Burkina Faso. This term seems to refer to a bundle of cattle health problems that includes trypanosomosis and other diseases with non-specific or protean manifestations. Indeed, Fulße appear to diagnose *wilsere* by a process of elimination of other named cattle diseases for which they do recognize particular patterns of occurrence and vital or post-mortem signs and lesions. These other diseases include streptothricosis (*gugna*), rinderpest (*caara*) and black-quarter (*baleeyel*). Twareg of Niger have an outstanding ability to describe many diseases of cattle and smallstock in terms that correspond closely with Western ones. But when it comes to camels, they struggle with a multifaceted syndrome (*azani*) that embraces the majority of ills that can befall this species. The remain-der of this article describes an epidemiological surveillance effort in Niger that drew upon pastoralists themselves as 'vetscouts' of disease. The author concludes that it is time to rethink animal health delivery to pastoral populations for whom, with the exception of control of a few viral diseases, Western veterinary models have done little. 'The crux is . . . building on multiple local initiatives' (p. 99).

Sollod, Albert E., Katherine Wolfgang and James A. Knight. 1984. Veterinary anthropology: Interdisciplinary methods in pastoral systems research. In: J.R. Simpson and Phylo Evangelou (eds). *Livestock Development in Subsaharan Africa: Constraints, Prospects, Policy.* Westview Press, Boulder, Colorado. Pp. 285–302.

Veterinary anthropology utilizes methodologies from both social science and epi-demiology and integrates findings from different fields such as ecology, biology and sociology. This chapter describes veterinary anthropological research on pas-toralists in Niger and Burkina Faso. A study of animal health in Niger [see also Sollod and Knight 1983] produced a number of significant findings. There were no noticeable differences in the health status of large and small herds. But endemic diseases reduce herd productivity and may thus increase the number of animals necessary for the economic security of the herder. Calf mortality was lower than usually reported for the Sahel. The type of production system influenced the inci-dence and prevalence of diseases. Because of high herd mobility and other man-agement practices, the provision of animal health services to pastoralists is difficult. The use of herders as veterinary auxiliaries could improve the situation. The study in Burkina Faso focused on ways to improve communication between Fulße (Fulani) herders and the government veterinary service. The Fulße classify localized and epidemic diseases as specific entities, while endemic, fatal systemic diseases are grouped together under the name *wilsere*. Women play an important role in maintaining herd health and in caring for calves. The authors recommend that veterinary agents should learn more about indigenous disease concepts, that pastoralists participate in animal healthcare extension and that livestock develop-ment specialists consider project impacts on women.

Sollows, John and Greg Chapman. 1990. Rice-fish culture. *The Sustainable Agriculture Newsletter* 2(1): 1–16.

Asia's integrated rice-and-fish farming systems have gained increasing scientific attention as a model for economically and nutritionally sound and environmentally friendly agricultural adaptations. Fish protein is produced in the rice paddies at low cost and in a sustainable way using biological pest controls in the form of natural pathogens, parasites and predators that are all safe for fish. However, some botanical pesticides, such as rotenone and tobacco, may be highly toxic for fish. Neem shows promise as an alternative choice, but further field studies are needed to establish its harmlessness for all farmed fish species.

Somopogul, Alfred Saki. 1998. Médecine vétérinarie traditionnelle: Note de synthése des activités. *Le N'Dama: Journal du Sous-Réseau PRELUDE Santé, Productions Animales et Environnement* 11, 12(1&2): 4–7.

In 1995, the National Livestock Direction of the West African republic of Guinea-Conakry added a section of Traditional Pharmacy and Veterinary Medicine to its structure, in recognition of the political-economic, scientific and cultural importance of the nation's EVK resources. At the same time, it established a methodology for collecting and handling EVK data, spanning: literature reviews of plant utilization, including forages as well as plants of veterinary pharmacological value; sectoral studies to identify problems that can be addressed with EVK; inter-institutional field research using surveys to inventory medicinal plants and their veterinary applications; creation of a corresponding herbarium; species identification; and detailed description and, if indicated, improvement of traditional preparation and preservation methods. In support of this initiative, efforts are being made to mobilize all possible human resources. These span: extensionists; target populations, i.e. stockraisers and traditional healers; key personages such as authorities and administrators; and other decision-makers and actors like international donors and scientific institutions. In this process, the National Livestock Direction has coordinated with other agencies like the Ministry of Health, the Faculty of Botany of the national university, the National Agricultural Research Center, international networks like PRELUDE and multilateral donors like the African Development Bank. Via survey sheets distributed in various parts of the country, to date the Direction has gathered information on 422 plants used in EVM. This information has been entered into a central registry according to numerous variables. In the registry effort, however, problems have been noted in linking vernacular with scientific plant names and in clarifying what parts of the same plant are used for treating different livestock ills. This article presents an illustrative table of 23 scientifically identified medicinal plant species along with their general veterinary uses, e.g. as anthelmintics, anti-diarrhoeals, parasiticides, febrifuges, wound treatments, purgatives and so forth. In conclusion, the author reiterates the importance of inter-institutional collaboration. Further, he underscores the need for legislation to ensure that ER&D is put to work rather than being merely 'empty words'.

Sonaiya, E.B. 1992. An assessment of extensive and intensive systems of pig and poultry production in the tropics. In: G. Tacher and L. Letenneur (eds). *Proceedings of the Seventh International Conference of Institutions of Tropical Veterinary Medicine, Yamoussoukro, Ivory Coast: Volume I.* Pp. 265–273.

About 80% of all poultry and pigs in the tropics are raised under traditional, extensive systems of smallholder production, which rely mainly on indigenous breeds. Extensive poultry production can be divided into two types: free range systems, which entail virtually no investments beyond the birds themselves; and part-confined 'backyard' regimes, which provide the birds with proper overnight shelter, grain supplements and ethnoveterinary care. The main production obstacle in the latter is Newcastle disease. Modest inputs of Western veterinary healthcare into traditional smallholder poultry systems can make for significant improvements. With such inputs in Uganda, for example, between 1980 and 1989 duck meat production was increased from 600 to 2500 tonnes annually, with 3500 tonnes projected for 1992. During the same period, average mortality rates for backyard ducks decreased from 40% to a mere 8%. Also noted are ducks' traditional role as biological controls on snails in Filipino rice–poultry farming systems. With regard to traditional practices in pig raising, this conference paper notes Burmese farmers' use of homemade rations prepared from a wide range of ingredients such as household scraps, corn, rice byproducts, groundnut meal, wild rice, dried fish and prawn meal. The author concludes by cautioning that, before attempting to maximize productivity in village poultry or pigs, it is imperative first to conduct exhaustive baseline studies and detailed system analysis of the specific regime. Only thus can workable, system-specific technologies and inputs be developed.

Songwe, Omer. 1998. Feature: Improving animal health with plants. *La Voix du Paysan English* 35: 11.

This English-language version of what appears to be a Cameroonian farmers bulletin presents a collection of press-release-style articles and interviews on the EVM efforts of HPI and collaborating individuals and groups in Bui Division, Northwest Province. The feature introduction gives tips on medicinal plant collection and handling and it emphasizes the importance of being sure about which plants are used in EVM, so as to avoid poisonous ones.

Soukup, Jaroslav. n.d. *Vocabulario de los Nombres Vulgares de la Flora Peruana y Catálogo de los Géneros.* Editorial Salesiana, Lima, Perú. 436 pp.

This compendium lists more than 2700 genera and approximately 6300 local names of plants used in human ethnomedicine in Peru, along with their contemporary and historical applications. Perhaps a score of entries mention ethnoveterinary aspects. Examples span plants employed to combat parasitism (pp. 65, 95), improve hunting dogs' performance (pp. 88, 215), serve as a purgative (pp. 181, 215) or affect reproduction (pp. 222, 236). Plants that poison animals or retard their growth are also noted (pp. 71, 121, 173, 181, 186, 206, 222, 248).

Spittler, Gerd, Kurt Beck and Georg Klute. 1990. Die Kontrolle von Kamelen im Sahel. In: Horst S.H. Seifert, Paul L.G. Vlek and H.-J. Weidelt (eds). *Tierhaltung im Sahel. Symposium 26–27 Oktober 1989.* Göttinger Beiträge zur Land-und Forstwirschaft in den Tropen und Subtropen, Heft 51. Forschungs- und Studienzentrum der Agrar- und Forstwissenschaften der Tropen und Subtropen, Georg-August-Universität Göttingen, Germany. Pp. 23–37.

This paper from a conference on Sahelian animal husbandry discusses how Kel Ewey Twareg in Niger, Kel Adagh (Ifora) Twareg in Mali, and Hawawir and Kawahla Arabs in Sudan manage their camels' grazing. The authors distinguish three grazing patterns. The first is wild grazing, in which camels roam at will and their owners merely round them up as needed. About 10% of Kel Ewey camels graze wild. More common, however, is free grazing, in which the animals are allowed to wander, but sometimes with hobbled forelegs to restrict their ranging; and owners always keep tabs on the camels' whereabouts. Third is controlled grazing, in which people stay with the herd and help keep it away from grazing grounds that are dew-ridden or infested with pests or toxic plants; the herders also ward against straying and rustling. Ifora Twareg follow this third system. In contrast, the other three groups believe that 'the camels know best'; the people see themselves more as following rather than leading the herds. In any given group of camel pastoralists, the choice of grazing management system is influenced by a number of variables, including: household structure, production goals (e.g. Ifora keep camels mainly for milk, El Ewey for transport and Kawahla for meat), economic and market considerations, and the larger social and political context of the countries the pastoralists inhabit.

Statescu, C. 1981. Plantele medicinale úi aromatice utile în terapia veterinară. *Revista de Creúterea Animalelor* 31(8): 61–62.

This article describes the preparation and dosage levels for a selection of medicinal and aromatic plants used in Rumanian ethnoveterinary medicine. Examples include the following. An infusion of *Tussilago farfara* (coltsfoot) works as an antispasmodic with expectorant properties. *Hypericum perforatum* (St John's Wort) is used as a diuretic, an antiseptic and for liver diseases. *Polygonum bistorta* is employed for enteric diseases or externally for sores.

Statescu, C. 1983. Plantele medicinale úi aromatice úi utilizările lor în terapia veterinară. *Revista de Creúterea Animalelor* 33(3): 63–64.

Additional plants of veterinary importance in Rumania are noted here. *Filipendula ulmaria* (meadowsweet) has anti-inflammatory properties, *Rahamus fragula* acts as a purgative and *Digitalis lino* is used for cardiac problems. The leaves and roots of *Digitalis purpurea* can be boiled to make a diuretic or prepared as a tincture for subacute and chronic heart problems. Dosages of some of the ethnomedicines discussed are cited for a variety of animals including fish.

St Croix, F.W. de. 1972 [1945]. *The Fulani of Northern Nigeria.* Gregg International, Westmead, Farnborough, UK. 74 pp.

Pages 22–27 of this classic ethnography outline animal husbandry and ethnoveterinary practices among Fulani in northern Nigeria. Topics include breeding, nutrition, vaccination against CBPP, bonesetting, castration, wound care and cauterization. Pages 65–66 describe superstitious beliefs relating to cattle. For example, herders give cattle preparations made from trees and shrubs containing a milky sap because they believe that this will increase the number of animals and their milk yield. Fulani also spread salt on termite hills so that cattle will gnaw at these hills and increase in numbers as the termite mounds also grow.

Steedman, Elsie Viault. 1927–28. Ethnobotany of the Thompson Indians of British Columbia: Based on the field notes by James A. Teit. *Forty-fifth Annual Report of the Bureau of American Ethnology to the Secretary of the Smithsonian Institution.* Smithsonian Institution, Washington, DC, USA.

Traditionally, Canada's Thompson Indians prepared and administered the same plants in the same ways for their horses and dogs as for themselves when treating swellings, sores, bruises and cuts. [See also Teit 1930.] For these purposes, they employed washes, powders and ointments (pp. 513–514). Three prescriptions for sores are given: a decocted wash of *Valeriana sylvatica* and *V. sitchensis* roots; dried and powdered *Leptotaenia dissecta* root, sprinkled thickly on the sores; and, particularly for running sores, an ointment of melted *Pinus ponderosa* gum and deer fat. Medicines to be administered internally to animals consisted of decoctions of the same plants that the Indians used as tonics and laxatives for their own ailments. Also, valuable hunting dogs were steamed, sweated and bathed in the same way as their human masters.

Stem, Chip. 1996. Ethnoveterinary R&D in production systems. In: Constance M. McCorkle, Evelyn Mathias and Tjaart W. Schillhorn van Veen (eds). **Ethnoveterinary Research & Development.** Intermediate Technology Publications, London, UK. Pp. 193–206.

This chapter overviews ER&D studies, methods and lessons learned based on mini-case studies of the experiences of Tufts University's Program of International Veterinary Medicine in livestock (ruminant) development among Fulani in Burkina Faso, Samburu of Kenya, Mexican peasants, Moroccan stockraisers, and Twareg and WoDaaße in Niger. ER&D can be a crucial component of any sustainable program of livestock development. When conducted early on in a project or policy initiative, ER&D encourages mutual trust and respect between development workers and livestock producers. The knowledge thus gained is vital to the success of livestock development projects because it pinpoints stockraisers' own, often very astute, views of the primary constraints to their animal production system. In both Morocco and Niger, for example, the importance of enterotoxaemia was masked by its difficult scientific diagnosis under field conditions; but in ethnoveterinary interviews, pastoralists' ability to describe its symptomology and occurrence in great detail convinced the government of their need and desire for manufacture of an enterotoxaemia vaccine. In Niger, herders avowed that it is not worth the expense for an individual routinely to dose his whole herd against gastrointestinal parasites, given that the animals must subsequently be turned out on communally grazed pastures; double-blind trials to investigate this claim later showed that, in fact, the cost of such an anthelmintic programme made the treatment group less economically productive than the controls. In both Kenya and Niger, another lesson learned is that, to ensure maximum accurate information on the production system, women as well as men in stockraising families must be consulted, because the sexes have different ethnoveterinary knowledge and deploy livestock products differently. If developers are not careful, they may end up harming rather than helping household economies overall. In Niger, for instance, diverting chaff used in women's crafting of items for market sale to livestock feed instead might reduce household income as a whole. Key inputs of stockraiser knowledge are also vital to the design of appropriate, and the avoidance of inappropriate, technology. Throughout the African Sahel, for instance, vitamin A deficiency is an annual dry-season problem that leads to blindness and even death in cattle and sheep who cannot find their way to wells or keep up with the rest of the herd. Herders have various effective, but usually only temporary, traditional ways to counteract this problem; but the materials are not always available. Likewise for the vitamin A injections and boluses recommended by the livestock service, which in any case are generally too expensive for pastoralists. In response to this express need, Tufts researchers successfully field-tested a much cheaper, water-soluble vitamin powder, which pastoralists then adopted. Moreover, the powder was a far safer and more appropriate technology than injections. It obviated the need for syringes. In the Sahel, this means non-disposable syringes, which under pastoral conditions are virtually impossible to keep sterile; but disposables are economically prohibitive. Also in the Sahel, dry-season forage bottlenecks are a well-known constraint to animal production. An oft-suggested solution is haymaking. But this turns out to be an equally often inappropriate technology in view of the multiple and intense herding, husbandry and social demands on stockraisers' time that fall just when haying must be done. For some problems, appropriate indigenous technology already exists and needs only to be extended more widely. Examples from Tufts research are Fulani's and Twareg's homemade but effective CBPP vaccines and their successful bonesetting techniques. Finally, ethnoveterinary intelligence can provide a basis for epidemiological investigations and long-term animal health and production monitoring, and for mounting cost-effective programmes of animal disease control through the training and supervision of paraveterinarians. This application of ER&D is illustrated in a Tufts-assisted 'vetscout' programme in Niger, which incorporated Twareg and WoDaaße pastoralists in these tasks. Armed with their indigenous veterinary savvy, some modest training and simple pictographic reporting forms, the scouts were able to track, treat and periodically report back on livestock diseases for even the most remote and nomadic of their peers. Tufts' experiences illustrate how, drawing upon stockraisers' own knowledge, skills and lifeways, both research and extension can sift out, reinforce and design and promulgate viable strategies that producer groups find acceptable and that hard-pressed developing-country livestock services can afford.

Stem, C. and A.E. Sollod. 1994. Rapid reconnaissance in animal health planning for pastoral production systems. *The Kenya Veterinarian* 18(2): 51–54.

This paper outlines a field methodology that draws on anthropology, economics and veterinary medicine in order to facilitate the design and implementation of low-cost and sustainable animal-disease-control programmes for pastoral peoples. The methodology embodies a multiphase approach consisting of ethnoveterinary surveys, eco-epidemiological investigations, field trials and targeted healthcare interventions. Based on their experience from previous projects and studies, the authors discuss these different phases, parts of which may be implemented simultaneously. The ethnoveterinary surveys should cover not only disease factors but also epidemiological, cultural and ecological aspects of animal health and production. If women perform any animal healthcare tasks, then they must be included in the surveys. Survey findings should generate a list of constraints to be verified and refined later through epidemiological studies based on clinical observations, physical examinations, analysis of blood and tissue samples and other data-collection methods. The results of the ethnoveterinary surveys and the eco-epidemiological studies then feed into the development of cost-effective interventions and a delivery system for them. Different cures, treatments and preventive measures can be tested through field trials. Products and techniques of proven efficacy may even be tested at the herd level.

Stewart, Miller J. 1978. Veterinary practices of the plains Indians. *Modern Veterinary Practice* Feb: 99–102.

The veterinary skills of various nations of North American plains Indians centred on horses and included castration, bonesetting, surgery and phytotherapy.

Castration and bonesetting were typically practised by specialists, while other members of the community were known to be particularly adept at curing colic and distemper. Horses gored by wild animals such as buffalo were treated surgically, for example by sewing up the wound with deer sinew. Other kinds of wounds (including bullet wounds) might be cauterized, or implanted with a burning yarrow stalk, or rubbed with sage ash.

Stiles, Daniel and Aneesa Kassam. 1986. An ethno-botanical study of Gabra Plant Use, Marsabit District, Kenya. Unpublished manuscript. Desertification Control PAC, UNEP, Nairobi, Kenya and Department of Literature, University of Nairobi, Kenya. 26 pp.

In this ethnobotanical study among Gabbra pastoralists of Kenya, some eight plants of ethnoveterinary value are identified. Examples are: *Blepharis* sp., ashes of which are spread over camel wounds; *Heliotropium albohispidum* leaves, which are chewed and applied to snakebites to reduce swelling; *Commicarpus helenae*, which is chewed and spat into the nostrils of a calf as a decongestant; and chewed *Pseudosopubia hildebrandtii* leaves, the saliva from which is put in an animal's mouth to protect it from the evil eye.

Storrs, A.E.G. 1982. *More about Trees (a Sequel to 'Know Your Trees'): Interesting Facts & Uses of Some Common Zambian Trees including a Selection of Honey Recipes.* The Forest Department, Ndola, Zambia. No. of pages not available.

The section of this volume on medicinal uses of trees found in Zambia notes two explicitly veterinary applications. An anthelmintic for livestock can be made from *Diospyros mespiliformis* roots; and parts of *Ficus capensis*, the fruit and leaves of *F. sycomorus* and a bark decoction of *F. ingens* are used as galactagogues for cattle (and sometimes humans). The author repeatedly warns against non-experts' use of herbal medicines, noting that it is essential to know exactly the species required and the method of preparation. This is because plant properties vary even between closely related species, poisons that are absent in ripe fruit are sometimes present in unripe fruit, and dangerous byproducts can ensue during preparation.

Sule, Alhaji Eggi. 1998. Alhaji Eggi: Ethnovet encyclopaedia. *La Voix du Paysan English* 35: 14.

A participant in the HPI/Cameroon EVM project, the 60-year-old Alhaji Eggi Sule is a walking encyclopaedia of ethnoveterinary know-how, based on knowledge he acquired from his father and on his own. The Alhaji keeps a botanical garden from which he draws the plants he uses in his ethnoveterinary practice. Other stockraisers come to him for advice and treatment for their animals, in exchange for small gifts. If he is called on to give outpatient care, the client must pay for his transport and food meanwhile. The Alhaji notes that he also uses modern medicines for some diseases 'because not all diseases can be treated through Ethnovet ... The Rinderpest is one of such diseases'.

Sumano López, Héctor, Ana Auró Angulo and Luis Ocampo Camberos. 1988. Comparación del efecto cicatrizante de varios preparados de la medicina tradicional y la medicina de patente. In: Luz Lozano Nathal and Gerardo López Buendía (coordinators). *Memorias: Primera Jornada sobre Herbolaria Medicinal en Veterinaria.* Universidad Nacional Autónoma de México, Facultad de Medicina Veterinaria y Zootecnia, Coordinación de Educación Continua, México DF. Pp. 80–84.

This experiment sought to compare the relative effectiveness of three different veterinary traditions in healing wounds of animals: several patent medicines; Mexican folk treatments, including an extract of *Aloe vera*, a certain oil, powdered *Mimosa tenuiflora*, and an infusion of *Desmodium plicatum*; and electro-acupuncture. Evaluated across a variety of parameters, findings suggest that electro-acupuncture is the most effective, followed by all of the traditional Mexican medicaments except the infusion. The patent medicines and the infusion showed no difference in healing ability vis-à-vis controls. The authors conclude with some thoughts on possibilities for marketing the traditional treatments.

Sutton, J.E.G. 1970. Cattle keeping in the Kenya highlands. Paper presented to the School of Oriental and African Studies (SOAS) Seminar on African Cattle-Keeping, London, UK, June 1970.

Unavailable for review.

Sutama, I-K. and A. Djajanegara. 1992. Traditional medicine: A feed additive. *The Newsletter of SRUPNA* 3(3): 3.

Feed supplements in the form of purchased concentrates and vitamins are too expensive for most stockraisers in the developing world. Yet supplementation is vital at certain points in animal growth and reproduction. Thus, farmers have created various supplements of their own, as reported in this article for Asian raisers of small ruminants. To fatten small ruminants in Indonesia, farmers feed 150 g of cooked, salted fish with 50 g of tamarind. A mixture of turmeric rhizome, tamarind, egg and salt increases milk production. Inappetence is cured with a combination of tamarind, *Paederia foetida* leaves, *Curcuma xanthorrhiza* rhizome, ginger, salt and water. In India, pre-parturient ewes are given a tonic of 250 g of *gur* in a jug of water topped with *methi* or another additive known as *bajra*. Also noted in this article are some remedies for general small ruminant ills. For example, fresh papaya and bamboo leaves or ground guava leaves mixed with 2 glasses of boiled water combat diarrhoea. Bloat may be alleviated with a drench of ground ginger and a teaspoon of ground coffee boiled in salt water. Examples of prophylaxes and remedies for endoparasites are, respectively: in India, dosing lambs with a spoonful of mustard oil at 3 and 6 days after birth; and in Indonesia, drenching small ruminants once every 3 months with 0.5 kg of *Curcuma aeruginosa* rhizome in 1 l of water. Other ingredients commonly used for gastrointestinal parasites are cashew-fruit skins, cucumber seeds and tobacco leaves.

Swallow, Brent M. 1993. The role of mobility within the risk management strategies of pastoralists and agro-pastoralism. Paper presented to the Commonwealth Secretariat's Research Workshop on 'New Directions in African Range Management and Policy', Woburn, UK, 31 May–4 June.

In addition to the well-known benefits of pastoralists' herd movements for ensuring good nutrition and avoiding disease threats are less-well-documented 'group insurance' strategies. These disperse livestock across the landscape in varying environments or micro-environments on a longer-term basis than seasonal or annual movements. This conference paper describes several such strategies traditionally found among African pastoralists and agropastoralists. One is bridewealth, in which livestock are paid by a prospective groom to his future father-in-law, who may well reside in a different locale. Another is tenancy or entrustment arrangements, whereby a stockowner contracts with a herder or another stockowner to care for all or a part of his herd elsewhere. An example is the 1.5-centuries-old institution of *mafisa* in Lesotho, in which a chief lends out stock to commoners who give him their fealty in exchange for the use of the animals under their care. *Mafisa* is practised nowadays between wealthy patrons and their poorer clients. These different dispersal arrangements may be motivated by a range of reasons, including marriage, power and charity. But nevertheless, they all reap the benefits of access to additional range resources plus decreased risk of an epidemic's wiping out all an individual's or a family's herd.

Tadjbakhsh, H. 1994. Traditional methods used for controlling animal diseases in Iran. *Revue Scientifique et Technique de l'Office International des Épizooties* 13(2): 599–614.

Based on an on-going study of 2200 ancient books and manuscripts, this article overviews traditional veterinary controls and practitioners of pre-Islamic and Islamic Iran. Early practitioners served both animals and humans, and they had well-developed theories of contagion. Beginning centuries ago and on into the 1800s, vaccinations were given against infectious diseases like CCPP and poxes in both livestock and children. For CCPP, lung tissue from diseased goats was ground with vinegar and garlic; the mixture was then passed through a fine cloth, applied to a thread, and sewn through the ears of healthy goats. Children were vaccinated against smallpox between the thumb and index finger using a needle dipped in a suspension of dried, ground smallpox scabs or by encouraging children with wounds on their hands to touch the lesions on an animal with cowpox. Along with other treatments, a kind of serotherapy was practised for rabies, in which the liver of a rabid dog was pressed against a dog bite, such that some antibodies might enter the wound. Diseases deemed non-communicable were classified by the organ or body part they mainly affected. For example, diseases of the nose included coryza, strangles and intranasal hyperaemia. In general, treatments of non-communicable diseases relied by preference on pharmacotherapy involving plant, animal and mineral ingredients. While plants were 'too numerous to list here' (p. 609), some of the *materia medica* of animal origin included sheep tail fat, tallow, eggs, milk, honey, donkey urine, wild animals' gall bladders, sheep leather, bovine bone marrow, goat brains, powdered human skulls and earthworms. Examples of mineral ingredients are lime, salt, sulphur, ammonium, alum, ferrous sulphate, zinc and dust. If pharmacotherapy failed, then cauterization and surgery in the form of bloodletting were essayed. Other surgical procedures included castrating, lancing purulent wounds, excising bone tumours and fibromas, and for laminitis, paring the hoof and applying a hot brick. Examples of manipulative and mechanical treatments were: to evacuate intestinal gases, pulling tight on bands tied around the head and back or inserting a reed into the rectum; to relieve bladder obstructions, massaging the urethra through the rectum or vagina; and up to the 1960s, to protect colts from insects carrying African horse sickness [trypanosomosis], covering the colts with cotton dresses. Also described are a variety of treatments for camel ills.

Talbot, N.T. 1972. Incidence and distribution of helminth and arthropod parasites of indigenous owned pigs in Papua New Guinea. ***Tropical Animal Health and Production*** 4: 182–190.

Villagers in the southern highlands of New Guinea singe off the bristles of pigs that are heavily infested with lice. Although this practice temporarily controls the lice, it 'invariably leads to severe burns with later secondary bacterial dermatitis and cellulitis resulting in retarded growth or death' (p. 188).

Tall, Amadou Mamadou. 1994. Synthèse des fiches sur la pharmacopée vétérinaire traditionnelle en Mauritanie. In: Kakule Kasonia and Michel Ansay (eds). ***Métissages en Santé Animale de Madagascar à Haïti: Actes du Séminaire d'Ethnopharmacopée Vétérinaire 'KAGALA', un Partage de Savoirs Burkina-Faso, Ouagadougou, 15–22 Avril 1993.*** Presses Universitaires de Namur, Namur, Belgium. Pp. 147–151.

Based on surveys conducted in the early 1990s by the Pastoral Division of Mauritania's Ministry of Rural Development and Environment, this chapter describes traditional treatments for six diseases of herd animals (cattle, sheep, goats, horses and donkeys) in Mauritania. Four plants are cited as endoparasiticidal: *Acacia scorpioides* for cattle, *Anogeissus leiocarpa* for calves, *Ceiba pentandra* for horses and donkeys, and *Cordyla pinnata* for equines. Apart from *A. scorpioides*, which is administered for trypanosomosis, herders did not detail which parasites could be treated with these plants. Constipation is relieved by a variety of methods, but especially by herbal drenches of plants that yield a viscous solution when their leaves and/or bark are crushed and macerated, such as *Corchorus tridens*, *Corchorus trilocularis* and *Grewia bicolor*. Any vegetable oil (e.g. from groundnuts or from watermelon seeds) may also be administered orally every 6 to 8 hours until relief is obtained. Colic in calves is relieved by a 1 l drench of decocted *Guiera senegalensis* leaves and sugar, given morning and evening for 2 days. For digestive pasteurellosis, a handful of *Lezernia inermis* leaves collected before flowering are macerated and 2 l of the liquid are drenched intra-nasally. For retained placenta, 0.5 l of decocted *Sclerocarya birrea* bark is orally administered morning and evening for about 2 days. Poultices of *Datura metel* or of sweet potatoes are applied to inflammations. The article concludes with a table summarizing 11 plants utilized in Mauritanian EVM, along with the pertinent botanical and veterinary procedures for each prescription.

Tanner, J.C. 1996. The role of livestock in nutrient cycling: A case study of upland farming in Indonesia. In: Karl-Hans Zessin (ed.). *Livestock Production and Diseases in the Tropics: Livestock Production and Human Welfare. Proceedings of the VIII International Conference of Institutions of Tropical Veterinary Medicine held from the 25 to 29 September, 1995 in Berlin, Germany.* Volume II. Deutsche Stiftung für Internationale Entwicklung, Zentralstelle für Ernährung und Landwirtschaft, Feldafing, Germany. P. 477.

Javanese smallholders traditionally rear their small ruminants in backyard barns with slatted floors built over pits, where the animals are fed indigenous forage collected from roadsides and field margins. Stock are purposely given excessive quantities of forage. Rejected vegetation is placed in the pit beneath the animals, where it becomes soaked with urine and mixed with faeces. Later, this rich refuse material is composted. By varying feeding as well as composting practices, Javanese farmers manufacture different qualities of manure or compost to suit particular soil types or crops. Using PRA ranking, matrix-scoring, seasonal diagramming and mapping techniques, the study reported here found that, among upland farmers of West Java, livestock feeding strategies are driven as much by people's need for compost as by considerations of animal productivity. Indeed, 90% of the fertilizer used on smallholdings is manure-compost, and farmers rank it as one of the most important outputs from stockraising.

Tanner, J.C., S.J. Holden, M. Winugroho, E. Owen and M. Gill. 1995. Feeding livestock for compost production: A strategy for sustainable upland agriculture on Java. In: J.M. Powell, S. Fernández-Rivera, T.O. Williams and C. Renard (eds). *Livestock and Sustainable Nutrient Cycling in Mixed Farming Systems of Sub-Saharan Africa. Volume II: Technical Papers.* Proceedings of an International Conference held in Addis Ababa, Ethiopia, 22–26 November 1993. ILCA, Addis Ababa, Ethiopia. Pp. 115–128.

This conference paper constitutes an earlier but more technical version of the information presented in Tanner 1996.

Tear Fund. 1992. The editor's scrapbook: Tips from around the world. *Footsteps* 10(Mar): 16.

Farmers and aid workers share animal management tips in this newsletter. A farmer discovered he could save his crop-bound chickens by cutting open the crop using a razor, removing the blockage, and then sewing up the incision. The same farmer was able to hatch eggs by wrapping them in cotton and putting them in a warm corner of his hut. A Nigerian farmer dyes his chicks with gentian violet to protect them from hawks (see Ajayi 1990). Oral rehydration therapy can be administered to diarrhoea-stricken calves, goats and piglets just as effectively as to children. Finally, Muscovy ducks feast on flies, thus providing effective fly control services.

Teit, James A. 1930. Ethnobotany of the Thompson Indians of British Columbia. In: ***Forty-fifth Annual Report of the Bureau of American Ethnology to the Secretary of the Smithsonian Institution 1927–1928.*** United States Government Printing Office, Washington, DC, USA.

Pages 513–514 of this study describe several treatments for horses and dogs used by Thompson Indians in Canada during the early 20th century. The Indians apply the same plant preparations to their animals as they use for themselves. Most applications are in the form of washes, ointments and powders, while internal medicines are only occasionally administered to horses and dogs. Fresh saddle sores are washed with human urine. Other remedies for wounds and swellings are preparations of *Valeriana sylvatica*, *Leptotaenia dissecta* and *Pinus ponderosa*.

Telanga, Ambaji. 1998. Who cares for the knowledge-rich economically poor workers? ***Honey Bee*** 9(1): 10.

Ambaji Telanga is a local veterinary healer who serves some 10 villages in one Kannada-speaking area of India. In this article, he shares his remedies for five common livestock problems. He dresses wounds with a mixture of 21 drops of juice from the *Calotropis* plant, 100 g of camphor and 400 g of fresh butter. For coughs and colds, powdered turmeric mixed with butter is placed on the tip of a *Calotropis* stem, which is then inserted into the patient's nostrils several times. Thereafter, crushed *Solanum* leaves mixed with the patient's urine are smeared over its body. Mr Telanga cures yoke galls with 100 g of *Pistacia lentiscus* plant that has been fried and mixed with 1 kg of butter in a brass vessel and then stirred every day for a week, until the mixture turns green. A wash of decocted *Pandanus tectorius* leaves keeps off ectoparasites. For sprains, the affected area is repeatedly painted with a mixture of soap chips and eggwhite; each time the mixture hardens, it becomes uncomfortable, causing the patient to kick its legs and thus 'set right the sprain'.

Tenetiga. 1997a. Garlic for diarrhoea and amla improves digestion. ***Honey Bee*** 8(2): 9.

Reprinted here from *Tenetiga*, the Teluga-language version of *Honey Bee*, are 12 local livestock treatments. Two cattle dewormers are: powdered *Holarrhena antidysenterica* seeds or bark mixed with rice bran or gram; and *Aristolochia bracteolata* leaf extract. To combat diarrhoea from harmful weeds or pesticide-contaminated fodder, the filtrate of decoctions of ground garlic, *Sinus vitazonia*, *Cajanus indicus* and *Piper nigrum* or of ground *Soymida febrifuga* and *Terminalia belerica* is fed to cattle. Bovine indigestion can be cured with a special 'salt wood treatment' mixed into the feed along with salt; the ingredients are equal proportions of *Acacia pennata*, *Pterololium hexapetalum*, *Capparis sepiaria* and *Attantia monophylla* bark mixed with *Emblica officinalis* fruits, *Ocimum sanctum* leaves and *Cissus quadrangularis* stems. Yanadulu tribals instead use ground *Aloe vera* and garlic; other groups recommend a peppered filtrate of boiled *Cassia fistula* mixed with garlic. Two galactagogues for cattle are: an infusion of 4 to 5 *Semecarpus anacardium* fruits that have been soaked in a mud pot for 2 days and then ground and mixed with rice or rice bran; and a mixture of *Algeria nervosa* and *A. pylosa* roots with palm jaggery, turmeric and *Ajma*. Snoring and coughs can be cured by feeding the extract of boiled *Alangium souifolium* bark or, alternatively, equal proportions of *Melyna arjoria, Holoptelea integrifolia* and *Lucas spiphora* leaves mixed with garlic or pepper. A treatment for pain and inflammation is *Euphorbia neriifolia* latex and turmeric boiled together and filtered. Inflamed legs are wrapped with *Calotropis* spp. leaves smeared with castor oil.

Tenetiga. 1997b. Polythene prevents pests! *Honey Bee* 8(4): 11.

From the Telugu version of *Honey Bee* comes a unique method for preserving colostrum (albeit for human rather than neonate consumption). A clean piece of muslin is dipped in the raw colostrum milk each day for the first few days after parturition. Thereafter, the cloth is stored in a clean polythene bag. To reconstitute the colostrum, the cloth is dipped in normal, raw milk and then wrung out over another container. People say the cloth can be kept and used for up to 6 months.

Thaker, A.M., S.K. Bhavsar, J.G. Sarvaiya, B.M. Jani, M.P. Venna and J.K. Malik. 1997. Ectoparasticidal [sic] activity of *Annona squamosa* in animals: Clinical and experimental evaluation. In: Anil Gupta (ed.). *International Conference on Creativity and Innovation at Grassroots for Sustainable Natural Resource Management, January 11–14, 1997: Abstracts.* Indian Institute of Management, Ahmedabad, India. P. 76.

Experiments were conducted to evaluate the ectoparasiticidal activity and subacute dermal toxicity of *Annona squamosa* seeds. In brief, topical applications of seed extracts of varying concentrations were found to be highly effective against fleas in dogs and sarcoptic and psoroptic manges in buffalo. Further studies to evaluate dermal toxicity of *A. squamosa* extracts as compared with saline applications on calves found the former safe for use as an ectoparasiticide for cattle.

Thaker, A.M., S.K. Bhavsar, J.G. Sarvaiya, R.K. Mishra and M.P. Verma. 1998. Oral toxicity of oil of *Annona squamosa* in chicken. In: E. Mathias, D.V. Rangnekar and C.M. McCorkle, with M. Martin (eds). *Ethnoveterinary Medicine: Alternatives for Livestock Development – Proceedings of an International Conference Held in Pune, India, 4–6 November 1997. Volume 2: Abstracts.* BAIF Development Research Foundation, Pune, India. P. 57.

Ancient Indian literature and traditional folklore claim insecticidal or parasiticidal properties for many plants. Research in the Department of Pharmacology at India's College of Veterinary Science and Animal Husbandry bears out some of these claims. For example, laboratory tests have demonstrated that *Annona squamosa* seed preparations can kill lice, while clinical studies have revealed their acaricidal activity. Subsequent trials entailing repeated topical application of *A. squamosa* seed extract to evaluate possible subacute dermal toxicity demonstrated that topical applications are safe. This paper reports on a further toxicological screen of an oral preparation of the seeds in which 5-week old broiler chicks were divided into: a treatment group that was orally administered hexane extract of *A. squamosa* seeds at a dose of 2.5 ml/kg bw daily for 3 weeks; and a control group that received refined cottonseed oil according to the same treatment schedule. For both groups, live body weights were recorded weekly; and all birds were observed for any toxicological signs. In brief, the birds showed no toxic manifestations; and there was little difference in weight gain between the two groups.

Thaker, Bharat R. 1998. Therapeutic use of acupuncture in dairy cattle. In: E. Mathias, D.V. Rangnekar and C.M. McCorkle, with M. Martin (eds). *Ethnoveterinary Medicine: Alternatives for Livestock Development – Proceedings of an International Conference Held in Pune, India, 4–6 November 1997. Volume 2: Abstracts.* BAIF Development Research Foundation, Pune, India. Pp. 57–58.

Acupuncture and moxibustion are ancient healing arts. Although the mechanisms of their action and effect in disease treatment are not yet understood, many practitioners around the world nevertheless employ these techniques. In 1940, scientists of the former USSR developed a type of acupuncture known as novocain blockade. It proved an effective therapy for inflammatory conditions. Nowadays, a number of animal and human ills are successfully treated with it, including peritonitis, gastritis, spasmodic colic, ruminal atony, pancreatitis, hepatitis, cystitis, orchitis, udder oedema, mastitis and other acute visceral inflammations. Because little information on this technique is available in India, however, the study reported here was mounted to investigate the efficacy of novocain blockade in clinical cases of primary ruminal dysfunctions, udder oedema, and mastitis in dairy cattle and buffalo. In 98 cases of primary indigestion (PI) and 58 cases of udder oedema and mastitis (UOM) three treatments were tested: acupuncture (ACP) in the form of an epipleural novocain blockade; conventional method (CM); and conventional method supplemented with ACP. Of the 98 PI cases, 28 received ACP. After 48 hours, these animals showed clinical improvements in the form of increased appetite, rumination and milk yield. Of the remaining 70 animals, only 18 showed clinical improvements within 3 to 8 days. The 52 that did not respond to CM were treated subsequently with ACP. Within 24 hours after blockade, 34 of these 52 improved. The last 18, who did not respond to either treatment, were found to have chronic digestive disturbances. Six of the seven UOM cases treated with ACP showed clinical improvement within 48 hours of blockade. Of the remaining 51 animals with UOM, who all received CM, seven showed improvement within 4 to 6 days. The 44 animals that did not respond to CM within 72 hours received ACP; and after 2 to 3 days, 37 of them improved. In sum, results indicate that epipleural novocain blockade enhances the recovery of PI and UOM cases.

Thakur, D.K., S.K. Misra and P.C. Choudhuri. 1983. Trial of some of the plant extracts and chemicals for their antifungal activity in calves. *Indian Veterinary Journal* 60(10): 799–801.

Tests of *Allium sativum*, *Curcuma longa* and *Leucas aspera* indicated that the last two show effective antifungal activity against calf dermatophytosis.

Thakur, R.P., S.N. Mahato and R. Rai. 1992. Use of *Sihundi* for the treatment of roundworms in pigs. In: IIRR (ed.). *Regenerative Agriculture Technologies for the Hill Farmers of Nepal.* IIRR, Silang, Cavite, Philippines. 2 pp.

Produced by IIRR and the Nepal Rural Reconstruction Association, this loose-leaf information kit mentions Nepalis' traditional use of the wild shrub *Euphorbia roylcana* as a treatment for gastrointestinal worms in humans. The kit goes on to describe an experiment in which pills prepared from *E. roylcana* latex were fed to pigs to combat roundworms. The pills were found to be 100% effective for this purpose. Moreover, they proved to be completely safe for pregnant sows, producing no side effects in the sow or piglets.

Theves, G. 1994. Remèdes de maladies animales au Luxembourg pendant les XVIIe et XVIIIe siècles. *Revue Scientifique et Technique de l'Office International de Épizooties* 13(2): 513–528.

This article describes aspects of 17th- and 18th-century veterinary medicine in Luxemburg. The veterinary pharmacopoeia of the time can be divided into three types: popular medicine; dating from the Middle Ages, blacksmiths' remedies; and magico-religious treatments, including sorcery and invocations to healing saints (*saints guérisseurs*). Popular medicine was practised on horses, cattle, sheep, dogs and poultry. Treatments made use of animal, vegetable and mineral ingredients. For cattle that had ceased to ruminate, salted beef was fed. Ash tree was a particularly popular cure-all, e.g. for lethargy in oxen, horses with damaged withers, and wounds and burns of all species. Ash contains tannins, essential oils, vitamin C, malic acid and mannitol; thus it can be used as an astringent, diuretic, laxative, soporific and stimulant. An example of an old blacksmiths' remedy for internal inflammation and external sores is a potion of *Ruta graveolens* L., *Salvia officinalis* L., *Hyssopus officinalis* L., *Levisticum officinale* Koch, *Anethum graveolens* L., *Solanum dulcamara* L. and *Ledum palustre* L., all of which contain volatile oils and other ingredients of known medicinal benefits of many sorts. Blacksmiths' medicine tended toward polyprescriptions. For example a cure for horse colic was an enema of milk and salt and a drench of apple vinegar with parsley filtered through a clean cloth.

Thiam, Abou and Moumouni Ouattara. 1994. Contribution à l'étude des plantes médicinales et alimentaires du Sahel. In: Kakule Kasonia and Michel Ansay (eds). *Métissages en Santé Animale de Madagascar à Haïti: Actes du Séminaire d'Ethnopharmacopée Vétérinaire 'KAGALA', un Partage de Savoirs Burkina-Faso, Ouagadougou, 15–22 Avril 1993.* Presses Universitaires de Namur, Namur, Belgium. Pp. 167–175.

Plants used in foods and drugs for both people and livestock of the African Sahel can be categorized as medicinal, eco-pathological, magico-therapeutic, and other. Plants in the first category are used to treat respiratory disorders, cutaneous diseases, wounds, oedemas and abscesses. Those in the second category serve to control insects. For example, *Guiera senegalensis* is burned in the kraal to ward off flies. Magico-therapeutic plants may include species believed to be galactogenic, such as *Annona senegalensis*, *Euphorbia hirta* and *Cucumis melo* (melon). The 'other' category embraces plants with indirect food or drug applications, like the fish poisons *Fagara zantoxyloides* and *Balanites aegyptiaca*. A concluding table summarizes the documented uses of 14 plants of veterinary interest.

Thill, Georges. 1994. Ethnopharmacopée vétérinaire, écosanté, ecodéveloppement global durable. In: Kakule Kasonia and Michel Ansay (eds). *Métissages en Santé Animale de Madagascar à Haïti: Actes du Séminaire d'Ethnopharmacopée Vétérinaire 'KAGALA', un Partage de Savoirs Burkina-Faso, Ouagadougou, 15–22 Avril 1993.* Presses Universitaires de Namur, Namur, Belgium. Pp. 57–61.

This brief essay argues for a more integrative concept of 'ecohealth' that addresses not just pathologies but 'pathological structures'. The latter are defined as the ensemble of environmental (including social and cultural) conditions that negatively affect human and livestock health and well-being. From this viewpoint, the cross-cultural study of ethnopharmacology is more than just an exchange of technical experience. Even though technology must be evaluated according to some technical norms and standards, it must also be contextualized in terms of the milieu in which it is to be applied. The goal in such initiatives as ER&D should be not merely technology transfer but rather the hybridization of technological knowledge. In this regard, the author draws some conceptual distinctions among knowledge, know-how, and knowing how to know, as it were. He also underscores the importance of traditional healers and of the users of local knowledge such as EVK as veritable 'kitchens of creativity' and a source of methodological knowledge for inspiring hybridization.

Thompson, Henry. 1895. *Elementary Lectures on Veterinary Science for Agricultural Students, Farmers, and Stock Keepers.* Brakenridge, Whitehaven, UK. 273 pp.

This 19th-century book is a compilation of lectures delivered to farmers and stockraisers at various county-council centres in Britain, focusing mainly on veterinary medicine for cattle and horses. In addition to informing people about ways to prevent livestock disease, the goal of such lectures was to caution against the many quack medicines advertised at the time, and to give stockraisers the alternative of treating their animals themselves with simple on-farm remedies. Although at the time, the latter idea was greatly criticized by the veterinary profession at large, the author argued that this approach is preferable to people's using treatments about which they know nothing and which may be ineffective or even harmful. An example of one such on-farm remedy recommended for mastitis in cows is to lance the infected teat(s) to expel the pus and then rub the site with carbolic oil. Feverish animals can be fed a treacle gruel that includes Epsom salts, saltpetre and a few ounces of aromatic cordials such as ginger, gentian or aniseed, until the bowels respond.

Thompson, K.C., J. Roa E. and T. Romero N. 1978. Anti-tick grasses as the basis for developing practical tropical tick control packages. *Tropical Animal Health and Production* 10: 179–182.

Six grass species found in the USA, Australia and Colombia were analysed for their tick-deterrent properties. *Melinis minutiflora* (molasses grass) proved the most effective in this regard, while *Andropogon gayanus* (Gamba grass) maintained a constantly low level of initial-host infestation plus a low-to-moderate tick population. 'Packaging' and disseminating these grasses with other methods of

512 *Ethnoveterinary medicine*

tick control would provide stockraisers an effective and low-cost way to manage tick-borne disease and thus enhance cattle production and productivity.

Tillman, Hermann J. 1983. Planificar el futuro de la comunidad. *Minka* 11(Jun): 21–25.

The author makes brief mention of the use of *tarwi* water as a dip to combat mange and other ectoparasitic infestations in Andean ovines and camelids. *Tarwi* (*Lupinus mutabilis*) is a bitter, alkaloid-laden but protein-rich legume native to the Andes. It must undergo prolonged steeping before it is suitable for human consumption. The resulting infusion is an effective ectoparasiticide of long-standing use in the region. [See also Avila Cazorla et al. 1985a&b, Jiménez J. et al. 1983, and PRATEC 1988b.]

Timaffy, László. 1961. Das Hirtenwesen auf den Donauinseln (Szigetköz, Westungarn). In: László Földe (ed.). *Viehzucht und Hirtenleben in Ostmitteleuropa: Ethnographische Studien.* Académiai Kiadó, Verlag der Ungarischen Akademie der Wissenschaften, Budapest, Hungary. Pp. 609–645.

In Szigetköz in western Hungary, cattle have for centuries been kept on islands in the Danube River. The herders regularly provide the animals with salt. They know when a cow is about to give birth and help her when necessary. They are skilled in caring for wounds, dressing them with soot or cattle dung, old spider webs and herbs to hasten the healing process. For some diseases the herders bleed the animals. In humid years, the herders use smoky fires day and night to protect the cattle from mosquitoes and other biting insects.

Toigbe, Emile Godonou. 1978. *Contribution a l'Étude de la Médecine Vétérinaire Africaine: La Pharmacopée des Peuls du Bénin et du Senegal.* These pour Docteur Vétérinaire, Faculté de Médecine et de Pharmacie, Ecole Inter-Etats des Sciences et Médecine Vétérinaires de Dakar, Dakar, Senegal. 115 pp.

According to numerous reports, approximately 50% of Africans lack sufficient protein in their diets. Hence the importance of productive livestock in Africa, which means good nutrition, healthcare and genetic control for animals. Traditional veterinary and husbandry practices have an important role to play in these regards. This thesis reports findings from field research on pharmacological and toxicological EVK for ruminants, equines, camels and poultry among 37 and 9 camps of Fulani (Peul) stockraisers in, respectively, Benin and Senegal. For the nearly 111 medicinal plants that interviewees identified, the following information is presented: Latin name; common names in Fula, Bariba (Benin) and Wolof (Senegal); plant collection locales in Benin, or habitat in Senegal; botanical description; and traditional use(s). The first half of the thesis presents this information in two parts: one for non-toxic (57) and one for toxic (54) medicinal plants. Some examples of treatments prepared from the former that interviewees deemed particularly effective are: a decocted drench of natron and *Anogeissus leiocarpa* root- and trunk-bark against intestinal worms, and one of papaya fruit and roots or of cotton seed (also given women) against agalactia; for snake venom in the eye, sheanut (*Butyrospermum papadoxum*) branch-tips, which the herder chews and then spits the saliva into the affected eye; to cause wounds to scar over, leaf juice of *Detarium microcarpum* dripped into the wound; for infertility and inappetence, feeding *Khaya senegalensis* bark pounded together with a certain salt from Niger that contains multiple minerals; a cold infusion of mashed *Parkia biglobosa* roots as a prophylaxis for epidemic diseases in poultry; for poultry with cholera, a drink of macerated *Pterocarpus santalinus* bark and kaolin (a fine clay) in water; the dried and powdered parts of five different plants as an antidote for poisonous snakebites in both livestock and humans. Herders keep such snakebite cures with them at all times. The author offers a personal anecdote about another such anti-dote, consisting of powdered seeds of the *Uapaca togoensis* Pax tree, ground together with the dried carcass of an *Echis* viper. Presented with two cows of the same race and age that were simultaneously bitten by a serpent in the pasture, the author watched while one cow was given this traditional preparation and the other was injected with a polyvalent antivenom serum by a veterinarian. The traditional remedy produced improvements within 2 hours, whereas the serum took 5 hours. Also described are herbal preparations for: synchronizing oestrus in a herd; bring-ing a female into heat by inserting ground *Gladiolus psittacimus* bulb into the vagina; restoring fertility by feeding decocted trunk-pith of the sheanut tree with an egg and a flea; and much more. One botanical + supernatural treatment is noted. Before administering a certain drench for dystocia, the owner of the labouring cow walks down a path leading away from his camp, striking the plants left and right along the way and uttering *barké Allah* ('in God's name') at each stroke. Toxic plants used in Fulani EVM span almost every livestock ill imaginable. A few examples are as follow. A pomade for sore or injured udders consists of baobab-seed ash in cream. To stimulate fertility, the pounded and macerated fruits of *Ficus glumosa* are administered via massages, baths and, very sparingly indeed, drenches. *Securidaca longipedunculata* roots macerated in water provide an antiseptic wash and an ectoparasiticide. Although considered highly toxic, macerated *Tinospora pakis* root may be given as a drench to camels with digestive disorders or skin erup-tions. An all-purpose poultry prophylaxis is to scatter bits of *Harungana mada-gascariensis* bark around the birds' drinking places. *Balanites aegyptiaca* has a multitude of uses, too numerous to describe here. Besides the non-botanical ingre-dients already noted, the Fulani ethnopharmacopoeia includes milk, butter, smoked fish, chicken droppings, horse urine and donkey hooves. The second half of the thesis lists 35 poisonous plants that herders know but do not employ in EVM because they are too dangerous. When consumed by livestock, these plants produce symptoms of poisoning recognized by herders: intestinal upsets, signalled by, e.g. vomiting and/or profuse diarrhoea; sweats and fever; uncoordinated move-ment; paralysis; photosensitization; abortions; accidents; and of course death. Herders' knowledge of these plants' effects on varying animal species and of their post-mortem signs are detailed, along with author notes on the chemical basis of their toxicity. In summary, this thesis' findings are striking for Fulani's over-whelming preference for using botanicals in the form of powders or ashes, which are then administered orally or sometimes intranasally in an aqueous solution. An alternative mode of administration, mentioned twice and only for calves, is placing pinches of the powdered medicament on calves' tongues just before suckling. Massages, shampoos and washes also appear to be a fairly common mode of administration. Also, the thesis is notable for detailing a great many prophylactic, as well as therapeutic, livestock treatments. Another plus is its many references to the equivalent human uses of the veterinary medicines described. Occasionally, additional plant applications are noted, e.g. in deterring pests, building fences, weaving, etc. In conclusion, the author makes a plea for safeguarding and developing this EVK 'treasure . . . for the greater health and protection of our animals' (p. 105). To this end he recommends three measures: more ethnobotanical surveys; work with herders to educate them about better hygiene in their EVM and to 'objectify' their dosage indications; and applied chemical, pharmacodynamic and clinical research to confirm and refine traditional remedies that, thanks to their cost-effectiveness, could then be extended to stockraisers everywhere the plant ingredients are to be had. Such efforts are especially important in view of the fact that formal veterinary services in Africa fail to reach so many; and when they do, they often have few medicines to offer.

Tolossa, Ayalew. 1996. Ethnoveterinary knowledge in [the] central highlands of Ethiopia. Paper presented to the Tenth Annual Conference of [the] Ethiopian Veterinary Association, 6–7 June, Addis Ababa, Ethiopia. 43 pp.

This detailed study is based on a survey of 236 Amharic and Oromo farmer-stockraisers belonging to 20 Ethiopian peasant associations that, among them, keep cattle, sheep, goats, horses, donkeys, poultry, dogs and bees. Farmers ascribe diseases to six kinds of causes: sunlight, sunfever, grass, dew, frost and supernatural aetiologies like the anger of God or guardian spirits. Interviewees also distinguish diseases as being sudden, acute or chronic. A table lists the international, Amharic, and Oromic names of 36 disease conditions. Local disease names generally reflect the species and ages of affected animals and/or the clinical signs. However, for some diseases (e.g. rabies) people will not speak the 'real name' for fear that it may attract the disease to their animals; in such cases, a metaphorically 'opposite' term may be employed. For instance, rinderpest is called 'happiness' in Amharic, and FMD is 'kindness' in Oromo. Ethiopians' ethnoveterinary practices can be grouped into five categories. First is mechanical/physical interventions such as exercise, massage and manual removal of ticks. Second are pharmacological remedies made from plants, animal products, minerals and industrial products. A table lists the vernacular and botanical names of 80 medicinal plants along with the plant parts used and the remedies' indications. Examples of some of the animal products in the Ethiopian pharmacopoeia are: mesenteric fat or butter and human urine for wound dressings; aged tail fat, butter, eggs and milk for bloat; also for bloat and other digestive problems, dung mixed with barn urine; honey for treating the oral lesions of FMD; poultry waste, burned as a fumigant for strangles in donkeys; and powdered hyena dung for saddle sores. Mineral-based treatments are: urea and kerosene for bloat; kerosene for tick and lice infestations; also for ticks plus leeches, salt mixed with pepper and butter; sulphur for skin infections; and saline for foot-rot. Among industrial products, farmers treat bloat and other digestive disorders with detergents, edible oils, Coca Cola, and the sediment from beer brewing. They use alcohol and burned cloth for disinfecting and dressing wounds. Third is surgery by farmers and/or specialized healers. It includes: wound treatment; castration, performed in a variety of ways by traditional healers; likewise for bloodletting, performed on the tongue for cattle and the wing vein for poultry; scarification; lancing of abscesses and excision of tumours; rumen trocarization; cauterization, typically with a hot sickle; obstetrical operations such as correction of dystocia and retained placenta, performed by healers known as *awwalags*; penile amputation; hoof trimming and dehorning; superficial keratectomy, done by healers specialized in this delicate operation; and cutting queen bees' wings to prevent escape. Traditional orthopaedists known as *wagesha* are considered better than their Western counterparts; along with standard fracture treatments, they know how to replace broken cattle bones using grafts from goats or hens. Fourth are management interventions. Some examples are: annual fumigation of the barn, during which all 'dirty materials are collected and burned, having smoke to keep animals from disease' (p. 29); strategic grazing on hillsides rather than in water-logged areas, to prevent liverfluke disease; maintenance and cleaning of animal shelters, including fumigating new beehives with medicinal plants and plastering hives with fresh cow dung to provide insulation and protection from disease; tracking animal age by teeth growth, to determine when to castrate, breed or begin using young animals for ploughing. Dam-calf relations are promoted by allowing neonates to suckle alone for up to 3 days. Weaning is achieved by smearing dung and aloes on the dam's teats or tying a leather muzzle studded with thorns on the calf; alternatively, calf and dam may simply be separated. To keep a cow that has lost her calf in milk, the cow is presented with a straw dummy dressed in the deceased calf's skin and sprinkled over with salt. Women are the experts in poultry management. They are astute in recognizing signs of disease, such as a blackened comb, shaggy feathers, yellowed skin, and darkened wing veins. And they know various techniques to encourage broodiness. Another part of management is dietary supplementation, like extra rations and salt for lactating cows and plough oxen or grain for chickens each morning. To prevent bloat, salt and dry feed may also be given ruminants before they are turned out to pasture in the morning. Other prophylactic management measures span isolating sick from healthy animals, slaughtering suddenly ill animals, and killing dogs and horses suspected of being rabid. Fifth are rituals and magico-religious practices, although 'the natural and super natural may be closely related' (p. 27). For example, 'church' healers known as *dabtaras* and *qallachas* perform chants over salt, salt bars, black teff bread and barley; these items may then be fed, e.g. to decrease aggression in oxen and cows or to prevent hyena attacks. Healers also prepare amulets consisting of pouches of medicines or enchanted religious, numerical, etc. writings that are tied around animals' necks or horns to prevent abortion, gentle aggressive animals, and ward off the evil eye. Farmers may tie red threads or metallic items like bells, keys or copper wire on calves, dogs and other animals to fend off diseases and the evil eye. Solemn religious vows, church donations and feasts may be indicated for birthing problems or sudden illness in cattle. Holy water from certain Coptic churches is used in myriad ways. For instance, it may be hung up in a bottle on the fence of animals' quarters, as a fetish to fend off the ill wishes of others. Or it may be administered as a drench for sudden illness, retained placenta and bloat. In such cases, the author wonders whether any special mineral content of the water may be helpful. Oromo animists sacrifice a sheep once or twice a year to promote herd fertility and productivity. Most of these magico-religious procedures are used for human ills as well. Indeed, a wide variety of both male and female healers often treat both livestock and people. For their veterinary services, they are paid in cash, kind or labour. Besides those already noted above, healers include herbalists and sorcerers. Although the latter are highly respected, they are usually called upon to solve social rather than medical problems. The author notes that ethnomedical information about livestock seems to circulate more freely than that for humans. Finally, he outlines future R&D needs in EVK as follow: further study to validate ethnoveterinary practices, inventories of village healers, the formation of healer associations, instruction of healers in modern medicine, establishment of a national committee for the study and development of traditional medicine, promotion of backyard gardens for medicinal plants, and preparation of an extension package to educate farmers on disease causes and preventive measures.

Topacio Jr., T.M. and M.L. Jovellanos. 1994. Traditional animal disease control methods in the Philippines. *Revue Scientifique et Technique de l'Office International des Épizooties* 13(2): 465–470.

In the Philippines' Benguet Province, popular ethnoveterinary practices include sacrifices, rituals, incantations, prayers, charms, incense and fumigation to ward off evil spirits that bring disease or accident. To keep 'evil spirits' away from animal sheds and water holes [places where pathogens are prone to build up and spread], a witchdoctor (*mambonong*) may be called upon to sacrifice a special albino breed of chicken or a young, black-skinned native pig. *Mambonongs* also perform sacrifices for therapeutic and livestock-fertility ends. When stock are sick or an epidemic threatens, owners tie red collars or ribbons on their animals. Sometimes such supernaturalistic practices are combined with practical health and husbandry measures. For instance, after the sign of the cross has been drawn on the foreheads and bodies of feverish pigs and cattle, the animals are rubbed down with a towel soaked in vinegar. For some diseases, an *arbularyo* 'herb doctor' may be brought in to chant incantations while burning *Arcangelista flava* stems or roots in the patients' quarters every night until the animals are cured. A practical precaution against evil spirits [at least those in the form of predators] is to fence pens, corrals and barns with thorny bamboo slats. Finally, as a charm to ensure neonate survival but also as a record of births, the owner of a newly-farrowed sow ties together a number of sticks equalling the number of piglets born.

Toyang, Ngeh J. 1997. General comments on paravets and ethnoveterinarians. *FAO Electronic Conference on Principles for Rational Delivery of Public and Private Veterinary Services.* 1 p.

This contribution to a worldwide electronic conference on the delivery of veterinary services notes that ethnoveterinary medicine was hardly mentioned during the conference, yet it is critical to solving healthcare delivery problems. The author informs that Cameroonian stockraisers interviewed about their ethnoveterinary practices reported that 60% of the livestock diseases they confront can be adequately prevented or treated with indigenous methods only, and another 31% by a combination of indigenous and orthodox medicines. According to farmers, only the remaining 9% are best treated with orthodox veterinary medicine.

Toyang, Ngeh J., Mopoi Nuwanyakpa, Christopher Ndi, Sali Django and Wirmum C. Kinyuy. 1995. Ethnoveterinary medicine practices in the Northwest Province of Cameroon. *Indigenous Knowledge and Development Monitor* 3(3): 20–22.

In a survey of EVM among Fulani of Cameroon, respondents claimed 33 out of 55 (60%) of their cattle's ills could be treated solely by ethnoveterinary medicines. Another 31% respond to a combination of EVM and orthodox veterinary medicine. According to Fulani, the remaining 9% (anthrax, blackquarter, bovine tuberculosis, CBPP and rinderpest) must be dealt with by Western medicine. More than 90% of local *materia medica* came from plants. This brief communication lists 14 of these plants. Some examples include: *Annona senegalensis* as an antiseptic for wounds and an anti-diarrhoeal; *Kigelia africana*, administered for brucellosis, retained placenta and mastitis; *Ficus elastica* for fertility enhancement; *Kalanchoe crenata* for ear problems; and *Tephrosia nana* for mange and ticks. [No precise prescriptions are given, however.] Since 1989 HPI/Cameroon's EVM and Fulani Livestock Development Project has promoted two local medicines, prepared from *Terminalia schimperiana* or *Vernonia amygdalina*, as the sole or principal drugs against helminthosis in cattle. This strategy has resulted in huge savings on annual project expenditures for commercial dewormers. Also, many poultry and most rabbit health problems are now being treated or controlled mainly through EVM. The authors strongly recommend that, in view of declining resources for veterinary care in many developing countries, governments should support the use of such local resources. Not only do they save money; they may also lead to the discovery of new and more natural drugs. To date, HPI/Cameroon has documented indigenous treatments for 55, 17, 12 and 21 ailments of cattle, horses, small ruminants and rabbits, respectively. Both on-farm and on-station testing of selected traditional remedies has been initiated, following Fulani prescriptions for plant harvesting, preservation, processing and storage. Using this information as a foundation, HPI is helping train and equip stockraisers themselves as the primary deliverers of animal healthcare, with support from trained veterinarians and with vaccines and other treatments for the 9% of ills that EVM cannot address. It is also helping people and institutions to establish backyard gardens and herbaria of medicinal plants, to ensure both *in situ* and *ex situ* conservation of these valuable species. So far, some 190 of the nearly 400 medicinal plants identified through the project have been classified scientifically and ethnotaxonomically, the latter in 10 major Cameroonian languages. Of the 190 plants identified to this point, most are multipurpose. They are used in human medicine and milk preservation and processing, as insecticides and rodenticides, and in soil amendments.

Trail, J.C.M. 1981. Merits and demerits of importing exotic cattle compared with the improvement of local breeds. In: A.J. Smith and R.G. Gunn (eds). *Intensive Animal Production in Developing Countries.* Occasional Publication No. 4. British Society of Animal Production, Thames Ditton, Surrey, UK. Pp. 191–231.

Existing indigenous populations of cattle in sub-Saharan Africa are generally well-adapted to their environment. Under harsh conditions, they demonstrate exceptional mothering behaviours, long-distance trailing abilities, water economy, heat and disease tolerance, and survival on low-quality feeds. Particularly noteworthy is trypanotolerance in the humpless N'Dama, the West African Shorthorn, and their zebu crosses. 'Trypanotolerant' is not a precise term however, as such cattle can become infected with trypanosomes to adverse effects. The author suggests that the term 'reduced susceptibility' would be more precise.

Tran DinhTu and Leigh Nind. 1998–1999. Duck health and welfare in Vietnam. *ACIAR Newsletter* 33: 7–8.

Vietnamese rice farmers raise ducks for eggs, meat, much-needed income and as biological controls on crop pests. In seeking ways to improve diagnosis of duck plague (duck virus enteritis) and to produce more effective vaccines for it, scientists from the University of Queensland, Australia and from Vietnam's National Veterinary Research Center spent time in the field learning about traditional duck-rearing techniques and their possible epidemiological implications. Vietnamese hatcheries prefer traditional incubation and duck-care methods because, despite their labour intensiveness, they are so cheap. Incubation begins by spreading 10 000 to 20 000 eggs to warm in the morning sun for 2 to 3 hours. During this time the eggs are turned several times. Next, each egg is touched against the face to test whether its temperature has reached the desired level, akin to that 'of a child with fever' say hatchery operators. Eggs that pass the test are stacked in deep bamboo baskets that hold up to 1200 eggs in layers of different-aged eggs alternated to maintain a constant temperature. Each day all the eggs are turned twice by transferring them back and forth between a full and an empty basket. Candling is done at 5, 10 and 15 days to remove infertile eggs and dead or inferior embryos. Finally, the eggs are placed on shelves, where they still must be turned by hand several times daily. All together, incubation takes about 27 days. In a typical hatchery, this process produces between 5000 and 7000 ducklings every 2 days, for immediate sale to farmers. From the first day of life, ducklings are herded on paddy fields during the day and penned at night. Health problems of concern to duck farmers include not only diseases (plague, diarrhoea, salmonellosis and pasteurellosis) but also predation by eels and snakes. For plague, farmers routinely vaccinate with either an imported or a nationally produced vaccine; some do likewise for fowl cholera (a form of pasteurellosis). Duck raisers welcomed the idea of more strategic vaccination and other cost-saving controls. They also elucidated some of their epidemiological concepts. Farmers said they worry about disease transmission from: other flocks' using the same rivers and canals as their own birds; unsold ducks they bring back home to the farm from the marketplace; and workers from other duck farms who come to visit.

Tran Thanh Xuan. 1994. Using pharmaceutical product [sic] from *Enhydra flucturans* Lour to stimulate the growth of piglets. Paper prepared for the 11–25 July Workshop to Produce an Ethnoveterinary Information Kit. IIRR, Silang, Cavite, Philippines. 4 pp.

Enhydra flucturans is one of a number of medicinal plants used in Vietnamese EVM. In this study, *E. flucturans* leaves were gathered, washed, dried, mixed with saline and phenol, and administered to pigs. Pigs injected with the plant solution gained 13% more weight than a group of control animals. This paper also mentions five other medicinal plants in Vietnam's ethnoveterinary pharmacopoeia for pigs and large ruminants: *Eclipta alba* for wounds, *Talinum crassifolium* for increasing milk production, *Houttuynia cordata* for mastitis, *Capsicum annuum* for stimulating digestion, and *Artemisia vulgaris* for making the pregnancy safe 'when the fetus is influenced badly causing belly ache' (p. 4).

Trapsida, Jean-Marie. 1994. Développement d'une politique en matière de médecine et de pharmacopée traditionnelles. In: Kakule Kasonia and Michel Ansay (eds). ***Métissages en Santé Animale de Madagascar à Haïti: Actes du Séminaire d'Ethnopharmacopée Vétérinaire 'KAGALA', un Partage de Savoirs Burkina-Faso, Ouagadougou, 15–22 Avril 1993.*** Presses Universitaires de Namur, Namur, Belgium. Pp. 77–83.

This brief conference paper traces the need for and the evolution of a policy on traditional medicine and practitioners in Niger. The author argues that recourse to these endogenous resources is necessary in view of African nations' weak economic situation coupled with their burgeoning population. He describes how Niger began to set its policies in a 1990 seminar that brought together formal-sector medical and veterinary professionals, researchers and traditional practitioners. The resulting policy had two main objectives: incorporation of this last group into national healthcare systems, including establishment of an association of 'tradi-practitioners'; and creation of a National Research Institute on Traditional Medicine. To implement this policy, an inter-ministerial committee was created. Headed by the Ministry of Public Health, it also included the ministries for agriculture and livestock, education, culture and communications, and the interior. The committee's mission is multifold: to centralize existing information on ethnomedicine in Niger; to establish research, training and production thrusts in this field, and then encourage them; to validate the efficacy and safety of traditional remedies and then extend them to the public; to promote collaboration between traditional and modern medicine; to exercise appropriate control over the practice of traditional medicine; and to interface with larger, regional entities working in the same domain.

Tripathi, Hemi, M.K. Mandape and P. Khandekar. 1997. Traditional veterinary practices in northern plains of U.P. Paper presented to the International Conference on Creativity and Innovation at Grassroots for Sustainable Natural Resource Management, 11–14 January, Ahmedabad, India. 4 pp.

In India's Uttar Pradesh state, some 300 stockowning families from 60 villages were interviewed about their traditions of animal healthcare. The remedies and practices they reported were classified by general disease domains: respiratory, digestive, skin, foot and mouth, fever, urinary, swellings, evacuation of dead calf, limping and mouth blisters. Wherever possible, the researchers attempted to identify a scientific basis for the *materia medica*. Indeed, ingredients such as *Trachyspermum ammi* and pepper, given for respiratory disorders, have antispasmodic and sudorific effects. Other materials were identified as having known anthelmintic and carminative properties. Farmers employed a variety of FMD treatments. In one, a mixture of white alum, skimmed milk, mustard oil and *chapati* bread made of Bengal gram flour is fed to the afflicted animal, while its legs and hooves are washed with a decoction of *Acacia nilotica*. In another, water containing fish scales is poured on the affected hooves. Although not all reported here, in total 80 different treatments for animal ills were identified.

Trucios, Timoteo. 1982. Tecnología alpaquera. *Minka* 8(Aug): 17.

In this short article, the author denounces 'transnational chemical laboratories with huge advertising campaigns' who say their products are more 'scientific' while at the same time that they import raw materials like botanicals to process into expensive drugs to be sold back to the nations from whence the materials came, at extremely high prices. He then describes four traditional recipes: one for making candles from alpaca fat; one for jerking llama meat; and two for treating ectoparasitic infestations in livestock. One of the latter is a cure for lice, applied topically every day to infested sites until they are healed. It consists of soaking barbasco (*Lonchocarpus* sp.) root in water for 12 hours, pounding it into a milk-like consistency and then further diluting the liquid with water. The other prescription entails applying hot, melted llama or alpaca fat to mangey sites on these same camelid species. Two such applications are said to suffice to cure the mange.

Tsongo, Angelus Mafikiri. 1998. Aspects economiques du medicament traditionnel et du medicament occidental en Afrique. *Le N'Dama: Journal du Sous-
Réseau PRELUDE Santé, Productions Animales et Environnement* 11, 12(1&2):
14–19.

In eastern Zaire, stockraisers choose traditional versus modern veterinary medicine
according to a number of factors relating to the economic risk that a stockraiser is
able and willing to assume. The first factor is herd size. The larger their herds, the
more likely people are to employ modern medicines, in order to protect the greater
financial investment that large herds constitute. Herder income is a second factor.
The richer the herder, the greater his use of modern medicaments relative to traditional ones; and vice versa for poorer stockraisers. Third, substantial subsidies for
modern veterinary inputs obviously promote their use over traditional treatments.
Likewise for herder proximity to an urban area (fourth). In urban environs, modern
veterinary care may be sought even for small ruminants and poultry. Fifth and
relatedly is the existence of credit programmes to defray the costs of modern veterinary medicine. Sixth and last is herder education. The higher the educational
level, the greater the disdain for EVM. Further, as a rule of thumb, stockraisers
prefer modern medicines for epidemic diseases that EVM cannot cope with. The
latter include viral and protozoal diseases, such as rinderpest or swine fever and
ECF, respectively. In addition to the foregoing analysis, this article presents a
summary table comparing modern and traditional veterinary medicines along the
parameters of availability, cost, access, application, yield, efficacy and period of
utilization. The author also describes how development projects' widespread sub-
sidization of, on average, 25% of the market price of veterinary inputs for associations of smallholder stockraisers in eastern Zaire triggered a livestock population
explosion. In one representative area, for instance, cattle numbers more than tripled
between 1980 and 1990. This situation engendered increased conflicts over land
between stockraisers and cultivators. Other observations of interest are that local
healers (who also treat humans) traditionally were paid in the same coin as the
animals they were called upon to cure. For example, they received a chicken for
treating poultry, a cow for treating cattle, and so forth.

Tubiana, Marie-José and Joseph Tubiana. 1975. Tradition et développement au
Soudan oriental: l'Exemple Zaghawa. In: Théodore Monod (ed.). *Pastoralism
in Tropical Africa: Studies Presented and Discussed at the XIIIth International
African Seminar, Niamey, December 1972.* Oxford University Press, London,
UK. Pp. 465–486.

Zaghawa agropastoralists live at the southern boundary of the Sahara Desert on the
Sudan–Chad border, where they raise camels, sheep, cattle and goats under a transhumant system. They know which pasture plants are preferred by each livestock
species, and they wisely graze their camels and sheep together.

Tubiana, Marie-José and Joseph Tubiana. 1977. *The Zaghawa from an Ecological Perspective: Foodgathering, the Pastoral System, Tradition and Development of the Zaghawa of the Sudan and the Chad.* A.A. Balkema, Rotterdam, The Netherlands. 111 + pp.

Zaghawa agropastoralists raise camels and sheep under a transhumant system overseen by young herdsmen. Along with horses, two types of donkeys (tall and short), and chickens, cattle and both short- and long-haired breeds of goats are kept near the villages. The long-haired goats are preferred for their larger size and better meat and milk yields. Two kinds of sheep are kept: a 'red' fat-tailed and dewlapped breed prized for its meat production; and a black, long-haired short-tailed race that endures cold, poor forages, and rocky regions better. Zaghawa distinguish four types of camels according to colour: white 'pure-blooded' ones, the most highly prized; black ones, valued for their resistance to thirst and their stamina as mounts on long journeys; grey ones, reserved for short trips; and the small and little-prized Bideyat. There is a rich vocabulary for individualizing every animal of each species. Special feeds are provided for horses and camels. The former are given 2 l of milk almost daily and occasionally balls or porridges of millet flour. Also, women regularly prepare and feed certain leaves and seeds to horses. Sometimes, special fields are cultivated for equine fodder. Camels receive natron mixed with water and sometimes cow dung in the amount of 15 to 20 kg per animal across the year. Efforts are made to drive all animals to pastures with salty grass at least once a year. People are very careful about keeping sick animals away from communal wells; a breach of this rule can lead to fatal fights. At wells, each clan has its own hand-carved troughs, identified by the clan brand. Also, people try to avoid mixing their herds with others' on pastures. Zaghawa women train all cattle calves to come for suckling when they hear the women call out their dams' individual names. Tricks to prevent suckling include fitting the young with a muzzle, smearing the dam's udder with cow or goat dung, or tying a stick onto each of the dam's teats. Herdsmens' ethnoveterinary techniques span cauterization with a red-hot iron, bleeding, adding natron to the drinking water, smearing tar on open wounds, and castrating he-camels, bulls and rams.

Uebach, L.W. 1996. Le role des femmes dans l'élevage au Ouaddai-Biltine. In: Karl-Hans Zessin (ed.). *Livestock Production and Diseases in the Tropics: Livestock Production and Human Welfare. Proceedings of the VIII International Conference of Institutions of Tropical Veterinary Medicine held from the 25 to 29 September, 1995 in Berlin, Germany.* Volume II. Deutsche Stiftung für Internationale Entwicklung, Zentralstelle für Ernährung und Landwirtschaft, Feldafing, Germany. Pp. 604–607.

Based on the experiences of a livestock development project among nomadic pastoralists of Chad, this conference paper notes that women of such groups are responsible for the daily healthcare of dairy stock and also for training the child-herders whom they supervise in the detection of disease. However, it is men's job to administer most veterinary treatments.

Upadhyaye, R.C. 1997. Ethinoveterinary [sic] paractices [sic] of Bharud and Gawali animal raiser casts of Khargone District of Madhya Pradesh. Paper presented to the First International Conference on Ethnoveterinary Medicine: Alternatives for Livestock Development, Pune, India, 4–6 November 1997. 5 pp.

Members of the Bharud and Gawali castes in India's Uttar Pradesh State are long-time stockraisers who control considerable traditional veterinary knowledge. Thus they are traditionally the ones first called in to help when other groups' animals fall ill. Livestock healers of these two castes employ plant medicines, some surgical techniques, acupuncture, firing, and, particularly among Gawalis, witchcraft. Reportedly, their recovery rates surpass 50%. Other observations based on the author's field research among these castes are as follow. In the aggregate, healers can differentially diagnose about 110 livestock ailments, and they treat all but a few bacterial and viral diseases. However, no one man knows and treats all 110. Healers generally do not charge for their services, but they jealously guard their EVK from one another, and certain healers enjoy multi-village reputations. Due to deforestation in the region, it is becoming ever more difficult to find medicinal herbs. Consequently, healers are turning more and more to commercial allopathic drugs, including many antibiotics. At the same time, younger Bharud and Gawali men no longer use EVM. Instead, they take their animals to veterinary hospitals. Overall, both castes keep fewer livestock nowadays, due to several factors: deforestation, the two castes' sedentarization, and the need for money that forces them to sell off greater numbers of animals to butchers. In conclusion, the author (a vet) finds that Bharud and Gawali EVK is far from perfect, and there is much work still to be done in terms of identifying local disease definitions in terms of scientific ones. But he has found many of these healers' prescriptions useful in his own practice.

Vabi, Boboh Michael. n.d. Fulani indigenous veterinary practices and implications for extension service delivery. Unpublished manuscript. 25 pp.

Based on the literature plus the author's participant observations in northern Cameroon and his extensive interviews in southern Nigeria, ethnoveterinary understandings and techniques among sedentary Fulani agropastoralists of the humid savannas of West Africa are overviewed here. Findings reveal that EVK differs greatly between the two regions, as evidenced in Table 1's listing of 18 disease names by region and Table 2's detailing of treatment responses to 14 of these diseases. However, Fulani EVK is everywhere quite rich and varied. And both Cameroonian and Nigerian Fulani agree on an overall bipartite categorization of diseases into those they can treat by themselves versus those that are best treated by the livestock extension service. The latter category includes brucellosis, heartwater, trypanosomosis, babesiosis and infectious keratoconjunctivitis. Even in such cases, however, before calling in an extension agent, both groups of Fulani almost always try first to treat their animals themselves, using traditional and/or modern veterinary medicine. Also, Fulani in both regions share common, traditional management practices that pertain to animal health. One is herd movement to avoid disease. In marketplaces and cattle camps, herd owners and their scouts gather information from other Fulani about disease prevalences and locations weeks or even months before making a move. Although the interlocutors in such conversations may use different disease names, via description of clinical signs they are able to communicate clearly. A second set of management strategies focuses on 'risk bearing' (p. 15). They span: for families with ample pastoral labour, breaking one's herd into several parts and grazing them separately; quartering part of one's herd with relatives; not camping close to others' herds; buying new stock only from relatives or others whose animals are known to the purchaser to be disease-free; and keeping large numbers of animals. A third management technique is the daily morning regimen of manually removing ticks from all animals in a family herd. The sight of even a single tick-ridden animal engenders 'Great scorn' (p. 17) for its owners and earns them a reputation as lazy and neglectful. Burning of areas where diseases like rinderpest and CBPP are known to have occurred or re-occur is a fourth strategy, along with a two-year prohibition on grazing any areas where blackquarter or anthrax has broken out. Fifth is seasonal dietary supplementation, notably of salt, *kanwa* (a traditional mineral supplement), and occasionally concentrate. Sixth are magico-religious practices, designed to ward against supernatural agents of disease such as various deities, evil spirits, both living and deceased ancestors, enemies and the wind. These practices span recitations and suspension of amulets with Koranic verses inscribed on them, fetishes and bouquets in kraals. Overall, the author considers that the major constraint to livestock production in the humid savannas is policy disorganization, such that appropriate research and extension services fail to reach Fulani or respond to their needs, especially as concerns the most troublesome diseases, which are linked to the humid-zone vegetation. Thus he concludes that, on the whole, 'Fulani descriptions and treatment of cattle ailments as well as health based management techniques support the argument that indigenous knowledge systems and practices are viable resources for directed change programmes' (p. 1) and suggests an R&D approach that takes off from this EVK. Additional recommendations include: whenever possible, using vernacular terms in extension work; distinguishing between innovations centred on adaptations of existing practices versus innovations intended to replace them; and responding to people's desire for modern as well as traditional veterinary medicines.

Valdizán, Hermilio and Angel Maldonado. 1985 [1922]. *La Medicina Popular Peruana: Contribución al Folklore Médico del Perú,* 3 vols. Imprenta Torres Aguirre for the Consejo Indio de Sud-América, Lima, Perú. Vol. I – 475 pp., Vol. II – 529 pp., Vol. III – 487 pp., with indices of 3, 93 and 39 additional pages, respectively.

This three-volume compendium is the classic source on human ethnomedicine in Peru. However, Volumes II and III occasionally mention ethnoveterinary applications. Examples from Volume II include the use of: sulphur to treat ectoparasitism in alpaca; a pomade of coarse brown sugar, garlic and wax to harden horses' hooves; the root of *Rumex patientia* L. to cure mange in general; *huamanripa* flowers to promote herd fertility; *Hura crepitans* L. as a purgative for horses; various cures and feeds to ward off disease and increase egg-laying among chickens; manure plasters to relieve saddle sores in horses; and many others (e.g. pp. 120, 255, 280, 419, 487, 494, 500). Perhaps the preponderance of entries emphasize ectoparasitism. Volume III notes that a mixture of llama fat and sulphur cures mange in camelids and *arestín* (an ailment of the heel). Also, rubbing a bit of the loco *mio garbansillo* (*Astragalus* spp.) on horses' lips stops them from eating it.

524

Valenciano, Lester A. and Basito S. Cotiw-an. 1980. The anthelmintic activity of betel nut (*Areca catechu*) against *Toxocara canis*. ***Mountain State Agricultural College (MSAC) Research Journal*** 6/7: 30–38.

Betel nut is widely cultivated in the Philippines, where it has long been valued in both human and livestock ethnomedicine for its purgative and vermicidal properties. The study reported here investigated the effects of a decoction of 5 g of dried, powdered betel nut (about 1 teaspoonful) in 8 g of water against common roundworms in dogs, along with tapeworm and hookworm. Naturally infested mongrel puppies were classified as slightly or severely infected, based on pre-treatment faecal egg counts. The puppies were then administered 2 cc of the decoction per kg of liveweight, and pre- and post-medication faecal egg counts were compared. A single such dose appeared sufficient to cure slight infections; severely infected animals required a second dosing a week later to become egg-free. Depending upon the amount and frequency of medication, the decoction also cured tapeworm and hookworm. Adverse effects such as emesis, salivation and ataxia were found to be linked to an animal's cachectic condition and severity of infection upon medication. The authors recommend the regime of 2 cc once or twice weekly, depending upon the infection, as a viable alternative to commercial dewormers for puppies and other animals.

Valette, G., et al. 1984. Hypocholesterolaemic effect of fenugreek seeds in dogs. *Atherosclerosis* 50(1): 105–111.

Both normal and diabetic dogs fed fenugreek seeds experienced reductions in their cholesterol and glucose levels.

Valle Zárate, Anne (ed.). 1987. *Condiciones Actuales y Potencial de la Producción Porcina para Mejorar la Situación del Pequeño Productor en la Provincia Gran Chaco – Bolivia.* Schriftenreihe des Fachbereichs No. 95. Technische Universität Berlin, Berlin, Germany.

A publication of Berlin's Technical University, this booklet reports the results of an interdisciplinary field study elaborated by a seminar group in livestock development. The focus is on the sad state of pig raising among smallholders of Bolivia's Gran Chaco Province, and ways to improve it. Husbandry conditions are extremely rustic. Pigs forage on their own by day. By night, they may be quartered in uncovered, uninclined corrals that are rarely bedded or mucked out; but 30% of the producers do not bother to corral their animals even at night. Consequently, road accidents, dog attacks, thefts, and deaths of young from cold are common. Since animals are rarely separated by sex or age, piglets also die from being rolled on by adults. Castration is asystematic. Maize is sometimes given as a dietary supplement, but often it is merely thrown down in the muck of corrals. And so forth. When it comes to veterinary care, swine-raisers of the Gran Chaco find themselves in even greater difficulties. Only 7% of interviewees had ever been visited by a veterinarian. At the time of the study, the majority of veterinarians in the area limited themselves to working with veterinary pharmacies in regional towns. Thus, producers are left to their own devices. They must provide their own diagnoses for the scores of diseases that afflict their swine, and then purchase drugs at the veterinary pharmacies or use home remedies. However, 'In many cases [their] diagnosis is mistaken and consequently [their] investment in [purchased] drugs is useless. The same result is seen when people vaccinate already-infected animals or use expired vaccines' (p. 123). The situation with regard to traditional remedies is equally grim. Unlike in other areas of Bolivia, due to the ethnic and social structure of the region, many traditional technologies have been lost. Those that remain include: treating wounds and ectoparasitism with gasoline, burnt engine oil, diesel fuel or lard; giving garlic, lemon, lime or hot chilli peppers for coughs and internal parasites; and for fevers, bleeding the ears. Faced with swine diseases, many producers simply do nothing at all. In short, they are left 'without access to modern medicine and uprooted from [their] traditional medicine' (p. 124).

Vandersmissen, Alain. 1992. PRELUDE Case Study IV. Rural Development in Ecuador and Kenya: Interrelating Health, Animal Production and the Environment. In: Georges Thill (ed.). *The Transfer of Scientific and Technological Skills and Expertise and their Appropriation: The Relevance of Associative Networks.* PRELUDE, Faculté Universitaires Notre-Dame de la Paix, Namur, Belgium. Pp. IV-7–IV-19.

A project to provide veterinary services to Quechua Indian communities in high-land Ecuador learned several important lessons in the course of attempting to intro-duce a [unspecified] commercial parasiticide. Project personnel found that Quechua still possessed a traditional pharmacopoeia. But much of the knowledge of its application for veterinary (as versus human) medical purposes had been lost, possibly due to a veritable fusilade of advertising by agroveterinary firms in Ecuador. In any case, introduction of the commercial drug represented yet another attack on Quechua's already-diminished corpus of EVK. This was true in another way too. With traditional remedies most people could treat their animals them-selves. But the commercial drug's toxicity and the complexity of calculating dosages by liveweight made it feasible to train only a few community members in its proper handling and administration. Thus introduction of such a drug consti-tuted a kind of 'de-empowerment' for local people generally. Project staff also came to realize that in the long run, the drug would probably create dependency on outsiders, who would have to be brought in again to train people in still newer drugs should chemoresistance develop. Meanwhile, it happened that the new drug doubled in price! These multiplying concerns led to a wide-ranging discussion between project personnel and stockraisers in which all came to acknowledge the value of certain traditional remedies and, on the part of Quechua themselves, the uselessness of others that they said were 'pure superstitions' (p. IV-14). Another lesson learned on this project was the value of intersectoral, human+livestock healthcare coordination. Two kinds of salt were sold in Ecuador: one with iodine and one without. The latter was intended for cattle, but because it was cheaper than iodised salt, people ate it themselves. Alerted by a health project that had been bat-tling endemic goitre in highland populations, the project noted a comparable iodine deficiency in Quechua's cattle. By instructing people in this problem and its simple solution in cattle, the project was able to 'kill two birds with one stone', as it were, to the benefit of human health as well.

Vania, Rustam. 1996. Duck rearing. *Pastures: The Newsletter about Pastoralists and Livestock Development in Asia* 1: 6.

Duck raising is big business in many parts of India, based on local varieties of ducks there. Transhumant duck herders move their birds from paddy to paddy as per carefully planned arrangements with farmers who want to garner the herds' many field services. The animals are released into paddy fields just after harvest. While feeding on fallen rice grains, insects, snails, crabs and frogs in the field, the ducks loosen and 'till' the soil, weed and manure the fields, and damp pest populations. Traditionally, herders made per-hectare egg-sales contracts with the host farmers. Today, however, they sell directly to egg dealers. Moreover, Indian duck herders now practise a truck- and train-based variant of their traditional transhumance that allows them much greater mobility and increased access to forage resources. They range as far afield as 850 km, using specially designed trucks to haul their ducks to different regions, especially those where feed is plentiful during the dry periods.

Vásquez Manríquez, Leticia, Héctor Sumano López and Luís A. Calzada Nova. 1988. Evaluación comparativa de un remedio de la medicina tradicional para el tratamiento de la traqueobronquitis en caninos. In: Luz Lozano Nathal and Gerardo López Buendía (coordinators). *Memorias: Primera Jornada sobre Herbolaria Medicinal en Veterinaria.* Universidad Nacional Autónoma de México, Facultad de Medicina Veterinaria y Zootecnia, Coordinación de Educación Continua, México DF. Pp. 85–89.

Using two groups of dogs, this experiment assessed the relative efficacy of a conventional versus a traditional treatment for bronchitis. The latter consisted of an infusion of bougainvillea, *Verbascum thapsus*, *Crataegus mexicana*, eucalyptus, cinnamon, lemon and honey. Findings showed equal outcomes for both treatments as measured by temperature, presence or absence of cough, and pulmonary sounds; however, the traditional treatment was superior in diminishing mucus and other secretions. The authors suggest that, with the exception of antibiotics, traditional remedies may often be able to substitute for orthodox ones. Moreover, such remedies are cheaper and more readily accessible. The authors opine that ethnomedical knowledge is a great patrimony of Third World countries and can play an important role in their technological and economic development.

Vedavathy, S. 1999. Ethnomedico-botany and its sustenance. In: E. Mathias, D.V. Rangnekar and C.M. McCorkle, with M. Martin (eds). *Ethnoveterinary Medicine: Alternatives for Livestock Development – Proceedings of an International Conference Held in Pune, India, 4–6 November 1997. Volume 1: Selected Papers.* BAIF Development Research Foundation, Pune, India. Pp. 99–102.

India boasts about 450 000 plant species, of which as many as 20 000 possess known medicinal properties. Yet in India as well as most of the world, plant species are disappearing at a frightening rate. This conference paper sounds a clarion call for the conservation of this invaluable biodiversity along with the ethnomedical knowledge about it. Immediate actions needed are to: update information about the present extent and distribution of medicinal plant resources; establish a network of protected areas to preserve these plants' ecotypes and gene pools; investigate ways to cultivate the plants, especially species under acute pressure; accelerate inventorying and screening of plants for pharmacological activity. The author also offers thoughts about the need for: national health policies and financial support for ethnomedical systems; communication and collaboration across indigenous medical systems; the rights of indigenous peoples with regard to their ethnobotanical knowledge base; and international patenting. Also, she introduces the notion of 'paramedicines' i.e. traditional medicines prepared with enhanced quality controls but without subjecting them to excessive research to isolate all their active ingredients.

Veena, T. 1997. Punya-koti [sic] test to diagnose pregnancy in cattle: An indigenous bioassay based on the ancient Egyptian practice. In: Anil Gupta (ed.). *International Conference on Creativity and Innovation at Grassroots for Sustainable Natural Resource Management, January 11–14, 1997: Abstracts.* Indian Institute of Management, Ahmedabad, India. P. 79.

According to papyri excavated from the pyramids of Kahun, ancient Egyptians employed a simple pregnancy test for women, based on the response of wheat and barley seeds soaked in the subject's urine. In a unique re-application of this technique to modern-day cattle, the author reports that cow pregnancies can be predicted with more than 80% probability when seed germination and seedling growth are inhibited by at least 70% and 60%, respectively, after exposure to the suspect animal's urine. Although research remains to be done on the mechanism behind these responses, preliminary results suggest the involvement of abscisic acid, a plant hormone known to inhibit seed germination.

Veena, T. and R. Narendranath. 1993. An ancient Egyptian pregnancy test extended to cattle. *Current Science* 65(12): 989–990.

Based on clues provided in ancient Egyptian papyri of 2100 to 2200 B.C., researchers attempted to devise a simple diagnostic test for pregnancy in cattle. The test relies on the differential response in germination and shoot growth of wheat seeds to the urine of pregnant and non-pregnant cows. Results showed that germination and shoot growth are suppressed by the urine of pregnant cows, whereas the urine of non-pregnant cows causes no growth inhibition. This differential response is probably due to the presence or absence of auxins (plant hormones) in the urine.

Veena T., R. Narendranath and P.V. Sarma. 1996. The reliability of ancient Egyptian pregnancy diagnosis for cows/buffaloes. *Advances in Contraceptives and Delivery Systems* 13: 49–53.

This article reports on a re-run of the experiment reported in Veena and Narendranath 1993, and reconfirms the earlier findings.

Vega, Belita. 1994. Indigenous crop cultivars in central and eastern Visayas. In: *Proceedings of the Seminar-Workshop on IK in Agriculture.* Visayas State College of Agriculture, Baybay, Leyte, Philippines. Unpaginated.

This article includes a 6-page table of 'Botanicals for Indigenous Control of Pest [sic] and Diseases in Crops and Livestock'. For each such plant species, the table notes: Latin, local and, where known, English names; plant parts used; crop or livestock species to which applied; for which pest or disease; and locations in the Philippines where the plant is thus employed. Treatments are listed for wounds, dog bites, swollen limbs, intestinal parasites, skin diseases, footrot, ticks and other ectoparasites, diarrhoea, castration, coughs, abscesses, fevers and fowl cholera in, variously, cattle, buffalo, sheep, goats, pigs and chickens. A total of 45 plant species are employed for livestock. Many are food plants like avocado, banana, beans, bitter gourd, citrus fruits, coconut, garlic, ginger, guava, hot peppers, mango, onion, papaya, pineapple, squash and sweet potato. A few other examples are: *Derris elliptica* for intestinal worms of buffalo and footrot in sheep and goats, and *Derris philippinensis* for larval ticks of cattle; *Leucaena leucocephala* for internal parasites of pigs; and *Spondias pinnata* for colds and coryza in chickens.

Veluw, Kees van. 1987. Traditional poultry keeping in Northern Ghana. *ILEIA Newsletter* 3(4): 12–13.

The Mamprusi tribe of northern Ghana see themselves mainly as cultivators. However, they also raise livestock, especially chickens and guinea fowl, because of the animals' high earnings. The birds are raised under a free-range system, although they are nightly supplemented with a handful of grain before retiring to their quarters underneath granaries. A young boy accompanies the flock during the day, to keep it out of cultivated fields and to protect it from predators. Occasionally he also collects pieces of termite hills for the poultry to feast on the insects. Because guinea fowl are bad brooders, Mamprusi use chickens to hatch the guinea fowl's eggs. Mortality is high among both species, with an overall rate of 75%. In rank order, death is due to: disease, especially Newcastle; predators, including snakes, raptorial birds, dogs and cats; and road accidents. Nevertheless, Mamprusi households annually harvest about 110 eggs, 65 young birds and 7 old ones; and 15% of a family's cash income derives from sales of eggs and birds. Red, white and black roosters fetch double the normal price because each of these colours is required for certain types of ritual sacrifices during key religious, social and juridical events. Moreover, only indigenous roosters can be used for these purposes. The author concludes with a discussion of the inadvisability of introducing exotic species.

Venkataramaiah, P. and Arati V. Marathe. 1998. Veterinary medicinal plants of Nandurbar Taluka. In: E. Mathias, D.V. Rangnekar and C.M. McCorkle, with M. Martin (eds). *Ethnoveterinary Medicine: Alternatives for Livestock Development – Proceedings of an International Conference Held in Pune, India, 4–6 November 1997. Volume 2: Abstracts.* BAIF Development Research Foundation, Pune, India. P. 58.

More than 70% of the population in the Taluka region of India are tribals such as Bhils, Gamits, Gavits, Kokanis, Mavchis, Tadvis, Valvis and Vasaves, spread over 95 villages west of Nandurbar town. A preliminary survey of ethnoveterinary medicinal plants used in the area was conducted, focusing on the five most common livestock diseases. About 30 such plants were recorded. For each, this paper presents the following information: details of plant parts used; preparation and dosage of medicines; vernacular names in Marathi, the local tribal language, and, wherever possible, English; and herbarium voucher number.

Verma, M.R. 1967. *Dairy Husbandry of Nomadic Gujjars in Six South-East Himachal Forest Ranges.* MS thesis, Haryana Agricultural University, Hissar, India.

Besides dairy practices, this thesis describes post-partum measures taken for cattle by Gujjar nomads of India (pp. 36–93). Once a newborn calf begins breathing, herders cut the umbilical cord with a sickle or scissors, tie off the cord with a thread, and cauterize it with a dusting of powdered charcoal. Meanwhile, the dam is prevented from eating the placenta at all costs, as this is believed to cause digestive and lactation problems. If the animal manages to ingest the placenta nevertheless, decoctions of ginger, soya and other plants are given to ensure good milk yield. [Abstract based on Gupta et al.'s 1990 annotated bibliography.]

Verma, M.R. and Y.P. Singh. 1968. Veterinary therapy in a nomadic setting. *Punjab Veterinarian* 7: 78–82.

Nomadic Gujjars of India's Himachal Pradesh region are famed throughout northern India for their cattle breeding. With no access to formal veterinary services, Gujjars have devised many veterinary treatments of their own. For the lice and ticks that pose serious production problems, Gujjars take mainly a prophylactic approach. Knowing that lice eggs attach to cattle's coats where they later mature, herders regularly clip the animals' hair. This method greatly reduces lice infestation. Ticks are manually removed and destroyed. Flies and mosquitoes, which disrupt peaceful rumination, are driven off by smoke screens created by burning wet tree leaves, straw and dung throughout the night and morning. Mange is treated with topical applications of powdered sulphur in sarson oil. To ward against land leeches, people avoid camping in areas where these pests abound and/or they smear cattle's legs with salt. For aquatic leeches, which attach to the animals' mouths and throats when they drink at pools, prophylactic measures are to close off the infested pools with bushes or to add crushed *Bauhinia vehlii* plants to the water. This homemade pesticide is said to kill the leeches while leaving the water safe for animals to drink. One therapy is nasal drenching with copper sulphate solution or with the leaf extract from a bitter shrub, both of which cause violent sneezing and thus ejection of the leeches. Another is to withhold water for a day and then, when animals are finally allowed to drink, to pull out the leeches, which poke their heads out of the nose in search of water. Treatments for conjunctivitis, keratitis and thread worms are varied: dusting the eye with potassium nitrate powder; applying an ointment of copper sulphate in butter; or spitting or blowing salt into the eye. However, the authors doubt that any of these eye treatments are effective. In an attempt to prevent blackquarter, which is believed to signal supernatural displeasure, Gujars brand young cattle with a red-hot horseshoe on the shoulder joint or the thigh. But this technique sometimes produces dirty, recalcitrant wounds. In any case, Gujars today prefer modern vaccines for this pernicious disease. Wounds are classified as 'wet' (bleeding) or 'dry'. The former are plastered with cow dung or dry mud; the latter are dressed with hot ghee and *methi*. Bites by snakes and wild animals are cauterized with a hot iron in order to 'kill' the poison. Examples of cough cures are having the animal inhale the smoke from a smouldering cloth soaked in sarson oil or feeding a fistful of paddy rice and chillies. A general treatment for plant poisoning is to drench with milk or, if that fails, ghee. To prevent abortions, Gujars forbid pregnant cows feeds like linseed, cottonseed, *Quercus dilatata*, *Q. incana*, oil and ghee; and they prescribe feedings of certain plants, like *Grewia oppositifolia*. They also guard the cows against bull teasing; and sometimes local healers remove the false membranes on the *os uteri* of repeater cows.

Verma, M.R. and Y.P. Singh. 1969. A plea for studies in traditional animal husbandry. *The Allahabad Farmer* 43(2): 94–98.

This article questions many of the practices of nomadic Gujjar herders of India. Does *Grewia oppositifolia* and mustard soaked in water and administered to cows after service help implantation of the foetus? Is there a relationship between linseed, *Quercus incana*, and *Q. dilatata* leaves fed to dairy cattle and the quality of butter produced? The authors make a plea for validation, as well as simple reporting, of such ethnoveterinary techniques. [Abstract based on Gupta et al.'s 1990 annotated bibliography.]

Vetaid. 1989. Special article: Using expatriate volunteers to establish training schedules for primary livestock health workers. *Vetaid News* 2: 3–4.

This short article makes two points of interest for EVK. First, to set up effective CAHW programmes, 'it is essential . . . to have knowledge of the local disease picture i.e. the most common diseases and . . . their local names and treatments that are known to be effective locally'. Because national disease data hardly ever provide such information, it is best collected directly from local stockraisers. Second, it is not necessary for stockraisers or CAHWs to be able to make definitive diagnoses before treatment. They need only differentiate among, e.g. diarrhoea that should not be treated with antibiotics, that should be treated with anthelmintics, or that should be referred to a professional veterinarian. Thus, they can be trained to work from clinical presentation to appropriate treatment through a path of simple yes/no questions, analogous to flow-chart diagnosis procedures used in medical computers. [This same approach could be used as a methodology for encoding local ethnodiagnostic and treatment knowledge, as well.]

Vetaid. 1991. Tim makes tracks to Afghanistan. *Vetaid Newsletter* 6: 2.

This short report announces the plan to identify 'local experts' with considerable knowledge of traditional animal healthcare in Vetaid's Afghani project. To build sustainable healthcare institutions, the work of such experts can be promoted and enhanced by training them in appropriate new techniques such as the use of modern medicines and vaccines or of crop byproducts as fodders.

Vetaid. 1994. What's next for Vetaid! *Vetaid Newsletter* 11(Winter): 3.

Here, Vetaid notes its intent to research traditional healers' medicines and traditional husbandry practices to avoid or control livestock diseases in Tanzania, so as to identify 'ways in which the debilitating trend to dependence on imported Western medicines may be reduced'.

Vetaid. 1997a. A dip tank attendant's story. *Vetaid Newsletter* 16(Winter): 2.

This brief article tells the story of one among many dip tank attendants in Mozambique who contracted arsenic poisoning from the livestock dipping compounds used for many years in that country. Dealing with these dangerous chemicals led to the man's early retirement from his job due to uncontrollable shaking and, ultimately, an almost complete paralysis. Vetaid is now training Mozambican attendants in the proper use of more environmentally friendly insecticides.

Vetaid. 1997b. Ethnoveterinary development project. *Vetaid Newsletter* 16(Winter): 1.

Vetaid announces its garnering of funds for a two-year project in Tanzania, for this nation to develop and maintain its ethnoveterinary knowledge and corresponding resource base. The project's goal is to document and validate alternative treatments for common animal ailments that are too expensive for pastoralists to treat with modern medicines.

Vetaid. 1998. The 1998 Arusha agricultural show. *Moredun News* 8: 2.

Vetaid work on EVK has revealed a number of local plants used by Simanjiro pastoralists of Tanzania to treat their livestock. A Vetaid display at the 1998 Arusha agricultural show featured pressed botanical samples of these plants plus details of their application for FMD, pyometra, mastitis, worms, calf scours, babesiosis, ephemeral fever, tick infestation and poisoning. In this last case, for example, poisoned stock are drenched with a tobacco solution; in addition, they may be bled and a handful of mud placed in their mouths. For FMD, non-botanical as well as botanical materials may be employed. For instance, a common treatment is to smear salt and ash on the buccal sores of FMD while applying the same materials, but mixed with cattle urine, to the hoof lesions.

Vetaid and CTVM. 1992. *The Daye Chopan Community Animal Health Care Project: First Phase Mid Period Report & Second Phase Proposal.* VetAid and CTVM, Edinburgh, UK. 55 pp.

The above-referenced community animal healthcare project included attention to local livestock experts among farmers in Afghanistan's Daye Chopan District, where 'government veterinary services are nonexistent' (p. 32). These experts were all men, usually Koochi pastoralists who had settled in farming communities. Experts were all well-respected; and farmers regularly consulted them *gratis* on what is locally termed *yunani* medicine, i.e. firing, bleeding, and the use of medicinal plants. Farmers themselves were adept at giving their animals injections, even intravenously, thanks to clinics' dispensing injectible drugs for humans. Research revealed that 'the livestock experts within the community were quite good at diagnosing diseases with definitive symptoms and all these diseases had specific names' (ibid.). But understandably, per-acute diseases or non-specific, chronic ailments sometimes stumped expert diagnosis. Experts' diagnostic knowledge was further constrained by the fact that only ritually slaughtered stock can be eaten. If an animal dies from disease before it can be administered the proper 'last rites', so to speak, its meat is tabooed for human consumption. Consequently, people rarely see a disease run its full course.

Villemin, M. 1984. L'empirisme, une necessité ou un anachronisme? *Ethnozootechnie* 34: 25–39.

This article is primarily devoted to tracing the evolution of veterinary medicine in France from a tradition of empiricism to a legalized, scientized profession. In the process, however, the author notes the continuing importance of a number of 'veterinary saints' specific to different species or types of disease (p. 29).

Vivekanandan, P. 1997. Personal communication to M. Martin of 8 May 1997. 1 p.

In India's Tamil Nadu State, anoestrous dairy cattle and buffalo traditionally are fed *Aloe vera* and *Cicer arietinum*. An on-farm trial to test this treatment was conducted using two cattle and eight buffalo cows. For 3 days, the animals were fed the flesh extract of a single *A. vera* leaf. This was followed by 2 weeks' feeding of 200 g of sprouted *C. arietinum* daily. Nine of the ten cows conceived after the treatment.

Vivekanandan, P. n.d.a Sri Muthu Servai's Herbal Medicine for Cattle Diseases. SEVA, Madurai, Tamil Nadu, India. 2 pp.

Seven ethnoveterinary treatments used by a renowned 90-year-old healer (Sri Muthu Servai) of humans and animals in India's Tamil Nadu State are presented in this short article, as collected and documented by SEVA staff. Pounded together and mixed with water, the plants *Acorus calamus*, *Clerodendrum phlomidis*, *Foeniculum vulgare*, *Helicteres isora* and *Piper nigrum* are administered to cattle with alimentary problems or swollen faces. The same mixture is also applied to fractured bones. Hypothermia in cattle is relieved by burning a burlap bag soaked in rice water or paddy straw on top of pebbles. Stiffness is alleviated by a fomentation using a burlap bag soaked in a certain plant extract. In buffalo with swollen tongues, the tongue tip is bled to release toxic blood. For cattle with white spots on the cornea, *Barberea cuspidata*, pepper seeds, betel nut and leaves, and tobacco are chewed, spat into a cloth, and then the extract is squeezed through the cloth into the eye. Finally, 2 fruits and 4 leaves of *Strychnos nux-vomica* are pounded together and fed for indigestion. The article notes that, while the 90-year-old healer's son has chosen to follow in his footsteps, his grandson has not.

Vivekanandan, P. n.d.b Traditional Cattle Treatments in Dharmapuri District, Tamil Nadu. SEVA, Madurai, Tamil Nadu, India. 1 p.

This paper describes traditional prescriptions for the relief of dysentery, stomach problems, infertility, calf scours, diarrhoea, retained placenta and fractured bones in cattle in one part of India, as reported by a traditional healer to SEVA staff and documented by the author. To take one example, *Pergularia daemia, Abrus precatorius, Diospyros montana*, cumin, pepper, garlic, *Aristolochia bracteolata*, asafoetida and *Tinospora cordifolia* are finely ground, mixed with hot water, and given morning and evening to assuage shivers in fevered cattle.

Vivekanandan, P. n.d.c Traditional Veterinary Practices in Pattukkottai and Perauvarani areas of Tamil Nadu. SEVA, Madurai, Tamil Nadu, India. 2 pp.

As reported to R.S. Narayanan and documented by the author, this paper lists a number of traditional veterinary prescriptions from a father–son pair of healers in India's Tamil Nadu State. The pair also treat humans. Diseases treated include bloat, diarrhoea, bloody diarrhoea, FMD, stiffness and shivering, fever and poisonous snakebites. Bloat, anorexia, cachexia, anaemia, swelling, arthritis, paralysis and dermatitis in cattle are treated with various preparations involving a total of 64 ethnopharmaceuticals and/or natural ingredients. The latter include cumin, garlic, ginger, turmeric, pepper, nutmeg and copper sulphate. The ingredients are purified, powdered with palm sugar, and mixed with hens' eggs before they are fed to cattle. FMD and fevers are treated with Avuri leaf tablets (*Indigofera tinctoria*). For snakebite, the patient's forehead is branded with a hot sickle and then sprinkled with the kern powder of *Strychnos nux-vomica*. An internally administered snakebite remedy consists of the dried, calcined, powdered (and thus de-toxified) fruit-flesh of *S. nux-vomica*.

Vondal, Patricia J. 1987. Intensification through diversified resource use: The human ecology of a successful agricultural industry in Indonesian Borneo. *Human Ecology* 15(1): 27–51.

This article thoroughly describes the successful evolution of an indigenous industry in commercial duck egg production in South Kalimantan, Indonesia. The shift from allowing flocks to forage in swamp to caging and feeding them with high-quality, low-cost homemade rations is detailed. The rations are prepared from 'concentrate', a multivitamin-protein additive manufactured in Java, combined with a variety of local materials. The latter include chopped sago palm, swamp vegetation, dried fish, snails and rice bran. Research suggests that this mix is 'equal to the maize-based diets used in Western countries in terms of growth and development of the bird' (pp. 37–38). Along with other innovations [see Vondal 1989], these changes markedly increased egg production and family income.

Vondal, Patricia J. 1989. Poultry management experimentation and productivity in a native Indonesian agroindustry. Paper presented to the Annual Meeting of the American Association for the Advancement of Science, San Francisco, California, USA, 14–19 January. 9 pp.

This paper reports on the successful application of local knowledge to the development of a rural duck hatchery industry in South Kalimantan, Indonesia. Duck farming is an ancient activity in many parts of Southeast Asia. In addition to experimenting with feeding and caging systems [Vondal 1987], farmers in South Kalimantan also successfully adopted an ancient Balinese incubation technique to replace expensive and hard-to-manage Muscovy brood hens. The method consists of packing rice hulls among layers of fertile eggs in cylindrical containers. The layers are shifted consistently to maintain precise temperature control. The resulting hatchability rate of 80% to 85% is the same as that derived from brood hens, but with great savings in production costs. When the success of this system was demonstrated, the current (1979) president of Indonesia proclaimed it a 'modern' improvement, and US aid officials rushed to offer farmers a loan for purchase of an electric hatchery. In view of the general lack and great expense of electricity, the loan was refused. As the author sums up, '. . . the Balinese system afforded the mass production methods needed. The technology involved has the additional virtue of being entirely appropriate for the rural economy of South Kalimantan where rice hulls are abundant, and electrical outlets are not' (pp. 6–7).

Vondal, Patricia J. 1996. Banjarese management of duck health and nutrition. In: Constance M. McCorkle, Evelyn Mathias and Tjaart W. Schillhorn van Veen (eds). *Ethnoveterinary Research & Development.* Intermediate Technology Publications, London, UK. Pp. 158–166.

Ducks have been raised in Southeast Asia for at least 2000 years. Today, in areas like the interior swamplands of Indonesian Borneo, duckraising continues to play a key role in the farming systems of the native Banjarese inhabitants. For well over 100 years, Banjarese have pursued an active commercial trade in duck meat, eggs and hatchlings. This chapter describes how – as populations exploded, household landholdings shrank, and consumer demand for poultry products surged – Banjarese shifted from their traditional, extensive regime of herding ducks to a self-designed intensive regime entailing confinement of the birds and greater specialization in eggs. A signal feature of contemporary Banjarese duckraising is its emphasis on disease prevention rather than cure. Significantly, no formal veterinary services for ducks exist in the area. Farmers take measures to protect the birds against sharp climatic fluctuations and extremes. Any sick birds are immediately quarantined. Also, flocks are divided by age, size and health status, so as to provide more specialized care. The latter includes tailored feeding schedules and age-specific rations mixed from locally available and highly nutritious materials (e.g. bran and cooked snail meat, fish and rice) technoblended with a commercially produced multivitamin protein supplement. Banjarese religiously practise good hygiene in: feed preparation, handling, storage and presentation; cage construction and cleaning; and watering. They also emphasize the importance of exercise, especially for the healthy development of young birds. Thus, up until age 6 months, ducklings are allowed periods of free foraging; and farmers furnish their cages with exercise equipment in the form of dangling items for the ducklings to jump at and peck. Banjarese farmers continue to experiment with low-cost ways to improve duck health and nutrition. Many of their management practices might serve as a model that farmers in other developing countries could adopt or adapt to increase their poultry enterprises' productivity and profitability.

VSF/Switzerland. 1998. Ethnoveterinary workshop – Malual Kon, Sudan, 9–12 November 1998. Unpublished manuscript received electronically. VSF/ Switzerland, Nairobi, Kenya. *Ca.* 17 pp.

This document reports on the structure and results from an ethnoveterinary workshop jointly convened by VSF/Switzerland and Save the Children Foundation/UK in order to follow up on findings from a 1996 UNICEF consultancy on EVK for the Operation Lifeline Sudan (OLS) livestock programme. The workshop brought together VSF and SCF staff with eight respected *atet*, traditional Dinka healers of livestock and people. Workshop objectives embraced: sharing knowledge and information between *atet* and OLS; further documenting ethnoveterinary practices and their efficacy; and exploring how to assist healers in their work without undermining or disrupting it. Participants were divided into two groups and asked to list the most important diseases of livestock in the region along with corresponding variables like: each disease's signs, traditional treatments, and recognized treatment side effects; immunity, seasonality and transmission aspects of each disease; opinions as to each treatment's efficacy, including recovery rates and treatment costs where known; and application of these same treatments to humans. This exercise produced information on 22 ailments of cattle, small ruminants and chickens, along with additional descriptions of surgical operations performed by *atet*. A sampling of findings includes the following. Besides botanicals, *materia medica* include honey, baking powder, alcohol, cattle urine, mud and crow feathers plus modern commercial medicines. Healers claim a good success rate from driving cattle through running water to cure *akuet kuet* (possibly hypomagnesaemic tetany). Likewise for various smoke inhalation treatments for *dony dony* (possibly avitaminosis A or ephemeral fever) in combination with withholding drinking water. Quite a few treatments involve spitting, blowing or otherwise introducing the *materia medica* into the patient's ears and especially nostrils, instead of or as well as the mouth. People know not to handle or eat the meat of stock dead of anthrax; but sometimes they do so anyway, adding *Acacia albida* fruit and/or leaves to the stewpot. Occasionally, deathly ill animals are handed over to another specialist, the spearmaster (*bany bith*), for him to dispose of them at his own risk however he sees fit. The spearmaster is also called upon to cast faecal samples from diarrhoeal animals into the river, so as to carry away the illness. A third type of specialist, an *apeth*, is engaged for cases of poisoning. An *apeth* is a person with evil eye who can remove poison from dogs, cattle and people. Surgical interventions span: castration; lancing abscesses and excising growths on the skin and bones, often followed by suturing; amputation, as in cropping bulls' ears; insertion of medicinal plant materials under the skin; cauterization; and various obstetric procedures, for which some *atet* take care first to wash their hands and trim their nails. *Atet* backgrounds and professional practices were also discussed at the workshop. All eight healers in attendance had had *atet* fathers; however, they noted that an aspiring healer can apprentice himself to someone other than his father for a fee. Women are not trained as *atet*. Healers reported that they acquire new EVK from their travels to other areas and from exchanges with colleagues. They also observed that the success of even the best of treatments is dependent on healer skill. In rank order, *atet* scored their most reliable ethnotreatments as those for castration, retained placenta, dystocia, *dony dony*, skull injuries and amputations. Asked about their views on actual and potential OLS veterinary interventions, *atet* responded that: some major diseases had been better controlled as a result of OLS paravets, with concomitant reductions in both livestock and human deaths; paravets did cut into *atet* business somewhat, but not in remote areas or in surgical cases; *atet* would welcome OLS assistance to help them in treating five diseases that they find particularly difficult (anthrax, blackleg, CBPP, haemorrhagic septicaemia and trypanosomosis); relatedly, they would also like access to Western medicines generally, and specifically to anaesthetics for surgery and to injectable drugs, plus basic equipment like burdizzos, better splints for fractures, and bicycles, the latter to cover the long distances entailed in gathering botanicals. Appended to the workshop report are: a table of Dinka and presumed English names of common livestock diseases, plus the scientific aetiologies and the animal species affected; and a table of local and Latin names [where known] for the medicinal plants mentioned at the workshop. Also noted in the text is the existence of a World Food Programme database on plants of southern Sudan.

Vučevac-Bajt, V. and M. Karlović. 1994. Traditional methods for the treatment of animal diseases in Croatia. ***Revue Scientifique et Technique de l'Office International des Épizooties*** 13(2): 499–512.

This article details scores of popular veterinary treatments for non-contagious diseases of horses in 17th- and 18th-century Croatia, as recorded in a specialized genre of early medical texts on healing for both livestock and humans. Both natural and supernatural treatments were employed, singly or in combination. For instance, in an act of sympathetic magic, anuria might be treated by feeding the air-bladder of a herring (i.e. treating like with like); but along with the bladder, the patient would also be given bread and *Artemisia abrotanum* L. leaves and flowers.

A few among many examples of treatments the authors deem to have been helpful include the following: also for anuria, placing a louse under the foreskin, where the irritation provokes urination; applying salt and hot lard to traumatic exostoses on the legs of horses, thus inducing local inflammation; rubbing areas with skin diseases with a mixture of oats and *Urospermum picioides* or with lentil-bean ashes; fitting hobnailed hooves with a piece of felt dipped in wheel grease before re-shoeing; plastering a hoof that has become detached from the muscles with a cast of hemp cloth, quicklime, and eggshells; for overfed horses, giving laxatives in the form of an anal suppository of soap, a soapy drench, or a drench of salt and human urine; deworming by feeding with dried *A. abrotanum* L., which has known anthelmintic effects; for aches and bruises, massaging horses with wine vinegar; washing injuries with distilled wine, which helps dissolve necrotic tissue and serves as a mild disinfectant; cooking *Atropa belladonna*, jimsonweed (*Datura stramonium*), or black henbane (*Hyoscyamus niger* L.) into an antidote for poisoning. Although they pose a risk of secondary infection, certain aspects of 'dirty pharmacy' were also helpful. Some examples are: poultices of cattle and swine faeces for bruises in both animals and humans; or, still in use today, hoof ointments of charcoal and cow dung. Likewise for other kinds of treatments that, like mercury-based preparations for pediculosis, can be beneficial but can lead to intoxication. Also noted are various running, riding and flogging prescriptions that, depending on the ailment, may have been helpful or harmful. The authors judge that most treatments for eye disorders were harmful. These consisted of: blowing any of a variety of powders into the patients' eyes, such as ground *Agrostemma githago* L. or *Aconitum napellus* L., or crushed oyster- or snail-shell; or applying ointments made from honey and quail grease, from willow cream and ashes, or from roasted and crushed snail, ginger and copper sulphate. Examples of indifferent treatments include: for anuria, feeding 'sea dust' (pulverized *Sepia officinalis*) between meals; for inappetence, a topical application or intranasal drench of powdered *Artemisia arborescens* L. cooked in strong vinegar and filtered. A number of traditional Croatian treatments for non-contagious diseases remain in use today. This is especially the case for fractures, inflammations and organic diseases. In contrast, many 'cures' for infectious diseases ultimately fell into disuse because they proved unsuccessful. This was particularly the case for rabies, glanders, rinderpest, anthrax and classical swine fever. Overall, the authors estimate that: while many folk medicines were helpful, many also were of dubious value and sometimes even harmful; purely magical rituals were 'devoid of therapeutic effect' (p. 500); and the best traditional practices were those related to surgical interventions. A number of the relatively effective practices remain in folk use today and/or have been adapted and introduced into scientific medicine.

Vyas, A.P. 1998. Ethnoveterinary practices among pastoralists of the Indian Thar Desert. In: E. Mathias, D.V. Rangnekar and C.M. McCorkle, with M. Martin (eds). *Ethnoveterinary Medicine: Alternatives for Livestock Development – Proceedings of an International Conference Held in Pune, India, 4–6 November 1997. Volume 2: Abstracts.* BAIF Development Research Foundation, Pune, India. Pp. 59–60.

Both sedentary and migratory herders of India's Thar Desert earn their living by raising livestock under extremely stressful and remote conditions. In the absence of any formal veterinary institutions and infrastructure, EVM is key to sustaining the desert peoples' stockraising systems. They treat their animals with a wide array of methods, e.g.: firing; plant medicines; special feeds for newborns, pregnant animals and stud bulls; and careful selection and breeding of livestock that maintains herds' genetic diversity. These peoples' age-old stockraising knowledge could be of value to modern animal scientists seeking to devise improved herding, feeding and breeding techniques.

Waffenschmidt, V. 1996. Traditional veterinary practice in northern Zambia. Handout for farmers, extension and veterinary staff. Farming Systems Research Team, Northern Province, Zambia. 17 pp.

Farmers of northern Zambia identified 20 local livestock diseases (seven for cattle, six for goats, four for pigs and three for poultry), their signs and occurrence, plus 87 different treatments for them. For instance, local treatments for ECF spanned: cauterizing the inflamed lymph nodes with a hot axe, followed by drenching with a teacupful of bean ash suspended in water; drenching with sisal soaked in water for one hour; or snipping off the tips of the patient's ears and allowing the blood to flow freely.

Wagner, Günter. 1970. *The Bantu of Western Kenya with Special Reference to the Vugusu and Logoli. Vol. II: Economic Life.* Oxford University Press, London, UK. 184 pp.

Pages 39–53 of this ethnography deal with animal husbandry and ethnoveterinary medicine. The Vugusu Bantu bleed their oxen, heifers and bull calves to obtain blood for human consumption and as a treatment against leanness. They use a special bow and arrow for this purpose. Another form of curative bleeding is cutting the ears of cattle. The herders select bulls but not cows with certain attributes for breeding. The remaining bulls are castrated by specialists who dress the castration wounds with ashes. Herders aid their cows in giving birth. The Vugusu have a good knowledge of livestock anatomy, as their extensive vocabulary for body parts and organs demonstrates. Wagner describes 13 disease conditions in cattle and their native treatments. Blackquarter is prevented by mixing the blood of a diseased animal with pounded roots and sprinkling it on the backs of the healthy animals. Magic is used for barren cows and for protection against evil and theft.

Wagner, Wilhelm. 1926. *Die chinesische Landwirtschaft.* Paul Parey, Berlin, Germany. 668 pp.

Chapter 4 of this treatise on Chinese agriculture describes the husbandry of silkworms, horses, donkeys, mules, cattle, buffaloes, yaks, camels, pigs, small ruminants and poultry. Wagner discusses ethnoveterinary practices for some of these animals. Alum plays an important role in Chinese ethnoveterinary medicine. In mules, mild cases of lameness remain untreated. In severe cases, the coronet or other parts (depending on the cause of the lameness) are pierced with a needle several times up to 1 cm deep. This treatment provokes the formation of a haematoma and, according to the Chinese, improves blood circulation to the affected area. Piercing is also used for colics and other ills. Periodic eye infection in mules is treated by bleeding or by spitting a concentrated salt solution into the animals' eyes. If a camel has a wound in its hoof, a piece of hide is wrapped around the hoof or sutured to the camel's skin. Other cases of lameness are treated as described for mules. Mange is widespread in camels; treatment consists of the application of a rhubarb preparation or burning the wounds with acidic substances. The Chinese castrate male and female piglets. In the latter, the ovaries are removed through an incision 1.5–2 cm long made with a special instrument and pinched off between thumb and forefinger. Although the wound is not sutured and no disinfectants are applied, mortality among the sterilized females is very low. Artificial hatching of chicken, duck and goose eggs has a long tradition in China. The author describes two different methods.

Wahua, T.A.T. and U.I. Oji. 1987. Survey of browse plants in upland areas of Rivers State. In: *Browse Use and Small Ruminant Production in Southeast Nigeria. Proceedings of a Symposium Held at the Federal University of Technology, Owerri, Imo State, 4 May 1987.* ILCA Humid Zone Programme, Ibadan, Nigeria. Pp. 23–33.

Tables 1 and 2 of this paper list about 40 browse and herbaceous species recognized and exploited by goat and sheep raisers in Rivers State, Nigeria. For many of these species, medical uses are also indicated.

Wahyuni, Sri, Tri Budhi Murdiati, Beriajaya, Harini Sangat-Roemantyo, Agus Suparyanto, Dwi Priyanto and Evelyn Mathias-Mundy. 1991. *The Sociology of Animal Health: Traditional Veterinary Knowledge in Cinangka, West Java, Indonesia – A Case Study.* SR-CRSP Working Paper No. 127. Balai Penelitian Ternak, Pusat Penelitian dan Pengembangan Peternakan, Bogor, Indonesia. 43 pp.

This working paper reports the results of a study on traditional animal healthcare for small ruminants in Cinangka village in West Java, Indonesia. A multi-disciplinary team consisting of veterinarians, social scientists and an ethnobotanist systematically interviewed 33 men and 35 women (often husband and wife) from 36 households, using an EVM interview guide. The interviews were complemented with participant observation, inspection of animals and their sheds, and faecal samples from 200 animals to test for parasites. Results indicate that the local management system keeps parasite numbers low and prevents infectious diseases. Sheep and goats are confined in raised barns with slatted floors, where they are fed under a cut-and-carry regime. Examples of other healthy management practices include sprinkling salty water on the feed and giving prophylactic herbal drenches. Farmers distinguish at least 20 different small-ruminant diseases. But scabies in goats appeared to be the only major health problem, although pink eye, diarrhoea, and some other diseases also occur. Home remedies span a wide range of drenches, ointments and other medications made from plants and other ingredients such as shrimp paste and kerosene. Farmers' decision whether to treat, sell or slaughter sick animals is influenced by whether or not they perceived the disease in question to be acute and directly life-threatening. For example, poisoned animals generally are sold or slaughtered because treatment is rarely successful. For scabies, on the other hand, farmers dispose of sick animals only if home remedies fail. Traditional scabies treatments and certain other village practices could be improved, however. But any efforts to improve the local system must take into account local beliefs and practices. Appendices to this working paper list 19 diseases defined and described by interviewees, plus the corresponding local remedies, which involve a total of 46 medicinal plants.

Wakeel, Ahmed S. El and Abuelgasim Yousif Gumaa. 1996. Some traditional husbandry and ethnoveterinary practices of the Messerya Humr Baggara trans-humants of southern Kordofan. *Nomadic Peoples* 39: 147–154.

In Sudan, 67% or 14.6 million of the nation's cattle are raised by Baggara Arabs. The Messerya Humr are one of the largest Baggara tribes of Sudan. They have been herders since time immemorial, first of camels and later also of cattle. This tribe has sustained larger numbers of livestock than most others, implying greater husbandry and healthcare skills. This paper documents these skills in hopes that researchers and planners 'may investigate their validity, improve them where and when necessary and eventually disseminate some among other . . . pastoralist societies' (p. 147). Husbandry practices are grouped into four categories. First is herd mobility, e.g. to avoid biting flies and mud. Second is grazing and herd management. Examples of healthy practices in this regard include grazing all species together when forage and water conditions permit, and keeping pre-weaned calves, lambs and kids indoors. Third is feed supplements. Crushed millet or sorghum bran in sour milk is fed to emaciated or otherwise unthrifty calves and to animals that fail to graze due to health problems during the late dry season. All animals receive salt at least twice during the dry season. Fourth is breeding strategies to ensure that births coincide with times of plentiful forage and water. One technique, unique to Messerya, is synchronization of breeding by controlling suckling. This is accomplished by attaching double rows of thorns to a cloth or rope tied around calves' muzzles. The accumulated milk in the dams' udders brings them into heat. Drawbacks to this technique are that the cows in question become dry soon after conception, and their calves obviously are suckled for a shorter period. However, it offers an alternative to modern veterinary medicine's expensive hormone treatments, which traditional stockraisers cannot possibly afford. And Messerya have other mechanical synchronization techniques consisting of tying off the male organ or covering it with an apron. The authors discuss Messerya EVK by disease categories. For CBPP and rinderpest, they note the Messerya habit of isolating the infected animals. Retention of placenta is infallibly treated by drenching with the juice of crushed *Gardenia lutea* nuts. Jaundice in young calves is aptly treated by temporarily weaning the calf from its dam's whole milk and placing it on a diet of sour or de-fatted milk. This technique is accompanied by branding along its flanks. Chronic pack-animal wounds are successfully and rapidly cured with applications of ashes, bull's urine, fresh cattle dung or diesel oil. Bloat is also successfully alleviated by drenching with a solution of soap and oil or, if this fails, piercing the rumen with a knife. Diarrhoea is treated by branding around the root of the tail. Excessive exercise and fatigue following a long rest period – or Monday Morning Disease, in Western parlance – is treated with a thrice-weekly drench of human urine and sometimes animal oils mixed with sesame. In addition, the fatigued animals may be fed high-energy items like grains and oils. Finally, to combat fly worry and infective flies, Messerya build smokey fires of cattle dung in the evening, when these pests are most active. The herd is divided into various groups so that each group can cluster close to a fire of its own.

Walker, Anthony R. 1986. *The Toda of South India: A New Look.* Hindustan Publishing Corporation, New Delhi, India. 371 pp.

The buffalo is the centre of Toda life in the Nilgiri Hills of South India. In addition to extensive socio-organizational information, this ethnography details almost every aspect of buffalo management, with emphasis on dairying. However, discussion of ethnoveterinary practices is notably lacking, with the exception of a lengthy exposition on salt feedings, both ritualized and secular (p. 173 ff.), and early care of calves' watering patterns to prevent illness (p. 112). Deceptions to keep a cow in milk after the loss of her calf are also described.

Walker, Anthony R. 1989. Toda society between tradition and modernity. In: Paul Hockings (ed.). *Blue Mountains: The Ethnography and Biogeography of a South Indian Region.* Oxford University Press, Delhi, India. Pp. 186–205.

The Toda people of India's Blue Mountains raise a unique breed of hardy 'long-horned, short-legged and rather ferocious buffaloes' (p. 189) famed for the high fat content of their milk. Toda class their buffalo into two broad categories: the sacred or 'temple' animals, and the ordinary domestic beasts that are the mainstay of Toda livelihoods. The pedigree in the female line sets the sacred animals apart. They are tended only by dairymen-priests, who undergo special, purifying rites of ordination. Their milk is processed in dairy-temples according to a strict, ritually defined routine; and the products are distributed for household consumption. In contrast, the milk of ordinary Toda buffalo can be sold raw or processed, without ceremony, at the farmgate. However, *all* female buffalo are sacred to some extent. Numerous religious pro- and pre-scriptions thus pertain to animal management and milking, such as: locating some dairies far from settled areas; stipulating particular transhumant routes and water sources to be used; and requiring dairiers to sweep up the dairy-temples and to wash themselves and put on special clothing before milking. [Also see Rivers 1906.]

Waller, R. 1988. *Emutai*: Crisis and response in Maasailand 1883–1902. In: D.H. Johnson and D.M. Anderson (eds). *The Ecology of Survival: Case Studies from Northeast African History.* Crook Academic Publishers, London, UK and Westview Press, Boulder, Colorado, USA. Pp. 73–112.

A classic case of how local knowledge can initially be stymied when a new disease strikes is Maasai pastoralists' response to rinderpest when it first appeared in their area. Rinderpest is a viral disease usually transmitted via close and immediate contact. Traditionally, all families of a given Maasai camp grazed and corralled their cattle together. But this practice provided ideal conditions for the rapid spread of rinderpest. It took some time before Maasai recognized this epidemiological pattern and took steps to disperse their animals more widely and to institute quarantine measures whenever rinderpest threatened.

Wanyama, Jacob. 1995. Animal health options for the poor. *Appropriate Technology* 21(4): 14–16.

For the past decade, ITDG has been working with pastoralists in northern Kenya to improve the animal healthcare available in this remote and impoverished region. One of the best ways to do this is by investigating, improving as needed and promoting ethnoveterinary treatments, folding them into contemporary veterinary service programmes. The latter task has been limited by the lack of credible research on EVM, however. This article overviews the steps that, across a decade, led up to a comprehensive R&D programme on EVK by ITDG/Kenya among Samburu and Turkana pastoralists to sift out their 'best' ethnoveterinary practices.

[For greater methodological detail, see later publications by Wanyama.] A particularly significant finding was that some of the diseases that pastoralists ranked as most important and as most confidently treated with home remedies were also the ones for which modern medicines have been advised in paravet training. In other words, in some cases training was adding little to pastoralists' existing knowledge. The author argues that it would be better to highlight such home remedies in training so that trainees can move on to learn about Western treatments for problems that traditional medicine cannot address adequately. In this way, 'Herders who feel pressured to buy the modern drugs because they want to do the best thing for their animals may no longer waste time and money buying modern drugs when their own are just as effective' (p. 16). Understandably, there are slight differences in plant use between plains- and mountain-dwelling groups of the same ethnicity, due to differential plant availability. But knowledge of botanicals is widely, freely and equally shared among men and women; and there is great consistency in plant nomenclatures, preparations and administration within ethnic groups, as attested by random checks of remedies with passersby. In contrast, only a few experts among Samburu and Turkana are skilled in surgical and manipulative procedures, although they are happy to train younger people in these skills.

Wanyama, Jacob. 1996a. A look at the on-going EVK research in Samburu. *IT-Kenya Newsletter* 12: 2–4.

This article outlines the methodology that ITDG/Kenya devised to research ethnotherapeutic knowledge among Samburu pastoralists of the northern frontier. The methodology had five steps. First, each of the six communities involved in the research generated a list of local names of livestock diseases known to them. Second, informants ranked these diseases in order of how confidently or successfully they could be treated with traditional techniques. Third, detailed semi-structured interviews on the treatments reported as most successful were conducted. Fourth, the results were analysed and a list was made of the plants or procedures used to treat each of the top ten diseases ranked as the most confidently treated ones. In the fifth and final step, socioeconomic issues, such as who owns and uses treatment knowledge, were investigated. Findings revealed that, unlike specialists' knowledge of manipulative procedures such as bonesetting or dystocia, traditional phytotherapies are generally known and shared by all. A noteworthy observation was that Samburu prepare mostly mono-prescriptions, suggesting that they may be knowledgeable in highly specific plant actions and have exceptional skills at empirical bioassay. [Also see Wanyama 1996b.]

Wanyama, Jacob Barasa. 1996b. Ethnoveterinary knowledge and practices among the Samburu: A case study. Paper presented to the 17th African Health Sciences Congress, Nairobi, Kenya. 18 pp.

This study of Samburu EVK used a five-step approach involving: (1) generating a list of livestock diseases known to pastoralists generally, and then selecting especially knowledgeable key informants; (2) ranking the diseases according to how confidently they are treated with traditional remedies, and then analysing the responses to determine the top ten such diseases; (3) eliciting treatment details for the ten diseases from the key informants; (4) researcher investigation of the most commonly used or cited remedies for the ten diseases; and (5) socioeconomic study of the use and distribution of knowledge about the remedies and other kinds of ethnoveterinary savvy. Steps 1, 2 and 5 used focus groups and other participatory group approaches. Altogether, herders identified and described some 60 livestock diseases, but the ten most confidently treated with local remedies were, in rank order: retained placenta, fleas, calf rejection, streptothrichosis, lice, fracture, eye infection, tumour, leeches and birthing difficulties. These disorders were treated using a total of 46 plants plus six non-herbal treatments as well as three manipulative techniques. In contrast to other communities, Samburu generally prepare their medicines from single rather than multiple plants.

Wanyama, Jacob B. 1996c. *Ethnoveterinary Research and Development Guidelines for Kajiado District. Report of a Consultancy.* Veterinary Department ASAL Liaison Office, Ministry of Agriculture, Livestock Development and Marketing, Kajiado District, Kenya. 53 pp.

This consultancy had the following objectives: to develop guidelines for ethnoveterinary R&D for Kajiado District's veterinary department; to test these guidelines with selected Maasai communities; to train department staff in the collection and analysis of ethnoveterinary field data; and to recommend future actions with regard to EVM. The guidelines are designed to be implemented in two phases. The first serves to identify and collect baseline data on successful ethnoveterinary interventions and perceptions using a combination of both key-informant and group interviews. The latter employ such techniques as brainstorming and ranking. The second phase entails scientifically validating, techno-blending, and adding value to the ethnoveterinary treatments and perceptions identified. Steps in Phase 2 include: scientific identification and collection of samples of remedies' ingredients; field and on-station trials; feedback of all findings to participant communities, for example as part of paraveterinary packages, local school curricula or agricultural extension programmes; and the wider documentation and dissemination of all R&D findings. In-field data collection methods during the consultancy followed the methods outlined above for Phase 1. Appendices present the results of the field study, i.e.: signs, causes and detailed treatments for ten diseases; a list of 56 diseases of Maasai livestock, with their English names; and lists of diseases ranked according to how confidently they can be treated with traditional remedies. In addition, the appendices contain an ethnoveterinary question list and guidelines for the collection of botanical samples.

Wanyama, Jacob. 1996d. *Existing Animal Health Practices in Maragwa: Visit to Tharaka Nithi (20–23 May 1996).* In-house report. ITDG, Nairobi, Kenya. 36 pp.

This study used group and key-informant interviews to learn about the livestock diseases that the Tharaka know and how they treat the diseases. The Tharaka differentiated 50 livestock disorders and classed them according to whether they were: important and treatable with local remedies; important but not treatable with local remedies; or not important and treatable with local remedies. For some 20 of the 50 conditions, the following details are presented: livestock species affected; disease occurrence, signs, source and transmission; and traditional methods of treatment, control and prevention. For training farmers and paravets (*wasaidizi*), the author recommends focusing only on those problems ranked as important, and emphasizing reliable local remedies whenever these exist. Modern medicine should be introduced only for conditions having no effective local methods of treatment or control.

Wanyama, Jacob. 1996e. Traditional medicines at [sic] crossroads. *IT/Kenya Newsletter* 11(Sep): 7–8.

This article recounts an interview with a traditional healer from Kenya who treats both humans and animals. He describes how different healers specialize in different animal diseases or techniques, such as dystocia and surgery. He laments young people's lack of respect for herbal medicines. He fears that traditional medicine use will die.

Wanyama, Jacob B. 1997. *Confidently Used Ethnoveterinary Knowledge among Pastoralists of Samburu, Kenya: Book 1 – Methodology and Results, Book 2 – Preparation and Administration.* ITDG/Kenya, Nairobi, Kenya. 82 pp. and 109 pp.

The lives of Samburu and Turkana pastoralists in semi-arid northern Kenya centre around their livestock. Through observation and trial-and-error, these pastoralists have developed a range of treatments for their animal health problems. Their EVK is a rich resource, especially where modern veterinary medicine is too expensive or unavailable. As part of the ITDG/Kenya and Oxfam Samburu Livestock Programme, IT Kenya conducted an applied ethnoveterinary study to: (1) gauge the level of understanding and use of traditional remedies among Samburu and Turkana communities; (2) identify treatments that the pastoralists were confident worked; (3) assess whether these treatments could be recommended more widely 'as is'; (4) determine whether their availability, efficacy and safety could be improved; and (4) share all these findings with other organizations. Book 1 of the resulting publication focuses on the study methodology and findings. First, focus groups of pastoralists compiled a list of about 60 livestock diseases. Second, key informants ranked the 60 in three ways: diseases considered most important in the area; those informants felt could be effectively treated, presumably with either modern or traditional medicine; and those that could be adequately treated with traditional remedies alone. Third, the key informants gave details of the traditional treatments. Fourth was tabulation of the most frequently cited remedies, and collection of information on who holds this knowledge, how it is shared, and who uses it. Book 2 gives details of common treatments for: retained placenta, fleas, calf rejection, leeches, streptothricosis, fractures, eye infection, dystocia, bloat and wounds (Samburu); and leeches, streptothricosis, lice, retained placenta, bloat, eye infection, diarrhoea, mange, wounds and jaundice or anaplasmosis (Turkana). For each remedy, the text describes: harvesting, availability and storage of *materia medica*; their methods of preparation, administration, dosages and time of application; side effects and effectiveness; and use in humans. Appendices list additional remedies and the medicinal plants used. Although little scientific information on the different plants and treatments is given, the author suggests that pastoralists' high regard for certain treatments indicates their possible effectiveness. In its next phase, the project plans to validate some of the remedies scientifically and re-apply them in community-based animal health programmes.

Wanyama, Jacob Barasa. 1999. Ethnoveterinary knowledge and practices among the Samburu people: A case study. In: E. Mathias, D.V. Rangnekar and C.M. McCorkle, with M. Martin (eds). ***Ethnoveterinary Medicine: Alternatives for Livestock Development – Proceedings of an International Conference Held in Pune, India, 4–6 November 1997. Volume 1: Selected Papers.*** BAIF Development Research Foundation, Pune, India. Pp. 88–98.

This paper describes the methodology and preliminary results of ethnoveterinary research and development by ITDG among semi-nomadic Samburu and Turkana pastoralists of northern Kenya, where disease is a major constraint to livestock production. Due to recent declines in livestock markets and to structural adjustments leading to cutbacks in government veterinary services, like many other pastoralists in arid and semi-arid areas, these two groups are finding it increasingly difficult to access modern veterinary services. As a result, they are perforce relying more on their traditional veterinary treatments to keep their livestock healthy. However, due to the lack of scientifically validated information on the preparation and effectiveness of such treatments, development professionals are hesitant to integrate ethnoveterinary practices into their animal healthcare programmes. This paper describes the design, testing and application of a methodology to scientifically validate, improve and promote the use of effective ethnoveterinary practices. The methodology relies on PRA to identify the most confidently used local remedies and to elicit details of their preparation and administration. With this methodology, information on more than 41 plant-based remedies was collected. This paper discusses how certain of these remedies are now being promoted among Samburu through a value-added and a source-community feedback process, and also how this experience is being used to win support for ER&D from national research institutions, development organizations and veterinarians.

Wanyama, Jacob and Sammy Keter. 1996. Ethnoveterinary knowledge and practice in Kenya (a comparative analysis). Paper presented to the 5th International Congress of Ethnobiology, 4 September 1996, Nairobi, Kenya. 10 pp.

ITDG's work among Samburu pastoralists and Kamba farmer-stockraisers of Kenya suggests that the former have more detailed ethnoveterinary knowledge. Among the reasons for this difference are: pastoralists' greater economic dependence on, and thus more intimate dealings with, livestock; farmers' relatively greater access and acculturation to modern veterinary medicines and services; and pastoralists' greater willingness to share ethnoveterinary knowledge freely among themselves. Among pastoralists, ITDG used group approaches to identify and rank livestock diseases known by the herders and to learn about traditional treatments for each disease. The results were supplemented and validated with key-informant and random interviews. In farming areas, a different approach was taken in which researchers organized meetings among livestock healers to help the healers exchange and improve upon their EVK and blend it with outside information.

Ward, David E., Roger Ruppanner, Philippe J. Marchot and Jørgen W. Hansen. 1993. One medicine–practical application for non-sedentary pastoral populations. ***Nomadic Peoples*** 32: 55–63.

This paper examines both theoretical and practical aspects of delivering human and animal healthcare at the same time to remote rural peoples. The use of satellite imagery and modelling, sentinel cases and ethnoveterinary research for delivering integrated healthcare are discussed. Healthcare providers with some knowledge of ethnomedicine will be better equipped to diagnose a complex disease syndrome (for example). They are also encouraged to declare an unknown diagnosis, or one based on best judgement, than to misdiagnose using a Western cultural bias.

Warrier, P.K. 1999. Animal protection: Indian tradition. Paper presented to the International Seminar on Integrated Approach for Animal Health Care, 4–6 February 1999, Calicut, Kerala, India.

This paper overviews the historical and religious relationship between people and animals in India. The Ayurvedic 'science of life' prescribes how to live and how to treat people and animals by paying attention to patients' internal and external environments alike. The Mrigayurveda and Adharvaveda hold references to the treatment of animals and their protection. In Ashoka's edicts there is a proclamation on the setting up of hospitals for people and animals along the trade routes. From Vedic times onwards, integrated healthcare delivery was practised, physicians were expected to treat both humans and animals. The sages Shalihotra and Palakapya wrote discourses on horse and elephant anatomy and physiology and included treatments for them. Life in its totality is observed in Ayurveda and today these observations are as important as ever.

Waters-Bayer, Ann. 1988. *Dairying by Settled Fulani Agropastoralists in Central Nigeria: The Role of Women and Implications for Dairy Development.* Farming Systems and Resource Economics in the Tropics, Vol. 4. Wissenschaftsverlag Vauk, Kiel, Germany. 328 pp.

Pages 92–96 deal with general cattle husbandry and milking. At irregular intervals, Fulani give their animals *kanwa*, a traditional mineral supplement. The herders often place this supplement in heaps on old termite mounds. They also pound leaves of certain plants and mix them with *kanwa* in order to improve the animals' condition. The Fulani regularly remove ticks by hand from their cattle. All herders know some traditional treatments; for unfamiliar treatments, they obtain help from other stockowners.

Waters-Bayer, Ann and Wolfgang Bayer. 1995. Entwicklung von Technologie in Zusammenarbeit mit Tierhaltern in Nigeria. In: S. Honeral and P. Schroeder (eds). *Lokales Wissen und Entwicklung. Zur Relevanz kulturspezifischen Wissens für Entwicklungsprozesse.* Special issue of *Landwirtschaft und Ernährung.* Pp. 141–149.

Despite several decades of livestock research in West Africa, the adoption of researcher-led innovations has been very limited. Therefore ILCA scientists tried a new approach, 'Technology Development in Cooperation with Livestock-Keepers in Nigeria' (the title of this article). Discussions with Fulani agropastoralists plus other investigations identified dry-season animal nutrition as the major stockraising constraint. Based directly on Fulani commentary and observation, scientists then recommended introducing the legume *Stylosanthes* to create small, improved pastures for increasing the dry-season condition and milk production of pregnant and lactating cows. However, the 20 collaborating stockraisers saw fit to modify scientists' models as follows. They used the fodder banks only during the second half of the dry season and only to feed weak animals because ensuring livestock survival was more important to them than increasing milk production. Furthermore, herders replaced the introduced fences with living fences because the latter were far cheaper to maintain; and they moved their crop-growing into the areas with project-introduced fencing, so as to benefit from the increased soil fertility. Subsequent studies showed that the herders' decisions made sound scientific sense in that: during the first half of the dry season, crop byproducts provided sufficient nutrients for pregnant and lactating animals; and roughly half of a herd that received no additional dry-season feed would die, whereas herds with access to a fodder bank experienced hardly any losses.

Wau. n.d. *Socio-anthropology Survey Interim Report Volume 2.* Planning Department Report No. 64. Ministry of Agriculture and Natural Resources, Juba, Sudan. 34 pp.

This report's Volume 2 consists of an appendix to Volume 1's socio-anthropological survey of Rek Dinka agricultural practices in southern Sudan. The appendix discusses several health-related aspects of Dinka sheep, goat and especially cattle husbandry. Only some 2% to 3% of bulls are selected as stud animals, based on their dams' superior milk performance; all the other bulls in a herd are castrated to make them better beef animals. A complex cosmetic horn operation is performed on animals chosen on the basis of horn colour and size to become 'song oxen' (most of which are in fact bulls). The appendix also notes that sheep are regarded as more sacred than goats and thus are preferred for sacrifices.

Wayne, Bruce. 1993. A comparison of ethnomedical and ethnoveterinary practices among pastoralists in sub-Saharan Africa with substantial background into development, FSR, and veterinary anthropology. Unpublished student paper. Department of Anthropology, University of Tennessee, Knoxville, USA. 29 pp.

This student paper reviews and interlinks some of the literature on veterinary anthropology, medical anthropology and farming systems research in relation to development. Selected case studies from sub-Saharan Africa are reviewed. The author notes that veterinary anthropology parallels the more established subfield of medical anthropology in many respects, but particularly their holistic and multidisciplinary approach.

Weeratunga, Ajantha Shanthekumara. 1992. Animal healthcare management in Sarvodaya-assisted dairy cattle projects in Sri Lanka. In: John Young (ed.). *A Report on a Village Animal Health Care Workshop – Volume II: The Case Studies.* ITDG, Rugby, UK. Pp. 108–116.

The Sarvodaya Shramadana Movement is the largest NGO in Sri Lanka, where it works in 5248 villages. Through its Rural Enterprises Development Services (REDS), it supports all aspects of extension for dairy (and many other) enterprises among the rural poor. In this regard, the REDS has recognized the valuable veterinary and extension services that traditional livestock healers provide. Their 'indigenous medicines, kept as secrets . . . have an impressive effect on curing diseases' (p. 116). Indeed, the majority of rural Sri Lankans – including participants in the NGO's dairy cattle projects – prefer traditional to modern medicine for most common livestock diseases. However, people are also interested in modern drugs because of their faster action. REDS agents seek to help farmers decide when to use one or the other, recognizing that Western treatments are effective if and when drugs are readily available at pharmacies but that low-cost traditional techniques like herbal medicines should also be encouraged. Thus, for example, the Dairy Cattle Projects commonly rely on traditional medicine for healing accidental injuries. The REDS has also made note of a number of other local remedies. For bloat and inappetence, cattle can be drenched with the juice from equal quantities of crushed ginger, garlic and *Moringa pterygosperma* bark, along with the local drug *perumkayam*. For worms, animals are given fresh *Althefolia swaris* leaf juice. Footrot is treated by washing the foot with freshly crushed coconut husks in water and then dressing it with neem oil mixed with coconut-husk ash. A complex treatment for mastitis is to mix the following ingredients in equal quantities in a clean cotton cloth: smoked coconut fruit and castor-seed kernels, cotton seeds and two other plants [no Latin name given]. This mixture is tied in a cloth bag, which is then steamed and pressed warm on the udder. Afterwards, honey is applied to the udder. Additional remedies for mouth infections are given.

West, Terry L. 1981. *Alpaca Production in Puno, Peru.* Sociology Technical Report No. 3. SR-CRSP, Department of Rural Sociology, University of Missouri-Columbia, Columbia, Missouri 65211, USA. 109 pp.

This report outlines the production of alpaca, and to a lesser degree of llama and sheep, in the department of Puno, Peru. It includes data on livestock statistics, pasture rotation, herd management and marketing of animal products. Traditional husbandry practices in two different locations are also discussed. Herders in Tolapalca control breeding of llama and alpaca, while sheep are allowed to mate freely. Selection of males is practiced in all three species. Herders differentiate between several types of mange and treat it with sulphur. Mites in sheep are treated with a mixture of lemon juice and cactus spines or with a preparation of *retama* leaves. The proliferation of *Astragalus* locoweeds on pastures is a major concern for Tolalpacans. In Cojata, herders select males for breeding but do not control mating. They use open surgery to castrate, and rub salt on the wound.

White, F.N. and P. Rowlinson. 1998. Use of both modern veterinary and traditional treatments by Samburu pastoralists in northern Kenya. In: E. Mathias, D.V. Rangnekar and C.M. McCorkle, with M. Martin (eds). *Ethnoveterinary Medicine: Alternatives for Livestock Development – Proceedings of an International Conference Held in Pune, India, 4–6 November 1997. Volume 2: Abstracts.* BAIF Development Research Foundation, Pune, India. Pp. 61–62.

This paper reports on semi-nomadic Samburu's use of modern and traditional treatments for their mixed-species herds of cattle, sheep, goats and camels. In cooperation with SAIDIA (Samburu Aid in Africa), a Kenyan NGO that provides human health services, Samburu were surveyed in 1996 and 1997 about their livestock treatments, as well as other production-system topics, using semi-structured questionnaires and interpreters. A large proportion of the interviewees relied on herding as their sole source of income; and overall, they ranked animal health as their number-one production concern. *Ndiss* (a complex of symptoms associated with contagious hepatitis, anaplasmosis and jaundice), pneumonia, malignant catarrhal fever and trypanosomosis were cited as the most important livestock diseases. People reported a marked increase in their use of modern medicines in recent years, although traditional remedies still played a major role in their animals' healthcare. Remedies relied on, e.g.: medicines made from the roots, bark, gum, fruits, seeds or leaves of local herbs and trees, sometimes in combination with giraffe hides, donkey dung, cows' urine and ant-hill mud; and hot metal pokers. Although many interviewees said they preferred modern drugs, 70% also said they often use traditional remedies. Generally, elders demonstrated greater knowledge of such remedies' preparation and administration, and of where to locate the necessary *materia medica*. The younger generations expressed no interest in expanding their knowledge or use of such remedies, and were sceptical about their efficacy, instead preferring modern drugs. Indeed, little is known about the efficacy of traditional treatments, and views about the value of specific treatments ranged from 'harmful' through 'useful' to 'surpasses modern equivalents'. Interviewees expressed a desire for assistance with modern drugs in terms of both provision and training. In fact, a number of problems with Samburu's use of modern veterinary drugs were noted: uncertainty about which drugs to use for which diseases; incorrect drug administration and dosages; the unavailability and high cost of commercial drugs; and ignorance of disposal and withdrawal periods for animals treated with modern drugs, before the animals or their products are consumed by people. As a result of these problems, modern veterinary medicines are often unsuccessful; and human health may be threatened. Coupled with livestock's vital role in Samburu survival, these problems suggest that it is important to evaluate and promote traditional treatments before they are forgotten.

White, Gilbert. 1977 [1788–89]. *The Natural History of Selborne.* Penguin Books, Harmondsworth, Middlesex, UK. 283 pp.

This 'parochial history' of the environs of a single English village is comprised of letters written by a clergyman of the community concerning local flora, fauna, farming systems and other ecological aspects of the area. A number of the letters touch on animal management and health issues (pp. 14–15, 27, 43, 153, 177–178, 185–186). For example, mention is made of how sheepgrazing on manor farms was managed in such a way as to be compatible with and maintain local deer populations. The author also notes how, to escape summer heat and flies, cattle took hours-long refuge in ponds, where their manure provided much-needed fish food. Another of his observations was the striking phenotypic differences in what might be termed 'micro-races' of sheep, even from one side of a river to the opposite bank: one horned, white-faced and uniform-coloured and the other hornless (poll sheep), black-faced and speckled. Also noted are animals' strong gregariousness, such that a lone horse will leap out of a stable-window to be with other horses, cattle will neglect the finest pastures if not accompanied by other cattle, an orphan deer will attach itself to a herd of cattle, or a lone horse and chicken will bond together. A village belief was that shrew-mice's running over the limb of a herd animal caused great pain or even loss of movement in the limb. This condition was remedied by striking the affected limb with twigs or branches of an ash tree, into a hollow of which people had entrapped a shrew-mouse and left it there to starve. Remarking on English grooms' and horsemen's belief that large nostrils are necessary for good breathing in hunt and race horses, the author describes the contemporary Maltese practice of slitting the nostrils of work-donkeys so as to admit more air to the lungs.

Wickens, G.E. 1980. Alternative uses of browse species. In: H.N. Le Houérou (ed.). ***Browse in Africa: The Current State of Knowledge.*** ILCA, Addis Ababa, Ethiopia. Pp. 155–182.

The flora of tropical Africa is estimated at 30 000 species, of which 7000 to 10 000 are trees or shrubs. This publication presents a textual and mainly tabular overview of numerous African trees and shrubs reported in a selection of readily available literature as being utilized for non-fodder purposes by cattle, sheep, goats, camels, horses, or donkeys. These woody plants are discussed according to six use categories: human food, agriculture, fuel, timber, domestic economy and medicine. Specifically for EVM and animal husbandry, Table 4 lists 28 browse species from 16 families exploited for all the foregoing livestock species plus poultry and dogs, along with the plant parts and purposes for which they are employed. Interesting additions to the plant parts typically given in such lists are sawdust (of *Diospyros mespiliformis* to treat canine mange) and twigs and charcoals of various species employed in a variety of medicaments. Other health problems treated include endo- and ecto-parasitoses, skin and eye conditions, fevers, colds, colics, fatigue, poisoning, flatulence, infertility, agalactia, fly worry, and epizootic lymphangitis in horses. Specific examples of medicinal browses are: *Annona senegalensis* bark and root, and *Carissa edulis* berries, from which vermifuges for horses and cattle are respectively made; *Saba florida* sap as a galactagogue for cattle; and *Euphorbia balsamifera* and *Grewia carpinifolia*, both of which are said to enhance livestock fertility. Uses as chicken feed, contraceptives for mares and tranquillizers for fractious cattle are also mentioned. No precise prescriptions are given, however. The author warns that some ethnomedicines may be of value and others worthless. Therefore medical-veterinary expertise should be brought to bear on which is which. He also cautions that 'information regarding the various uses to which plants are put is widely scattered and . . . it is quite clear from the literature already studied that a great deal of the information has been passed on from one author to another, sometimes without acknowledgement or in a garbled form. [Moreover] Much of the information is now out-dated' (p. 155).

Willoughby, Sharon. 1998. Chiropractic care. In: Allen M. Schoen and Susan G. Wynn (eds). ***Complementary and Alternative Veterinary Medicine: Principles and Practice.*** Mosby, Inc., St Louis, Missouri, USA. Pp. 185–200.

The veterinary profession should not consider drug and surgical interventions as the only valid approaches to animal healthcare. Chiropractic and other modalities are part of a holistic trend that complements conventional veterinary medicine, which itself is not purely allopathic. Chiropractic, from the Greek words for 'hand' and 'praxis', is a drugless form of treatment based on spinal manipulation and adjustment, applied in accord with the same anatomical and physiological facts used by all medical practitioners. Although practised on humans since at least the 3rd century B.C. in China, the first mention of veterinary chiropractic techniques in English appeared only in 1656, with the publication of a text on bonesetting. Not until 1995 did chiropractic care for animals receive some professional recognition, at least in the USA. This book chapter briefly describes chiropractic's basic approach, the theories behind and experimental validation for it, its anatomical and biomechanical foci, and examination and treatment techniques. The author notes that chiropractic is perhaps particularly appropriate as a complement to conventional veterinary medicine for 'athletic' and work animals, whose performance may place more stress on spinal structures.

Wilson, Gilbert L. 1924. The horse and the dog in Hidatsa culture. *Anthropological Papers of the American Museum of Natural History* 15: 127–311.

Hidatsa Indians of North America rubbed dried dung of antelope, elk or jack-rabbit on newborn colts to dry their bodies quickly, presumably thereby preventing chills. The dung of such fleet animals was chosen in preference to other species' because Hidatsa believed it would help colts to become equally fleet as adult racing and hunting mounts. Castration was performed by specialists in this craft, using a knife. After the operation, the wound was cleansed with wild sage and prairie turnip and sutured with elk sinew, the latter to give the colts the strength and endurance of elk. Dogs were also castrated by drawing the teste out of the cut scrotum. This operation was done to gentle and fatten dogs.

Wilson, R.T. 1980. Population and production parameters of sheep under traditional management in semi-arid areas of Africa. *Tropical Animal Health and Production* 12: 243–250.

Population structures and production parameters of sheep raised under traditional management systems were studied among five groups: Fulani of Mali's Niger River delta, with their unique wool breed of Macina sheep; Bambara of central Mali, with their West African Fellata or 'Sahel' sheep; Afar of Ethiopia, with their African Fat-tails; Baggara Arabs of western Sudan; and Maasai of Kenya (the latter two groups with mixed-breed sheep). While flock demographics were broadly similar across the five groups, they did reflect owners' interventions as per product emphases and cultural norms. Afar had the highest proportion of females in their flocks, as they are almost entirely dependent on milk for subsistence. Since Macina sheep are raised mainly for their wool, sex ratios in Fulani flocks were slightly more balanced. Because of their liking for fat, Maasai kept a higher proportion of wethers. Among the Islamicized groups (Fulani, Bambara and Baggara), the percentage of young male animals in flocks was lower than for Afar and Maasai due to offtakes required for Moslem holidays or for the satisfaction of Islamic canons of hospitality.

Wilson, R.T. 1983. Livestock production in central Mali. The Macina wool sheep of the Niger inundation zone. *Tropical Animal Health and Production* 15: 17–31.

'Macina' is the Fulani word for the deepest part of the Niger River's inundation zone. There, possibly for hundreds of years, Fulani have husbanded the only true wooled race of sheep raised under traditional management in tropical Africa. When bred pure, the Macina sheep presents a very distinctive appearance. But Fulani have often crossed it with the larger Sahel sheep, possibly to increase the Macina's meat and milk yields or to improve its endurance on long transhumant cycles that take the animals through drier areas. Twenty-year-long French colonial efforts to cross Macinas with Merinos and Merino derivatives failed utterly, however. The crossbreeds could not survive the harsh climatic and management conditions. Furthermore, Fulani rejected them because the crossbreeds' finer wool was unsuitable for the local spinning and weaving industry and technology. Traditionally, this unique breed is associated with a unique forage, the *burgu* (*Echinocholoa stagnina*) that flourishes well into the dry season on the Niger flood-plains. Macina sheep also exploit the monospecific meadows of wild rice and vetiver grass in their eponymous region. During the brief rainy season of the Sahel, flocks migrate a short distance away, where they graze on lands with salty soils until the flood waters recede. Selected management aspects of Macina husbandry include the following. When lambs cannot be weaned simply by removal to a flock subdivision, their dam's teats are blocked with mud or tied with a cord. Bloodless castration is the norm, performed by beating the spermatic cord with two sticks. With a double-bladed knife, a sheep may be sheared as many as four times per year, whenever wool is needed and fleece growth is deemed sufficient. Lambing also occurs throughout the year, with a fairly high rate of twinning. Overall, 'Present traditional management practices are quite sophisticated' (p. 30). Macina sheep represents a unique genetic resource that potentially could be exploited in other parts of Africa such as the Lake Chad basin or the floodplains of the Nile.

Wilson, R.T. 1984. *The Camel.* Longman, London, UK. 224 pp.

The vast majority of camels in the world are maintained under traditional hus-bandry systems, where they are often raised mainly for two purposes: milk pro-duction; and transport of the goods and (among moors and Kababish Arabs) women necessary for the nomadic or transhumant lifestyle that allows camels to seek out sparse forage across vast expanses of arid land. Herders take care to match a camel's pack to its age and abilities. Most camel-raising peoples have a complex vocabulary for camel age and sex, and they pay considerable attention to breeding. Castration is widely used except in certain Muslim countries. People are also well-aware of camels' need for salt. Thus Twareg of northern Mali and southern Algeria drive their herds to places with salty wells and earths twice a year; at other times of the year, they transport mineral-rich earths and salt slabs from distant areas to their animals. Camel raisers in Tunisia have the opposite problem, however; their home range and water resources are often too salty; thus they move the animals elsewhere every spring. Whether in North Africa or Kenya, camel owners are quick to detect metabolic disorders in their camels, which they often attribute to 'poi-soning' by new forages or an imbalance of forages in the diet (p. 131). Stiffness, lameness and arthritis are treated by firing the site of the problem. Only in East Africa are camels bled for blood for human consumption.

Wilson, R.T. and S.E. Clarke. 1975. Studies on the livestock of southern Darfur, Sudan: I. The ecology and livestock resources of the area. *Tropical Animal Health and Production* 7: 165–185.

Among other things, this article debunks the myth that Baggara Arab pastoralists of Sudan have a non-commercial attitude towards their cattle and retain large sur-pluses of mature males in their herds. To the contrary, offtakes of non-work-animal males are so great that Baggara probably have a problem of cattle-herd sub-fertility, even though bulls are allowed to run with the females continuously, and herds are not subdivided by age during daytime grazing. At night, however, calves and lambs are tethered separately, as are all the goats. Among sheep also, few males are retained until mature breeding age. Apparently, Baggara have struggled to keep pure their own strain of sheep, which consists of a modified Sudan Desert type. For instance, Baggara refuse to buy animals from other flocks for breeding purposes. Nevertheless, there has been outcrossing with Fulani sheep (known locally as Umm Bororo) at shared water sites. Also noted is the fact that Baggara's annual movements are designed to steer their herds clear of biting flies, with their associated risk of trypanosomosis, and of wet, muddy conditions.

Wilson, R.T., H.G. Wagner, E. Chalon, C. Ly and B. Sauveroche. 1992. Regional Project for the Promotion of Trypanotolerant Livestock: Objectives and progress. In: G. Tacher and L. Letenneur (eds). *Proceedings of the Seventh International Conference of Institutions of Tropical Veterinary Medicine, Yamoussoukro, Ivory Coast: Volume II.* CIRAD-EMVT, Yamoussoukro, Ivory Coast. Pp. 541–546.

Vaccination alone cannot control trypanosomosis in African livestock because of the variable antigenic properties of the trypanosomes. Among other non-pharmacological and/or non-polluting methods of control, one of the most important is increased exploitation of Africa's indigenous trypanotolerant breeds. Small ruminants in the tsetse-infested areas are all generally resistant to trypanosomosis, and they are thought to have a high resistance for other prevalent diseases of the region. West and Central Africa have 9.8 million trypanotolerant cattle of various indigenous breeds. The N'Dama accounts for 4.9 million of these. Other less-studied trypanotolerant cattle are the Borgou, Baoulé, Lagune (Benin), Kapsiki and Namchi (Cameroon), Somba (Benin and Togo), and West African Shorthorn (Ghana). All but the first two in the list are endangered, however. This conference paper reports on a major project to study and preserve these invaluable genetic resources.

Wirtu, Gemechu. 1995. Traditional veterinary medicine: Gathering base-line information. *Indigenous Knowledge and Development Monitor* 3(2): 27.

This brief article describes how data on Ethiopian EVM are being gathered in and around Addis Ababa, Nazareth and Debre Zeit, beginning with the collection of baseline information on traditional veterinary practices and beliefs in order to identify and characterize medicinal plants or other agents of veterinary importance and to establish a garden of medicinal plants for further experimental work and for exhibition.

Wirtu, G., G. Adugna, T. Samuel, E. Kelbessa and A. Geleto. 1999. Aspects of farmers' knowledge, attitudes and practices (KAP) of animal health problems in central Ethiopia. In: E. Mathias, D.V. Rangnekar and C.M. McCorkle, with M. Martin (eds). *Ethnoveterinary Medicine: Alternatives for Livestock Development – Proceedings of an International Conference Held in Pune, India, 4–6 November 1997. Volume 1: Selected Papers.* BAIF Development Research Foundation, Pune, India. Pp. 41–52.

ER&D could significantly enhance livestock development if the knowledge, attitudes and practices (KAP) of stockraisers were properly investigated and considered. Actions could then be taken to avoid or modify harmful traditional practices, to promote beneficial ones, and to develop realistic 'technology packages' of healthcare and husbandry interventions. To this end, in early 1995, a survey of 104 farmers (both literate and illiterate) of three central Ethiopian ethnic groups was conducted to collect baseline KAP information on their EVM. EVM provided the bulk of healthcare for the livestock of 41% of the farmers, while 85% of intervie-wees said they had utilized EVM alternatives at least once. In central Ethiopia, EVM is mainly comprised of herbal preparations, but surgical, managerial and magico-religious elements are also involved. KAP information for six livestock diseases was collected and assessed: endoparasitism (which 77% of the farmers complained about), blackquarter (67%), anthrax (50%), rinderpest (11%), rabies (10%) and FMD (6%). For endoparasitism and anthrax, the majority of intervie-wees said they used modern medicines, although 29% of those who complained about anthrax did not know that it could be so treated. Among interviewees who mentioned blackquarter, 73% preferred traditional therapies; a high proportion also relied on such therapies for FMD. Regarding prophylaxes, 73% of endoparasitism complainers were unaware of modern strategic deworming measures, which were employed by only 20% of interviewees. Across all six diseases, only for rinderpest did more than half the farmers (67%) know about prophylactic measures such as vaccination. In contrast, interviewees were generally quite knowledgeable about the epidemiology of certain diseases (e.g. fasciolosis), and took valid healthcare measures accordingly. However, a number of beliefs and practices were difficult to interpret scientifically. For example, since blackleg is thought to result from ingest-ing water, affected animals' water intake is restricted. The KAP study included an analysis of 130 Oromo and Amharic vernacular names and descriptions of animal health problems. This analysis revealed that names were based on nine factors, mainly clinical signs (48%), other effects of disease (11%), ethnoaetiologies (20%) and affected organs (11%). Farmers were careful not to utter certain disease names in the vicinity of animals for fear of attracting infection. Based on all the study results, the authors make specific recommendations for future research and farmer training needs in central Ethiopia. They also note that their recommendations may not apply to other areas, as the region studied enjoys relatively good modern vet-erinary services; in more remote areas, the extent and importance of EVM is prob-ably greater.

Wiryoshuhanto, Dadi. 1997. Field application of traditional veterinary medicine in Indonesia. Paper prepared for the First International Conference on Ethnoveterinary Medicine: Alternatives for Livestock Development, Pune, India, 4–6 November 1997.

Despite the incursions of Western medicine, a majority of Indonesian farmers still use traditional veterinary medicine. Medicinal plants play a particularly important role in their ethnopharmacopoeia, such that people cultivate them in their gardens. But other ingredients also figure in livestock remedies, e.g. eggs, honey, coconut oil or milk, cow's milk, sugar, soybean catsup and charcoal. *Jamu* (traditional Indonesian medicine) for livestock consists of both mono- and polyprescriptions for tonics, anthelmintics, pyretics, anti-toxins, antiseptics, galactagogues and much, much more. Herbal preparations also exist for maintaining animal colour and weaning. This article overviews the findings from a number of field studies on EVK in Indonesia and provides the following tabular summaries: more than 50 medicinal plants by local, Latin and English names along with their veterinary uses; 6 illustrative *jamu* polyprescriptions (2 composed of 9 ingredients each); and 24 bibliographic references on EVK in Indonesia.

Wiysenyuy, Evelyne. 1998. Give the right dosage. *La Voix du Paysan English* 35: 14.

In Cameroon, HPI gives an annual Golden Talent Award to an outstanding project participant. In 1998 the winner was Mrs Wiysenyuy for her success in raising HPI-distributed chickens and rabbits using EVM. In this brief interview, Mrs Wiysenyuy describes how HPI introduced her and her husband to EVM, encouraged them to establish a herb garden, and taught them specific treatments. She offers the further observation that, especially for large flocks of poultry, identification and diagnosis of sick birds is difficult, no matter what treatment is envisioned.

Woillet, J.C. 1979. A survey of traditional technology: A basis for development programmes (activities). *African Environment* 3(3–4): 207–213.

A number of development programmes in Mali have initiated activities to identify traditional technologies. This short article tells how the Office of Animal Husbandry and the OMBEVI Project already depend on herders' knowledge to implement their livestock development and meat marketing efforts. For example, by drawing upon herders' familiarity with traditional vaccination techniques, the project facilitated their understanding of, move to, and correct use of modern vaccines.

Wolfgang, Katherine. 1983. *An Ethno-veterinary Study of Cattle Health Care by Fulße Herders of South Central Upper Volta.* Thesis, Hampshire College, Amherst, Massachusetts, USA. 100 pp.

This study of animal healthcare among Fulani herders is based on scheduled and open-ended interviews with herders, field observations, and discussions with members of the livestock service in Upper Volta (now Burkina Faso). It reports on the veterinary delivery system and its problems, and details the Fulße system of categorizing, diagnosing and treating cattle diseases. Veterinary laboratory facilities in Burkina Faso are briefly surveyed. Lack of training, equipment and medications reduce the effectiveness of the delivery system. Because of poor communication with the livestock service, herders often misuse medications and vaccines and then blame the resulting failure of the treatments on Western medicine. The livestock service, on the other hand, does not understand indigenous disease concepts and regards herders as ignorant. The Fulße classify diseases into two main categories: diseases that are brought from afar, such as rinderpest and other highly contagious diseases; and *wilsere* or 'bush diseases' i.e. syndromes that are contracted in the region through infected water and pastures. Traditional treatments and practices include surgery, bonesetting, cauterization, castration, obstetrical procedures, vaccination and the application of home remedies. But the herders generally regard Western medications as more effective and easier to use than traditional medicines. Women play an important role in maintaining herd health. The Fulße have a wide-ranging and sophisticated understanding of disease diagnosis, treatment and aetiology, but this understanding is different from the Western one. The author recommends increased study of disease problems in Burkina Faso, improved healthcare delivery infrastructure, and education programmes for both herders and the livestock service. The interview questions and response frequencies are given at the end of the study.

Wolfgang, Katherine and Albert Sollod. 1986. *Traditional Veterinary Medical Practice by Twareg Herders in Central Niger.* Integrated Livestock Project, Ministry of Animal Resources, BP 85, Tahoua, Niger, and Tufts University School of Veterinary Medicine, North Grafton, Massachusetts, USA. 29 pp.

This report is based on interviews with Twareg herders and traditional healers. It briefly describes these pastoralists' drought strategies and their inadequate interaction and poor communication with the livestock service, and then details Twareg concepts of livestock health and disease. Twareg believe that goats are the hardiest stock in droughts and that they destroy pasture to a lesser degree than cattle. During droughts, herders sell off their weak and ailing animals. Traditional animal health specialists are herders who are acknowledged to be particularly adept at treating animals and humans. They perform surgery for abscesses and bloat, castration, bloodletting, bonesetting and compounding and administering medication. Branding is a frequent treatment. The authors list 11 cattle, 17 camel, 21 goat and three donkey diseases as described by the herders, including the disease symptoms, classification systems, treatments and local beliefs about their causation. In many cases the authors suggest a scientific counterpart for the indigenous diagnosis. They conclude that the veterinary service must gain a better understanding of Twareg concepts of health and disease in order to improve communication between these two groups and thus make animal healthcare more effective. The authors also stress the importance of small ruminants to pastoralists' survival. They recommend that certain traditional medicines be analysed, that traditional medical practices be evaluated for beneficial and harmful effects, that identification of Twareg disease concepts be continued, and that increased attention be given to small ruminant production, training for veterinary auxiliaries and education for herders.

Worcester, Don. 1987. *The Texas Longhorn: Relic of the Past, Asset for the Future.* Texas A&M University Press, College Station, Texas, USA. 97 pp.

This book extols the many virtues of an antique but vigorous cattle breed, the Texas Longhorn. Longhorns arose from a mix of wild, creolized Spanish Retintos with smaller northern European races introduced by Anglo settlers in the US southwest. The breed is noteworthy for its natural immunity to tick fever and for its great hardiness. The latter is evidenced by the Longhorn's ability to survive on marginal pastures where most other cattle starve. With good forage, Longhorns could actually put on weight even during their hundreds-of-miles-long trek to market.

Wosene, Abebe. 1991. Traditional husbandry practices and major health problems of camels in the Ogaden (Ethiopia). *Nomadic Peoples* 29: 21–30.

Among camel pastoralists in Ethiopia's Ogaden region, newborn camel calves' suckling of colostrum is restricted because pastoralists fear it may bring on diarrhoea and death. Camels are not given any supplemental feeds; but they are fed salt every 2 or 3 months and, especially during the rainy season, are grazed on salty soils and grasses to fatten them. Pastoralist knowledge of the epidemiology of *Trypanosoma evansi* is appreciable.

Wu, Ning. 1998. Indigenous knowledge of yak breeding and cross-breeding among nomads in western Sichuan, China. *Indigenous Knowledge and Development Monitor* 6(1): 7–9.

Sichuan is the third most important yak-raising area of China. The various breeds of yak found there today have been selected across generations by their transhumant and nomadic masters to meet differing environmental conditions and stock-raising emphases. The two main breeds are: the high-valley or *jiulong* yak, which is the superior meat, hair and draught animal; and the plateau or *maiwa* yak, which is the better dairy animal. Their distribution largely coincides with the traditional homelands of the Kham and Amdo Tibetans. For both cultural and geographic reasons, the valley yak is rarely crossbred. This reflects longstanding Kham preferences and the difficulty of exchanging animals among the rugged and remote mountain valleys. Just the opposite is true for plateau yak. But for both, the selective breeding system is essentially the same. Females are chosen mainly for their reproductive prowess. Criteria for males are more stringent. Their dams must have a history of high milk yield, large bodies, tameness and fertility (measured by having produced at least two previous calves). Their sires must also have demonstrably high fertility plus rich, thick hair. As to the stud calf itself, a complex constellation of horn, head, body, limb and tail conformations plus coat colour are sought. Stud selection proceeds in three stages, at age 1 year, 3 to 4 years, and after first mating. At each stage, rejects are castrated, after which they serve as draught or meat animals. Herders try to keep several successors to an outstanding bull. Sichuanese also have a tradition of sophisticated inter- and back-breeding between yak and cattle that is designed to produce even more fine-tuned improvements on animals' ecological adaptiveness and performance characteristics. Across the past three decades, many government-directed breeding programmes have been mounted to cross 'improved' races of meat, dairy and dual-purpose cattle with yaks. But when these hybrids were mated with local yak, their progeny were disappointing. Often the young did not survive the harsh climate; and without supplemental feeding, milk yields were low. In sum, research-driven interventions in yak breeding have so far been unable to improve upon the traditional Sichuanese breeding system in terms of enhancing herder livelihoods. In large part, this has been because scientists do not take sufficient account of the harsh, hostile environment yaks inhabit and do not directly involve yak raisers themselves or their wealth of local knowledge in breeding research.

Wynn, Susan G. and Michael D. Kirk-Smith. 1998. Aromatherapy. In: Allen M. Schoen and Susan G. Wynn (eds). *Complementary and Alternative Veterinary Medicine: Principles and Practice.* Mosby, Inc., St Louis, Missouri, USA. Pp. 561–578.

Aromatherapy can be defined as the medicinal use of volatile essential oils to effect psychological or physiological responses. It is part of herbal medicine, in that natural plant substances are used with a health purpose in view. In today's Western world, aromatic oils are typically administered by diffusion/nebulization or topical massage. However, the international trade and use of fragrant vegetation, spices and oils for medicinal purposes is ancient, as is the prophylactic or therapeutic burning of aromatic plants (fumigation). Significantly, the word *perfume* derives from the Latin words for 'through' and 'smoke'. Aromatherapy is currently experiencing a renaissance in the developed world. This is especially in France, where it sometimes appears in medical-school curricula, and in England. The name 'aromatherapy' comes from a 1937 publication of Gattefosse, who concluded that 'besides their antiseptic and bactericidal properties ... essential oils possess antitoxic and antiviral properties, have a powerful vitalising action, an undeniable healing power and extensive therapeutic properties' (p. 561). Interestingly, the technique is now gaining a commercial as well as a medical reputation in the USA. There, it has been successfully used to spur customer purchases in stores by as much as 45%, and to stimulate productivity in factories or offices. Although aromatherapy's veterinary applications are so far largely unexplored scientifically, references to animal fumigation are found in veterinary history as early as the 4th century. An early example is causing horses with glanders and respiratory symptoms to inhale burning oregano from an earthen pot set over a charcoal fire. Similar techniques have been reported for elephants in Sri Lanka (Piyadasa 1994). Illustrating with selected plant species, this chapter discusses various aspects of essential oil chemistry plus general clinical, behaviour-modification, and aversive-conditioning uses of aromatherapy in humans and animals. A lengthy section on 'Pharmacopeia' lists 35 pungent plants in general clinical use by aromatherapists, along with the plants' constitutents and toxicity or contraindications. Familiar species include, e.g., aniseed, basil, camphor, cardamom, cedar, chamomile, cinnamon, citronella, clove, eucalyptus, fennel, fir, garlic, ginger, juniper, lavender, lemongrass, marjoram, orange, peppermint, rosemary, tarragon, thyme, turmeric and valerian. The authors conclude that the veterinary use of aromatherapy is promising, given that animals depend so heavily on scent to communicate. However, they warn against confounding scents that are pleasant and evocative for humans with those that best 'speak to' animals, as it were. 'One has only to watch dogs investigate stools, urine and decayed food to realise that human standards do not apply to animals' (p. 575). If it proves out, aromatherapy would allow veterinary practitioners to reduce the dose or frequency of more expensive or potentially toxic drugs, and it would permit trainers to use less harsh techniques of behaviour correction.

Xie, Huisheng and Jianxin Zhu. 1998. Veterinary herbal therapy in China. In: Allen M. Schoen and Susan G. Wynn (eds). ***Complementary and Alternative Veterinary Medicine: Principles and Practice.*** Mosby, Inc., St Louis, Missouri, USA. Pp. 405–435.

Traditional Chinese veterinary medicine (TCVM) dates from the Neolithic, when people first began to domesticate animals. The earliest writings on the subject are references to dental disease and endoparasites of livestock, as inscribed on bones from the Shang Dynasty (16th to 11th centuries B.C.). The next dynasty witnessed the advent of full time veterinarians; and during the Warring States period (475 to 221 B.C.), veterinary specialization arose in the form of 'doctors of horses'. The classic text on traditional Chinese medicine was also written during this period. The first herbal book, which described 365 Chinese medicinals for humans and animals, appeared during the Han Dynasty (106 B.C. to 220 A.D.). Modern university education in TCVM was first offered in 1947. Since then, undergraduate and graduate programmes in the subject have proliferated. This book chapter overviews the components and theory of TCVM, and then lists several score of

TCVM medicines and formulae, their actions and indications, clinical applications, dosages for different livestock species, contraindications, and so forth. TCVM uses plant, mineral, and animal *materia medica*, although plant materials predominate. Hence the common label 'Chinese herbal medicine'. Technically, however, 'medicines' are distinguished from 'formulae' in that the former involve only a single plant whereas the latter are combinations of the former. Today about 800 medicines are typically used to treat animals, and out of some 2000 recognized veterinary formulae approximately 200 are commonly employed clinically. The complex theory behind TCVM revolves around four properties – cold and cool (Yin) versus hot and warm (Yang) – as assigned to different symptoms and medicines plus five tastes – pungent, sweet, sour, bitter, salty – as assigned to different medicines' effects. Further complicating this picture are the 'seven features' achieved by applying multiple medicines: single action, potentiation, enhancement, antagonism, suppression, counterdrive and incompatibility. In this chapter, all of these elements are illustrated and, where possible, translated into rough Western-medical equivalents. For the interested reader, the conclusion lists TCVM research organizations, professional associations and periodicals.

Yilma, Tilahun D. 1989. Prospects for the total eradication of rinderpest. *Vaccine* 7(Dec): 484–485.

Despite a vigorous campaign begun in 1962 to eradicate rinderpest in much of Africa, the disease is once again rampant on that continent, due mainly to problems in the production, preservation, and delivery of the tissue-culture vaccine used [see also Yilma 1990]. However, a new vaccinia-virus-based rinderpest vaccine is now being developed along the lines of traditional vaccines used by African pastoralists. The new vaccine can easily be administered and propagated by methods similar to those employed in the world-wide eradication of smallpox. A calf is extensively scarified and the wounds are seeded with the vaccinia virus; the resulting scabs are then collected and administered to other animals merely by scratching them into the skin, just as herdsmen have already been doing for hundreds of years. Thus there is no need to purchase huge quantities of vaccine nor to invest in expensive needles, syringes, and sterilization materials for them. Together, these considerations mean that African herders can readily adopt the vaccine and independently inoculate their herds themselves. Moreover, the vaccine works against goat plague (PPR) as well.

Yilma, Tilahun. 1990. A modern vaccine for an ancient plague: Rinderpest. *Bio/Technology* 8(Nov): 1007–1008.

Rinderpest (German for 'cattle plague') has been a recognized scourge of millions of cattle and buffalo since the great European epizootic of A.D. 376–386. The need to combat this dread viral disease, which produces mortality rates in excess of 95%, led to the establishment of the first veterinary school in Europe, in 1762. Rinderpest's introduction to Africa via three infected Indian cattle as a form of germ warfare during the Italian invasion of Ethiopia in 1888 wiped out 90% of that country's cattle, along with vast numbers of wild ruminants, and led to death by starvation of as much as 60% of Ethiopia's human population. Rinderpest then spread to the rest of Africa, killing hundreds of millions of animals. Since then, conventional vaccine technology has failed to control the disease in Africa because the technology has not been adapted to Third World problems of cost, foreign exchange, and sustained manufacture and delivery of vaccine in the field. This article describes the on-going development, using bioengineering, of a thermostable vaccinia-virus recombinant vaccine for rinderpest, reminiscent of the vaccine used in the WHO-sponsored global eradication of smallpox. Rinderpest is a member of the *Paramyxoviridae* family, which also includes the viruses that cause human measles, dog distemper and PPR. Such a vaccine offers dramatic advantages over earlier ones for several reasons. It can be safely stored without refrigeration for years; thus it requires no costly cold chains, which in any case have proven essentially impossible to sustain under African political-economic and infrastructural conditions. It is administered in the same, simple way as smallpox immunizations, which all nations already have experience in giving. After age 6 months, cattle of all ages can be vaccinated at the same time. Best of all, for countries that cannot maintain a tissue-culture facility, more than 200 000 doses of the new vaccine can be made merely by scarification of a single, vaccinated calf, in the same way that African pastoralists have been doing for centuries with their indigenous livestock vaccines. This lessens developing-country dependency on external inputs. Ultimately, the vaccine can free countries suspected, rightly or wrongly, of harbouring rinderpest from current livestock export embargos that deny them access to world markets. This is a critical consideration for nations that, like Somalia, rely on livestock sales for as much as 90% of their foreign exchange earnings.

Young, John. 1992. How to collect ethnoveterinary information. In: John Young (ed.). *A Report on a Village Animal Health Care Workshop – Kenya, February 1992.* ITDG, Rugby, UK. Pp. 12–15 of Appendix 5.

During the above-referenced workshop, participants visited ITDG/Kenya programme sites and themselves experimented with applying a 12-question version of an ethnoveterinary interview instrument pioneered by ITDG/Kenya. Sample data from the instrument's application in Somalia and Zambia for one disease and one informant each are presented here, to illustrate the instrument's flexibility. Also presented are participants' field findings from their training application of the instrument to two other diseases. Together, these illustrate the range of response types researchers can expect. Also discussed are ways to record and code the information thus gathered. [For greater detail, see Grandin and Young 1996.]

Young, John. 1993. *Intermediate Technology Kenya Annual Report 1993.* English Press Ltd, Nairobi, Kenya, for ITDG. 16 pp.

ITDG's work to establish locally based paravet training and service programmes among Kenyan farmers and pastoralists is highlighted in this annual report. ITDG found that, in contrast to farmers, pastoralists traditionally diagnose and treat their herds themselves. Many Samburu pastoralists, for example, can recognize over 40 diseases without difficulty and treat many of them effectively. In pastoral areas, therefore, ITDG opted for training herders directly rather than, as in farming areas, training selected individuals. For pastoralist training, traditional as well as modern medicines were included in the curricula. ITDG has also begun a study of pastoralists' ethnobiological knowledge, focusing on their understanding of disease-bearing ticks in their environment.

Yuan-Chang, Chou. 1978. The experiment on *Glynus lotoides* (*amika*) toxicity to the sheep and the effectiveness for the treatment to the sheep's cestodes, [and] gastro-intestinal tract nematodes. Unpublished manuscript. No place of publication or publisher given. 6 pp.

Ethiopians have long used preparations of *Glynus lotoides* seeds to expel cestodes in humans. This paper reports on an experiment to assess such preparations' effectiveness against cestodes and nematodes of sheep in Ethiopia. For the experiment, *G. lotoides* seeds were formed into a bolus with teff meal, honey and water, and administered to groups of naturally infected local sheep in the following dosages of grams-of-seed per 1 kg of animal weight: 0.0 for a control group and 0.25, 0.5, 0.75 and 1.0. After a week's observation and faecal examinations, the sheep were sacrificed and the types and rate of worm infection identified and calculated. During observation, some animals were seen to expel worm segments within 5 hours of bolus administration; expulsion peaked between 24 and 48 hours and continued strong for another 1 to 2 days. Faecal examination revealed that immature, mature, and gravid segments were expelled. Upon necropsy, reduction in worm burdens was found to be greatest for the 0.75 g test group, followed by the 0.25 group. So treatment effectiveness was not stable. *Glynus lotoides*' effectiveness against different worm species also varied considerably by dosage. Nevertheless, treatment reduced infection from all worm species except scolex. But dosages of greater than 0.5 proved seriously, and in some cases fatally, toxic to the sheep.

Zalla, Thomas M. 1982. *Economic and Technical Aspects of Smallholder Milk Production in Northern Tanzania.* Doctoral dissertation, Department of Agricultural Economics, Michigan State University, East Lansing, Michigan, USA. 334 pp.

Smallholder farmers in northern Tanzania decide whether or not to use Western veterinary medicine on their milk cattle depending upon breed. Pure zebu cattle receive very little, if any, Western treatments (mostly vaccines). 'Grade' cattle receive more, reflecting three variables: these cross-bred animals' greater susceptibility to certain diseases in the Tanzanian environment, such as tick-borne ills; the greater awareness and sophistication about Western veterinary medicine among owners of grade cattle, who tend to be wealthier than average; and grade cattle's higher value as compared to zebu. Most farmers know whether their animals have been vaccinated; but less sophisticated farmers are not always sure what the vaccinations were for. People have devised a cheaper way to apply acaricides by using their coffee-spraying equipment instead of the very expensive, high-pressure spraying units recommended by the veterinary service.

Zessin, Karl-Hans and Tim E. Carpenter. 1985. Benefit-cost analysis of an epidemiologic approach to provision of veterinary service in the Sudan. *Preventive Veterinary Medicine* 3: 323–337.

Conventional veterinary services are inadequate for healthcare delivery in pastoral systems. An alternative is a comprehensive animal disease surveillance network. Such a system would make use of existing veterinary infrastructure and resources (e.g. slaughterhouses, field personnel), foreign aid personnel and facilities, and a heretofore untapped resource: traditional healers such as the Dinka *atet*. The epidemiological data supplied through such an information network can be the basis for selective disease control efforts. Benefit-cost analysis of the two approaches for CBPP reveals that a network system would not only be economically superior to a mass vaccination campaign but would also have the advantage of gradually improving the veterinary infrastructure by establishing, via healers, a field-level link between herders and government veterinarians.

Zeutzius, Isolde. 1990. *Literaturrecherchen – konventionell und online - zur ethnobotanischen Veterinärmedizin. Aufbau einer strukturierten Bibliographie.* Diploma thesis, Studiengang Biowissenschaftliche Dokumentation, Fachhochschule Hannover, Hannover, Germany. 77 pp. plus extensive, unpaginated annexes.

This thesis sought to generate a bibliography of ethnobotanical veterinary medicine using three different search methods: an online search, analysis of reference lists in documents and professional contacts. The thesis outlines and evaluates the three methods and their results. For the online search, the author used the DIALOG information services in California, which gave access to some 300 online databases. The online search proved useful for rapidly generating a 'starter' base of literature. But it did not result in many new items once a certain stage was reached. In contrast, the other two, conventional search methods continued to produce steep increases in new finds beyond that stage. The thesis also compares its search results with the *ca.* 250 references of the 1989 annotated bibliography on ethnoveterinary medicine by Mathias-Mundy and McCorkle. Only 38 references appeared in both. While the percentages of references from Africa, Australia, Europe and North America were relatively similar in both bibliographies, those for Asia and Latin America were reversed; i.e. Zeutzius found 40% and 10% citations for Asia and Latin America whereas these figures were 14% and 37% in the 1989 bibliography. Three reasons may explain this difference: online services cover Asia better than Latin America; the authors of the 1989 bibliography had personal contacts and field experience in Latin America; and Zeutzius confined her search to ethnoveterinary botanicals whereas Mathias-Mundy and McCorkle took a holistic approach to EVK, including surgical techniques, traditional vaccinations, management practices, sociocultural aspects, and so forth. The author concludes that, if subject-matter specialists and experts in online searches collaborate, the combination of conventional and online searches will yield the best bibliographic results. The thesis' eight annexes contain examples of the different search strategies, selected databases, and a structured bibliography of about 300 references with different indices.

Zolla L., Carlos. 1989. Enfoques de la medicina tradicional y la importancia de su estudio. In: Gerardo López Buendía (ed.). *Memorias: Segunda Jornada sobre Herbolaria Medicinal en Medicina Veterinaria.* Universidad Nacional Autónoma de México, Facultad de Medicina Veterinaria y Zootecnia, Coordinación de Educación Continua, México DF, México. Pp. 4–8.

When academics speak of 'herbal medicine' often they confound the resource with the system. Although plants constitute the bulk of *materia medica* in traditional systems, of equal importance are the human resources (e.g. herbalists, curers, midwives), disease classifications, ethnomedical rituals, and empirical techniques surrounding the use of botanicals. In other words, traditional medicine constitutes a complex of elements that together make up an alternative 'medical model', one that, moreover, is subordinate to the hegemonic conventional model. Illustrating from the common Latin American complaint of evil eye, the author emphasizes that a multidisciplinary, scientific, clinical understanding of traditional medical models must be complemented by an equally sensitive understanding of how they may condition health perceptions and behaviours on the part of patients, therapists and societies. Along with reductionism, he warns against observer's paradox in the study of traditional medicine, and praises the new horizons opened by such evolving fields as medical anthropology, ethnobotany, transcultural psychiatry and especially ethnoveterinary medicine. With regard to this last field, the author notes that it offers a fresh stance from which, critically and comparatively, to re-evaluate past perspectives on traditional medicine for humans.

Zuberi, M.I. 1999. Present state of the ethnoveterinary system in northwestern Bangladesh. In: E. Mathias, D.V. Rangnekar and C.M. McCorkle, with M. Martin (eds). *Ethnoveterinary Medicine: Alternatives for Livestock Development – Proceedings of an International Conference Held in Pune, India, 4–6 November 1997. Volume 1: Selected Papers.* BAIF Development Research Foundation, Pune, India. Pp. 53–56.

Traditionally, livestock have been a key component of Bangladesh's national and village economies. Across centuries, rural Bangladeshis have relied on botanicals for livestock healthcare. But during the 20th century, widespread deforestation, erosion and over-exploitation of biodiverse plant resources have greatly diminished the availability of these botanical *materia medica*. Moreover, government, NGO and private enterprise have so far made no attempt to research, develop and promote traditional veterinary systems in Bangladesh. No surveys exist on veterinary herbal medicines or the animals treated with them, the related plant materials, or the problems and prospects of EVM. This paper reports what is thus a groundbreaking pilot survey, in which 19 veterinary herbalists (*kaviraj*) from six villages in two districts of northwestern Bangladesh were interviewed about their treatments for cattle ills. The herbalists described treatments for 17 such ills, utilizing as many as 39 local plant species (of which 16 have so far been identified botanically). All *kavirajs* reported good success and client satisfaction with their treatments, but they complained of an acute shortage of several important plant species. They also commented that poverty and lack of any official support, training and recognition for their work was seriously eroding their profession. Currently, therefore, the author is assisting herbalists to organize themselves in order to better their situation. In addition, he is working with *kavirajs*, village groups and local NGOs to help them document, conserve and use plants of veterinary value, and to grow the plants in village homesteads and on under-utilized lands.

Index

A Mdo Pa, Tibetan people 224
abdominal inflation *see* bloat
Abelmoschus moschatus, for rumination 480
abomasum, worms of 255
aboriginal people, Madhya Pradesh (India) 489
abortion
    after-treatment 110, 211
    causes of 189, 230, 481
    prevention 238, 329, 529
Abrus precatorius 161, 402, 532
    for placenta expulsion 202, 234, 399, 480
abscess 110, 222, 272, 281, 371–2
absinth buds, for liver fluke 461
Acacia, pods 235, 449, 450
Acacia albida fruit/leaves 535
Acacia amythethophylla Steud 374
Acacia arabica 234, 292
Acacia brevispica 278
Acacia catechu 65–6, 213, 414
Acacia cyanophila (mimosa tree) 461
Acacia ehrenbergiana root bark 91
Acacia leucophloea 399
Acacia melliphera bark and pods 169
Acacia nilotica 237, 261, 415, 519
Acacia nilotica bark 212, 236
Acacia nilotica pods 39, 91
Acacia nilotica seeds 169, 429–30
Acacia pennata 507
Acacia scorpioides 505
Acacia senegal 282
Acacia seyal 282
Acacia stulhmannii Brenan root 374
Acacia sundra stem bark 455
Acacia tortillis roots 157
Acalypha indica leaves 400
acaricides 79–80, 118, 197, 217, 385
    see also ectoparasites; mange; mites; ticks
accana medicinal plant 130, 380–1
ACCOMPLISH paravet project 174–5, 183
acetone, in insecticide preparations 150
Achillea millifolium 207
achiote 238, 434
Achyranthes aspera leaves 409
Achyranthes aspera roots 448
Achyranthes indica 300
acidosis, in goats 417
aconite (wolfsbane), deterrant training 14–15, 87–8
Aconitum napellus L. 536
Acorus calamus 432, 482, 532
Acorus calamus leaves 231
Acorus calamus rhizome 379, 409
acriflavin, natural fungicide 66
ACROSS Project, paravet programme 485
Action for Food Production (AFPRO), in India 267, 467

acupuncture 309, 311, 474
    for anaesthesia 246
    for diarrhoea 235, 314
    for lameness 38
    for mastitis 169–70
    for oestrus induction 25, 149, 244, 343
    novocain blockade 509
    post-surgery 311
Adansonia digitata 50, 209
adappan syndrome, in cattle 263
Adenia gummifera, for FMD 373
Adenia volkensii 373
adenitis, horses, Peru 316–17
Adenium obesum, for lice 379
Adhatoda vasica 412, 458
Adiantum capillus veneris L. 111
Adonis vernalis 207
adorning the patient, medico-religious act 17
adzuki beans, for wounds 277
Aegle marmelos 129, 202, 213
Aerva tomentosa crushed 212
Aesculus indica 486
Afar (Ethiopia) 48–9, 333, 370, 550
Afghanistan 78, 313, 530
    see also Daye Chopan; Koochi; Pashtun
AFPRO (Action for Food Production) 267, 467
Africa 68–9, 96–9, 206–7, 364, 372–3, 434
    disease control 13, 95–6, 187, 194, 462, 504
    feed 82, 128, 549
    husbandry 140, 289, 326–7, 376, 495, 512–14
    livestock 457, 474
        beekeeping 183–4
        camels 16
        cattle 137, 155
        piglet mortality 393
        poultry 208–9
        small ruminants 406
    pharmacopoeia 273–4, 439
    writing on EVK 96, 112, 154, 412
    see also East; Northern; South; West and individual countries
African horizontal beehives 18
African horse sickness 505
African locust beans, *see also* locust beans
African locust beans (*Parkia filicoidea*) 50
African marigold (*Tagetes erecta*) 458
Afrikaander cattle, tick-resistant 184
Afromum melegueta rhizome or seeds 439
Afrormosia laxiflora 282
agalactia 396, 512
    see also contagious agalactia; galactagogues
Agave americana 202, 458
Agave spp. 167
aggression reduction 515, 557
aggressiveness, of French bouquets 112, 114
agitation, in calves 135

Agriculture and Natural Resources, VSO 173–4
Agrimonia eupatoria L. 111
Agroforestry Technology Information Kit 149, 253
Agrostemma githago L. 536
agugu fern (dried) 157
ajana ajana 125, 437–8
ajenjo/maize-beer, for liver fluke 317
ajma, used in India 235, 507
Akamba stockraisers (Kenya) 251–2, 353–4
akota tree bark 238
akuet kuet (hypomagnesia) 334–5
Akwasasne Indians, Canada 210
Alabama, American Indians 306
Alangium souifolium bark 507
Alangium sp. 449
Albizia almara leaves and bark 458
Albizia anthelmintica 169, 223, 278
Albizia odoratissima L., fish poison 86
Alchemilla orbiculata juice 228
alcohol, *see* ale; beer; brandy; gin; liquor (country);
    palm liquor; rice water (fermented); rum; sugar-
    cane; wine
alcohol drench 114, 183
alder (*Alnus incana*) bark 306
ale, in EVM 156
alfalfa, mineral-rich feed supplement 64
algarrobo (*Ceratonia siliqua*) 65–6
Algeria, *see* Twareg
Algeria nervosa 507
Algeria pylosa roots 507
alhucema in liquor, for bloat 317
Alka-seltzer, for conjunctivitis 228
allergic oedema, skin problem 281
alligator-pepper in gin, in Nigeria 62
Allium cepa see onion
Allium sativum see garlic
allopathic medicine 6, 217, 226, 228
    and EVK 113, 206–7, 239–41, 286, 298, 311,
        520
    disadvantages of 147, 362
    in holistic livestock healthcare 152, 456
    misuse
        camel herders 229
        Fulani herders 68, 108–9, 554
        in India 59, 290
        in Kenya 203, 206, 223–4, 254, 548
        in Somaliland 109
        in Sudan 443
almonds, for energy and agility 127
Alnus incana (alder) bark 306
Aloe 380, 386, 486
Aloe barbadensis juice 402
Aloe barteri 250
Aloe cooperi 138
Aloe ferox juice 371
Aloe fibrosa (aloe) leaf sap 198
Aloe kedongensis (aloe) leaf sap 198
Aloe vera 300, 400, 401, 503, 507, 532
    immune system boost, chicks 298, 301
Alor island (Indonesia) 340
alpaca 120–1, 130, 245, 437–8
    sarcoptic mange in 66–7, 265, 523
    see also huacaya; Macusani
alpaca fat, uses of 120–1, 201, 519

Alstonia, in health tonic 209
Alternanthera sessilis leaves 202
alternative therapies 146–7, 150
    see also acupuncture; chiropractic; homeopathy
Althaea (marshmallow) 485
Althefolia swaris leaf juice 546–7
altitude tolerance, Sichuanese yak 16
alum 273, 465
    appetite stimulant 237
    for FMD 261, 492, 519
    for sore mouth/throat 306
    for wounds/injuries 64, 213, 380
    in Chinese EVM 537–8
    milk stimulation 284
Alysicarpus spp., fodder plant 47
amaranthus, in bouquets, for poultry 148
amaro (*Webebaueri* sp.) 437–8
ambuta (*Lantana camara*) leaves 164
Amdo Tibetans, yaks of 556
America *see* USA
American Indians
    horses of 13, 153, 282, 304–6, 462, 501–2
    see also Alabama; Apache; Assiniboine;
        Blackfoot; Catawba; Cheyenne; Comanche;
        Cree; Crow; Hidatsa; Navajo; Nez Percé;
        Ogalala Sioux; Omaha; Piegan; Potawatomi;
        Sioux; Teton Sioux
Amharic hammer, bull castration 196
Amharic peoples (Ethiopia) 514–16
Amish, North American farmers 118
ammonia 64, 65, 76, 114
ammonium chloride, expectorant 213
Amorphophallus campanulatus tuber 236
amputation, of tongue tip 366, 367
amulets 41, 124–5, 142, 156, 285, 515, 522–3
Anabasis syriaca sap 73
anabolic medicinal plants 201–2
anaemia prevention, piglets 340
anaemia treatment, zebu cattle 159
anaesthetic, acupuncture in 246
anal route for medicines 11, 536
analgesia
    Ayurvedic medicine 297
    electroacupuncture 280–1
Ananas comosus 176
anaplasmosis, Samburu pastoralists 258
anatomical dissection, Dinka healers 476
Ancash Department (Peru) 126
ancient history, EVK overview 445
Andes 14, 125, 213–14, 435, 437
    camelids
        alpaca 120–1, 245
        ectoparasitism 66–7, 117, 466, 512
    cattle, bloat 315
    guinea pigs 104–5, 192
    poultry breeds 116–17
    sheep 191, 512
    see also Canchis Province; Bolivia; Peru
Andhra Pradesh (India) 58–60, 217–18, 437, 455–6
Andrographis alata leaves 400
Andrographis paniculata 281, 458
Andropogon gayanus (Gamba grass) 68, 511–12
Anethum graveolens 416–17, 510
'anger of the gods', in Sri Lanka 433

angiosperms 141
angry people, disease caused by 226, 227
animal and human medicine *see* integrated health care
animal health assistants, in Kenya 259
animal health services *see* veterinary health services
animal husbandry *see* livestock husbandry
animal names, Sahel, Twareg 459
animal oils, in drench for fatigue 539
animal products, used in Ethiopia 514
animals/insects, toxic agents 248–9
animist rituals, in Bolivia 126
aniseed, uses of 114, 303, 511
Anisopappus africanus leaf juice 354–5
Ankole cattle, ECF resistant 137
ankus, in elephant management 378, 433
Annand (India) 262–3
Anne, HRH the Princess Royal, anecdote 57
Annona senegalensis 14, 250, 282, 510, 517
    roots 209, 549
Annona squamosa
    leaves 129, 235, 236, 237, 281, 491
    seeds 150, 508
anoestrous *see* oestrus induction
Anogeissus leiocarpa 250, 505, 512
anorexia *see* inappetance
antacid drench 401
antacid eye medicine 228
antelope, in zoo, plant medicines for 461
antelope dung, for neonatal colts 550
anthelmintic evaluation 219, 247, 468
anthelmintic EVM
    in Africa 39, 97, 388
        Fulani 50, 157, 250, 512
        Gambia 133
        Ghana 279
        Kenya 192, 254–5, 259
        Tanzania 373, 463
        Zambia 502
    in Andes 50, 83, 125, 317
    in Arab medicine 198
    in India 141, 231, 385–6, 448, 468, 486–7
    in Italy 339
    in Philippines 149, 162, 174, 176–7
anthelmintics
    camels 278
    dogs 264, 303, 524
    horses 118, 536, 549
    pigs 436, 510
    poultry 209, 394
    rabbits (baby) 412
    ruminants 26, 300, 493
        calves
            buffalo 77, 273, 418
            cattle 140, 212, 237, 273, 486
        cattle 141, 172, 213–14, 507–8, 517, 547, 549
        small ruminants 73, 256, 396
            goats 57, 88, 243, 273, 449
            sheep 54, 61, 360–2, 560
    see also tapeworms; worms
Anthemis nobilis 65–6
ANTHRA, Indian women's NGO 58–60, 197
anthrax

knowledge of 151–2, 154, 159, 214
    prevention 96, 407
    treatments 91, 142, 183, 459, 465
anthropology, and EVK 252, 281, 501
anti-inflammatory agents 216–17, 339, 499
antibacterial agent 464, 492
antibiotics (commercial) 39, 57, 228, 318, 395–6
anticancer agent 97
antifungal ointment, in India 147
antimalarial agent 97
antimony, in mix for liver fluke 461
antiseptic agents 147, 287, 491, 499, 513, 517
antispasmodic, in Rumania 499
antler velvet, Saami Lapps 52–4
anuria, horses, in Croatia 535–6
anus, cauterization for diarrhoea 86–7
Apache, American Indians 305, 306
apeth (evil eye), Dinka healers 535
aphrodisiacs 158, 173
appetance, appetite stimulant 237
appetite stimulant *see* inappetance
apprenticeship *see* training
appropriate technology
    importance of 500–1
    see also inappropriate technology
apron
    male contraception 418, 474, 539
    ram 155, 187, 264, 302, 474
Apurimacia incarum Harms 225
aqua camphor, for colds, caged birds 303
aqua-acupuncture, for diarrhoea 314
aquafortis, in astringent 132
aquatic grass (*chopattia*) 261
aquavitae, for glanders (farcy) 156
Arabs 198
    camel pastoralists 139, 289, 457, 498–9
    sheep pastoralists 78
    see also Baggara; Hawawir; Kababish; Kawahla
arbularyo, 'herb doctor' 516
Arcangelista flava 516
Archibaccharis hirtella, var. *taeniotricha* Blake 193
Areca catechu 172, 174, 256, 411, 486–7
    in Wopell 455
    see also betel nut
areca nut, anthelmintic 213, 303, 385–6
areca nut (*Piper betle* L.) shoots 129
Arequipa Department (Peru) 134, 200, 201
arestín (heel ailment), Peru 523
Argemone mexicana 237, 281
arid areas, camels in India 284
Arid Lands Information Network website 419
Arisaemia tortuosum root/seeds 141
Aristolochia albida bark 466
Aristolochia bracteata 237, 468
Aristolochia bracteolata 236, 260, 399, 507, 532
Aristolochia indica 160–1, 281
armadillo fat, for hoof problems 395
arnica, turkey feed supplement 321
aromatherapy, veterinary, USA 556–7
arsenic poisoning, livestock dips 530
Arsenicum album 166
artemisia, mugwort leaves 388
Artemisia abrotanum L. 535–6
Artemisia absinthiul 317

Artemisia annua 97
Artemisia arborescens L. 536
Artemisia herba-alba shoots 169
Artemisia moxa 277
Artemisia vulgaris 338–9, 518
arthritis, in camels 237
artichoke (*Cynara scolymus*) 61, 84, 360–2
artificial incubation *see* incubation
Artocarpus heterophyllus leaf juice 491
Artocarpus lakoocha R. bark 102
Arundo phragmites, medicinal teas 110
asafoetida 235, 260, 416–17, 532
   for tympany 449, 450, 485–6
ash tree 156, 510
ashes 114, 126, 531, 536
   for ectoparasites 77, 386, 396, 410, 437–8
   for footrot 257–8
   for locoweed poisoning 130
   for wounds 116, 386, 395, 537, 539
   in medico-religious rites 118, 402
ashes (baobab-seed) 513
ashes (bean), for ECF 537
ashes (coconut husks) 546–7
ashes (cow manure) 317
ashes (date pits) 132
ashes (dung) 231
ashes (Islamic hat) 383
ashes (kitchen) 349
ashes (leather shoe) 235, 236–7
ashes (lentil-bean) 536
ashes (onion) 415
ashes (*Polyporus fungus*) 491
ashes (sage) 501–2
ashes (*Sesamum indicum* stalks) 414
ashes (stove) 130
ashes (wood) 88, 118, 137
Asia 56–7, 170, 349–50, 368–9
   camels, specialised for desert 16
   feed supplements 503
   horse, colic 369
   poultry, in pest control 14, 432
   rams, contraception 369
   weaning techniques 369
Asparagus racemosus 329, 468
Asparagus sp. roots 237
aspergillosis, poultry 301
Aspidium Filix-mas (*helecho macho*) 119
Assam, India, Nepalis of 107
Assiniboine, American Indians 306
asthma, in India 231
Astragalus sp., *see also* locoweed
Astragalus sp. (locoweeds) 437–8, 547
astringents, in India 213
atet Dinka healers 326–7, 334–5, 475–7, 560–1
Atropa belladonna 207, 536
Attantia monophylla bark 507
Atylosia scarabaeoides Benth. 491
Australia, parasite control 155, 511–12
autogenous vaccines *see* vaccines, traditional
automotive lubricant, for mange 214
auyama leaves, for ectoparasites 434
Avena sativa (oats), in feed 167
Avuri leaf tablets (*Indigofera tinctoria*) 533
awwalaga, Amharic/Oromo healers 514

axe-hammers, in horn shaping 115
Axonopus scoparius (imperial grass) 365–6
Aymara Indians
   Bolivia 89, 120, 296
   Peru 317, 410
Ayurvedic medicine 13, 352, 455, 488, 545
   in Asia 170, 349
   in India 56, 352, 408, 455
   in Nepal 172
   in Sri Lanka 55, 432–3
   in Trinidad and Tobago 298
   prescriptions 129, 161, 256, 297
   principles of 171, 456, 489–90
   ritual, in remedies 148
Azadirachta indica (neem) 203, 234, 396
   for ectoparasites 173–4, 197, 301, 458
      mange 262–3, 281
   for endoparasites 209
   for wounds/sores 129, 329
   pest control 47, 50, 429
azani disease syndrome 496
azawak zebu cattle, of Fulani 158–9

Ba-Hema, Great Lakes people 274
baby oil, for ear mites, cats/dogs 233
bacterial infections 120, 231
   herbal ointment 330–1
   see also braxy
bacteriostat, pastoralists Ethiopia 370
bad blood, as diagnosis 251, 481
Baggara Arabs (Sudan) 82–3, 197
   livestock 474, 539, 550, 552–3
      EVM 96, 138, 197
BAHAs *see* barefoot animal health assistants
Bahia (Brazil), goat production 439–40
BAIF, Indian NGO 447–8
bajra (millet) 234
   feed 212, 234, 400, 416–17, 503
Baktaman (New Guinea), pigs 78
Baladi cattle, FMD resistant, Arab 214
Balanites aegyptiaca 510, 513
Balanites aegyptiaca bark 189
Balanites aegyptica fruit pits 91
Balanites aegyptica leaves 430
Balanites spp. bark 414
Bali, banana stem in feed 393
Balkans, EVK, historical review 152–3
ball (tennis), for flatulence 233
Bambara (Mali), sheep breeds 550
bamboo grass, temple charms, Japan 277
bamboo leaves 383, 400, 503
   for retained placenta 126, 213, 300, 449
bamboo splints 281, 443–4, 482
Bambusa bambos leaves 415
banana juice, for diarrhoea 212
banana leaves, for ectoparasites 448
banana stem, fodder 393
bananas 127, 172, 400, 456
bandage, for fractures 238
Bangladesh 89, 170, 282, 385
   herbalist (*kaviraj*) 562
   livestock husbandry 242, 443
   see also Noakhali

banifoo leaves, abortion caused by 230
Banjarese people (Borneo), ducks 533–4
Bantu, Vugusu (Western Africa) 537
bany bith (spearmaster), rituals 535
banyan tree (aerial roots) 235
baobab 50, 106, 513
   see also Adansonia digitata; *Combretum* spp.
Baoulé cattle, disease-resistant 471, 552
Barabaig people, (East Africa) 286–7
Barabaig (Tanzania), mange treatment 480
Baragoi District (Kenya) 253–5
barbasco (*Lonchocarpus* sp. root) 380, 519
Barberea cuspidata, for eyes 401, 532
Barberi goats 55
barberry root juice, for digestion 232
Bare Center of Traditional Medicine (CMTB) 464
barefoot animal health assistants (BAHAs) 217
barefoot animal health services 215
barefoot doctors, treatments 309
barefoot technicians (BFTs) 267
barefoot veterinarians 204, 397–8
barley 125, 212, 527
   forage 41, 330
   see also Hordeum vulgare
barley flour 65–6, 261, 295, 414
barley water, for urinary disorders 234
barn fumigation, in Ethiopia 515
barns, *see* raised barns
Basella alba L. green leaves 277
Basic Veterinary Workers 310–11
Basque shepherds, in California 60
Bassia latifolia, for milk yield 449
Bassia longifolia leaf extract 202
Basuto (South Africa) 12, 63
bathing, for pack horses/mules 156
battery acid, for skin conditions 24
battery acid (spent), for wounds 334
battery carbon powder, for wounds 231
Bauhinia, leaves 157
Bauhinia purpurea L. 102
Bauhinia racemosa 400
Bauhinia reticulata 92
Bauhinia vehlii plants 14, 529
Bawadra (Sudan), camel pastoralists 44–5
be:koko (mouth disease), in India 232
beaks, sores on, cashew nuts as cause 301
bean ash, drench for ECF 537
bean juice, for myiasis 157
bean leaf, for digestion problems 232
beans 64
   see also adzuki; locust
bears, sheep predators, in Bulgaria 334
beating sick animal, as cure 226, 229
beda bark, in poultry remedies 237
Bedouin
   livestock husbandry 41–2, 73, 160, 214–15, 289
      EVM 14, 132–3, 214, 245, 471
beef (salted), medicinal use 510
beekeeping 135–6, 400
   in Africa 18, 183–4, 234
      Ethiopia 18, 40, 514–15
   in Europe 77, 310
beer brewing, by witch doctor 183
beer froth, to bait beehives 234

beer residue, for digestive disorders 514
beeswax, in egg preservation 76
behaviour modification 118, 377, 557
behavioural signs, in disease 75, 152
bejuco, feed supplement, turkeys 321
beleño negro seeds, in horse feed 327
Belgium, bovine plague (contagious typhus) 329
beliefs, in cattle breeding, India 199–200
belladona, in poultice for mastitis 323
bells, medico-religious practices 89, 110
Bengal (India), medicinal plants 261, 409–10
Benguet Province (Philippines) 516
Beni plateau (Bolivia) 239–40
Beni-Amer pastoralists 38, 188–9
Benin, stockraisers 256, 307–8, 379–80, 512–14,
   552
ber bush, for retained placenta 295
Berberis aristata, in Himax 330–1
Berberis vulgaris roots and stem 142
betel, for colon/caecum impaction 128
betel leaf 202, 532
betel nut
   anthelmintic 174, 388, 409, 524
      tapeworms 264, 486–7
   for eye instillation 401, 532
   see also Areca catechu
Betula nigra (birch tree) buds and bark 306
bezoar stone (yak), in Chinese EVM 311
BFTs *see* barefoot technicians
Bhaca people (South Africa) 219
Bharat (India) 88
Bharud caste, Uttar Pradesh (India) 522
Bhat, caste/class, Rajasthan (India) 453
BHC (benzene hexachloride), for mange 290
Bhil tribal peoples (India) 86, 480, 528
bhopa, healer/spirit medium, India 453
Bhuddhism, illness and 221–3
Bhutan 13, 297, 312, 313, 486
Bibliography, An Annotated, India 444–5
'big belly'
   hydatidosis 326
   see also tapeworm
Bihar (India) 261, 375–6, 409–10
   see also Santal people
Bikaneri red camels, in India 287
bioprospecting and conservation 285
biotechnology, EVM as form of 342
birch tree (*Betula nigra*) buds/bark 306
bird nests as food strainers, India 486
birds (caged), colds, herbal remedies 303
birth control *see* breeding control; contraception
Bishariin (Sudan), camel pastoralists 38
bites (animal), firing/branding for 189
bitter leaves, used by Fulße 106
Bixa orellana, anthelmintic 176
Black Head Persian rams, introduced 208
blackberry root tea, for diarrhoea 118
Blackfoot, American Indians 305, 306
blackleg, in Turkey 153
blackquarter 334, 402, 458, 529
   prevention 375, 537
blacksmiths' remedies 132, 323, 510
bladder obstruction, Iran 505
bladder (yak), in Chinese medicine 311

bladderworm removal, for camels 229
bleach drench, for meteorism, France 114
bleeding
    Africa 132–3, 200, 514, 531, 537
        Fulani 159, 397
        Kenya 51, 115, 187, 253, 386–7
        Sudan 183, 334
        Turkana/Twareg 51, 91, 96
    Americas 64, 298, 396, 525
    Arab technique 215
    Asia 134, 222, 277, 369–70, 537
    Europe 318, 323, 334
    India/Sri Lanka 263, 448, 532
    for food 134, 163, 200, 287, 306, 537, 551
bleeding (internal), diagnosis 233
bleeding (wounds), South Africa 371–2
Blepharis linariifolia, galactogogue 91
Blepharis sp, ashes for wounds 502
blessings, in treatments 103–4, 264
blindness, aetiologies of 189
'blisters', for throat problems 323
bloat 13
    Afghan Koochi pastoralists 183
    Africa 39, 86–7, 91, 277, 514, 515, 539
    Asia 141, 148, 149, 383
    Europe 75–6, 110, 114, 148, 485
    in goats 417
    India 77, 211, 213, 328, 485–6
        treatment by women 449, 450
        cattle 102, 283
        small ruminants 503
    Iran 505
    South America
        Andes 125, 315, 437
        Bolivia 126
        Mexico 148, 423
        Peru 200, 317, 380–1
    Sri Lanka 273, 546–7
    see also eructative (antibloat)
blood and fat, for sore mouths 98
blood clotting (failure), in anthrax 154
blood collection, at ritual slaughter 184
blood eye drops, for conjunctivitis 130
blood in milk, camphor for 453–4
blood supply, mixture for horses 127–8
bloodletting *see* bleeding
blows, 'diverse charms' 158
boar dung, uses for 157–8
bodily humours, in Ayurvedic medicine 432
Boerhavia diffusa roots 415
Bogor (Indonesia) 43–4, 349, 384
boils, treatments 65, 237
Bolivia 13, 122, 220, 239–41, 465
    guinea pig 377–8
    women, EVK 125–6
    see also Aymara; Gran Chaco Province;
        Trinitarios
Bombax ceiba, for broken horns 236
Bombax costatum, for fever 103
bone brittleness, feed supplements for 64
bone marrow, as energizer 8
bone meal and salt 64
bonemeal 8, 91
bonesetters, healers 12, 310, 320, 370

Book of Home Remedies, cats/dogs 233
Boran cattle, indigenous 216
Borana pastoralists (Ethiopia/Kenya) 208, 216,
    370, 393–4, 397
Borgou, trypanotolerant cattle 552
Borneo (Indonesia) 13, 18, 533–4
borona, for dermatophilosis 446
Bororo (WoDaaße) pastoralists 158–9
bororoji zebu cattle 158–9
Borreria verticillata 282
Borreria verticillata leaves 209
Boscia coreacea unripe fruit 104
Boscia senegalensis 68, 90, 91–2
bot larvae, removal 214–15, 461
botanical nomenclature, in EVK 166–7, 202
botany *see* ethnobotany; medicinal plants
Botswana 457, 458–9
bottle gourd 260, 399, 453
bottle jaw, treatment in Bolivia 126
bouganvillea, for bronchitis, dogs 526
bouquets
    medicinal 40, 148
    medico-religious 110–15, 135, 156, 310, 330,
        522–3
Bouzou people, camel specialists 157–8
bovine plague (contagious typhus) 329
bovines 169–70, 290, 376, 486
    parasites 42, 308–9, 508
    see also buffalo; cattle
box leaves (blessed), in bouquets 135
brain concussion, camels, Mongolia 368
brain damage, risk in horn shaping 115
brake fluid, for ectoparasitism 386
bran
    feeds 64, 65, 129, 449
    in egg preservation 76
    poultice for mastitis 323
branding 12, 215, 433
    Africa 91, 159, 189, 366
        Baggara (Sudan) 138, 539
    India 235, 284, 290, 529, 533
brandy, in wash for ectoparasites 461
Brassica campestris oil 261
Brassica juncea (mustard) 458
braxy, clostridial infection 75, 483
Brazil 12, 343, 468
    see also Bahia
bread
    blessed, disease prevention 111
    for anuria, in horses 535
breath smell, disease diagnosis 471, 486
breathing (stimulation to), calves 397
breeding 15–16, 137
    in Africa 62, 188–9, 474, 539
    in India 447
    camelids 120, 225, 228
    camels 92, 292–3
        Somalia 165, 232–3, 246, 396
    cattle 158–9, 200, 470, 471, 546, 560
    goats 417–18
    pigs 193
    sheep 225, 228, 302
    yaks 312, 556
breeding ceremony, camelids, Peru 410

breeding control, *see* contraception
breedstock exchange 184–5, 287, 425–6, 427–8, 429
brewer's yeast, medicinal use 118, 233
Brickellia spp. (calf's herb) leaves 120
Bridelia ferruginea bark 466
bridewealth, livestock, Africa 504
brinjal, galactagogue in India 400
Britain 13, 148, 342, 511
    see also England; Scotland
broken bones *see* fractures
bronchitis 245, 526
broom (*Retama duraeginista barbara*) 132–3
Brosimum alicastrum, tonic 167
browse plants 81, 479, 538, 549
browsing goats, parasite-avoidance 391
browsing sheep, Caussenarde breed 111
brucellosis 79, 466, 481, 517
bruises, remedies for 198, 536
Brunei, Malay people 284–5
Bryophyllum leaves 212, 401
Bryophyllum pinnatum juice 301
buccal abscess, in camels 132–3
bucks, *see also* goats; rabbits
bucks (goat) 262, 468
Buddleia longifolia 317
buffalo 133, 390–1, 442, 509
    in India 142, 211
    in Philippines 77, 143, 162
    breeding
        fertility 77–8, 211
        milk yield 55, 127, 415, 492
        oestrus induction 127, 532
        retained placenta 126
    ectoparasites
        mange 262–3, 436
        tick control by poultry 432
    endoparasites 191, 528
    feed/fodder supplements 237
    ruminal dysfunction 283, 480
    sacred herds, of Toda people 459–60, 539–40
    see also bovines
buffalo calves *see* calves (buffalo)
Bulgaria, Karakatshan shepherds 334
bullet wounds, horses 501–2
bullocks 211, 400, 414, 415
    injuries 231, 414, 491
    yoke galls 210, 234, 238
bulls 63, 200
    castration *see* castration
    contraception *see* apron; contraception
bulls (yak), in Himalayas 312
Bunaji white cattle, Fulani 80–2, 470
burgu (*Echinocholoa stagnina*) 551
Burji peoples, in Kenya 208
Burkina Faso 103, 294, 495
    Fulani herders in 88–9, 256, 323–5, 494–5
Burma 136, 168, 498
burning, disease control 13–14, 82, 522–3
burning cloth, smoke cure for cough 529
burning (parotid lymph nodes) 183
burning with acid, for mange, camels 538
burns, remedies 198, 371
burrs, cats/dogs, home remedies 233

Burundi 69–72, 273–4
Bushi region, Zaire 131
Butana (Sudan) 37–40, 44–5, 169
Butea frondosa 455, 468
Butea monosperma 234, 284, 414, 449, 458
Butea sp. resin 261
butter 202, 370, 399
    for abscesses 91, 281
    for digestive problems 232, 514
    for ectoparasites 91, 132–3, 370, 441, 514
    for wounds 8, 295, 415, 488, 507, 514
    intranasal 139, 159
butter quality, feed and 530
buttermilk 129, 211, 231, 458, 486
Butyrospermum papadoxum (sheanut) 512
Butyrospermum parkii (sheanut) 209
buzzards, predators, in piglet loss 395
byne, galactagogue for cows 230

Cabrits area, Dominica 262
cactus, parts of 211, 220, 237, 547
Cadaba glandulosa leaves 209
caesarean operation, in sows 395
CAH *see* community animal healthcare
CAHW *see* community-based animal health worker
Cajamarca Department (Peru) 200, 437–8
Cajanus cajan L. leaves 411
Cajanus indicus 507
calabashes, beehives in Ghana 234
calcareous soil, for mange 214
calcium deficiency, milk fever 75, 211, 414, 416–17
calendar
    seasonal disease 83, 123, 215–16
    traditional, in India 199–200
calf hepatitis, Kenya 250
calf rejection, by cow, Kenya 379
calf's herb (*Brickellia* spp.) 120
California, Basque shepherds in 60
Calliandra spp. 404
callouses, treatments by Twareg 91
Calotropis 40, 507
    leaves 237, 453, 508
Calotropis gigantea 283
Calotropis gigantea leaves 126, 212, 432, 491
Calotropis procera 157, 160–1, 192, 282, 379, 480
Calotropis procera leaves 55, 214, 234
Calotropis procera root/branch 91
calves 72, 95, 253, 397, 502, 505, 539
    diarrhoea 118, 506
    ectoparasites 223, 441
    endoparasites 158, 211, 466, 505
        worms 140, 212, 230, 237, 273, 486
    fungal infection 310, 509
    indirect vaccination 220, 287
    mortality 118, 458, 482
    neonatal care 64, 135, 232, 403–4, 528–9
    see also weaning
calves (buffalo) 232, 262, 273, 418
calves (camel) 92, 232–3, 278–9, 555
calves (yak) 312
calving aid, for cows, in India 230
Cambodia 307

camel breeds 16, 521
  see also Bikaneri; Jaisalmeri; Marwari; Mewari
camelids 117, 207, 466, 512, 519
  Aymara Indians 296, 410
  in Peru 201, 410, 523, 547
camels 90–1, 478–9, 498–9, 551
  in Ethiopia 555
  in India 151, 237, 284, 287–94, 453
    breeders 287–8, 289–91, 293
  in Kenya 103–4, 277–9, 386–7
  in Mongolia 366–7, 369
  in North Africa 132–3, 289, 377
  in Somalia 79, 165–6, 232–3, 246
  in Sudan 37–40, 169, 292–3, 457
  Bedouin remedies 73, 214–15
  bloodletting 51, 551
  breeding 90, 92, 396
    control of 13, 138, 479
  cough 379
  diseases 139, 229, 245, 367, 496
    camelpox 229, 288
  fattening, in Kutch 325
  husbandry projects 177–8, 289–90
  lameness, firing for 38, 44–5
  overheated 414
  pack/draught 132, 287, 288
  scarification ritual cure 157–8
  skin lesions 90, 91, 212, 502, 513, 538
  zoo animals 461
Cameroon
  Fulani pastoralists 157–8, 333, 376
  HPI 37, 99, 397–9, 498, 502
    Ethnoveterinary Council 151
    Golden Talent Award 554
  livestock 15, 147, 209, 391, 552
  mange, acaracides 79–80, 322
  see also Bouzou; Fulani
camomile drench 114, 225, 226, 228
camphor
  for cold/cough/fever 223, 303, 388
  for ectoparasites 161, 262–3, 277
  for FMD 234, 458
  for joint problems 132, 211
  for mastitis 110, 323, 453–4
  for skin lesions 65, 283, 507
camphor oil 65
Camphora officinarum see camphor
Canada *see* Akwasasne Indians; Thompson Indians
Canchis Province (Andes) 104–5
Canna indica L. 409–10
cannabis 335, 400
Cannabis indica seeds 160–1
Cannabis sativa 168, 329, 330, 446
Capparis brevispina leaves 231
Capparis decidua 189
Capparis decidua wood charcoal 234, 415
Capparis sepiaria 507
Capraria biflora (ground) 262
caprine *see* goats
Capsella bursa-pastoris 110, 207
Capsicum 209, 303, 433
Capsicum annuum 518
Capsicum frutescens, chilli 129, 176, 458
capuli-wood ash 380

CAR *see* Central African Republic
carabao 162, 191
  see also buffalo
Caralluma somalica sap 379
carbolic acid 65, 323
carbolic oil, rub for mastitis 511
carbon powder from batteries 231
carcinoma, third eyelid, removal 386–7
cardiac system 64, 207, 400, 485, 499
Cardiospermum halicacabum leaves 399
Carica papaya 192, 209, 282, 463, 468
  see also papaya
Carica papaya leaves 448
Carica papaya shoots and seed oil 97
Carissa edulis berries 549
Carpathian mountains (Poland) 294–5
carrier ingredients 8
carrots 212, 233
Carthamus tinctorius oil 491
Carum copticum seeds (boiled) 126
Cascosán (commercial drug) 395–6
cashew nuts 143, 301, 503
cashew-nut oil 143
cassava, in feed 440
cassava leaves, for ectoparasites 14
Cassia alata (*ketepeng*) 383
Cassia auriculata 415
Cassia fistula 491, 507
Cassia occidentalis 250, 262
Cassia senna leaves 169, 401
Castanea vulgaris (chestnut) 65–6
Castella texanum L. 167
castor leaves, poisoning by 102, 236
castor oil 237, 400, 508
  antidote to toxic plants 64, 386
  for ectoparasite control 212, 415, 417
  for indigestion 202, 295
  for poultry distemper 238, 240
  for wounds 210, 211
castor seeds 400, 546–7
castor-bean (*Ricinus communis*) wash 417
castration 12, 13, 18, 51
  techniques 13, 333, 403–4, 455
  buffalo 133
  camelids 120–1, 220, 225, 228
  camels 38, 90, 92, 246, 479
  cattle
    in Africa 86, 92, 306, 335, 366, 397
      ceremonial 196, 314
    in Asia 89, 137, 399, 486
    in South America 239
  dogs 89, 550
  elephants 433
  female animals 63, 538
  horses 89, 90, 224, 474
    American Indians 304, 462, 550
  pigs 16, 89, 380, 395, 538
  poultry 89
  reindeer 52–4
  small ruminants 51, 90, 183, 335
    goats 93, 306, 418
    sheep 88, 92, 225, 228, 551
  yaks 312
catagua (*Hura crepitans* L.) 50

cataract *see* eye
catarrh, cure by American cattlemen 64
catarrhal fever, of goats, in Nigeria 62
Catawba, American Indians 306
catheter (indigenous), for camels 132
catnip, behaviour modification of cats 377
cats 14, 118, 166, 233, 303, 311, 377
cattle 229–30
  in Africa 102, 117–18, 191
    Botswana 457, 458–9
    Fulani 80–1, 102, 190, 302, 466, 471, 545–6
      WoDaaße 158–9, 328
    Kenya 143–5
    Mandari, Horn of Africa 117–18
    South Africa 219
    Sudan 168–9, 268, 326–7, 521, 552
    Tanzania 560
    Uganda 163, 200
    Zambia 86–7, 429
  in Bangladesh 282
  in England 156
  in Europe 482–3, 512
  in India 237, 409–10, 415, 416, 442, 528–30
    Andhra Pradesh 455
    Chotanagpur 491
    Hissar farmers 283
    Kannada-speaking region 230–1, 507
    Rajasthan 480
    Tamil Nadhu 401–2, 443–4, 532
    Tamil-speakers 260, 399, 400–1
    Teluga-language people 507–8
  in Indonesia 153, 172
  in Italy 338–9
  in Luxemburg 510
  in Mexico 414
  in Nepal 329, 330
  in North America 64–5
  in Pakistan, Afghan Koochi 183
  in South America 279–80, 317, 365–6, 437–8
  in Sri Lanka 263–4, 273
  bloat 75, 148, 200, 315
  constipation 432
  diarrhoea 282, 330, 491
  diseases
    dermatophilosis 444, 462
    ECF 287
    malignant catarrh 326–7
    rinderpest 326–7
    syndromes 211, 246, 495–6
    trypanosomosis control 88–9
  feed supplements 199, 237, 393, 455, 481–2, 549
  fever 103
  flies 102, 548
  fumigation 63, 102
  hoof protection 277
  hypothermia, India 482
  immunity stimulation 102–3
  joint problems 282
  neem (*Azadirachta indica* A. Juss.) tree 396
  parasites
    anaplasmosis 258
    ectoparasites 133, 173–4, 200, 265
      ticks 203, 528
    endoparasites 84–5, 133, 141, 213–14, 505

  pneumonia, in Europe 75
  rumenal dysfunction 109, 202, 342
  skin lesions 162, 294
  see also bovines; bullocks; bulls; calves; cows;
    dairy cattle; horns; oxen
cattle breeding
  in Africa 16, 40, 187, 190, 253
    Fulani 107–8, 470, 471
  in India 199–200
cattle breeds 471, 517
  ECF resistance 137, 355
  tick-resistant 184
  trypanotolerant 255, 310, 385, 552
  see also Afrikaander; Ankole; azawak zebu;
    Baladi; Baoulé; Boran; Borgou, bororoji zebu;
    Bunaji white cattle; Kapsiki; Keteku; Lagune;
    Mashona; Muturu; Namchi; N'Dama; Nguni;
    Nuba dwarf Koalib; Raja; Sanga x zebu;
    Somba; Szigetköz; Texas Longhorn cattle;
    Tswana; West African Shorthorn; zebu
cattle dung *see* cow dung
Caucasus Mountains, yak imports 312
Caussenarde, sheep, in the Cévennes 111
cauterization 12, 157, 339–40, 397, 514
  for bullet wounds 501–2
  for diarrhoea 86–7, 429
  for ECF 537
  for eye infections 86–7
  for footrot, with gunpowder 343
  for hydatidosis, Turkana 326
  for lameness 38–9, 132–3, 339, 429
  for rabies (after amputation) 366, 367
  for skin diseases 132–3, 292, 369–70
  for snake/wild animal bites 529
  see also firing; moxibustion
cayenne pepper, for poultry houses 76
Caylloma Province (Peru), alpaca 134
CBAH *see* community-based animal healthcare
CBPP
  quarantine 326–7
  traditional vaccination 96, 106, 302, 366, 370
    indirect, calves 220, 397
    technique 332
  treatments 50, 159, 183
CCPP
  prophylaxis 183
  traditional vaccination 78–9, 96, 183, 504
  treatments 96, 328
Cedrela odorata leaves 301
Cedrus deodara wood (oil) 451–2
Ceeldheer, Somali pastoralists 165–6
Ceiba pentandra 489, 505
Celosia schweinfurthiana 379
Celosia stuhlmanniana 379
Centella, in health tonic 209
Centella asiatica 444
Central African Republic (CAR) 96, 107–9
Central Java, small ruminants 209
central nervous system signs 158, 431
Central Rangelands Development Project 79
century plant *see Agave americana*
Ceratonia siliqua (algarrobo) 65–6
ceremonies 196, 304, 314, 427
cestode infestations 455

Cestrum hediondinum juice 135
Ceterach officinarum Willd. 111
Cévennes, France 110–15, 135
Chad 48, 54–5, 105, 521
    Ishtirak, paravet programme 73–4, 329,
      429–30
    SECADEV, paravet training 218–19
    see also Salamat; Zaghwa
chalk, uses of 76, 211, 213
chancarro leaves, fumigation 321
chanting, medico-religious 306, 317
chapati bread, as carrier 211, 519
charcoal 76, 415
    as digestive 75, 244, 417
    for wounds 91–2, 234, 536
charms, medico-religious 96, 157–8, 277
Charvah pastoralists (India) 442
chawlla lago, for liver fluke 410
cheetah skin, for fever 103
Chenopodium ambrosioides 83, 262, 485
Chernobyl explosion 52–4
chestnut (*Castanea vulgaris*) 65–6
Cheyenne, American Indians 306
Chhotanagpur (India), medicinemen 491
Chiapas highlands (Mexico) 420–30
chicken (albino), sacrifice 516
chicken droppings, medicinal 211, 395
chickens 164, 239, 310, 528
    crop-bound 76, 506
    feed supplement 265
    lice in coops 262
    parasite control by 243, 387
    weed control by 243
    see also chusca; criolla; eggs; incubation; snake-
      fighting
chickpea *see* gram
chicks 209, 297, 301
    gentian violet dye, protection 506
chickweed, for colds, caged birds 303
chilca, in Peru, as purgative 50
chilcúan (*Helosis longipes*) 464
Chile 173
chilli 335
    see also Capsicum
chilli pepper 103
chilli pod 401
chilli powder 232, 400, 458
chillies
    dried red 295, 529
    green (*Capsicum frutescens* L.) 129, 400
Chim-Shaullo (Peru) 175–6
China 246, 285, 537–8
    bovine mastitis control 169–70
    dairy-goat husbandry 309
    duck fattening 325
    pig husbandry 137, 149, 314
    yak husbandry 311, 312–13
    Yin versus Yang theory 371
    see also acupuncture; Hangzhou; Sichuan; Taihu
      pig
Chinese medicine 56–7, 128, 311, 314, 349, 557–8
    herbal 315, 477–8, 558
    ritual in diagnosis 148, 371
Chinese rice-husk incubation system 65

CHIP (Camel Husbandry Improvement Project)
    289–90
chiqollo, for endoparasites 410
chirimoya fruit, for ectoparasites 437–8
chiropractic care, for animals 549–50
chlamydiosis (*qange*) 339–40
chlorinated lime, disinfectant 65
cholera, poultry 513
cholesterol levels reduced, dogs 524
chopattia (aquatic grass) 261
Christianity 298, 420–1, 428, 515
    Church lamp oil 152–3, 465
chronic diseases 188, 288, 477–8
Chrozophora brocchiana, poisoning by 91
Chrysomya bezziana, for screw worm 191
Chrysophyllum cainito, anthelmintic 177
Chumbivilcas (Peru), stock raising 418–19
chusca, poultry breed, Andes 16, 116–17
Cicer arietinum, oestrus induction 532
cicihuataa, for pleurisy 381
Cinchona pubescens 201–2
cinnamon, uses of 118, 433, 526
circulatory problems, hypertension 132–3
Cissampelos mucromata roots 373
Cissus cactiformis G. 459
Cissus quadrangularis 133–4, 202, 282
Cissus quadrangularis stems 231, 507
citronella grass stems and leaves 243
Citrullus colocynthis 55, 212, 283
Citrus aurantifolia 431
Citrus aurantium 409, 463
citrus fruit/juice, for poultry 301, 436
Citrus lemonum (lemon) 161
Citrus mitis B. 45–6
Citrus quadrangularis 324
civet dung, for coenurosis 158
civets, sheep predators 107–8
clam shells (ground) 334
clay
    in mineral mixes 168, 237
    see also kaolin; red clay
clay tablets, in ancient Mesopotamia 445
clay (wet) poultices, foot problems 65
cleavers (*Galium aparine*) 485
Clematis hirsuta leaf juice 354–5
Clematis hirsutissima 282
Clematis spp. root 378–9
Cleome icosandra L. seeds 126
Cleome pentaphylla leaves 202
Clerodendron phlomoides leaves 399
Clerodendrum inerme 281, 458
Clerodendrum multiflorum leaves 234
Clerodendrum phlomidis 482, 532
Clerodendrum phlomidis leaf juice 235
Clitoria ternatea 176
clostridial infection, braxy 75, 483
cloth dipped in pig blood (burnt) 400, 402
clover, mineral-rich feed supplement 64
cloves, for calf scour 118
cloves (oil of), in sheep dip 303
CMTB (Bare Center of Traditional Medicine) 464
coal-oil/coal-tar, for parasites 64
coat colour (red), cattle 172

cobwebs, wound dressing 8, 371–2, 512
coca, for cold, in newborn care 134
coca leaves, offerings/rituals 126, 317
CocaCola, drench 431, 514
coccidiosis 108, 167, 209, 245
Coccinia grandis 55
Cocculus spp. 166
Cochiospermum tinctorium 308
coconut 149, 273, 453
coconut fruit 260, 546–7
coconut husk 162, 210, 231, 546–7
coconut milk 77, 172, 191, 210, 301, 318
coconut oil 162, 172, 340, 383, 399, 402
    for wounds 162, 401, 448, 452
coconut palm, pollination 400
coconut palm leaves, feed supplements 237
coenurosis (tapeworm cyst) 88, 110, 111, 158, 316,
    334
coffee, uses of 281, 299–300, 503
coherence/convergence/concordance analysis
    273–4, 275
coin (penny), for copper deficiency 342
Coix lacryma-jobi thorns 281
cold, agent of disease 134, 228, 229
cold water, uses of 13, 76, 77–8, 183
colds 235, 303, 528
    livestock 91, 111, 262, 415
Coleus aromaticus leaves 176
colibacillosis *see Escherichia coli*
colic 111, 282, 367, 380–1, 485
    in India 141, 480
    calves 505
    horses 133–4, 369, 480, 510
Colocynthis sp. ashes 288
Colocynthis vulgaris seeds/tar 169
Colombia 365–6, 377–8, 511–12
colon/caecum impaction 128
colonial veterinary interventions 372–3
Colonos, from Andes, in Bolivia 239–40
colorado, feed supplement 321
colostrum 335, 397, 416–17, 508
    for retained placenta 76, 126
    intake restricted 24, 40, 55, 278, 309
colour, chick protection 48
colts, neonatal care, Hidatsa Indians 550
coltsfoot (*Tussilago farfara*) 485, 499
Columellia obovata decoction 83, 84
Comanche, American Indians 305
Combretum 106, 209
Combretum glutinosum 55, 282
comets, livestock diseases and 120
comfrey (*Symphytum officinale*) 148, 485
Commelina forskalei 68
Commicarpus helenae 502
Commicarpus plumbagineus 379
Commiphora africana gum 91
Commiphora erythraea 370–1, 386
Commiphora incisa gum 386
Commiphora madagascarensis J. 459
Commiphora mukul bark 234
communication, the seven 'C's for effectiveness
    389
communication failure, and cultural diferences
    226–9

Communication for Technology Transfer in
    Agriculture Project 363
community animal healthcare (CAH) projects
    98–9, 531
community livestock care programme, Sri Lanka
    263
community livestock development project, Uganda
    201
community vaccinators, for rinderpest, in Sudan
    100
Community Veterinary Agents, in Ethiopia 215
community-based animal health worker (CAHW)
    123–4, 269, 334–5, 337, 530
community-based animal healthcare (CBAH) 37,
    63, 99–100, 204, 205–6
community-based application of EVK, Conference
    working group 347
community-based EV research, Zaire, 'local
    research brigades' 330–1
community-based health-care, in Kenya 48–9
community-based research, ANTHRA in India
    59–60
community-based vaccination programmes 333–4
community-organized approach, Recording and
    Using Indigenous Knowledge: A Manual 252
compresses, in European treatments 76
computerized database, HERVET 10 319
conception promotion 211, 236, 401, 453
conception rates, and compass direction 199–200
conditioner, for horses, herbal remedies 303
condors, predators on llamas 126
Conference on EVM, First International 344–8
congestion, scarification for 157
conjunctivitis 130, 176, 223, 225, 226, 228
    contagious 191, 483
constipation 149, 198, 235, 303, 400, 505
    buffalo 126
    cattle 237, 264, 432
    elephants 433
contagious agalactia, in goats 417
contagious bovine pleuropneumonia *see* CBPP
contagious caprine pleuropneumonia *see* CCPP
contagious diseases, prevention 106, 188
contagious ecthyma 79, 167, 277
contagious kerato-conjunctivitis 191, 483
contagious skin necrosis 103–4, 278, 279, 292
contagious typhus (bovine plague) 329
contraception 13, 90, 92, 474
    camel 138
    goats 418
    sheep 155, 264, 369
    see also penis
contraceptive, herbal agents 97, 203
contraceptive devices 18, 343
    see also apron
cooking oil 238, 240, 360–2, 381
copper, in navel cauterization 64
copper container, for mix for worms 486
copper deficiency, copper coin 15, 342
copper sulphate 142, 212, 273, 372
    for eye disorders 372, 529, 536
    for parasitic diseases 213, 461, 529
    for skin lesions 244, 401
copper vitriol, for foot problems 88

copper-containing 'green' salt 175
coptis, in Chinese medicine 314
coquera, digestive system disease 420
Corchorus spp. leaves 236
Corchorus tridens 505
Corchorus trilocularis 505
Cordia curassavica leaves 301
Cordia dichotoma 486
Cordia gharaf leaves 238
Cordia sp. 211, 238
Cordyla pinnata 439, 505
coriander, ground seeds 127
corn, as feedstuff 498
corn syrup, for ketosis 462
corncobs, infusion 228
Cornell Peru Project 392
corrals 225, 228, 253, 524
    disease prevention 193–4, 232–3, 257–8
coryza, poultry infection 176, 528
Coryza balsamifera L. 45–6
cosmological classification of elements, China 371
cost effectiveness, assessment of 149
cottage cheese, for vomiting 233
cotton ball, for milk production 415
cotton bolls and roots 237
cotton dresses, as disease prevention 505
cottonseed 40, 103, 512, 529, 546–7
    feed supplement 64, 199
cottonseed oil 64, 169, 292–3
cougars, llama as alarm-givers 14
cough 318, 329, 388, 399, 448, 485
    camels 367, 379, 386
    cattle 129, 376, 402, 507, 529
    horses 103, 306
    pigs 432, 525
    poultry 209, 335
    small ruminants 142
Council of Experts, HPI Cameroon 397–9
counter-magic, sorcery 286
cow dung 282, 536, 539
    for skin infections 288, 396
    for wounds 334, 512, 529
cow dung ash 212, 283, 317
cow pox, neem tree treatments 492
cowpea, mineral-rich feed supplement 64
cows 127, 129, 138, 230, 265
    abortion, risk 230, 529
    calf rejection 379
    infertility 137, 415, 459, 537
        medico-religious practices 286
        oestrus induction 77, 127, 147, 211, 486
        vaginal cauterization 12
    milk production 253, 415, 515
        galactagogues 55, 338, 409, 502
    parturition 64, 328
        placenta expulsion 77, 138, 195, 287, 415, 489
        postpartum care 135, 414, 416
    pregnancy test 413, 527
    sexual maturity delayed by oil cakes 77
    sterilization 63
    trolls/goblins, protection from 430
    udder
        mastitis 195, 323, 447–8, 511
        swollen 415, 437

see also other conditions/infectious diseases
cow's milk, medicinal uses 91–2, 401
coyotes, predators 14, 238, 395
crab (field, live), for foot injuries 400
cranberry juice 233
Crataegus mexicana 526
'craziness' 91, 306, 316
cream of tartar, in anthelmintic 118
Cree, American Indians 305, 462
creolene, for demodicosis 240
creosote 64, 76, 228, 303, 396
cresol, disinfectant 65
Crinum sp. bulb and tuber 138
criolla, poultry breed 116–17
criollo, pig breed 395
criollo, sheep 61
Croatia, horses 535–6
cropping and stockraising interactions 82
Crossopteryx febrifuga 282
Crotalaria linifolia L. 491
Croton macrostachys leaves 373
Croton tiglium L. 45–6
Crow, American Indians 305, 306
cucumber seeds 503
Cucumis melo (melon) 510
Cucumis prophetarum 195
Cucumis pseudo-colocynthis 491
Cucumis pustulatus 209, 466
Cucurbita maxima (giant pumpkin) 421
Cucurbita maxima seeds 61, 110, 111, 427
Cucurbita moschata seeds 493
Cucurbita pepo seeds 448
Cucurbitae evaluated 455
cud feeding, for ruminal dysfunction 8, 109, 342
culén (*Psoralea glandulosa*) 465
cults
    Fulani, Nigeria 157, 190
    horse medicine, American Indian 304
    veterinary saints, France 56, 372
cultural impact of FMD, in Peru 392
culture
    in communication failure 226–9, 291–2
    in EVM 298, 300, 304–6, 321–2, 342
    in livestock management 229–30, 241, 247–8, 278
    of ethnopharmacology 511
cumin 399, 400
    cattle 129, 416–17, 455, 532
    horses 118
Cuminum cyminum see cumin
Curculigo orchioides Gaerin tuber 491
Curcuma 209, 237
Curcuma aerginosa rhizome 503
Curcuma longa 129, 161, 409, 458, 509
Curcuma phaeocaulis 172
Curcuma xanthorrhiza rhizome 503
curds, medicinal uses 236, 400, 414, 486
curers *see* healers
CURPHAMETRA, drug trials 441–2, 464–5
curse, disease caused by 136, 240
Cuscuta reflexa 237
custard apple tree 413, 418
cut-and-carry fodder 440, 538
cutaneous streptothricosis *see* dermatophilosis

cuttlefish powder, for eye problems 138
'cuy sickness', guinea pigs 104–5
Cuzco (Peru) 225, 380–1
cyanide poisoning 440, 455
Cyanotis tuberosa 491
Cymbopogon giganteus 158
Cymbopogon nerrvalus 169
Cymbopogon proximus 91
Cymbopogon schoenanthus 103
Cynara scolymus (artichoke) 61, 84
Cynodon dactylon 399, 400, 482
Cyperus alternifolius bark 104
Cyperus rotendus rhizomes 260

dabtaras, church healers, Ethiopia 515
Daedalacanthus roseus T. 409–10
dairy cattle 188, 283, 509, 528–9, 546–7, 560
dairy goats, China 309
dairy-temples, Toda people 459–60, 540
Dalbergia sissoo 211, 212, 216–17, 296
'Damascus' goats, Syria 387
dancing, medico-religious 17, 157–8, 306
dandelion 169–70, 485
Darfur, Sudan, Arab tribes 63
database, computerized 56, 319, 413–14
date pits ashes, for pack sores 132
date syrup, for mange/scabies 132–3
datepalm nuts (dried), feed supplement 237
datura, as pain killer 168
Datura metel 202, 236, 400, 401, 439, 505
Datura stramonium (jimsonweed) 129, 536
Daye Chopin District (Afghanistan) 531
days of the week, conception rates 199–200
DDT, use of 24, 132–3, 189, 228, 288
decongestant, for calves 502
deer hair (scorched) 369–70
deer horn, medicinal use 191
deer sinew, suture material 502
deficiency diseases 213
  see also calcium; copper; magnesium;
    phosphorus
dehydration 233, 318
demodicosis, of dogs 240
Dendrophthoe spp. 235
dermatitis, mycotic *see* dermatophilosis
dermatological conditions
  Himax for 330–1
  see also ectoparasites; mange; skin; specific con-
    ditions
dermatomycosis 386
dermatophilosis 55, 129, 444, 446, 462
dermatophytosis 437, 509
Derris eliptica 528
Derris philippinensis 528
desi ghee see ghee
Desmodium maxonii 193
Desmodium plicatum 503
destiny, in sudden death 188
Detarium microcarpum 513
detergent 138, 265, 371–2, 386, 437–8, 514
development projects, inappropriate 100, 241–2,
  520, 525
dew avoidance 81, 96, 306, 334, 391, 461

Dewasis *see* Raika
Dhami healers, Nepal 148
Dhangars, Indian stockraisers 59
diabetes, diagnosis in cats/dogs 233
diagnosis 8, 139, 148, 158, 233, 307, 486
DIALOG on-line search methods, EVM 561
diarrhoea 24, 54, 65–6, 97, 134, 197–8, 201, 245
  in Africa 39, 41, 50, 91, 429–30, 539
    Fulani people 108, 157, 517
  in Asia 149, 222, 253
  in Ecuador 228
  in Europe 338–9, 485
  in India 202, 235–6, 296, 400, 448, 491
    Gujarat 210, 212
    Rajasthan 414, 416
  bovines/buffalo 77, 458, 486
  calves/kids/piglets 118, 279, 314, 506
  camel 104, 279, 461
  camelids 134, 201, 245, 410
  cattle
    in Africa 86–7, 117–18, 159
    in India 237, 329, 330, 507–8
    North America 64, 118
  pigs 69, 314, 431
  poultry 55, 209, 335, 436
  rabbits 120, 200
  small ruminants 142, 391, 458, 503
    goats 417
    sheep 111, 119, 193–4, 295, 423, 437
diarrhoea (bloody) 410, 480–1
diarrhoea ('green') 55
Dichrostachys cinerea 466, 480
Dictyocaulus filaria 128
diesel oil 119, 288, 395, 525, 539
dietary specialization, in sheep 16
digestive disorders 152–3, 207, 338–9, 492, 514
  camels 132–3, 513
  cats/dogs 233
  goats 420
  see also ruminal dysfunction
digestive pasteurellosis 505
digestive stimulant 396, 518
Digitalis lino 499
Digitalis purpurea (foxglove) 485, 499
Digitaria horizontalis 482
Dinka 44, 99–100, 136, 268, 546
  healers (*atet*) 326–7, 334–5, 475–7, 560–1
Diola pastoralists, Senegal 418
Diospyros cordifolia fruits 235
Diospyros melanoxylon 284
Diospyros mespiliformis 250, 502, 549
Diospyros montana 532
dipping, in disease control 120, 134
direction animal is facing, in conception
  199–200
disbudding, cauterization for 397
disease avoidance 14–15, 107–8, 229, 538
disease characteristics, of bouquets, in France 112,
  114
disease concepts 380, 494–5
  evil spirits as cause 89
  genies as causes 157–8
  transference to inanimate object 156
disease control 39, 250, 317, 375, 386–7, 469–73

disease increase, use of wells and 381
disease names, linguistic difficulties 144–5, 205
disease patterns, epidemiology 404–5, 494, 560–1
disease prevention
    in Africa 124–5, 206–7, 521, 522–3
    in France, bouquets 111
    NGOs in 197, 217
    poultry in 513, 534
    see also pest control
disease resistance 16, 209
    livestock breeds 80, 387–8, 471
        cattle 198, 216
    poultry breeds 116–17, 249–50, 404
    small ruminants 406
    see also cattle breeds; sheep breeds
disease scoring, for EVM study 122, 125
disease susceptibility 560
disease syndromes, anthropology 495
disease-ranking tool, BVW training 311
disinfectants (commercial) 65, 396
disinfection (indigenous) 88, 329
distemper
    in horses 306
    see also strangles
distemper (*moquillo*), in poultry 238
distomatosis *see* fasciolosis
diuretics 264, 402, 499
Djallonké sheep 255, 471
doddi vines 210
Dodonaea viscosa 281, 400
dog faeces 103, 369–70
dog-rose, in bouquets, France 310
dogs 47, 74, 233, 524, 526
    in Asia 206, 277
    in India 264
    in Mexico 321
    in North America 155, 239–40, 499–500
    in South America 240, 317
    as predators (sheep/piglets) 108, 395
    castration 550
    ectoparasites 118, 265
    electroacupuncture for 280–1
    hunting, breeding by Twareg 90
    mange 140, 549
    motion sickness 166
    mycotic dermatitis 129
    predator control by 14
    puppies, anthelmintic 524
    rabies 96, 101–2, 237, 366
    roundworms 194, 303
    tapeworm 52–4, 486–7
        coenurosis 110, 111
        hydatidosis 60, 116, 255, 326
Dominican Republic 37, 262, 463
Donegal (Ireland) 482–3
donkey (black), droppings of 157–8
donkey faeces, for food poisoning 235–6
donkeys 91, 189, 254, 386, 514
    aconite (wolfsbane) 87–8
    endoparasites 181–2, 505
    evil eye, protection from 321
    skin lesions 212, 406
dony dony 334–5
Doroboro people, Kenya 250

Dorpner sheep, parasite-resistant 387
Dracaena steudneri leaf juice 354–5
draught animals *see* bullocks; camels; oxen; pack
    animals
drenching equipment 18, 300
dressings for fractures 18, 234, 238
drinking areas, disease prevention 124–5
dromedary *see* camel
droppings *see* dung
drought resistance, Boran cattle 216
drought strategies, Twareg herders 555
drumstick tree bark 485–6
Drymis spp. 173
Dryopteris filix, in Wopell 455
Dryopteris filix-mas Schott (male shield fern) 463
Duchesnea indica 141
duck plague (duck virus enteritis) 517, 518
ducks 301, 325, 497–8, 525–6
    duckling rearing 13, 18, 517–18
    egg incubation 65, 285, 437, 518, 533
    egg production 533–4
    pest control by 42, 308–9, 430–1, 498, 506
Dundi, in home-made mineral licks 168
dung 75, 76
    for digestive problems 514
    for wounds 8, 86–7, 231, 306, 539
    in horn shaping 115
    see also faeces; manure; under animal species
dung beetles, destroy nematode larvae 155
dung (cow), to bait beehives 234
dung extraction, in calf bloat 86–7
dung fires (smoky) 168, 187, 239, 268, 326–7, 385,
    529
dung on teats, weaning 392, 397, 515, 521
dust-baths, for poultry 13, 76, 77
dwarf small ruminants 255, 351–2
dysentery 129, 231, 376, 491
dystocia 142, 264, 292, 309, 513
    see also obstetric operations

ear bleeding (treatment) 159, 376, 525
ear disorders 65, 399, 517
ear notching (identification) 52–4, 184–5, 201
ear slitting (treatment) 87–8, 295, 366
ear ticks/mites 64, 233, 272, 317
ear tip cutting (treatment) 232, 283, 328, 537
earth, edible 78, 245
earthworm farming 365–6
earthworms (dried and powdered) 212
East Africa 135, 198, 375, 462–3
    camels, bloodletting 551
    horn shaping 115
    livestock husbandry 13, 137, 191, 479
    see also Barabaig; Turkana; WaSwahili
East Coast Fever *see* ECF
East Java 340, 394–5
ECF 162, 258, 472, 537
    cattle resistance 16, 137, 287, 355
    lymph nodes in 183, 251, 471
Echinacea angustifolia 306
echinococcosis *see* hydatidosis
Echinops echinatus 235–6
Eclipta alba Hassak roots 491, 518

eco-pathological plants, Sahel (Africa) 510
'ecohealth', concept of 511
economic advantages, of EVM 26–7, 84–5, 520
economic loss, ticks as cause 272
economic role
  livestock 41–3, 77, 123, 125
    camels 44
    cattle 86, 159, 168–9
ecthyma
  contagious 79, 167, 277
  lambs, bouquets for 111, 113, 115
ectoparasites 24–5, 461
  in Afghan women's knowledge 142
  in Africa 251, 253, 517
  in India 234, 281, 507
  in Mongolia 369–70
  in North America 64
  in South America 226, 434
    Peru 200, 317, 358, 380
  buffalo 143, 262–3, 390
  camelids 410, 466, 519
    alpaca 437–8, 523
    llamas 220
  camels 229, 386
  cattle 129, 437–8, 458, 529
  dogs 277
  paravet training, by ITDG for Gabbra pastoral-
    ists, Kenya 316
  pigs 317, 468, 525
  poultry 77, 209, 301, 308, 459
  sheep 85, 391
  see also fleas; ked; lice; mange; ticks
ectoparasiticides 352
  in Africa 115–16, 513, 514
  in India 173–4, 508
  in Peru 175, 463
  see also tarwi; tobacco
Ecuador 225–7, 228–9, 377–8
  see also Quechua Indians
eczema 212, 281
  skin problems, healers' therapies, in India 281
edible oil 234, 235, 514
Edinburgh Zoo, herb garden, Scotland 485
eels, predators on ducks, Vietnam 518
eggplant (*Solanum incanum*) 50
eggs
  hatching 17, 506, 533
  incubation 65, 285, 437, 518, 533
  medicinal uses 77, 118, 453, 514
    for fractures 238, 480
    in feed supplement 128, 399, 416–17, 503,
      513
  preservation 76
  production, ducks 75, 533–4
eggshells 76, 168, 536
eggwhite 231, 371, 443–4, 465, 507
Egypt (ancient), like Dinka healers 476–7
EIG (Ethnoveterinary Interview Guide) 205–6
eland hide collar, medico-religious 286
eland rinderpest, and cattle 326–7
elderberry (*Sambucus* sp.) 132, 264, 321
electrical stimulation, therapy 434
electroacupuncture 280–1, 503
elements, cosmological classification of 371

Elephantopus scaber leaves 129
elephants 168, 378, 433, 488, 557
  dung of, for coenurosis 158
Eleusine coracana flour 236, 238, 284
elk dung, neonatal care of colts 550
elk sinew, suture material 550
Embelia ribes 455, 468
Emblica officinalis 411, 507
embryotomy/fetotomy 38, 64, 386–7
  see also obstetric operations
emorong, Turkana healers 253
emotional rapport, with sheep 423
Enartocarpus clavatus 139
encepahalitis 64
encephalomyelitis (louping ill) 483
endoparasites 16, 197–8
  in Afghan women's knowledge 142
  in Africa 54, 73, 90, 439, 505
  in Ecuador 226, 228, 229
  in India 211
  in Kenya 223, 253
  in Mexico 419
  in North America 64
  in Peru 83
  in Philippines 411
  buffalo 191, 437–8, 528
  camelids 201, 410
  camels 169, 292–3
  cattle 396, 416, 437–8
  donkeys 181–2
  pigs 525, 528
  poultry 208–9, 508
  sheep 130, 383, 421, 437–8
  small ruminants 142, 503
enemas, medicinal uses 64, 317
energizers, in feed 8, 127
engine grease 220, 412
engine oil 24, 86–7, 396
  for mange 189, 322, 436
engine oil (burnt) 201, 417, 525
engine oil (spent) 75, 179, 235
  for ectoparasites 386, 391, 485
England, historical 132, 148, 156, 323, 548
Enhydra flucturans 518
Enicostema hyssoplifolium 237
Entada phaseolides M. 45–6
Entada pursaetha Benth. seed cotyledon 491
Entada sudanica 157–8
enteric diseases, in Rumania 499
enteritis, of livestock 453
enterotoxaemia 142, 152–3, 295, 417
environment 13–14, 137, 190, 197, 389–90
envy, and cattle disorders 118
ephemeral fever 159, 399, 400
epidemic, in Ayurvedic medicine 433
epidemics, sorcery as cause 232
epizootic ulcerative syndrome (EUS) 192
Epsom salts, uses of 64, 118, 511
equines 14–15, 47, 485, 486
  see also donkeys; glanders; horses; mules
Eritrea, Beni-Amer pastoralists 188
eructative (antibloat) *see* bloat; ginger
Erycibe paniculata Roxb. 491
Erythrina edulis 365–6

Erythrina variegta 433
Escherichia coli
  in poultry 452
  see also colibacillosis
ethics, veterinary bioethics 187–8
Ethiopia 48, 195, 209
  beehives, dung insulation 18
  Boran cattle, indigenous 216
  community-based veterinary medicine 215, 333
  ER&D 215–16, 466, 552–3
  traditional veterinary practices 196, 270, 370–1,
    560
  see also Afar; Amharic; Ogaden; Oromo; Sidama
ethnobotanical survey, in Burundi 70–2
ethnobotanical treatments 83, 84–5, 281–2, 373–4,
  451–2
ethnobotany 32–3, 49–50, 72, 75, 379, 489
ethnodentistry 12
ethnodiagnostic techniques 471–2
ethnology, overview 187
ethnomedical pharmocopoeia 273–4
ethnomedical techniques, intersectoral 364
ethnomedicine 6, 270–1, 380–1, 498
ethnopharmacology 186, 511
ethnopharmacopoeia (*materia medica*) 8–11
ethnoveterinary, defined 284, 290
Ethnoveterinary Council, in Cameroon 151
ethnoveterinary data collection 204, 205–6
ethnoveterinary drugs, commercial 56
Ethnoveterinary Interview Guide (EIG) 205–6
ethnoveterinary knowledge *see* EVK
ethnoveterinary medicine *see* EVM
Ethnoveterinary Medicine in Kenya: A Field
  Manual 256–7
ethnoveterinary perceptions 254–5
ethnoveterinary plants 139, 174
ethnoveterinary R&D 1, 56–7, 343–5, 350
  difficulties 247–8, 260–1
  literature review 350, 357
  management of 273–4, 275, 301, 500
  new directions 28, 257–60, 365
  principles of 259–60, 422, 423–4
  programmes 540–2
  status of 468–9
ethnoveterinary RD&E 359, 360–2
ethnoveterinary surveys, anthropology in 501
Eucalyptus 197, 209, 526
Eucalyptus grandis leaves 88
Eucalyptus leaves 225, 226, 228
Eucalyptus sp. leaf oil 370, 451–2, 485
Eupatorium amygdalinum Lam (chilca) 50
Eupatorium ligustrinum 50, 193, 423
Euphorbia balsamifera 549
Euphorbia cameroonica (kerenahi) 79–80
Euphorbia candelabrum T. latex 459
Euphorbia characias 111
Euphorbia hirta 510
Euphorbia lancifolia 338
Euphorbia neriifolia latex 508
Euphorbia pilulifera L. leaves 102
Euphorbia roylcana 509–10
Euphorbia somaliensis latex 333
Euphorbia sp. branches 330
Euphorbia sp. (roasted) 261

Euphorbia sp. roots 210
Euphorbia spp. 439, 468
Euphorbia spp. latex 250
Euphorbia thymifolia 491
Euphorbia tortilis latex 399
Euphorbia triaculeata 96
Europe 13, 15, 135, 148, 461
  herbal farming (book) 74–7
EUS (epizootic ulcerative syndrome) 192
evil, magic as protection from 537
evil eye 118, 298, 300
  livestock protection 41, 103–4, 321, 483
  magico-religious beliefs 41, 167, 268, 515
  protection against 129, 420, 502
evil eye (*apeth*), Dinka healers on 535
evil principle, in disease 96
evil spirits 120, 240, 285
  driven off 228, 229, 285
  protection from 17, 89, 335, 449, 516
evil winds, protection from 17
EVK 195, 285, 336, 346, 347, 452
  allopathic medicine and 206–7, 268, 297–8,
    299
  collection 103, 205, 217–18, 299, 336, 494
  commercialization of 347
  dissemination 106–7, 151, 210, 398
  global pharmacopoeia concept 285
  holistic nature of 99, 100, 101, 271
  pan-African conference proceedings 58
  projects 99, 164, 346
EVM 22–4, 162, 193–4, 341
  advantages/disadvantages 23–7, 68, 178, 179,
    341, 348
  An Annotated Bibliography 349
  bibliography, search methods 561
  books/manuals, local language 28
  commercial production 327
  databank 347
  First International Conference on 344–8
  healers 291, 354
  in Africa 364
  in Asia 349–50
  in India 388–9
  in Mexico 46–7
  information dissemination 27–9, 266, 389
  international conference 337
  interview instrument 559
  national-level needs 48, 69, 266, 341–2
  principles vii–viii 7–8
  validation 180
  veterinary medicine and 123–4, 146–7, 166–7,
    286
  veterinary training and 178, 180
  websites 30–2
ewes 42, 110, 199, 323
exercise 13, 65, 77, 129, 148, 534
expectorants 213
eye ailments
  in Africa 223, 334, 371–2, 374, 514
  in India 491
  in Philippines 318
  alpaca 201
  buffalo 232, 532
  camels 73, 132–3

eye ailments (*cont.*)
  cattle 65, 138, 232, 283, 529
  horses 536
  poultry 176
eye cataracts 132–3, 328, 401, 443–4
eye infections 86–7, 132–3, 156, 198, 399, 537
eye injuries 24, 189, 202, 512
eye protection 18, 289, 401
eyelid carcinoma removal 386–7
Eysenhardtia polystachya 338
Eysenhardtia texana 51

face, *see also* jaw; mouth
face swelling 532
facial neurectomy, as treatment 157
faeces, medicinal use 197–8
faeces (hard), in fasciolosis 471
Fagara zantoxyloides, fish poison 510
faith healing, for CCPP, Somali 96
FAO Electronic Conference, EVM overlooked 516
farcy *see* glanders
FARM-Africa, Pastoralist Development Project 177–8
farmer-to-farmer communication network 363
farmers and vetinarians, co-operation 376
farming, herbal management (book) 74–7
farriers (blacksmiths), England 323
fasciolosis 42, 45–6, 469, 471
  in Africa 370, 469, 471
  in Asia 42, 45–6
  in Europe 114, 482–3
  in Mexico 423
  in South America 83–5, 119
fasting, in European treatments 76
fat (animal)
  in topical dressings 8, 98, 223, 386, 519
  see also llama; mesenteric; sheep; whale; white rhinoceros
Fat-tail sheep (African) 62, 268, 282, 550
fate, concept of disease 105, 106, 223
fatigue, livestock 539
fattening livestock 327, 340, 380, 503
  cattle 437–8
  horses 327
  pigs 395, 518
feast ram, Islamic communities 15
feed supplements 244, 320
  in Africa 188, 199, 522–3, 539
  in India 447–8
  camels 165, 246
  cattle 237
  horses/mules 156, 521
  pigs 78, 116, 498
  poultry 148, 450
  pregnant animals 147, 503
  reindeer 54
  sheep 503
  tarwi (Lupinus mutabilis) grain, Andes 265
  minerals/salt 64, 147, 165, 245
  neem 47, 203
  probiotics 197–8
feeding
  cut-and-carry system 349, 351

dogs, herbal regime 74
ducks, disease prevention 534
feeding management, in Ireland 482–3
feeding strategies, in Africa 41–2, 47
feeds 65, 189, 237
  see also fodder; forage
feedstuffs, in medico-religious acts 17
feet *see* hooves
Fellah, glanders, Arab knowledge of 214
female prohibitions breached 118
fences, introduction of, in Nigeria 545–6
fennel 197, 237, 303
fenugreek 303, 416–17, 453, 524
  see also methi
feral goats 88
Feretia apodanthera 282
Ferlo (Sengal), Fulani in 105–7, 261–2
fermented foods, for weak animals 127
fermented rice water, for cattle 260
fertility
  in Africa 157, 282, 513, 517
  in Peru 523
  of American Indians 306
  feedstuffs for 77, 291, 320, 549
  medico-religious charms and talismans 157
fertility ceremony, alpaca, in Andes 120
fertility control *see* contraception
fertility problems *see* infertility
fetishes 89, 159, 201, 481, 522–3
fetotomy/embryotomy 38, 64, 386–7
fever 97
  in India 202, 235, 401, 491, 533
  in Philippines 149
  in Tibet 223
  camels 90, 91
  cattle 103, 260, 400, 402, 511, 532
  pigs 525
  small ruminants 396
Ficus benghalensis 212, 235
Ficus capensis 502
Ficus elastica 517
Ficus glumosa 282, 513
Ficus hispida roots 237
Ficus ingens bark 502
Ficus racemosus bark 212
Ficus religiosa 126
Ficus sp. 363, 459
Ficus sycomorus fruit and leaves 502
Ficus tinctoria 399
field beans, for ephemeral fever 400
field crab (live), for foot injuries 400
field workers' manual, workshops for 382
fierceness induced, dog, Peru 317
fig-tree oil, for castration wounds 395
Filipendula ulmaria (meadowsweet) 499
Filipino *see* Philippines
Finland, Saami Lapps, reindeer-herding 52
fires
  smudge fires 153
  see also dung fires
firing 12, 24, 342
  in Africa 91, 96, 104, 189
  in India 293
  camels 45, 290, 291, 386

firing (*cont.*)
    for joint problems 453, 551
    for ECF lymph nodes 251, 334
    for joint problems 251, 281, 416, 551
    for rheumatism/wry neck syndrome 453
    for wounds/skin infection 108, 151, 213, 322
    see also cauterization
fish
    diseases of 66, 192, 419
    medicinal uses of 214
fish (dried), for FMD 235, 399, 400, 432
fish dried/salted, for feed 340, 498, 503
fish farming, multi-species 435–6
fish (herring air-bladder) 535
fish poisons, plants 86, 115, 510
fish scales, in FMD treatments 234, 519
fish-and-rice farming, in Asia 496–7
fish-poison bean plant (*Tephrosia vogelii*) 485
flatulence 129, 233, 235, 416
flaxseed meal, conditioner for horses 303
flea, in fertility restoration mix 513
flea control 109–10, 214, 265, 415
    bouquets for, in France 112, 114–15
    cats/dogs 74, 233
    guinea pigs 104–5
    poultry 277
fly, biting 72–3, 366
fly avoidance, migration in 14, 82–3
fly control 243, 548
    by Muscovy ducks 506
    cattle management 173–4, 326–7
    for trypanosomosis 25, 552
fly repellents 97, 148, 385, 434
    for bovines/horses 191, 303, 529
fly strike *see* myiasis
flying insects, smudge fires in control 14
FMD 456, 467–8
    Arab knowledge of 214
    in Africa 183, 253, 325, 373, 514, 531
    in France 481
    in India 234, 235, 236, 449, 467–8, 492
        Gujarat 212
        Rabari people 296
        Tamil Nadu 453, 533
        Tamil-speaking people 399, 400, 432
        Uttar Pradesh 127, 261, 492, 519
    in South America 122, 392
        alpaca 201
        buffalo 126, 442, 458
        cattle 129, 183, 273, 282, 458
        sheep 295, 396
        yaks 313
    prophylaxis against 234, 235, 330
    vaccination (traditional) 214, 220, 397
fodder 279–80, 291, 443, 448–50
    cropping 365–6, 404, 545–6
    cut-and-carried 64, 440, 538
    environmental conditions 234, 389–90
    medicinal uses 237
    storage technique 399
    see also feeds; forage
Foeniculum vulgare 482, 532
folk botanical nomenclature 166–7, 202
fomentations, for elephants 168

food animal production, homeopathy in 487
food poisoning 222, 235–6, 416
foodstuffs, in rituals for prosperity 157
foot, *see* hoof; pad
foot and mouth disease *see* FMD
foot diseases, buffalo resistance to 390
foot problems 65, 108, 156, 400
foot protection, camel pastoralists 289
foot trimming, by Maasai 251
footbaths, for FMD prevention 481
footrot 110, 437–8, 528
    in Africa 91, 257–8, 371–2
    in Ecuador 228
    in Sri Lanka 546–7
    treatments 12, 88, 126, 343, 514
    see also hooves
forage 116, 330, 551
    migration for 53–4, 163–4, 379–80
    resources 13, 199, 218–19
    see also feeds; fodder
forehead wounds, herbal therapy 162
forest-dwelling people, in India 489
formaldehyde, disinfectant 65
fortune tellers, healers, Ethiopia 370
fostering techniques 92, 312, 479
four seasons, in Mongolian EVM 368
fowl cholera (pasteurellosis) 33, 518
fowl pox 130, 321
foxes, predators 126, 238
foxglove (*Digitalis purpurea*) 485
fractures 189, 222
    in Africa 63, 515
    in India 234, 238, 281, 399, 482
        Gujarat 211, 284
        Rajasthan 415, 480
        Santal District 102
        Tamil-language people 202, 401
    in South America 239, 433
        alpaca 130
        cattle 416, 443–4, 532
        goats 417
        sheep 130, 437–8
    see also splints
France 12, 109, 112, 113–14, 208, 338, 339
    veterinary saints 156, 531
    see also Cévennes; Normandy; Picardie;
        Provence; Pyrénées; Ubay
French West Africa, Fulani 302
fright, and soul loss, Aymara Indians 317
'frog disease', in cattle, India 399
frostbite, copper sulphate treatment 142
fruit and flowers in remedies 448
fruits, in rituals for prosperity 157
Fuerstia africana 373
Fulani 67–8, 307–8, 407, 512–14
    cattle 16, 190, 314, 397
    diagnosis/treatment 96, 471, 513
    disease control 25, 96, 102, 494–5
    see also Fulße (Fulani) ; Mbororo
Fulani (Benin) 307–8, 379–80
Fulani (Burkina Faso) 88–9, 323–5, 500, 554
Fulani (Cameroon) 157–8, 333, 376, 516–17,
    522–3
Fulani (Chad) 54–5

Fulani (French West Africa) 302
Fulani (Gambia) 47
Fulani (Kenya) 48–9, 403
Fulani Livestock Development Project, start-up 398
Fulani (Mali) 219–20, 314, 550
Fulani (Mauritania) 392–3
Fulani (Niger) 23, 157–8, 302
Fulani (Nigeria) 49–50, 138, 247, 522–3
  cattle 441, 466, 545–6
  herding strategies 80–1, 250, 307, 335–6
  poultry breeds 249–50
  superstitious beliefs 499
Fulani (Sahel) 90
Fulani (Senegal) 15, 67, 105–7, 133–4
Fulani (Sudan) 302
Fulani (West Africa) 470, 471
Fulani white cattle (Bunaji) 81–2, 441
Fulße (Fulani) 105–7, 194, 256, 261–2, 554
  disease concepts 380, 494–6
fumigation 324, 366
  in Ethiopia 40
  in Mongolia 367
  animal housing 250, 465, 515
  calves 158
  cattle 156, 400, 402, 491
  donkeys 514
  for FMD 127, 235, 238, 399, 402
  for fowl pox prevention 321
  magico-religious practices 110, 158, 516
Fung tribe of Sudan, nomadism in 82–3
fungal, *see also* mycotic
fungal infections 281, 330–1
  protection from 26, 111, 135, 310
  see also dermatophytosis

Gabbra 44, 256, 315–16, 386–7, 502
  beliefs about evil eye 268
  camel pastoralism 259, 277–9
Gabbra sheep/goats, breed introduction 208
galactagogues 55, 157, 510
  in Africa 91, 324
  in India 210, 468, 528–9
  for buffalo 492
  for cattle 338, 502, 507, 549
  for goats, in Mexico 167
  for pigs/large ruminants 518
  for small ruminants 503
Galium aparine (cleavers/sticky willie) 485
Galla bucks, goat breed introduction 208
gallstones, in bullocks, India 211
galsundha, throat swelling, India 235
Gamba grass (*Andropogon gayanus*) 511–12
Gambia 133, 310, 493
Gamits, Taluka (India), tribal people 528
gandraph 295
Garcinia indica fruit extract 236
Gardenia gummifera 412
Gardenia lutea nuts 539
Gardenia resinifera leaves 235
garlic 57, 161, 233, 423, 458
  for bacterial infections 231, 452
  for bloat 273, 546–7
  for cyanide poisoning 455

for dermatophytosis 437, 509
for diarrhoea 376, 507–8
for ectoparasites 140, 161, 468
for endoparasites 50, 172, 231, 264, 463, 525
  of fish 419
for fevers 260, 401, 532
for inappetance 301, 401, 546–7
for indigestion 260, 507
for respiratory diseases 399, 451–2, 508
for strangles, donkeys 386
for 'womb cleaner' 300
for wounds 231, 433
in poultry tonic 415
planted for worm-infested pastures 75
garlic cloves necklaces, against trolls/goblins 430
garlic smoke, against evil spirits 285
garlic (wild), in mineral licks 168
gasoline, in wound dressing 396, 525
gastroenteritis
  seasonal 214
  transmissible 164
  verminous 245
gastrointestinal disorders 212, 235, 532
gastrointestinal parasites *see* amthelmintics;
  endoparasites; worms
Gavits (India), tribal peoples 528
Gawali caste, Uttar Pradesh (India) 522
geese 243, 285, 445, 472
geld(ing) *see* castrat(e/ion)
gender, *see also* women
gender roles in stockraising 42, 490–1, 500
gender-based differences in EVK 21–2, 142
genetic diversity, African livestock 457
genetic selection, in Mexico 425, 427–8
genies, diseases caused by 157–8, 159
Genista saharae 132
genital region infection, *karachi* 296
gentian, in horse conditioner 303
gentian (cordial), for fever 511
gentian tonic, for eye problems 65
gentian violet dye, chick protection 48, 506
Gentiana lutea L. 396
Gentiana phyllocalyx 486
Gentianella thyrsoidea 83, 84
gentle veterinary remedies, Tamil saint 411
Gerbera gossypina root 486
Germany, bloat 13, 76
Geum quellyon Sweet 173
Ghana 234, 279, 294, 552
  see also Wenchi District
ghee
  as laxative 492
  for bloat 283
  for fertility problems 415, 529
  for fractures 234, 415
  for leg strengthening 128
  for placenta expulsion 236
  for plant poisoning 529
  for ringworm 288
  for sore throats, Uttar Pradesh, India 213
  for wounds 386–7, 529
  in feed supplements 246, 416–17
ghodakhundi bark 414
ghosts, religo-medical healing 118, 172

Ghrib Bedouin (Tunisia) 132–3
giant pumpkin (*Cucurbita maxima*) seeds 421
gid *see* coenurosis
Gikuyu (Kikuyu), (Kenya) 256
gin, alligator-pepper in 62
gingelly oil 202, 273, 443–4, 453
gingelly seed, for bloat 273
ginger
  for asthma 231
  for bloat 50, 449, 450, 485–6, 503, 546–7
  for eye disorders 65, 536
  for fever 260, 511
  for galactogogue 528–9
  for gastric symptoms 50, 260, 453
    diarrhoea in calves 118
  for inappetance 197, 416–17, 503, 546–7
  for post-parturition injuries 64
  for rabies 458
  for respiratory disorders 129, 409
  for toxic plants, antidote 409–10
  for wounds 149
  in health tonic 128, 209, 303, 455
ginseng root broth, for rabies 366, 367
girls (three-same name and age) 399, 402
Gladiolus psittacimus bulb 513
glanders (farcy) 101, 156, 214, 367, 557
Glinus lotoides 370
Gliricidia leaves 138
glossary, of livestock terms, Fulani 323–5
Glycyrrhiza glabra (liquorice) 213
Glynus lotoides seeds 560
Gmelina arborea Roxb. bark 102
Gnidia kraussiana root 115–16
goat breeds
  downy, in Turkmenistan 282
  introductions, in Kenya 208
  trypanotolerant 255
  Zaghwa agropastoralists 521
  see also Barbari; 'Damascus' goats; feral; Galla;
    Shami
goat bucks, foul smell, in Dominica 262
goat droppings, for wounds 415
goat hairs, for fractures, in India 234
goat kids 77, 167, 506
Goat Production in the Tropics, manual 417–18
goat-meat soup, for camel mange 367, 368
goats 307, 439–40
  in Afghanistan 142
  in Africa 92–3, 391
  in Bangladesh 443
  in India 399, 480
  in Indonesia 18, 43, 153
  in Peru 420
  in Syria 387
  anthelmintics 88, 256, 269, 273
    ipil-ipil (*Leucaena*) seeds 57, 163, 243
  castration 12, 183
  catarrhal fever 62
  CCCP 78–9, 183
  ectoparasites 102
  exercise for 13
  galactagogue 55
  horn shaping 115
  respiratory diseases 451–2

tick-born disease 214–15, 255
  vaccinations, traditional 152–3
  see also bucks
goblins, protection of cows from 430
God, cause of disease 253
'gods, anger of the', epidemic 433
gods, mountain-peak (*wamani*) 185
Godwara, Rajasthan (India) 453
goitre, treatment by American cattlemen 65
goose grease, for mastitis 323
Gossypium spp., contraceptive action 97
grain
  in mix for placenta retained 449
  see also barley; rice; wheat
grain husks, in mineral licks, Nepal 168
gram 507–8
gram (Bengal) 401, 402, 519
gram (black) 400, 443–4, 453
gram (horse) 399, 400
gram (sprouted) 77, 401, 402
Gran Chaco Province (Bolivia) 524–5
grass (fresh), for constipation 303
grass species, tick control 511–12
grasshoppers with chapati bread 211
grazing 128, 323, 342
  in Africa 41, 188
    camel herding 169, 246, 498–9
    Chad 105
    disease control 124–5, 188, 521
      CCCP 78–9
      fasciolosis 469, 471, 472
      trypanosomosis prevention 187, 289
      worms 169
    Ethiopia 515
    Kenya 394
    Nigeria 80–1
    Sahel 190–1, 498–9
    Somalia 78–9, 124–5, 246
    Sudan 62–3, 169
    West Africa 469, 471, 472
  in Himalayas, yak husbandry 313
  in Israel 214–15
  in Mexico 422
  migration and 52–4, 62–3, 190–1
  reindeer herding 52–4, 187
  tick control by chickens 387
  see also herd movements
grease, and gunpowder, for hooves 305
Greece (Ancient), beekeeping 135
green feed, for eye conditions 15, 65
green ointment, for swellings/wounds 132
Grewia bicolor 505
Grewia carpinifolia 549
Grewia flavescens root 400
Grewia oppositifolia 529, 530
grit, for poultry 76
groundnut hay, fodder resource, India 450
groundnut meal, in feed, Burma 498
groundnut oil 235, 414–15, 505
groundnut tops, fodder in Madagascar 482
groundnuts, foodstuffs 47, 157
growth promotion, turkeys 321
Guatemala 109–10, 156–7
  see also Petén

guava, in poultice for wounds 388
guava leaves 253, 503
Guiera senegalensis leaves 505, 510
Guinea Bissau 439
guinea fowl, in Nigeria 48
guinea pigs 104–5, 226, 227, 377–8
  commercialization 378
  flea control 265
  fluke susceptibility 85
  in ritual sacrifice 192
Guinea-Conakry 497
Gujarat (India) 147, 210, 212, 328, 447
  cattle/buffalo raising 262, 442
  cows, milk fever prevention 414
  horse husbandry 127–8
  tribal people 284
  women's EVK 450, 451
Gujjar nomads 14, 528–30
Gunnera perpense root 138
gunpowder
  for camel mange 367, 368
  for footrot 12, 343
  for horse hooves 305
gunshot, anthrax prophylaxis 142
gur
  for bloat, cattle 283
  for retained placenta 295
  in feed supplements 503
  see also jaggery
Gynandropsis pentaphylla leaves 231
gypsum, powdered, for lightening burns 157

haboub (wind) syndrome 39, 44
Hadendewa, Sudanese camel pastoralists 38
haemoglobinurea, Normandy (France) 481
haemonchosis 169, 466
haemorrhages, healers in India 281
haemorrhagic septicaemia 91, 316
haemostatic dressings, for wounds 128
hail, talismans against 111
hair, roseships for, Scotland 485
hair clipping, against ectoparasites 529
hair dressing for rotted horns 211
hair (horse), for warts 244
hair (human) 236, 283, 400
hair loss, livestock, in India 414
hairballs, cats, United States 233
Haiti, stockraising 431–2
Haloptelea integrifolia arjoria 508
hand washing, by Fulani (Peul) 308
handling of livestock, in Europe 77
Hangzhou (China), egg incubation 285
hantu (evil spirits), in Brunei 285
Haplopappus spp. 173
Harungana madagascariensis bark 513
Hausa (Nigeria) 138
  livestock 194, 289
  poultry breeds 249–50
Hawawir Arabs (Sudan), camels 498–9
hawks, predators on chicks 209, 238, 506
hay feed 65, 302
hay-making technique 399
haycha, bloat prevention 437

headache, in humans, American Indians 306
healers 19–22, 286, 359
  in Africa
    Fulani 157–8
    Maasai, East Africa 375
  in Cameroon 397–9
  in Ethiopia 370–1, 514
  in France 111, 113, 115, 310
  in India 196–7, 281, 454
    Bharad/Gawali caste 522
    Kannada-speaking area 507
    Kerala 408
    pasuvaidyulu, Andhra Pradesh 455–6
    Rabari people 296
    Rajasthan
      Godwara 453
      Raika pastoralists 288, 290, 291, 293
    Tamil Nadu 443–4
    use by women 451
  in Kenya 259
    Akamba 354–5
    Gabbra pastoralists 316
    Samburu and Turkana pastoralists 253
    WaKamaba farmers 257–8, 394
  in Mexico 320, 321–2
  in Nepal 172
    (*jhankries*), Tamang tribe 329–30
  in paraveterinary training programmes 364–5
  in Peru, Nazca Valley 481
  in Philippines 318
  in Sudan 560–1
    atet, Dinka 326–7, 334–5, 475–7
    camel pastoralists 38
  in Trinidad and Tobago 298, 300
  in Venezuela 433
  veterinary personnel and 257–8, 291–2
  see also curers; training
healing, and religion, in Africa 117–18
health training, participatory design 254–5
healthcare delivery, intersectorial proposal 57
healthcare initiatives, need for EVK 100
heart conditions 64, 207, 400, 485, 499
heartwater 272
  resistance to 16, 80, 81–2
heartwater bane, sheep tick control 191
heat *see* oestrus
heat stress, poultry 301
heat stroke, scarification for 157
heat tolerance
  Fulani white cattle 80–1
  small ruminants 406
hedgehog spines (burning), for FMD 296
heel ailment (*arestín*), Peru 523
Heifer Project International *see* HPI
heifers *see* cows
helecho macho (*Aspidium Filix-mas*) 119
Helianthemum glomeratum 193
Helianthus annuus W. 102
Helicteres isora 399, 482, 532
Heliotropium albohispidum leaves 502
Heliotropium indicum L. 176
hellebore (*Niger/Viridis*) rhizome 339
hellebore root (*Helleborus niger/H.viridis*) 101, 339, 465

Helleborus foetidus 110, 111, 481
Helleborus niger (hellebore) rhizome 339
Helleborus purpurascens 102–3
Helleborus spp. 264
Helleborus viridis (hellebore) rhizome 339
helminthoses *see* anthelmintics; worms
Helosis longipes (chilcúan) 464
hemp cloth, for plaster 536
henbane (*Hyoscyamus niger* L.) 369–70, 536
hepatitis, calf 250
'herb doctor', magico-religious 516
herb garden, Scotland, Edinburgh Zoo 485
herb garden (herbarium), Cameroon 398
herb gardens, Fulani pastoralists 376
Herbal Encyopedia, The Concise 303
herbal medicine 268, 269, 456, 463–4
    for bloat 125
    for oestrus induction 147
herbal medicines
    commercial 96–7, 268, 277, 436–7, 441–2
        for mastitis 150
        polyherbal preparation 127, 411
        production 268, 384, 436–7, 441–2
herbal ointment, commercial, Himax 330–1
herbalist-healers 394, 464, 515
herbicide (commercial), misuse 437–8
herd dispersal, Fulani 522–3
herd loss, inter-community co-operation 43
herd management 105, 140, 199, 323–5
    camels, Somalia 165–6
    disease control 148
    Quechua Indians (Peru) 356–7
herd movements 522–3
    ECF avoidance 162
    pasteurellosis control 157–8
    see also grazing
herd productivity, assessment 277–9
herd prosperity, charms for, Fulani 157
herd size, and environment 389–90
herding, EVK in 14–15
herding strategies 359
herring air-bladder, for anuria 535
HERVET 10, computerized database 319
Hibiscus surattensis L. leaves 277
Hibiscus trionium (wild okra) 39
Hidatsa (American Indians) 462, 550
hide patch stitched on, hoof wound 537
Himachal Pradesh (India) 529
Himalayas, yak husbandry 311–13, 461–2
Himax, commercial herbal ointment 330–1
Himba cattle herders, Namibia 287
hind-quarters pricked 87–8
Hindu priests, in EVK 298, 300
Hindus, camel pox inoculations 139
hinjo, for udder swelling 437
Hissar District (India) 72, 283
hog lard, in green ointment 132
hogs, *see* pigs
Holarrhena antidysenterica bark 235, 507
holistic animal healthcare 197, 456
holistic medicine 99, 148
    chiropractic care in 549–50
    preventive, need for 187–8
holly (*Ilex aquifolium*) 135, 310, 485

hollyhock/mallow, for FMD 201
holm oak (*Quercus robur ilex*) 65–6
holy water 152–3, 483, 515
holymen, healers, in Ethiopia 370
homeopathic healers, in Nepal 172
homeopathy 6, 143, 166, 185–6, 407, 467–8
    in food animal production 487
    in holistic healthcare 456
honey
    for bronchitis 526
    for eye ailments 156, 536
    for FMD lesions 514
    for fractures 234
    for inflammation 317
    for mastitis 546–7
    for wounds 8, 179, 303, 406
    in anthelmintic 560
    rabbits, mortality reduction 412
Honey Bee, India-based local-knowledge network
    210
hoof care, horses/mules 156, 305
hoof ointments, horses 536
hoof problems 387, 395–6, 536
    infections, tobacco for 50
    lesions 126, 200, 237, 402
    wounds 88, 537
hoof protection
    camels, shoeing 366, 369
    cattle/horses 277, 536
    moccasins and equipment 18
hoof trimming 51, 277, 505
hoof wash, for FMD 400
hooves
    horses 523
        rosemary for hardening 153
    medicinal uses of 238, 369–70
    rosehips for 485
    small ruminants 306
        growth between claws 306
    see also footrot
Hordeum vulgare (barley) 65–6
horn (deer), medicinal use 191
Horn of Africa 117–18
horns
    broken 236, 283, 284
    cancer 328
    dehorning/disbudding 251, 397
    ingrown 416
    rosehips for 485
    rotted 211
    shaping 115, 118, 268, 476, 546
Horro sheep, parasite-resistant 387
horse breeds *see* Turkmenistan; Yakut
horse doctors 277, 305, 306
horse medicine cult, American Indians 304
horse tail-hair noose, for leeches 297
horseradish tree (*Moringa oleifera*) 253
horses 445, 548
    in Africa 133–4, 302, 303, 439, 521
    in America, Indian tribes 153, 155–6, 304–6,
        378–9, 501–2, 550
    in Canada, Indian tribe 499–500
    in Croatia 535–6
    in East Java 153

horses (*cont.*)
  in England 132, 156
  in India 127–8, 329
  in Peru 316–17, 327
  in Tibet 224, 474
  in Venezuela 434
  aromatherapy for 557
  calming and taming 118
  castration 462
  colds/coughs 91, 103
  colic 369, 480, 510
  conditioner for, herbal remedies 303
  ectoparasites 76, 265, 303
  eczema 212
  endoparasites 118, 505, 549
  exercise for 13
  gastric troubles/inappetance 212
  homeopathy for 186
  leg ailments 76
  metritis 215
  pack animals 156–7, 406
  pasteurellosis 68
  physical therapy 434–5
  poisonous plants 15, 87–8
  purgative for 491
  rabies 366
  restorative 378–9
  tonic 303, 379
    immunity stimulation 102–3
    stimulant 282
  undescended testicles 239
  wood chewing, prevention 118
  wounds 173, 371–2, 406
  see also colts; glanders
horseshoe, lightening protection 310
hot iron, for chronic disease 288
hot iron spatula, for indigestion 202
hot sticks, for blackleg 152–3
hot stones on abdomen, for worms 221
hot/cold diseases 226, 228, 229, 298, 328
hot/cold treatments 434, 463
hotte bigiyalu (stomach swollen) 232
household animal management 140, 142
housing and handling structures 18
housing (livestock), nutrient cycling 506
housing (raised barns) 349, 351
Houttuynia cordata 518
HPI 37, 376, 397–9, 502
  Ethnoveterinary Council 151
  Golden Talent Award 554
  medicinal plant collection 498
  paravet programme 122, 406
  plant nurseries 99
huacaya alpaca 134, 201
huamanripa flowers 523
Huancayo (Peru) 120, 134–5
human and herd prosperity, charms 157
human hair oil, for bloat 126
human resources in EVM 18–22
humoral balances, in Greece (ancient) 445
humoral pathology, in Asia 349
Hungary 88, 512
Hura crepitans L. (catagua) 50, 523
husbandry *see* livestock husbandry

hydatidosis 60, 116, 245, 326–7
Hydnocarpus wightiana Blume 462
hydrogen peroxide wash, for footrot 228
hyena bites, treatment for 209
hyena dung, for skin disorders 168, 514
hyena hide collar, for infertility 286
hyenas, protection from 515
hygiene 75
  barn fumigation 515
  disease prevention, ducks 533–4
  dung burning 387
  hand washing 308
  parasite control, sheep 423
Hyoscyamus niger (henbane) 168, 207, 536
Hypericum perforatum (St John's Wort) 499
hypocalcaemia, milk fever 75, 211, 414, 416–17
hypomagnesia (*akuet kuet*) 334–5
hypothermia, cattle 482, 532
Hyptis suaveolens 77
Hyssopus officianalis L. 510

identification, ear notching 52–4, 184–5, 201
Ilex aquifolium (holly) 485
ilgoff, in camel calf mortality 278, 279
immunization, equipment for 18
immunostimulant 311
  commercial 95
  for chicks 297
  implant 102–3
imperial grass (*Axonopus scoparius*) 365–6
impotence, treatment by Basuto 63
inappetance
  in Africa 513
  in India 197, 202, 400, 453
  in Sri Lanka 546–7
  buffalo 126
  cattle 211, 260, 401
  horses 212, 536
  poultry 300–1
  small ruminants 503
    appetizers 50, 213, 416
    rehydration therapy 149
inappropriate technology
  in development projects 322, 520, 525
  in paravet training 541
  sheep in Mali 550–1
incantations
  for snakebite 110, 111
  in castration 314
Incas, ritual sacrifice, guinea pig 192
incense 516
  for soul lost by fright 317
  lightening cure 366
incisions, for lameness, in camels 132–3
incubation (artificial), China 285, 488
incubation/hatching, ducks 437, 518
India
  EVK 77, 99
  EVM 56, 448, 485–6, 489
    An Annotated Bibliography 444–5
    commercial production of 327
    indigenous medicines 55, 212
    indigenous remedies 385–6, 482

India (*cont.*)
  literature 57, 491
  overview (course) 160
  overview (FAO report) 170
  SRISTI, database 56
  buffalo 142, 232, 283, 459–60
    ectoparasites 262–3, 436
  calves, buffalo/cattle 418, 509
  camels 229, 284, 287–94
    see also Raika camelherders
  cattle 127, 129, 199–200, 211, 232, 283
    breeding 199–200, 412, 413
    dairy 283, 509
      milk fever 416
  diseases 160–1, 197, 296, 330
  dogs 264, 280–1
  ectoparasites 13, 151, 387, 508
    leeches 13, 297, 529
  fish diseases, neem treatments 192
  forages/feeding 330, 447–8, 503
  goats 93–4, 451–2
  healers 87, 281, 494
    learning and professional development 196–7
  healthcare delivery 215, 234–8, 454, 545
  homeopathy 467–8
  horses 127–8
  medicinal plants 57, 412, 443, 448, 526–7
    collection and database 56
    neem tree 26, 387, 492
    parasiticides 141, 413, 418
  NGOs 58–60, 197, 293–4
    AFPRO (Action for Food Production) 267, 467
  poultry 130, 486, 508, 525–6
  sheep 151, 503
  women, EVK of 58–60, 448–51
  yak husbandry 312, 313
  see also Andhra Pradesh; Assam; Ayurvedic medicine; Bengal; Bharat; Bhils; Bihar; Charvah; Dhangars; Gavits; Gawali caste; Gujarat; Gujjar nomads; Himachal Pradesh; Hissar; Jalpaiguri; Jammu and Kashmir; Kalbelia; Kannada-speaking; Karnataka; Kashmir; Kerala; Kokanis; Kondh; Kumhars; Kutch; Ladakh; Lodha; Maharashtra; Maldhari; Marwar; Mavchis; Mewar; Monda; Oraon; Orissa; Punjab; Rabari; Rajasthan; Rebari; Santal; Saurashtra; Taluka; Tamil Nadu; Thar Desert; Toda; Tripura; Uttar Pradesh; Uttrakhand; Yanadulu
India-based local-knowledge network, Honey Bee 210
Indian Herbs Anthelmintic (commercial product) 140
Indian laburnum (*Lassia fistula*) 415
Indian refugee camps, Tibetan medicine 87
indigenous, definition 6
indigenous clinical services 233
indigenous knowledge 87, 93, 182–3
  lack of in NGO strategies 293–4
indigestion 127, 198, 453, 532
  cattle 202, 260, 507
  elephants, self–medication 433
  sheep 295

Indigo articulata (indigo) 236
Indigofera tinctoria (Avuri leaf tablets) 533
Indonesia 42, 172, 384, 553
  endoparasites 242–3, 256, 308–9, 384–5, 493
  poultry 384–5, 394–5
  rabbits 383
  ruminants 308–9, 493
  small ruminants 18, 349, 382–3, 503
  sheep 242–3, 383
  see also Alor; Bogor; Borneo; East Java; Java; Malang; Nagrak; Pantar; South Kalimantan; West Java
Indonesian Thin Tail sheep 16, 242–3
infertility 286, 415, 456, 513, 529
  camels 38, 73, 92
  cattle 118, 260, 416, 459, 537
    evil eye as cause 118
inflammation 97, 317, 439, 505, 508
influenza, poultry, in Africa 209
infusion techniques, by Fulani 50
inhalation 103, 431
injections 128, 342
injuries 429–30, 481, 491, 536
inorganic materials, in EVM 8
insect bites 76, 168
insect control 243, 510
insect repellent 214, 539
  for cattle 268, 396, 512
  neem (*Azadirachta indica*) 50, 203, 396
insecticide 13–14, 118, 150, 352, 464
insecticide (commercial) 340, 396
insecticide (crop), for demodicosis 240
insects (nocturnal), Zaria, Nigeria 251
integrated disease management (IDM) 25, 359, 472–3
integrated healthcare 473, 544–5
intellectual property rights in EVK 99, 124, 298, 299, 526–7
intensive stockraising, USA 281
internet resources 30–3
  DIALOG on-line search methods 561
intersectoral healthcare 359, 363–4, 475, 477
intestinal disorders 50, 75, 412, 471, 485
intestinal microbial balance 8, 109, 197–8, 342
intranasal route, for medicines 11
intraocular route, for medicines 11
intrauterine injection, cows 64
iodex, in massage for fractures 211
iodine, dressing 134, 312
iodine supplementation, for goitre 65
iontophoresis, physical therapy 434
ipecacuanha, emetic 323
ipil-ipil (*Leucaena leucocephala*) 57
IPM (integrated methods of pest management) 284
Ipomoea asarifolia 91
Ipomoea cairica 68
Ipomoea vagans 324
Ipomoea verticillata 91
Iran 98, 504–5
Ireland, Donegal 482–3
Iris germanica L. 264
iron rod, in navel cauterization 64
iron sulphate 64, 65

iron-deficient anaemia in sows 393
Ishtirak, paravet programme 73–4, 218–19, 329, 429–30
Islam, *see also* Koran
Islamic communities, feast ram 15
Islamic culture, male sheep in 550
Islamic hat (ashes from), scabicide 383
Islamic priests (*malam*) 335, 429–30
Islamic verse, at castration 314
Israel 13, 41–2, 214–15
Italy 318, 389
    see also Sard
Ivory Coast 49, 77, 302
ivy (*Nepeta glechoma*) 156

jackal, sheep predators 219
jackal meat, medicinal use of 91
jackfruit leaves, for retained placenta 77
jaggery 211, 212, 234, 400, 480
    buffalo 126
    cattle 260, 400, 414
        cows 237, 416–17, 507
    dogs 237, 264
    for hoof/leg problems 234, 237
    for tumours 236
    for worms 385–6
    horses 127–8
    poultry 130, 401
    ruminants 458
    see also gur; palm; palmyra
jaguar bite, preventive medicines 206
Jaisalmeri swift camels, in India 287
Jalpaiguri District (India) 141
Jammu and Kashmir (India) 486
jamu medicine, in Indonesia 553
jamun fruit juice, in India 415
Japan 87, 277, 285, 430–1
Japotropha curcas seeds 169
jasmine flowers 448
Jasminum fluminense 379
Jasminum sambac flowers 318
Jat caste, Rajasthan (India) 453
Jatropha curcas 45–6, 448
Jatropha gossypifolia Linn. 491
jaundice 295, 298, 539
Java (Indonesia) 153, 340, 441, 506
    bees and beekeeping 136
    ruminants 13, 133, 209, 350–1, 466–7
jaw conditions 231, 245
jaya-shipita, for liver fluke 61, 120, 134
jhankries (healers), Nepal 329–30
jimsonweed (*Datura stramonium*) 536
jinjara leaves 210
John the Baptist, saint of sheep 428
joint problems 281, 399, 416, 551
    bovines 211, 414, 415–16
    camels 237, 551
Jordan, Bedouin pastoral systems 160
jowar flour 128
juniper 114, 156, 222, 295, 465
juniper oil 111, 465
Juniperus communis 151
Juniperus virginiana 306

Kababish Arabs (Sudan) 62–3, 551
Kaduna (Nigeria) 247
Kajaido District (Kenya) 542
Kalanchoe crenata 209, 517
Kalanchoe sp. leaves 195
Kalbelia castes/classes, in India 453
kalu, for increased blood supply 127–8
Kam Tibetans, yaks of 556
kamala (*Mallotus philippensis*) 269
Kamba stockraisers (Kenya) 102, 256, 543–4
kan:belle, eye ailment 232
Kannada-speaking area (India) 230–1, 507
Kansu-Tibetan frontier, Monguers of 474
kanwa (mineral supplement) 522–3, 545
kaolin 354–5, 513
Kapsiki, trypanotolerant cattle 552
karachi, alpaca disease 296
Karakatshan shepherds, in Bulgaria 334
Karamajong, Kenya/Uganda, CBAH 48–9, 333
Karamoja District (Uganda) 48
karanja (*Pongamia glabra*) oil 262–3, 417
karfa, plant mixture 102
Karimojong pastoralists, in Uganda 162, 269
Karina area (Sierra Leone) 72–3
karkka cane, smoke cure 316–17
Karnataka (India), ruminants 458
karval spines 235
Karwassa Pastoral Association of Mali 163
Kashmir, Ladakh, traditional health system 87
kasturi seeds 482
kaviraj (veterinary herbalist) 562
Kawahla Arabs (Sudan) 498–9
Kazakstan 13, 187, 282
Kedrostis foetidissima leaves 202
keds, sheep ectoparasites 83, 228, 229, 265, 360–2
Kel Adagh (Ifora) Twareg, Mali 498–9
Kel Ewey Twareg, Niger 498–9
Kenya 48, 136, 192, 251–2, 472
    development programmes
        CBAH projects 48–9, 98–9, 204
        ITDG 99, 257–60, 559
        Kenya Livestock Programme 204, 257, 488
        Marsabit Project 208
        paravets 255, 488, 559
    Ethnoveterinary Medicine in: A Field Manual 256–7
    pastoralists 206, 268, 277–9, 386–7
    traditional healers 259, 543
    see also Akamba; Baragoi; Borana; Burji peoples; Doroboro; Gabbra; Kajaido; Kajaido District; Kamba; Kikuyu; Kilifi; Kipsigis; Luhya; Luo; Maasai; Mbeere; Mijikenda; Pokot; Rendille; Samburu; Tharaka; Turkana; WaKamba
Kerala (India) 129, 407–8
keratectomy, eye disorders 514
kerenahi (*Euphorbia cameroonica*) 79–80
kerosene 122, 235, 400, 514
    buffalo 143
    cattle 64, 72–3, 283
    for ectoparasites 24, 234, 265
        demodicosis/scabies 240, 340
        keds 228, 229
        myiasis 449, 450

kerosene (*cont.*)
  ticks 214–15, 385
  for evil spirits 228, 229
  goats/sheep 214–15, 391
  pigs 118–19
  poultry 237
  rabbits 322
Keteku cattle 470
ketepeng (*Cassia alata*) 383
ketosis, in cows 127, 462
Khaya senegalensis 97, 439, 513
khechincha 381
kidney disease, diagnosis, cats/dogs 233
kidney stones 212, 401, 414, 415
Kigelia africana 517
KiKamba, disease names 205
Kikuyu (Kenya) 96, 256, 306
Kilifi District (Kenya) 143–5
king grass (*Pennisetum purpureum*) 365–6
Kipsigis people (Kenya) 256, 404, 405
kisal, or survival, Fulani 105–7
Kita, Mali, paravet services 132
kittens, respiratory infection 311
k'iwcha kururu (liver fluke) 120
kkayara cactus, burning 317
Klenia sp. wash 104
KLPP (Kenya Livestock and Pastoral Programme)
  488
Kokanis, Taluka (India) 528
Kondh tribes (India) 409–10
Koochi nomads 142, 183, 310–11, 531
Koran, *see also* Islam
Koranic readings/recitation 17, 96, 339
Koranic verses 41, 124–5, 152–3, 522–3
Kordofan, Kababish Arabs 62–3
Korea 285
Koshi Hills, Nepal 193
kraal hygiene 63–4, 124–5, 375, 510
kraal wall jumping, for impotence 63
kraals, fetishes/bouquets in 374, 522–3
Krishi Vigyan Kendram Badgaon (VBKVK) 93–4
kum, in earth infection by sorcery 452
Kumhars caste/class, in India 453
kundu, buffalo/cattle, India 232
kuntz (*Thysanolaena maxima* R) 443
kusmaylla juice 381
Kutch (India) 215, 325
Kwazulu, South Africa 138
Kyllinga flava 223

labour *see* parturition
Laccopetalum giganteum Wedd. flowers 320
Laciniaria scariosa L. 379
lactation enhancement 17, 157, 282, 400
lactogenic plants *see* galactagogues
Ladakh, Kashmir (India) 87
Lagenaria sciceraria (bottle-gourd) 260
Lagune, trypanotolerant cattle breed 552
Lahawiyin (Sudan), camel pastoralists 44–5
laibons, healers, East Africa 253, 375
lajamani root juice 211
lamas (holy men), in Tibet 367, 368
lambs 41–2, 75, 482, 503

mouth sores 98, 111, 113, 115
lameness 222, 251, 339, 537–8
  camels 38, 45, 132–3, 292, 386
laminitis, hoof paring for 505
lamp oil, for ritual (church-like) 481
lampers, horse's mouth 155–6
lancing, uses by Twareg 91
landless villagers, in India 442
language *see* linguistic difficulties
Languas Galanga roots 243
Lantana camara leaves 126, 164, 230, 262
Laportea aestuans 300
lard 201, 226, 228, 296, 536
  for ectoparasites 64, 410, 525
  for hoof lesions 220, 228
laser-beam irradiation, of acupoints 169–70
Lassia fistula (Indian laburnum) 415
latex-ful creeper, lactogenic 211
Latuka (Sudan), CAHW workshops 334–5
laundry detergent *see* detergent
lavender, to bait beehives 234
law of signatures, in EVK 297
Lawsonia alba seeds 448
Lawsonia inermis leaves 415
laxatives 50, 300, 396, 492, 536
laying on of hands, for snakebite 110, 111
lead (red), dressing for horn cancer 328
lead (white lead powder) 132
League for Pastoral Peoples (LPP) 291–2, 294
leather blinkers, for eye protection 289
leather (shoe) ash, in India 235, 236–7
leather shoes (moccasins) 289, 305
leaves (foodstuffs), in rituals 157
Ledum palustre L. 510
Leea robusta 491
leeches, removal of, in India 13, 297, 529
leeks, medicinal uses 114, 396
leg ailments 73, 76, 155, 491, 508, 536
legumes, in feeding practices 47
Lehwee, Sudanese camel pastoralists 38
lemon 161, 225, 226, 395, 525, 526
lemon and salt 214–15, 239
lemon drench, for whitlow 226
lemon juice 228, 238, 239, 240, 277
  for ectoparasites 116–17, 547
lemon water 234, 410
lentil-bean ashes 536
lentils 212
Leptadenia reticulata 55, 412, 468
Leptotaenia dissecta root 499–500, 507
Lesotho, *mafisa* 504
Leucaena 163, 404
Leucaena glauca L. seeds 411
Leucaena leucocephala 57, 174, 234, 243, 528
Leucas aspera 281, 399, 458, 509
Leucas lavandulifolia 441
Levisticum officinale Koch 510
Leyte, Philippines 176, 177
Lezernia inermis 505
libido stimulation 395, 468
lice 13
  in Africa 371–2, 379
  in America 64
  in Andes 265

lice (*cont.*)
  in France 112, 114–15
  in India 453
  in Philippines 138, 409
  calves, prevention 223
  camelids 410, 519
  dogs 74
  pigs 505
  poultry 116–17, 209, 210, 262, 277
  sheep 323
  see also pediculosis
lightening burns, caused by sorcery 157
lightning, protection from 111, 219, 310, 366
limb paralysis, superstition 548
lime 75, 76, 211, 329, 525
  for wounds 130, 321–2, 340, 395
lime juice 262, 307
lime water 234, 414
Limonium acidissima leaves 238
linguistic difficulties 79, 144–5, 205, 235, 245, 335
linseed 126, 213, 529, 530
linseed meal 65, 323
linseed oil 64, 151, 449, 450
linseed plants, toxic 102
Linum usitatissimum L. 396
Lipa City, Philippines, urban EVM 340
lipomas, tumours 65
liquid paraffin 386
liquor, *see also* alcohol
liquor (country) 436, 485–6
liquorice (*Glycyrrhiza glabra*) 213, 314
literacy training, and EVK booklets 106–7
Litsea glaucescens 193
liver disorders 233, 448, 485, 499
liver fluke 313
  in Bolivia 120
  in Ethiopia 515
  in Europe 461
  in Kenya 136, 257–8
  in Nepal 329
  in Peru 120, 134, 175, 225, 317
  bovines 308–9
  camels 410
  phantom, curse 136
  reindeer 52–4
  sheep 88, 294–5, 334, 360–2, 423
    resistance to 16, 242–3
  see also fasciolosis
livestock breeds 137, 255, 387–8, 457
livestock byproducts 365–6, 506
livestock development needs 208, 281, 286
livestock husbandry 155, 229–30, 348, 478–9, 492–3
  in Africa 177–8, 469–73, 498–9, 504, 512–14
    Beni-Amer pastoralists 188
    Benin 379–80
    Botswana 458–9
    Fulani 324–5, 522–3
    Kenya 253
    Nigeria 441
    Somalia 123, 125
    Sudan 539
  in America 304
  in China 149

  in Europe 156, 482–3
  in India, women 448–51
  in Indonesia 351, 440, 538
  in South America 435, 524–5
livestock terms, glossary, Fulani 323–5
lizard, *see also* monitor lizard
lizard (boiled in oil) 283
llama fat 104–5, 130, 201, 317, 523
llama herders, Quechua 184–5, 225, 228
llama meat, camelid recipes 519
llamas 14, 126, 356
local, definition 6
'local research brigades', Zaire 330–1
loco (craziness) 306
locoweed (*Astragalus*), for fractures 437–8
locoweed (*Astragalus*) poisoning 15, 130, 465, 523, 547
locust beans (*Parkia* spp.) 50, 55
Lodha tribes (India) 409–10
Lonchocarpus sp. root (barbasco) 519
Loranthus powdered 157
louping ill (ovine encephalomyelitis) 483
louse infestations, guinea pigs 104–5
louse under the foreskin for anuria 536
love potions, of Fulani 158
Lozi, of Zambia 13, 86–7
Lucas spiphora leaves 508
lucerne, in forages, India 330
luck, magical property, in cattle 159
Luffa cylindrica R. 491
Luhya, Kenya 251–2, 256
lunar influences 298, 300
lungworm infestation 128, 472, 482–3
Luo, Kenya 164, 256
Lupinus mutabilis (*tarwi*) 14, 66–7, 83, 200, 264–5, 466
Luri, nomadic pastoralists, Iran 98
Luxemburg, historical EVM 510
lye (sodium hydroxide), disinfectant 65
lymph nodes, in ECF 251, 334, 471
Lythrum salicaria 65–6

Maasai 187, 205, 251–2, 474–5, 540, 542
  allopathic drugs, misuse of 203, 206
  cattle 13, 203, 397, 474
  disease avoidance 148, 203, 405
  disease names (linguistics) 205
  healers 203, 375
  livestock husbandry 366, 404
  parasites 203, 326
  sheepraising 13, 51, 471, 474, 550
  women of 385
Macaranga tanatius juice 162
machine oil (black) 240
Macina wool sheep, Fulani (Mali) 550, 551
Macusani alpaca 201
Madagascar 444, 446, 481–2
  endoparasites 54, 97, 455
Madhuca indica broom 415
Madhuca indica cakes 432
Madhuca indica flowers 211, 235, 236, 237
Madhuca latifolia 234, 414
Madhuca longifolia kern oil 402

madhuca seed cake 237
madhuva flowers 450
Madhya Pradesh (India) 450, 451, 488–9
Maerua crassifolia bark 90, 91
mafisa, in Lesotho 504
maggots in wounds *see* myiasis
magic 141, 291, 295, 329, 537
  in France 111, 309, 310
magico-religious practices 167, 298, 300, 510, 516
  in Africa 339, 515, 522–3
magico-therapeutic plants, Sahel (Africa) 510
magnesium deficiency, *akuet kuet* 334–5
magnolia 128
Maharashtra (India), women of 58–60, 450
maize, feeding supplement 156
maize beer (residue) 317
maize cob tassels 210
maize stalks 399
majith, in drench for conception 211
makar, tobacco plant parasite 238
Malagasy system, pit beef 15
malam (Islamic priests) 335
Malang, East Java (Indonesia) 394–5
malathion, plant pesticide 290
Malawi 270–1, 309
Malay people, Brunei 284–5
Malaysia 147
Maldhari pastoralists (India) 442
male shield fern (*Dryopteris filix-mas* Schott) 463
Mali
  development programmes 132, 554
  disease prevention 96, 219–20
  Fulani in 67, 219–20, 256, 314, 397
  livestock 314, 392, 397, 498–9, 550–1
  migration, pastoral wisdom 163–4, 256
  poultry production 295
  see also Bambara; Fulani; Karwassa Pastoral
    Association; Kel Adagh (Ifora) Twareg;
    Twareg
malignant catarrh 148, 326–7
malignant oedema 281
Mallotus philippensis fruit 142, 269, 455
mallow/hollyhock drench 201
mambonong, witchdoctor 516
mammary acupoints, in China 169–70
Manchu (China), poultry 488
Mandari, Horn of Africa 117–18
Mandinka, in Gambia, N'Dama cattle 47
mane clippings (smoke inhalation) 386
mange
  in Africa 73, 91, 189, 197, 333, 480
  in Andes 265, 523
  in Europe 461
  in India 212, 235, 281
  bovines 262–3, 436, 441, 508, 529
  camelids 117, 410, 512, 519, 547
    alpaca
      in Andes 66–7, 120–1, 245
      in Peru 119, 130, 201, 265
    llamas 184–5
  camels 289, 366, 538
    in Africa 132–3, 214, 259
      Sudan 39, 40, 169, 292
    in India 151, 288, 290, 417

dogs 140, 240, 549
goats 417
horses 133–4, 303
pigs 161
psoroptic 184–5, 383, 436
rabbits 322, 383
sarcoptic 161, 169, 185, 265, 417
sheep 111, 130, 151, 264, 334, 512
Mangifera indica 176, 234
mango flowers 212
mango leaves 458
mango peel and kernels 237, 415
mango-tree bark 448
Manihot caculenta 308
manipulation, use in Sri Lanka 264
Mantaro Valley (Peru) 270
mantras, in Tibetan Buddhism 222
manure
  for cough/asthma 103, 231
  in leather shoes (moccasins) 305
manure plasters, for saddle sores 523
manure (sheep), fish steeped in 214
manure-compost, nutrient cycling 506
manzanilla 66, 191
Maori sheepraisers, New Zealand 116
mapping livestock disease 404–5
Mapuche Indians, Chile 173
marcioure, in bouquets 111
margosa oil/leaf juice 273
marigold 148, 213, 371–2
Maring Tsembaga (New Guinea) 452
marking cattle, festival in Peru 317
marking-nut tree kern oil 328
Marsabit Project 33, 44, 208, 315–16
marshmallow (*Althaea*) 485
Marsilea quadrifolia L. 102
Martynia annua L. 109–10
Marwar (India) 93–4
Marwari dark-brown camels, in India 287
Mashona cattle, tick-resistant 184
massage 129, 148, 309, 435, 505
masseurs, in Ayurvedic medicine 298, 300
mastication problem 491
mastitis 150, 453–4, 456
  in Africa 195, 223, 354–5, 386, 517
  in Ecuador 226
  in India, by women 449
  in Mongolia 141
  in Sri Lanka 546–7
  pigs 298, 396, 518
  ruminants 458, 509, 518
    cows 323, 467–8, 511
    goats 309
    sheep 75, 110, 264, 295, 323
materia medica, commonalities 22–3
materia medica (ethnopharmacopoeia) 8–11
matico 50, 380, 437–8
matorral rub 396
Matricaria chamomilla 207
Mauritania 67, 392–3, 439, 505
Mavchis (India), tribal peoples 528
Mawre herders, vaccination technique 220
Maya, religion 420–1, 423, 427
Mayan sacred number (9) 298, 300

maycha 50, 317
maygora, fowl cholera prevention 321
Mbeere tribe (Kenya) 102, 459
Mbororo Fulani 107, 380
meadowsweet (*Filipendula ulmaria*) 499
measure, in dosing for treatments 308
meat, as energizer 8
meat quality, goats, in India 399
meat storage/preservation, llama 519
Meau, in Thailand 89
Medicago spp. 323
medicinal plant insertion *see* pegging
Medicinal Plant Project, database 413–14
medicinal plants 351
  in Africa 543
    Cameroon 498, 517
    Kenya 192
    Madagascar 444
    Nigeria 402
    Somalia 147
    Tanzania 373–4
    Zaire 276–7
    Zambia 502
  in India 261, 526–7
  in India (booklet) 57
  in Indonesia (bibliography) 384
  in Mexico 321
  in Nepal 329, 330
  in Philippines 409, 410–11
  in South America 228, 365–6
  database, computerized, HERVET 10 319
  harvesting and storage 365–6, 498, 517, 543
  in Traditional Animal Health Care, An
    Information Kit 252
medicinal teas, in France 110
medicinemen, Chhotanappur (India) 491
medico-religious practices 16–17, 138, 226–9, 431,
  492
  in Africa 124–5, 157–8, 286–7, 335
medico-religious texts, in Tibet 221–3
Melia volkensii leaves 102
Melinis minutiflora 511–12
melon (*Cucumis melo*) 510
Melyna arjoria 508
Menispermum coculus L. 45–6
men's work, beekeeping 183–4
menstrual blood in water, for colic 480
Mentha piperita (mint) 207
Menz sheep, Ethiopia 387
Mercurialis annua L. 111
mercury 328, 461
mercury-based compounds 24, 65, 237, 296, 536
mesenteric fat 514
Messerya Humr tribe, in Sudan 539
meteorism *see* bloat
methi 330, 503, 529
  see also fenugreek
methylene blue 201
metritis 64, 215, 396
Mewar (India) 93–4
Mewari white camels 287
Mexico
  EVK 62, 155, 500
  EVM 46–7, 338

herbalism 26, 46
  Medicinal Plant Project, database 413–14
  medicinal plants 201–2, 321, 464
  aquaculture, endoparasites 419
  bloat 13, 76, 148
  cattle 148, 414
  ectoparasites 109–10
  healers 321–2
  rabbits 120
  wounds 406, 503
  see also Chiapas highlands; Nahua; Nayarit;
    Puebla; Puebla State; P'urhé; Rambouillets;
    Totonac; Totonac people; Tzotzil
Mexico City, urban EVM 319
Middle East, herd management 140
midge repellent, smoky fires 187
midwives, healers 87, 320, 370
migration 107–8, 163–4, 190
  see also nomadism; seasonal movements; tran-
    shumance
Mijikenda cattle-keepers, Kenya 143–5
milk
  brucellosis transmission by 481
  feeding supplement, for horses 521
  in fly repellent 385
  medicinal use
    bloat 283, 514
    colic 510
    FMD 234, 519
    intranasal 139, 159, 377
    lice prevention 223
    piroplasmosis 159
    plant poisoning 529
    respiratory diseases 139
    retained placenta 295
    worms 157, 264
    wounds 386–7
milk (buffalo) 415
milk (camels) 386, 551
milk (condensed), in mineral blocks 406
milk fever, hypocalcaemia 75, 211, 414, 416–17
milk (goats) 231, 399
milk (human) 130, 228
milk let-down 77, 92, 202, 211
milk powder, in feed/mineral blocks 210
milk production 284, 415, 453
  after calf death 121, 224, 286–7, 515
  economic role 168
  feeds/fodders for 237, 291
  medicinal plants 75, 127, 253, 409
  Tamil-language people 400–1
  Trinidad and Tobago 300
  see also galactagogues
milk quality, treatments in India 238
milk taste, in trypanosomosis 471
milk thickener 399, 480
milk yield 49, 50, 230, 237, 449, 450
  see also galactagogues
milk yield (poor), evil eye as cause 118
milk/oil feed, general prophylaxis 183
milking 165, 313, 329
millet 47, 90, 91, 302
  see also bajra
millet chaff 199

millet (crushed) 539
millet flour (porridge) 521
millet (pearl) 236, 415
millet (red) 103
Mimosa pudica 177, 230, 300, 400
Mimosa tenuiflora 503
mimosa tree (*Acacia cyanophila*) 461
mineral oil 61, 322, 360–2
mineral supplements 54, 168, 210, 406
    in Africa 124–5, 147, 270
        Fulani 335–6, 513, 522–3, 545
mineral-based treatments, in Ethiopia 514
minerals, forages and wells 8, 105
mint 207, 225, 226, 415, 485
Minthostachys andina (*muña*) 118–19, 463
Miombo woodlands, beekeeping 183–4
miot herbalists 404
Mirabilis jalapa L. 86
miscarriage, *see also* abortion
mistletoe (*Tapinanthus oleifolius*) 287
mites 112, 114–15, 138, 330–1, 547
mixed-species management 14, 42, 471, 472
Miyanmin (Papua New Guinea) 380
mocco-mocco (*matico*) 380
modern medicine *see* allopathic medicine
modlu tree pulp 284
mokko mokko, baths for bloat 317
molasses 237, 297, 301, 365–6
molasses grass (*Melinis minutiflora*) 511–12
Momordica charantia 191, 237, 301, 340, 411, 415
Monda tribes, in India 409–10
mondono (edible earth), New Guinea 245
Mongolia/Mongols 141–2, 366–7, 369–70
    livestock 13, 302, 313
    mineral blocks 210, 406
Monguers, of Kansu-Tibetan frontier 474
Moniezia see tapeworm
monitor lizard, *see also* lizard
monitor lizard fat 138
moon phases
    castration in 138, 395
    cattle breeding in 199–200
Moors, CBPP, traditional vaccination 96
moquera (rhinitis), horses 317
moquillo (distemper), poultry 238
Morantel Citrate 140
Morinda morindoides leaves and fruits 485
Moringa oleifera 140, 253, 340
Moringa pterygosperma bark 414, 415–16, 547
Moringa spp. 414, 432
Morocco 500
morphine, for diarrhoea 485
mortality rates 78, 188, 272, 395, 443
mortars, wood from, against *hantu* 285
Moschosma polystachym 415
mosquitoes 164, 173–4, 189, 529
moss, in splint for fracture 76
moth tubers, fodder, in India 234
motion sickness, dogs 166
motor oil, in pesticides 120–1, 132–3, 243
motsoso medicine, for impotent bulls 63
mouse (live), for cough 367–8
mouth

mix in cloth over tongue 400
    thorns in, for weaning 397
    see also jaw; palate
mouth bleeding, treatment for anaemia 159
mouth lesions 183, 213, 232, 292, 306
moxibustion 222, 263–4, 277
Mozambique 337, 388, 530
mucilaginous drinks 64
Mucuna pruriens 401
Mucuna prurita 468
Mucuna prurita leaves 212
mud 214, 429, 531
    for wounds 229, 231, 529
mud (putrefied) 396
mugwort (artemesia) leaves 388
mules 87–8, 156–7, 321, 367, 537
muña (*Minthostachys andina*) oil 118–19, 463
Mundari pastoralists, Sudan 174–5, 183
Mundri District (Sudan) 485
munduga sprouts 230
Murraya koenigii leaves 129
Musa paradisica stem juice 281
Musa textilis sap 191
musculoskeletal disorders 38, 45, 416
musk-deer scent glands, for fever 223
mustard 432, 458
    for worm-infested pastures 75
mustard (*Brassica juncea*) seeds 129
mustard oil 77, 376, 503, 519
    for wounds 213, 452, 486
mustard poultice, for metritis 64
mustard (*suero de vaca*) flowers 437
Muturu cattle 187, 471
Muyal kathazhai leaves 402
muzzle
    for weaning calves 515, 521
    sheep parasite control 18, 422
mycotic, *see also* fungal
mycotic dermatitis *see* dermatophilosis
myiasis 150
    in Africa 50, 157, 459
    in India 212, 415, 418, 450, 491
        by women 449, 450
        Tamil-speaking groups 399, 401
    buffalo 126
    camels 229
    cattle 283
    horses 76
    small ruminants 349
Myrica cerifera 193

Nagrak (West Java) 440
NAHAs *see* nomadic animal health auxiliaries
Nahua communities, Mexico 167–8
Namchi cattle, trypanotolerant 552
Namibia, Himba cattle herders 287
naphthalene 231, 282, 340
NAPRALERT, databank 147
nasal conditions 263, 292, 399
nasal drenching 377
natron (sodium carbonate) 157, 512
    feeding supplement 74, 105, 108, 406, 521
Navajo, American Indians 13, 155–6, 305, 306

navel treatments 64, 130, 134, 386
  lambs/kids 130, 228, 349
Nayarit State (Mexico) 146
Nazca Valley (Peru), healers 481
N'Dama cattle 47, 133, 155, 187, 470, 517
  disease-resistant 294, 471
    trypanotolerant 255, 267, 310, 387, 552
Near East, Semitic peoples 214–15
neck disorders 39, 44, 231, 292, 402
  wounds 234, 491
necklaces, therapeutic 399, 402, 430
necropsy, in Sudan, and anatomy study 39
neem 50, 203, 404, 429
  buffalo 262–3
  bullocks 400
  dogs 140
  elephants 433
  fish (care of) 192, 496–7
  for ectoparasites 14, 140, 173–4, 262–3, 387
  for endoparasites 140, 385–6, 449, 485
  for FMD 129, 236, 399, 432, 453
  for wounds 231, 429
  poultry 14
neem leaves 26, 47, 140, 485
  for myiasis/ticks 243, 418
neem oil 129, 399, 400, 453, 546–7
neem seedcake 47
neem tree (*Azadirachta indica*) 47, 396, 492
neem tree bark 130
Negev desert, Bedouin in 41–2, 73
Nelumbo nucifera 128
nematode larvae, dung beetles against 155
neonatal care, alpacas 134
neonatal care, by Afghan women 142
neonates, colostrum for *see* colostrum
Neorautanenia mitis roots 441
Nepal 170–1, 172, 221–3, 329, 330
  bloat 13
  diarrhoea 296
  pigs 193, 509–10
  Village Animal Health Workers 376
  yaks 312, 313, 461–2
  see also Dhami; Koshi Hills; Tamang
Nepal Rural Reconstruction Association 509–10
Nepalis, of Assam, India 107
Nepeta glechoma (ivy) 156
nervous disorders 207, 463–4
nettle bedding, medicinal 229
New Agriculturalist On-line 387–8
New Guinea
  pig keeping 15, 24, 245, 505
  see also Baktaman; Maring Tsembaga
New Zealand, hydatid disease 116
Newcastle disease, poultry 48, 50–1, 404
Nez Percé, American Indians 282, 378–9
Nguni cattle, Swaziland 198–9
Nicaragua 238, 239–40, 279–80, 395–6
Nicotiana glauca 209
Nicotiana paniculata L. (utashayli) 85
Nicotiana tabacum (tobacco) 45–6, 50
Nicotiana tabacum (tobacco) leaves 262–3
nicotine, parasiticide 64, 273
nicotine extract, *see also* tobacco
Nigella sativa L. 172

Niger 440–1, 456, 494, 495, 501, 518–19
  see also Bouzou; Fulani; Fulße (Fulani); Kel
  Ewey Twareg, WoDaaße (Fulani); Sahel;
  Twareg
Niger Range and Livestock Project (NRLP) 320–1
Nigeria 13–14, 43, 49–50, 60, 62, 402
  anthelmintics 87, 247, 487
  ethnoveterinary R&D 247–8, 260–1
  horses 303
  livestock breeds 80
    cattle 80–2, 190, 267, 441, 466
    small ruminants 351–2
  poultry
    breeds 249–50, 404
    raising 48, 209, 247–8, 506
  Rural Appraisal Methods 335–6
  ticks 81–2, 472
  see also Fulani; Hausa; Kaduna; Ogun; Rivers
  State; Zaria
night blindness 15, 23, 90
nitre, for sprains/strains 132
Noakhali (Bangladesh) 89
Nomadic Animal Health Auxiliaries (NAHAs) 51,
  78–9
nomadism
  in Chad 521
  in dry tropics 241–2
  in Ethiopia 209
  in Iran 98
  in Kenya 386–7
  in Sahel 190–1
  in Sudan 82–3, 138, 281
  in West Africa 469, 471, 472
  of Fulani 102, 105–7
  of Twareg 90
nomenclature *see* linguistic difficulties
Nong Pho, Thailand 139
Normandy (France) 309–10, 480–1
North America *see* American Indians; Amish;
  Canada; USA; Wa-Nande
North Ronaldsay sheep, in Scotland 137
Northern Africa *see* Africa
Northern Kenya *see* Fulani (Kenya)
Norway, Saami Lapps, reindeer-herding 52
nosodes, in homeopathy 487
nostril-slitting, therapeutic 153, 305, 366
novocain blockade (acupuncture) 509
NRLP (Niger Range and Livestock Project) 320–1
Nuba dwarf Koalib cattle, in Sudan 385
nuclear fallout (Chernobyl explosion) 52–4
Nuer pastoralists, Sudan 44, 99–100, 101, 474–5
nutmeg, for calf scour 118
nutrient cycling, Java (Indonesia) 506
Nutrospel, herbal immunostimulant 95
Nux vomica, for motion sickness 166
nyabende winy (*Lantana camara*) leaves 164
Nyctanthes arbor-tristis 160–1, 480

oath, to combat pasteurellosis 159
oatmeal, for skin disorders 65, 233
oats (*Avena sativa*) 64, 167, 461, 536
obe tree 259
obeahmen, skills against evil eye 298

obstetric operations 12, 38, 64
   see also embryotomy
Ochradenus baccatus 73
Ocimum basilicum leaves 409
Ocimum gratissimum 374, 463
Ocimum sanctum 411, 415, 507
Ocimum sp. leaves 401
ocular *see* eye
odour, in sympathetic magic 112, 114–15
oestrogenic agents, pigeon excrement 127
oestrogenic plants 55, 126
oestrus induction 343, 513
   in India 210, 212, 236, 401, 449
   bovines 127, 300, 532
      buffalo 211
      cows 147, 320, 402, 486
   by acupuncture 244, 343
   sheep 295, 300
   sows 149
   women's EVK 449
offerings, ritual healing 264, 317, 372, 420
offerings (burnt) 232
Ogaden (Ethiopia) 555
Ogalala Sioux, American Indians 306
Ogun State, Nigeria 60
oil
   abortion risk 529
   at parturition 416–17, 449
   for anthrax 465
   for bloat 417, 539
   for FMD 481
   for skin disorders (itching) 295
   for ticks 386
   see also animal; automotive lubricant; baby;
      brake fluid; camphor, *Carthamus tinctorius*;
      cashew-nut; castor; church lamp; cooking;
      cottonseed; diesel; edible; engine; fig-tree;
      gingelly; human hair oil; juniper; kerosene;
      linseed; machine; margosa; marking-nut tree
      kern; mineral; motor; neem; olive; palm;
      paraffin; peanut; python; red palm; *Ricinus
      communis* L. seed; sarson; turpentine oil; veg-
      etable; walnut
oil cakes, sexual maturity delayed 77
oil/milk feed, general prophylaxis 183
ojha healers, Ayurvedic medicine 298
okra
   in multipurpose prophylaxis 106
   see also wild okra
older animals, acupuncture for 311
oleum picis liquidae 330–1
olive oil 64, 132–3, 327
   in egg preservation 76
olive oil and charcoal 75
olives, soaking water 214
OLS (Operation Lifeline Sudan) 63, 123–4, 334–5
Omaha, American Indians 379
Oman, biting flies 366
one-medicine concept, and zoonoses 473
onion (*Allium cepa*) 76
   cattle 129, 415
   for bloat 114
   for diarrhoea 458
   for flatulence 129, 235

for rabies 458
for strangles 386
for worms 50
pigs 161
poultry 237, 395, 415
onion ashes 415
onion bouquets 156
onion (crushed, steamed) 402
onion juice 236, 436
onion leaves 210, 406
onion skin smoke, against *hantu* 285
onion (white) 211, 231
onion (wild) 448
Operation Lifeline Sudan (OLS) 63, 123–4, 334–5
opium 168, 232
OPP (Outreach Pilote Project), West Java 43
oral rehydration therapy, diarrhoea 506
oral route, for medicines 11
orange leaves 201
orange (roasted) 273
orange (sour) 128
Oraon tribes, in India 409–10
oregano 557
orf 279
organ tissue, home-made vaccines from 8
organizations interested in EVM 29
organizational issues, in paravet programme 320–1
Orissa (India) 409–10
Ormocarpum sennoides leaves 401
orobanche, for oestrus induction 338–9
Oromo peoples (Ethiopia) 514–16
orthopaedists, healers, in Ethiopia 515
Oryza sativa (rice) 65–6
osteomyelitis, jaw, alpaca 245
ostrich dung 168
ostrich intestines 91
otitis, firing for 108
Outreach Pilote Project (OPP) 43
ovine *see* sheep
Oxalis corniculata juice 129
oxen 72–3, 127, 152
   anthrax vaccination 152
   castration wounds 455
   display 118
   respiratory problems 236
   yoke wounds 195
oyster shell grit, for poultry 76
oyster-shell (crushed) 536

PA, *see also* participatory appraisal
pack animals 132, 156–7, 158, 287
   wounds/sores 132, 406, 539
   see also bullocks; camels; donkeys; horses;
      mules; oxen
PACKs (primary animal health-care kits) 215
pad problems in dogs, herbal care 74
Paederia foetida leaves 503
paico, bloat prevention 437
pain relief 485
   in cattle 508
   in elephants 168
   in horn shaping 115
pains (tick pyaemia) 483

Pakistan 171, 269, 313
  see also Koochi nomads; Punjab
palate swollen, mouth disorders 132–3
palm jaggery 400, 507
palm oil 79–80, 391
palm sugar 401
palm wine 62
palmyra jaggery 453
Panax pseudoginseng 128
Pandanus tectorius leaves 507
pangolin skin (burning) fumigation 402
Panicum miliare 400, 402
Pantar island (Indonesia) 340
panthers, sheep predators 107–8
Papaver somniferum (poppy) 65–6, 485
papaya, *see also Carica papaya*
papaya (*Carica papaya*), anthelmintic activity 468
papaya fruit 211, 383, 384–5, 512
papaya leaves 383, 503
papaya seeds
  anthelmintic 126, 141, 279
    small animals 230, 264, 412
Papua New Guinea, Miyanmin 380
paraffin, for ticks 317, 386
paralysis, goats, tick-born 214–15
parasite burden, seasonal estimate 83, 123
parasite control *see* countries; livestock husbandry
parasite control, *see also* paravet programmes
parasite resistance *see* livestock breeds
parasites *see* countries; livestock breeds; parasite type/species
parasitic gastroenteritis 130, 262
parasitic infection *see* individual infections
parasiticides *see* anthelmintics; ectoparasites; endoparasites; plant name
parasitism 332, 360–2
parasitology 461
paravet, definition 7, 36
paravet programmes 117, 218–19, 364–5, 402–3, 488
  Chad 218–19
    Ishtirak 73–4, 329, 429–30
  Kenya 255, 259, 403, 541
    Gabbra pastoralists 44
    ITDG 316, 382, 559
    Marsabit Project 208
  Mozambique 388
  Nepal 376
  Niger, NRLP, in Niger 320–1
  Philippines 325
    HPI 122, 406
  Somali nomads 51, 388
  Sudan 40
    ACROSS Project 485
Paraveterinary Medicine: An Information Kit (booklets) 137
paravets
  Kenya 203, 223–4, 394, 542–3
  Mali 132
  Pakistan, need for 163
  Sudan, *atet* Dinka healers and 535
PARC-VAC (Participatory Community-based Vaccination and Animal Health) Project 123–4
paresis, effect of electroacupuncture 280–1
Parkia biglobosa (locust beans) 55, 513

Parkia clappertononia bark 466
Parkia filicoidea (African locust beans) 55
parotid lymph nodes, in ECF 251, 334, 471
parsley infusion 201, 510
Parthenium hysterophorus flowers 160–1
participatory appraisal (PA) 122–3, 125, 336, 493
participatory approach
  to R&D 360–2, 420–9
  to vaccination programme 333–4
Participatory Community-based Vaccination and Animal Health (PARC-VAC) Project 123–4
participatory rural appraisal (PRA) 221, 310–11, 333–5
participatory workshops 382
parturition care 157, 264, 290, 403–4, 416–17
  see also animal species
Pashtun pastoralists (Afghanistan) 142
Pasir Gaok (West Java) 440
pasmo, overwork in water buffalo 77
Paspalum scrobiculatum 202, 235
pasteurellosis 68, 157–8, 159
pasteurellosis (digestive) 505
pasteurellosis (fowl cholera) 518
pastoral nomads, ethnology of 187
pastoralism 117, 376
Pastoralist Development Project, FARM-Africa 177–8
pastoralist dictionary, Somalia 124
pasture, migration and 82–3, 107–8, 136
pasture improvement, medicinal plants in 276
pasture selection, preventative care 106
pasuvaidyulu, healers, India 455–6
Pavonia spinifex 431
pawpaw *see* papaya
peach leaves 371–2
peacock feathers 283
peacock quills (ash of) 210
peanut oil 212
Pedalium murex 400, 480
pediculosis 118–19, 536
  see also lice
pegging (seton application) 11, 101, 110, 339, 465
Peltophorum ferruginaeum 209
penis tied
  contraception 13, 90, 539
    goats/sheep 418, 474
penis (yak), used in Chinese medicine 311
Pennisetum purpureum (king grass) 365–6
pennyroyal leaves 118
pepper
  for bacterial infections 231
  for coughs, in poultry 209
  for diarrhoea (bloody) 481
  for ectoparasites 514
  for endoparasites 158, 385
  for fevers 260, 532
  for FMD 481
  for indigestion/ bloat 260, 485–6
  for respiratory disorders 139, 231, 519
  for snoring/coughs 508
  for sore throats 213
  in anus of sick animal 228
  see also Capsicum; chilli

pepper (alligator-pepper) in gin 62
pepper (black)
  for crop-bound poultry 76
  for eye diseases 399
  for swollen throat 491
  in appetite stimulant 197, 416–17
  toxic plants antidote 409–10
pepper (crushed) 376
pepper fruits 455
pepper (ground) 132–3, 209
pepper (red) 367
pepper seeds 202, 401, 453, 532
peppercorns (black) 102
peppermint, for bloat 114
peppers, in feed for fractures 482
peppers (hot, chilli) 525
peppers (red and yellow) 412
performance, and management system 478–9
perfume, for pasteurellosis 157–8
Pergularia daemia 400, 432, 532
pericarditis 64
Peru 50, 83, 316–17, 357–8, 523
  ectoparasites 85, 175
  endoparasites 26, 61, 83–5
  guinea pig 377–8
  horses 15, 327
  medicinal plants 120, 201, 463, 498
  sheep 61, 83
  SR-CRSP in 358, 360–3
  swine, pediculosis 118–19
  see also Ancash; Arequipa; Aymara; Cajamarca;
    Caylloma Province; Chim-Shaullo;
    Chumbivilcas; Cuzco; Huancayo; Mantaro;
    Nazca; Piura; Puneño; Puno; Quechua; Usi;
    Vicos
perumkayam 546–7
pest control 60, 115–16
  by neem 47, 429
  by poultry 432
    ducks 430–1, 498, 517
pest management, integrated (IPM) 284
pest-repellents, traditional 13–14
pesticide handling 217
pesticides 264–5, 379
  in rice-and-fish farming 496–7
  plant pesticide, misuse 290
Petén region (Guatemala) 156–7
Petiveria alliacea 300, 301
petrol
  after castration 116
  for CCPP prophylaxis 183
  for ectoparasites 64, 111
  for footrot and FMD lesions 126
petroleum, medicinal uses 166, 191
petroleum jelly, for hairballs, cats 233
petroleum products, for mange 151
Peul, *see also* Fulani
Peul (Fulani) stockraisers 153–4, 281–2, 307–8,
  512–14
pharmacological evaluation 186
pharmacology, conference working group 347
pharyngitis, in cattle 400
Philippines 173, 244, 317–18
  anthelmintics 176–7, 524

buffalo (carabao) 77, 143, 191
coconut, many uses of 149
ducks, pest control by 498
medicinal herbs 161–2, 174, 409, 410–11, 480
paravet programme 37, 122, 325, 406
see also Benguet; Leyte; Lipa City; Visayas
Phoenix sylvestris bark 235
phosphorus deficiency, grazing for 342
Phylanthus 209
Phyllanthus emblica L. 102
Physalis alkekengi (wild tomato) 50
physical therapy, veterinary 434–5
Physostigma mesoponticum (Taub tubers) 270–1
Phytolacca dodecandra 370
Picardie (France) 156
Piegan, American Indians 306
piercing, for lameness, in China 537–8
pig (black-skinned, native), sacrifice 516
pig breed, *see also* Taihu
pig dung
  burning of in paddock 295
  in poultices 273, 536
pig fat 201, 453
pig flesh 488
pigeon droppings 127, 211, 486
piglets
  castration 538
  diarrhoea 314, 506
  female castration 538
  iron-deficient anaemia 393
  milk teeth clipped 138
  urban 340
pigs 14, 321–2, 497–8
  in Bolivia 524–5
  in Haiti 431–2
  in Nepal 193
  in Nicaragua 395–6
  in Papua New Guinea 78, 380
  in Peru 118–19, 317
  in Philippines 528
  in Senegal 116
  in Solomon Islands 190
  in Trinidad and Tobago 298, 299
  in Vietnam 518
  'bad blood', in France 481
  diarrhoea 69
  ectoparasites 118–19, 161, 468, 505
  endoparasites 174, 194, 509–10
  feed 393, 498
    supplements 15, 57, 245, 265
  gastroenteritis, transmissible 164
  immunity stimulation 102–3
  oestrus induction 25, 244
  viral encephalomyelitis 446
  see also boar; hog; piglets; sows
pilgrimages 111, 372
Pimenta racemosa leaves 301
pine tar and cotton seed oil, ear ticks 64
pine tar dressing 65
pineapple, bromelain plant enzyme 192
Pinus ponderosa gum 499–500, 507
Piper aduncum 463
Piper angustifolium R (matico) 50
Piper betle L. (areca nut) shoots 129

Piper elongatum (matico) 50
Piper guineense (pepper) 209
Piper longum 458
Piper nigrum 507, 532
Piper nigrum fruits 409, 451–2
Piper nigrum seeds 401
piroplasmosis 152–3, 159
Pistacia lentiscus 507
'pit beef system' 15, 481–2
pitcalu (watery dung), buffalo/cattle 232
Pittosporum sp., bark 54
Piura (Peru) 420
placenta, fears about, in India 528–9
placenta expulsion
  in Ethiopia 370
  in India 212, 234, 237, 399, 414, 415
  in Kenya 459
  in Latin America 489
  in Namibia 287
  in Sudan 539
  in Tanzania 373
  cows 237, 287, 399, 414, 415, 489
placenta retained
  Arabs 76
  in Bolivia 13, 220
  in Ethiopia 195
  in Fulani (Cameroon), use of EVM 517
  in India 77, 236, 443, 449
    Gujarat 210
    Rajasthan 295
    Tamil-speaking groups 202, 400
    Uttar Pradesh 126, 213
  in Italy 338–9
  in Mauritania 505
  in Peru 135, 201
  in South Africa 138
  in Sri Lanka 264
  in Tanzania 325
  in Trinidad and Tobago 300
  ruminants 300
    buffalo 126
    cows 77, 135, 138, 195, 220
    sheep 295
plant, *see also* medicinal plants
plant compendium, Peru 498
plant databases 32–3, 56
plant enzymes, anthelmintic activity 192
plant identification (book), Peru 120
plant nurseries, in Cameroon, HPI 99
plant pesticides, misuse 290
plant pharmacopoeia, of Fulani 308
plant tars, for mange/scabies 132–3
Plantago psyllium leaves 214
plantain leaves 132
plantain stems 365–6
plaster 38
  for fractures
    by Bedouin 73
    in India 202, 399, 401, 415
    in Latin America 125, 130, 239, 433
  for hoof disorders 536
  mud plaster, for myiasis 229
plastic bag ingestion 40, 222
pleurisy 381

Plumbago zeylanica 412
pneumoenteritis 225, 226
pneumonia 91
  cattle 75, 283
  goats/sheep 142, 152–3
poison, treatment by *apeth* 535
poisoning 50, 480, 531
  cattle 172, 466, 507
  horses 536
poisoning (shrimp), of dogs 277
poisonous bites, in India 400
poisonous materials *see* toxic materials
Pokot pastoralists (Kenya) 103–4, 204, 206
Pokot pastoralists (Sudan) 115
Polakowskia tacacco 148
Poland, Carpathian shepherds 294–5
political influences
  Negev Bedouin 41–2
  Saami Lapps 52–4
political power systems, and indigenous health
  systems 87
political-economic organization, of nomadic pastoralists 98
Polygala grinerisis leaves 400
Polygonum bistorta 65–6, 499
Polyporus fungus ash 491
pomade, camphorated 110
Pongamia glabra (*karanja*) oil 262–3, 417
Pongamia pinnata branch tip juice 235
ponies *see* horses
poppy (*Papaver somniferum*) 65–6, 485
pork meat, in feed for FMD 400
pork soup, for blackquarter 402
Portulaca oleracea 340
post-surgery, acupuncture in China 311
pot shards 40
  powdered 86–7
potash, oral use 282, 303
potassic-tartrate of antimony 323
potassium nitrate 213, 529
potassium permanganate 48
Potawatomi, American Indians 306
poultices 90, 91, 264, 536
poultry 497–8
  in Africa 208–9, 513
    Ivory Coast 77
    Mali 295
    Nigeria 48, 247–8
  in India 130, 237, 376, 401, 415, 416, 436
  in Indonesia 394–5
  in Mexico 321, 338
  in Nicaragua 238
  in North America 51
  in Philippines 176
  in Trinidad and Tobago 300–1
  crop-bound 76, 506
  diarrhoea 55
  E.coli infection 452
  ectoparasites 14, 54–5, 308, 459
    flea/lice killers 109–10, 210, 277
  egg-laying promotion 48, 55, 86
  endoparasites 279, 384–5, 486, 508
  feed supplement 148
  housing/hygiene 14, 76, 77, 118, 308

poultry (*cont.*)
  insect pest control by 14, 37, 214, 432
  locomotion problems 209
  marketing 242
  Newcastle disease 50–1
  protection of, snake repellent 60
  women in production of 335, 450, 515
  see also chickens; ducks; fowl; turkeys
poultry breeds
  indigenous 116–17, 249–50, 404
  introduction 208
  see also Rhode Island Red
poultry manure, fumigant 400, 514
pox
  camels 289
  indigenous vaccination 152–3, 183, 504
  sheep 91, 152–3
PPR, in Nigeria, treatments for 62
PRA (participatory rural appraisal) 221, 310–11,
  333–5
prairie turnip 550
prajana, for oestrus induction 147
prawn meal, in pig feed, Burma 498
prayer sticks, in Turkey 152–3
prayers
  for alpacas, disease prevention 201
  for goats/sheep 142, 183, 420
  in cattle rites 118
  in medico-religious acts 17, 516
predators 324
  charms/magic against 158, 159
  dogs in control of 14
  ducks 518
  on cattle 159, 163, 326–7
  on llamas 184–5
  on piglets 395–6
  on poultry 77, 238
  on sheep 219, 334
pregnancy detection, camel husbandry 165
pregnancy test, punyakoti, cattle 413, 527
pregnancy tonic, in Vietnam 518
PRELUDE databank 72, 121–2, 273–5, 439
Premna odorata leaves and flowers 318
preparation and administration of *materia medica*
  11
prescriptions
  defined, in Zaire 131
  in Traditional Animal Health Care, An
    Information Kit 252
preventive care 106, 435
preventive medicine 183, 187–8, 219–20, 394, 445
  cattle 457, 529
  dogs 206
  for FMD 481
prickly pear cactus 371–2
primary animal health-care kits (PACKs) 215
probiotics, in veterinary practice (product booklet)
  197–8
production losses (FAO report) 170
PROFOGAN livestock project 225–7, 228–9
proprietary information, in EVK 124
Prosopis cineraria 237
Prosopis juliflora 399
Prosopis juliflora juice 94

Prosopis juliflora seeds 237
Prosopis spp. pods 449
prosperity, charms for, Fulani 157
Provence (France) 264
Prunus armeniaca seed 222–3
Prunus persica 193
Pseudosopubia hildebrandtii 379
Pseudosopubia hildebrandtii leaves 502
Psiadia punctulata leaves 223
Psidium guajava 431
Psoralea glandulosa (culén) 465
psoroptic mange *see* mange
Psorospermum guineensis (sawoiki) 79–80
psychics/diviners, healers, Kenya 394
psychological support, for sick goats 418
psychosomatic medicine, ritual in 148
Pterocarpus marsupium bark 400
Pterocarpus santalinus bark 513
Pterololium hexapetalum 507
Pterospermum acerifolia bark 158
puberty rites, of Fulani 158
Puebla State (Mexico) 51–2, 129, 320, 337–8
pueraria, in Chinese medicine 314
p'uju usu (livestock ailment) 120
pulmonary congestion 412
pulmonary parasites 125, 381
pumpkin, *see also* squash
pumpkin-seeds
  anthelmintic 83, 213–14, 360–2
  tapeworm in dogs 110, 111, 487
Puneño, Peru, alpaca herders, Andes 121
Punjab (India), camel herders 245, 289
Punjab (Pakistan) 163
Puno (Peru) 130, 547
punyakoti, pregnancy test 413, 527
puppies, anthelmintic 524
purgatives 64, 90, 91, 157, 282
  camels 103–4
  cattle 64, 220
  horses 486, 491, 523
  sheep 111
  betel nut 524
  cactus juice 220
  catagua and chilca, in Peru 50
  Mercurialis annua L. 111
  Ricinus communis L. seed oil 97
P'urhé people (Mexico) 446
pus, home-made vaccines from 8
pus-filled lesions, treatments 91
pustules, possibly FMD, Mongolia 369–70
pyegrease, against ticks 272
pyosepticaemia, alpaca/sheep 130
Pyrénées Mountains (France) 93, 202
python oil, fly repellent 191

Q fever, infectious disease 339–40
qallachas, church healers 515
qange (chlamydiosis) 339–40
q'icha, livestock disease 358
quack methods, dangers of 149
quail grease, in eye ointment 536
quarantine 14, 220, 307, 326–7, 539
  buffalo 442

quarantine (*cont.*)
  camels 278
  cattle 117–18, 159
  for anthrax 465
  for bovine plague (contagious typhus) 329
  for diarrhoea 117–18
  for FMD 127, 214, 313, 400, 442
  yaks 313
Quechua Indians (Ecuador) 225–7, 228–9, 525
Quechua Indians (Peru) 14, 184–5, 356–7, 358
queen bee, tethering of 136
Quercus dilatata 529, 530
Quercus incana 529, 530
Quercus robur ilex (holm oak) 65–6
quicklime
  disinfectant 13, 65
  for hoof plaster 536
  in topical mange lotion 212
quince necklace, fetish 201
quinsy, throat infection 323

Rabari people (India) 93–4, 296
rabbits 299, 412
  bloat 277
  deramophytosis 437
  diarrhoea 120, 200
  ectoparasites 243, 265, 383
rabies 101–2, 237, 458, 504
  in Ethiopia 515
  in India 234, 237, 284, 458
  in Iran 504
  in Mongolia 366–70
racing animals 13, 288
ragi, for enteritis 453
Raika people, India 151, 287–8, 289–91, 293, 453
rainbow spirit, disease and 226, 229
rainy season, worm infestation in 255
raised barns, husbandry system 440, 538
Raja cattle, *adappan* syndrome in 263
Rajasthan (India) 293–4, 453, 486
  camels 414
  galactgogues 480
  sheep 295
  women's roles 450, 451
  see also Bhils, Bhat; Jhat; Raika; Rajput
Rajput caste, Rajasthan (India) 453
Rambouillets sheep breeding programme 426–7
rams
  breeding control 302
  contraception 264, 369
    aprons 155, 474
    penis tied 474
  feeding practices 47
rangeland burning, tick control 307
Rangeland Development Project, Ethiopia 466
rapid rural appraisal (RRA), in Nepal 221
RAPP (Rural Agricultural and Pastoral
  Programme) 358
Rashaida, camel pastoralists, Sudan 38, 44–5, 289,
  292–3
rati bhindi leaves 211
Rebari, camel pastoralists, India 289

Rebaris, *see also* Raika
Recording and Using Indigenous Knowledge: A
  Manual 252
rectal prolapse, in India 400
red ants, poultry pest, Africa 209
red clay, for anthrax 91
red cloth, to ward off bad spirits 173
red lead, dressing for horn cancer 328
Red Maasai sheep, Kenya 387
red palm-oil, for mange 322
red pepper, mule, colic, Mongolia 367
red ribbon, magico-religious 481, 515, 516
red soil, medicinal uses 281, 334, 453
redwater scourge, in East Africa 191
REDS (Rural Enterprises Development Services)
  546–7
redwater (haemoglobinurea) 64
reed inserted into rectum, for bloat 505
rehydration therapy, coconut water 149
reindeer
  Saami Lapp herders 14, 52–4
  Tungus herders 187
Rek Dinka (Sudan) 546
religious belief 87
  in American Indian tribes 304
  in Bolivia 241
  in France 111, 114, 310
  in Horn of Africa 117–18
  in Nepal, Tamang tribe 329
  in Peru, Quechua Indians 184–5
  in the Andes 207
Rendille people (Kenya) 208, 221, 277–9
Renealmia alpinea leaves 301
repeater cows *see* infertility
resin, in mix for wounds 295
resource, or system in herbal medicine 561–2
Resource Manual, Latuka agropastoralists, Sudan
  335
respiratory ailments
  Fulani 55, 158
  in India 236, 519
  in Philippines 409
  in Romania 207
  in Scotland 485
  in Somalia 124–5
    camels 132–3, 139
    cats (kittens) 311
    goats 451–2
    horses 557
    pigs 395
    poultry 238, 240, 301, 401
resuscitation, electroacupuncture 280–1
retama leaves 547
Retama raetam branches and leaves 73
Retrofraca 209
rheumatism 282, 453, 485
rhinitis (*moquera*) 317
rhino-laryngeal symptoms 367
Rhode Island Red poultry, introduced 208
Rhodesia (former) 128
Rhoicissus digitata bulb and tuber 138
rhubarb 128, 538
ribbons, magico-religious 111, 129
rice 400

rice *(cont.)*
  bulls, for castration wounds 137
  cattle 529
  cows 129
    for placenta expulsion 236, 300, 414–15
    in galactagogues 415, 507
    for diarrhoea 65–6, 295
    for oestrus induction 212
    in astringent 213
    poultry 237
rice bran 237, 507–8
rice by-products, in feed supplements 237, 482, 498
rice starch 295
rice water 409–10
rice water (fermented) 260, 402, 482
rice (wild) 498, 551
rice-and-fish farming 496–7
rice–duck farming 430–1, 498, 517–18
rice-husk incubation system 65
Ricinus communis (castor-bean) 417, 444
Ricinus communis L. seed oil 97
Ricinus communis root 409
rinderpest 370, 540
  cattle 129, 159
  disease control 96, 197
  treatments for 48–9, 152–3, 183, 326–7
  vaccination
    allopathic 96, 100, 312, 313, 373
    indirect for calves 220
    new sustainable 243, 558–9
    traditional 91, 333–4
  yaks, vaccination of 312, 313
ringworm 288, 306, 386
ritual
  buffalo/cattle, treatments India 232
  by Islamic priests 429–30
  for cattle 118
    in castration 196
  for llamas 184–5
  for sheep
    for mastitis 295
    for sadness 423
  in Ayurvedic medicine 148
  in bloat treatments 102
  in diagnosis, in Chinese medicine 148
  in disease prevention 201
  in FMD treatments 261
  magico-religious practices 148–9, 157, 516
ritual (church-like), for injuries 481
ritual healer, for soul loss 317
ritual sacrifice, guinea pigs 192
Rivea hypocrateriformis leaves 414
Rivers State (Nigeria) 538
rock traction, for retained placenta 220
Romania 207
rope burns, carabao/cattle Philippines 162
Rosa rugosa (rosehips) 485
Rosa sinensis leaves and flowers 307
rosemary (burnt-smoke and heat) 153
rosemary-artemisia fire 305
rotenone (pesticide), fish toxicity 496–7
RRA (rapid rural appraisal), Nepal 221
rubber (burning), inhalation 431

rue *(Ruta graveolens)* 156
Ruellia tuberosa 300
Rufa camel pastoralists, Sudan 44–5
rum, medicinal uses 228, 423
Rumania 102–3, 499
rumen perforation, for bloat 64, 539
Rumex acetosa 486
Rumex patientia L. 523
ruminal dysfunction 109
  cattle/buffalo 414, 480, 510
  cud feeding for 8, 109, 342
  medicinemen, in India 491
  novocain blockade 509
ruminants 299–300, 437–8, 458, 466–7
  anthelmintics 279, 493
  bloat 437, 485
  see also buffalo; camels; cattle; goats; sheep
Rural Agricultural and Pastoral Programme (RAPP) 358
Rural Appraisal Methods, in Nigeria 335–6
Rural Enterprises Development Services (REDS) 546–7
Russia *see* USSR
rustling *see* theft
Ruta graveolens (rue) 156, 193, 510
Rwanda 273–4, 354–5, 464
  CURPHAMETRA, drug trials 441–2
  scabicide, commercial 26

Saami Lapps, reindeer-herding 14, 52–4
Saba florida sap 549
sachants, definition 122
sacred dairies, Toda people, India 459–60
sacred value, medicinal plants, Somalia 147
sacrifice
  healers, Nepal 329
  magico-religious practices 172, 515, 516
  ritual, in Andes 192
  witch doctor, in Sudan 183
saddle sores 380–1, 514
  camels 90, 91
  horses 523
sadness, transmitted to sheep 423
saffron, in mix for anthrax 465
sage ash rub, for bullet wounds 501–2
sage (wild), for castration wounds 550
Sahara Desert, herders of 132–3, 138, 377
Sahel 42–3, 363, 510
  brucellosis in 481
  camels 498–9
  forage resources 199, 389–90, 498–9
  nomads, strategies 190–1
  see also Twareg
Sahel (West African Fellata) sheep, Bambara (Mali) 550
SAIDA (Samburu Aid in Africa) 547–8
saints
  in France 111, 156, 208, 310, 531
  in Luxemburg 510
  of sheep 420, 427, 428
  Tamil, gentle remedies 411
Sal Andrews 228
salamander, fetish 111, 112

Salamat region, Chad 48
saline *see* salt water
saliva
    for yoke galls 210
    home-made vaccines from 8
salivation (continuous), in *valo* 211
Salix alba leaves 200
Salsola spp. 124
salt 15, 91, 92, 108, 188, 491
    alpaca 130
    buffalo 77, 232
    camels 103–4, 233, 457
        feed supplement 165, 246, 555
        for skin diseases 169, 292–3
    cattle 200, 512
        for fever 103
        for poisoning 172
        for tonic 260
    cows 260, 416–17, 486
    for bloat 485–6
    for bottle jaw 126
    for diarrhoea 231
    for ectoparasites 434, 461, 514
    for endoparasites 61, 371, 461
    for flatulence 235
    for FMD 234, 235, 369–70, 531
    for fractures 130, 234
    for inappetance 202, 400
    for injuries 481
    for oestrus induction 401
    for pneumoenteritis 225, 226
    for purgative 157
    for stress, in fodder shortage 237
    for trypanosomosis 288
    for unthriftiness 282
    for wounds 317
    horses 302, 510, 536
    in feed supplements
        Fulani 106, 157, 522–3
        in Columbia 365–6
        in East Africa 287
        in Senegal 105–7
        in Somalia 332
        in Sudan 539
    in medico-religious acts 17, 90, 111, 157
    in sorghum/maize stalks storage 399
    pigs 116, 395
    poultry 238, 240, 436
    ruminants 300, 458
    sheep 130, 295, 360–2
    small ruminants 349, 391, 503
salt and lemon 214–15, 239
salt and whey feeding 262
salt bars, magico-religious practices 515
salt (black) 127–8, 213
salt (copper-containing 'green') 175
salt in incisions, for lameness 132–3
salt licks, home-made, Nepal 168
salt (rock), mineral supplements 270
salt rub, for *valo*, cattle disease 211
salt supplements, in Bulgaria 334
salt water 281, 396, 538
    for eye ailments 226, 228, 232, 283, 537
    for FMD 261, 325

    for ticks 127
salt water drench, for bloat 114
salt water enema 64
salt with cuttlefish powder 138
'salt wood treatment' 507
saltpetre 118, 461, 465, 511
salty soil 103, 386, 387
salty wells 105, 124, 551
Salvadora persica leaf juice 415
Salvadora spp. leaves 235
Salvia officianalis L. 510
Sambucus nigra 110, 111, 207
Sambucus sp. (elderberry) 264
Samburu (Kenya) 220–1, 223–4, 256, 260, 547–8
    cattle 268
    ECF diagnosis 471
    ER&D 500, 540–2, 543–4
    misuse of allopathic drugs 206
    paravet programme 559
    school booklets on EVM 419
    see also Baragoi District
san cap 111, 113
Sanaag region (Somalia) 124–5, 245
sand, for fertility problems 415
sand (hot), for FMD 234, 236, 261, 449, 450
sandalwood 432
Sanga × zebu cattle 355
Santal people (India) 102, 261, 409–10
saprolegniasis, in fish 66
sarcocystosis, in alpaca, Andes 245
Sarcophyte piriei H 459
sarcoptic mange *see* mange
Sard shepherds, Sardinia, Italy 318
sarna (mange), in alpaca 66–7, 119, 410
Sarothamnus scoparius L. 110
sarson oil 283, 529
Sarvodaya Shramadana Movement 546–7
sauerkraut juice 294
Saurashtra (India), forages 330
savants, definition 122
sawoiki (*Psorospermum guineensis*) 79–80
scabicides 26, 383
scabies 340
    camels 132–3, 139
    pigs 161, 396
scabs, home-made vaccines from 8
scarification 91, 96, 157–8
scheduled castes, donkeys, in India 453
Schima wallichi (DC) Korth. 329
Schinus molle leaves and stalks 200
schistosomosis, in Ethiopia 370
Schleichera oleos oil from fruits 235
school booklets on EVM, in Kenya 419
Scilla spp. bulbs 235
Sclerocarya birrea bark 505
Scoparia duleis leaves 491
scoring, livestock disease 122, 125
scorpion bites 272
Scotland 16, 137, 485
scour *see* diarrhoea
screw worm 16, 191
scute, in Chinese medicine 314
Scutellaria scandens Buch.-Ham. 329
sea dust (*Sepia oficinalis*) 536

sea water 39, 40
search methods, EVM bibliography 561
seasonal disease calendar 83, 123, 215–16
seasonal movements 14, 62–3, 88–9, 165
    see also migration; transhumance
seawater bathing, for ectoparasites 74, 169
seaweed eating sheep 137
sebadilla, for ectoparasites 380
Sebei pastoralists, in Uganda 200
SECADEV, paravet training, Chad 218–19
Securidaca longipedunculata 439, 513
sedentarization, in Senegal 381
seed germination, in pregnancy test 527
selenium, in feed/mineral blocks 210
self-medication 405, 433
Sema didymobotrya 270–1
semantic research, livestock terms 323–5
Semecarpus anacardium fruits 507
Semecarpus anacardium seed 236, 401
semen, Dinka belief on 476
Semitic peoples, Near East 214–15
Senecio akhana 130
Senecio huamanlipa 130
Senecio lyratipartius leaves 373
Senecio pseudotites Griseb (maycha) 50
Senecio serratuloides leaves 138
Senecio vulgaris (maycha) 50
Senegal 116, 208–9, 381, 439
    see also Diola; Ferlo region; Fulani; Peul;
        Toucouleur
Sepia oficinalis (sea dust) 536
septic toes, Uttar Pradesh, India 213
septicaemia 135, 278, 279
serpentaria, for conditioner 303
sesame 211, 416
sesame oil 211, 237, 414, 539
    buffalo 211
    camels 169, 237, 246, 292–3
    for FMD 235, 456
    pigs 161
    sheep 295
sesame seed tar 169
sesame seeds 290
Sesamum indicum stalks (ash) 414
Sesbania aegyptica seeds 115
Sesbania grandiflora 432
Sesbania sesban 234
Setaria pallidefusca 482
seton application (pegging) 101, 339, 465
settlement livestock carers (SLCs) 51
SEVA, EVM documented in India 532
sexual maturity delayed, by oil cakes 77
shamans 53, 159, 304, 366
Shami goats, Syria 387
sheanut butter 103, 251, 485
sheanut (*Butyrospermum papadoxum*) 512
sheanut (*Butyrospermum parkii*) 209
sheanut tree trunk and pith 513
sheanut tree bark 108
shearing 17, 120, 201, 551
sheep 303, 360–2
    in Afghanistan 78, 142
    in Africa 51, 219, 387, 552
    in Ecuador 225, 228–9

    in Europe 75, 264, 323, 334, 482–3
    in India 295
    in Java 43
    in Mexico 420–30
    in Peru 83, 130, 356
    anthrax 183
    bloat 141
    braxy 75
    breeding control 155, 187, 302
    castration 12, 183
    colds 262
    contagious kerato-conjunctivitis 191
    diarrhoea 437
    distomatosis 119
    ectoparasites 66, 85, 200, 265
        mange 151, 512
        ticks 191
    encephalomyelitis (louping ill) 483
    endoparasites 54, 61, 383
        hydatidosis 60
        liver fluke 61, 83, 84–5, 242–3
        lungworm 128
    feeding 47, 325, 503, 548
    footrot 437–8
    fractures 437–8
    galactagogue for 55
    immunity stimulation 102–3
    mastitis 75
    pox 152–3, 214–15
    predators 107–8
    tail docking 126
    see also ewes; lambs; rams
sheep breeds 208, 255, 471, 521
    see also Black Head Persian; Caussenarde;
        Djallonké; Dorpner; Fat-tail; Horro; Indonesian
        Thin Tail; Macina wool; Menz; North
        Ronaldsay; Red Maasai; Sahel; Sudan Desert
sheep droppings (boiled) 402
sheep fat 223, 268, 386
sheep horn, fumigation 367
sheep skin on rump, as cure 317
sheep's head (boiled) 104, 386
shepherd-healer, India 494
shepherds, in Europe 88, 202, 294–5
shipping fever, in cattle, China 246
shooting into the air, for anthrax 183
Shorea robusta trees, fungus from 491
Shorthorn cattle *see* West African shorthorn
    cattle
shoulder dislocation, horses 155–6
shrew, disease transferrence belief 156
shrimp poisoning, dogs, in Japan 277
Shukria (Sudan), camel pastoralists 38, 44–5
Siberia, Yakut horses 16, 137
Sichuan Province, China, dairy-goats 309
Sichuanese yak, altitude tolerance 16
Sida acuta 202, 432
Sida veronicaefolia 330–1
Sidama region (Ethiopia) 195
Siddha medical system, in India 56
Sidha healers, in Nepal 172
Sierra Leone
    work oxen in 72–3
    see also Karina area

Silphium lacinatum 379
silver nitrate solution 65
silver wire, for ear lacerations 65
Simanjiro pastoralists (Tanzania) 531
Sinai desert, Bedouin in 73
singeing, for lice removal 505
singing and chanting, medico-religious 17
Sinus vitazonia 507
sinusitis 91
Sioux, American Indians 147, 282, 306
sipda twigs 211
sisal water 537
Sisymbrium sp. seeds 234
sitaphalas, for sarcoptic mange 140
skin, insertion of medicine *see* pegging
skin disorders 179
   in Africa 50, 250, 373
   in France 112, 114–15
   in India 235, 236, 281, 448
   camels 132–3, 169, 386, 513
      necrosis 103–4, 278, 279, 292
   cats/dogs 233
   cattle 65, 168
   dry/itchy 233, 235, 253
   horses 306, 536
   infections 50, 514
   pigs 396
   sheep 75, 112
   see also dermatitis
skull (human), for ritual 481
sky, cause of disease 253
slaughter
   by Saami Lapps 52–4
   ritual, by Quechua Indians 184
SLCs *see* settlement livestock carers (SLCs)
sleeping sickness *see* trypanosomosis
slippery elm 303
small animal practice, in USA 477–8
Small Ruminant Collaborative Research
   Programme (SR-CRSP) 83
small ruminants 73, 277, 407
   in Cameroon 391
   in France 396
   in India 402, 503
   in Indonesia 349, 382–4
      Java 209, 350–1
      West Java 382–3, 440, 538
   in Philippnes 528
   disease tolerance 351–2, 406
   feed for 37, 503, 538
   weaning practices 392
   see also goats; sheep
smallholder farming, West Java 281
smelly substances, medicinal use 228, 229
smoke
   against *hantu* (evil spirits) 285
   household, guinea pig raising 104–5
smoke administration technique 432
smoke cures 342
   for adenitis 316–17
   for constipation 433
   for diarrhoea 222
   for *dony dony* 334–5
   for FMD 296

   for mastitis 264
   for pasteurellosis 68
   for respiratory conditions 55, 529
   for strangles 386
   for *valo* 211
smoke inhalation, paper with mantras 222
smoke tar, for ticks 127
smoky fires 102, 214
   insect repellent 188, 251, 512, 539
      midge/mosquito 187, 529
   trypanosomosis prevention 187, 289
smudge fires, as insect repellents 72–3, 153, 307
snail (roasted, crushed) 536
snail shell with cuttlefish powder 138
snail shell (crushed) 536
snails, disease vectors 42, 45–6
snake (eyeless), medicinal use of 183
snake flesh (dried) 437–8
snake repellent 14, 209, 282, 374
   tobacco plants 13–14, 48, 50
snake skin, for eye ailments 334
snake venom in eye 512
snake-fighting chickens 16
snakebite 13, 110
   in Africa 158, 439, 502, 513
   in Europe 110, 111, 264, 295
   in India 399, 529, 533
   in North America 65, 306
   in Surinam 206
   in Venezuela 433
snakes
   attacked by chickens 16
   predators on ducks 518
snoring, in cattle 507
snuff, medicinal uses 367, 368, 379
soap 64, 395, 536
   for bloat 114, 381, 539
   for sprains 231, 507
   for wounds 406
   insecticides 303, 379, 385
soap (black) 135, 175
soap (red) 189
social power, and indigenous health 87
social role in livestock ownership 42–3, 241
   cattle 41–2, 77, 86, 107–8, 159, 168–9
   llamas 184–5
   poultry 77
Society for Research and Initiatives for Sustainable
   Technologies (SRISTI) 56
socio-economic factors, in healthcare 47, 221–4,
   392
sociology, in Recording and Using Indigenous
   Knowledge: A Manual 252
Sociology and Veterinary Medicine Project 360
soda ash 104
soda drench 118
sodium bicarbonate 210, 213, 228, 236, 385,
   417
sodium carbonate *see* natron
sodium sulphate 65, 128, 273
soil, mineral supplements 270, 393
soil (red), medicinal uses 281, 334, 453
Solanum dulcamara L. 510
Solanum incanum (eggplant) 50, 439

Solanum indicum fruits 399, 400
Solanum leaves 507
Solanum nigrum 162, 455
Solanum sp. smoke 366
Solanum surattense fruit juice 235
Solanum xanthocarpum fruit 399
soldier ants, tobacco plant deterrent 48
Solomon Islands, pig production 190
Somali, paravet programme 388
Somali nomadic pastoralists 339–40
Somali nomads, paravet training 51
Somalia 57, 78–9, 109, 122–3, 256, 332–3
    camel husbandry 79, 232–3, 245, 396
    camel pastoralists 165–6, 246, 277–9, 289
    contraceptive apron 13, 474
    medico-religious practices 96, 147
    minerals feed supplements 147
    small ruminants 78–9, 474
    traditional vaccinations 78–9, 96, 332
    weaning, calf rearing 397
    see also Sanaag region
Somba, trypanotolerant cattle 552
'song oxen', cosmetic horn surgery 546
soot, medicinal uses 75, 391, 410, 512
sopladera (bloat), in Peru 317
sorcerer-healer, in France 310
sorcerers, practices of 157–8, 310, 515
sorcery
    illness/death caused by 106, 118, 232, 286
    protection against 115, 157–8, 208
sore throats, in India 213
sores 98, 198, 303, 499–500, 510
    see also saddle sores
sorghum
    feed supplement 47, 539
    plant poisoning by 91, 102, 236
sorghum stalks, storage 399
soul loss, fright as cause 317
souls, of sheep 420–1, 423, 427
sour and salty plants used by Bedouin 73
sour milk, use of 539
South Africa 138, 371–2
    see also Basuto; Bhaca; Kwazulu
South America 66, 489
    see also Bolivia; Brazil; Ecuador; Peru;
        Venezuela
South American Indians, Aymara Indians 317
South Kalimantan (Indonesia) 533
sows 149, 253, 395
soya 277, 528–9
Soymida febrifuga 234, 235, 236, 507
Spanish 'water bags' (submandibular oedema) 84
spearmaster (*bany bith*) 535
spells, used in Sri Lanka 264
Spermadictyon suaveolens Roxb. bark 329
spider bites 104–5, 239, 395
spider eggs, prophylaxis for FMD 127
spiders (long-legged), for fractures 102
spider's web, for wounds 8, 371–2, 512
spinal manipulation, chiropractic 549–50
spirit world/environment 354, 452
spirits, as cause of ills 329
spirits of wine, medicinal 323
spiritual healing 298, 370

spitting, for respiratory ailments 124–5
splints, *see also* fractures
splints for fractures
    Arab remedy 76
    in Africa 63, 386–7
    in India 102, 211, 281, 284, 443–4, 482
    in Nicaragua 239
    in North America 64
Spondias mombin branches 300
Spondias pinnata 176, 528
sprains/strains 132, 491, 507
squash
    giant (*Cucurbita maxima* Duch) 61
    see also pumpkin
squash-leaf juice 434
SR-CRSP (Small Ruminant Collaborative Research
    Programme) 61, 83, 358, 360–3
Sri Lanka 170, 173, 263–4, 429
    Ayurvedic medicine 55, 432–3
    cattle and buffalo 273, 546–7
    elephants 378, 557
    Rural Enterprises Development Services (REDS)
        546–7
    Sarvodaya Shramadana Movement 546–7
    sheep fattening 325
SRISTI (Society for Research and Initiatives for
    Sustainable Technologies) 56
St John's Wort (*Hypericum perforatum*) 499
stabbing, for bad blood 251
Stachytarpheta jamaicensis 300
standardized measures, in medicines 131
steam treatment 13, 386, 432–3
Stephania japonica root 401
Stereospermum kunthianum 108
sticky willie (*Galium aparine*) 485
stiffness, cattle 532
Stilboestrol, use in cattle 137
stinging nettle (*Urtica* spp.) 201
stinking hellebore 114–15
stock raising, breeding for conditions 37
stock-buying, small ruminants 402
Stockholm tar, for wounds 371–2
stockraising
    and cropping 82
    and over-grazing 323
    Aymara, in Bolivia 120
    strategies, in India 447
    women's role in India 59–60
stomach ailments 212, 282, 327
    pain 90, 91, 126, 129, 428
    swollen 232
stones 63, 111, 138, 221
    see also river pebbles
strains/sprains 13, 132
strangles
    donkeys/horses 133–4, 386, 439, 514
    see also distemper
straw shoes, hoof protection 277
streptothricosis 16, 294
stress
    commercial formulation 411
    in fodder shortage 237
    poultry 301
    probiotics for 197–8

stretching exercises, therapy 434–5
string, protection from hoof problems 396
stroking, in medico-religious acts 17
Strychnos nux-vomica 401, 409, 532, 533
Stylosanthes 545–6
suava, for placenta expulsion 414
sub-mandibular oedema, fasciolosis 84, 423
Sub-Saharan Africa, botanical survey 71–2
subcutaneous implant *see* pegging
suckling (stimulation to), calf 397
Sudan 48, 154, 281, 560–1
    allopathic medicine misused 443
    camel pastoralists in 37–40
    trypanosomosis 245, 385
    see also Arabs; Baggara; Bawadra; Beni–Amer;
        Bishariin; Butana; Darfur; Dinka;
        Hadendewa; Hawawir Arabs; Kababish;
        Kawahla Arabs; Lahawiyin; Latuka; Lehwee;
        Messerya Humr; Mundari; Mundri; Nuer;
        Pokot; Rashaida; Rek Dinka; Rufa; Shukria;
        Tibdawet; Zaghwa
Sudan Desert sheep, Baggara Arabs 552
sudden death, livestock of Beni-Amer 188
suero de vaca (mustard) flowers 437
sugar 143, 237
    for conception/fertility 211, 238, 415
    for eye conditions 201, 223, 443–4
    for fractures 130, 437–8
    see also jaggery, *gur*, molasses; palm
sugar and coconut milk 172
sugar crystal, for myiasis 212
sugar paste, in foot paint for FMD 282
sugarcane 126, 193–4
sugarcane alcohol 226, 228
sugarcane trash (bagasse) 230
sukku naripal grass 432
Sulfathiazol 238, 240, 321
sulphur 118, 296, 380, 514
    for ectoparasites 340, 523
        mange 184, 197, 212, 461
            camelids 523, 547
            camels 132–3, 214
            cattle 529
            horses 303
            sheep 111
sulphur in local rum, for diarrhoea 228
sulphur (volcanic), for mange 410
suñay, breedstock gifts, in Peru 185
sundarsol leaves 237
sunstroke 142, 434
supernatural causes of disease 120, 206–7, 514
supernatural forces
    Aymara Indians 89
    in Ethiopia 40
    Quechua Indians 226, 229
supernatural happenings, vaccination for 63–4
supernatural practices, for livestock 159, 325
supernatural treatment 513, 535
superstitious beliefs 499, 548, 552–3
supplemental feeds, provision 15
suppositories, in EVM delivery 342
surgical administration, for medicines 11
surgical equipment 18, 368–9
surgical operations 11–12, 64–5, 142

in Africa 132–3, 370, 386–7, 514
    see also castration; horn shaping
Suri alpaca 134, 201
Surinam, dogs, herbal medicines 206
surra see trypanosomosis
sustainability
    EVM in 37, 48
    parasite control 42, 155
sustainable development, and EVK 182–3
suture materials 65, 501–2
suture method, crop-bound poultry 76, 506
Swaziland 198–9, 307
Sweden 52, 109, 430
sweet potatoes, feed supplement 78
swellings, treatments 189, 366, 400, 532
Swertia chirata 213, 458
swine *see* pigs
Switzerland 57, 339, 465
sympathetic magic 112, 114–15, 286, 535
Symphytum officinale (comfrey) 485
syphilis, *karachi*, alpaca disease 296
Syria, grazing improvement 323
system, or resource in herbal medicine 561–2
Syzygium aromaticum buds 451–2
Syzygium cumini bark 234, 236
Syzygium cumini seeds 210
Syzygium cuminii bark 414
Szigetköz (Hungary), cattle on islands 512

Tabernaemontana pandacaqui 162
Tadvis, Taluka (India), tribal people 528
Tagetes erecta (African marigold) 330–1, 458
Tagetes minuta L. 97
Taihu, pig breed, in China 137
tail, bloodletting from 263
tail amputation, as cure 235, 366, 367
tail cutting, for enterotoxaemia 295
tail docking 126, 225, 228, 380
tail fat, for bloat 514
tail hair loss 414
Taiwan 244, 314, 343
Talinum crassifolium 518
talismans 110, 111, 157–8, 295
Taluka (India), tribal peoples 528
Tamang tribe, healers, in Nepal 329–30
tamarind
    feed supplement 340, 402, 503
    medicinal use 172, 273, 381
tamarind seeds 400–1, 402
Tamarindus indica 234, 416
Tamarix nilotica chewed bark 73
Tamil farmer, EVK of 202, 260
Tamil Nadu (India) 401–2, 443–4, 453, 532–3
Tamil saint, remedies 411
Tamil-speaking people (India) 399–402, 412, 432
Tanacetum annuum L. 111
tanatanamanga, for dermatophilosis 446
tantal, crop protection by fence of 120
Tanzania 325, 373–4, 530, 531
    CAHWs in 337
    cattle 287, 355, 560
    disease control 96, 197, 463
    see also Barabaig; Simanjiro

tapeworm 370, 371
  camels 169
  dogs 486–7
  goats 142
  hydatidosis 60, 116, 245, 326–7
  plant remedies 39, 54, 126
  sheep, gid (coenurosis) 482–3
  see also coenurosis;
tapeworm cyst *see* coenurosis
Tapinanthus oleifolius (mistletoe) 287
tapioca tubers, feed supplement 237, 400
tapioca-leaf poisoning 129
tar
  for ectoparasites 139, 214–15, 386
  for wounds 237, 521
Taraxacum officinale (dandelion) 485
tarwi (*Lupinus mutabilis*) 66–7, 83, 264–5, 317
  for camelids/ovines 437–8, 466, 512
tastes, elements in TCVM 558
Taub tubers (*Physostigma mesoponticum*) 270–1
Taverniera cuneifolia 237
Taxus brevifolia Nutt. 97
TCVM (traditional Chinese veterinary medicine)
  557–8
tea, medicinal use 210, 234, 415
tea (black) 39
tea (blackberry root) 118
tea (green) 55
tea leaves, medicinal use 132, 223
tea powder 234
teak seeds 212
teat damage, in cows 138
Tecomella undulata bark 288
teeth cleaning, for cats/dogs 233
teeth (loose), cattle disorder 416
teething pain, cats/dogs 233
teff bread 515
teff meal 560
Teloxys ambrosioides sprigs 421, 427
Teluga-language treatments 507–8
temperature resistance, Yakut horses 16
temu ireng, for poultry worms 394
tenancy arrangements, livestock dispersal 504
tendonitis, warming ointment for 412
teosán tree leaves 395
Tephrosia nana 517
Tephrosia purpurea 202, 260
Tephrosia vogelii (fish–poison bean plant) 116,
  270–1, 462, 485
Terminalia arjuna bark 400
Terminalia avicennioides 250, 466
Terminalia belerica 507
Terminalia chebula 129, 237, 486
Terminalia schimperiana 517
termite-mound soil 238, 402
testicles (undescended), horses 239
tethering, of queen bee 136
Teton Sioux, American Indians 282, 378–9
Tetradenia fructicosa Benth. 444
Texas Longhorn cattle 16, 555
Thailand 89, 136, 170–1
  see also Nong Pho
Thar Desert (India) 536–7
Tharaka (Kenya) 102, 542–3

tharakar, healer, in India 443–4
theft, deterrent 107–8, 184–5, 317, 379, 480
theilerosis, control of, Tanzania 197
Thespesia populnea tree latex 281
third eyelid carcinoma removal 386–7
Thompson Indians, Canada 499–500, 507
thorn wounds 162
thorns fixed to offspring, weaning 392
thorny plants, in bouquets 112, 114
three day sickness (ephemeral fever) 159
throat conditions 292, 323, 400
  sore 306, 410
  swelling 235, 491
thrush, treatments Cévennes 111
Thuya tetraclinislariks leaves 132–3
thyme, for FMD 396
Thymelaea hirsuta leaves 73
Thymus vulgaris 167, 277
Thysanolaena maxima 436, 443
Tibdawet, Sudanese camel pastoralists 38
Tibet 87, 128, 134, 312
  see also Kam Tibetans; Kansu-Tibetan frontier
Tibetan people
  in Indian/Nepal 14–15, 87, 221–3, 556
  see also A Mdo Pa;
tick avoidance 162, 165, 214–15, 229
tick control 134, 138, 189, 243, 379, 511–12
  in Africa 82, 115–16, 191, 197, 370, 485
    Kenya 223, 258–9, 394
    Nigeria 81–2, 251
  in India 387, 415
  in Nicaragua 239
  for camels 39, 40
  for cattle 173–4, 191, 265
  for goats 417
  for oxen 72–3
  for sheep 323
  see also acaricides
tick removal 86–7, 385, 529, 545
  in Africa 96, 108, 188–9, 522–3
  by poultry 214, 243, 387
  from camels 229
  from cattle 203
tick-born diseases 16, 81–2, 272, 483, 555
  cattle breeds, disease-resistant 16, 81–2, 184
ticks 13, 124
  in Africa 125, 307, 371–2, 462, 472
    nomadic pastoralists 340, 386
  in India 127
  in South America 126, 317
  in the ear 64
  on camels 169
    calf mortality 279
  on cattle 133, 230, 528, 529
  on poultry 209
  see also acaricides
Tilia cordata 207
Tinosperma cordifolia 449
Tinospora cordifolia 129, 297, 458, 480, 532
Tinospora pakis 513
Tinospora rumphii 177
Tinospora sp. 237
Tinospora tuberculata B. 172
TMWG (Transmara Western Group) 404–5

toads, fetish against disease 111, 112
tobacco 91, 115, 371, 531
  buffalo 143, 191, 232, 262–3, 532
  camels 90, 132–3
  cattle 283
  fish toxicity 496–7
  for ectoparasites 50, 175, 234, 358, 369–70,
    461
    lice 453
    mange 385
    ticks 272, 379, 385
  for eye ailments 132–3, 232, 401, 532
  for FMD 234
  for wounds 91–2
  horses 303
  insecticide/repellent 118, 385
  llamas 184
  pigs 321–2
  poultry 48, 54–5, 277
  sheep 83, 334, 360–2
  small ruminants 277, 503
  snake repellent 13–14, 60
  snakes, for snakebite 433
  see also nicotine extract
tobacco plant, parasite of 238
Tobago and Trinidad 297–301
Toda peoples (India) 459–60, 539–40
Togo 209, 552
tomato, *see also* wild tomato
tomatoes, medicinal use 76, 453
Tonga, Zimbabwe, trypanosomosis 381
tongo tongo, throat sores 410
tongue, amputation of tip 366, 367
tongue immobilised, weaning practice 392
tongue swelling, buffalo 532
tonic 209, 260, 311, 400
  horses 303, 379
  poultry 300–1, 415
tonsilitis, Jammu and Kashmir 486
tools and technologies 18
toothache 399
tortilla (charred), for diarrhoea 193–4
tortoise, protection from lightening 219
tortoise-shell ash 400
Totonac people, Mexico 224–5
Toucouleur pastoralists, Senegal 281–2
toxic plants
  in Africa 248–9, 282, 370, 513
  in India/Bhutan 102, 297
  in Peru 225
  avoidance 14–15
  camels 139, 386
  cattle 64, 129, 409–10, 529
  sheep 334, 383
  uses of 112, 114, 513
  see also Aloe vera; cassava; custard apple;
    Enartocarpus clavatus; *Glynus lotoides*;
    locoweed; papaya fruit; tapioca-leaf
toxic risks, in allopathic treatments 25
Trachyspermum ammi 234, 415, 519
Trachyspermum spp. seeds 127–8
traditional, definition 6
Traditional Animal Health Care, An Information
  Kit 252

traditional Chinese veterinary medicine (TCVM)
  557–8
traditional healers, Kenya 543
traditional medicine 49, 50, 384, 520
Traditional Veterinary Practice (compendium) 96
Tragia involucrata leaves 129
Tragia involucrata root 401
trainee selection, inappropriate 403
training, Samburu pastoralists 259–60
training healers 257–8, 259
  apprenticeship 38
  knowledge transfer 401–2, 502, 535
  professional development 196–7
transhumance 63–4, 256, 379–80, 381
  duck herding, India 525–6
  shepherds, France 110, 264
  see also seasonal movements
Transmara Western Group (TMWG) 404–5
transport camels, overview 551
trauma, treatments for goats/sheep 142
treacle gruel, for fever 511
treatment validation, ER&D 259–60
Treculia africana var. *africana* 485
trees, medicinal uses of, Zambia 502
Trianthema decandra juice 458
tribal healers, Somalia 147
tribal medicinemen, in India 491
Tricanthera gigantea 365–6
trichinellosis, in pigs, in Africa 194
Trichocerus sp. (*tullway*) 315
Tridas procumbens 281, 308
Trigonella foenum 127–8, 283
Trinidad and Tobago 297–301
Trinitarios, in Bolivia 239–40
Tripura (India) 435–6
Triumfetta rotundifolia 210
trolls, cows protected from, Sweden 430
trypanosomosis 24, 160–1, 429–30
  in Africa 91, 187, 316, 439, 494–5
    Gambia 493
    Zimbabwe 381
  camels 39, 90, 152, 293, 457
    diagnosis 151, 245, 288, 471
    prevention 79, 289
  control 25, 197, 373, 552
trypanotolerance 16, 80, 255
  cattle 155, 310, 385, 517, 552
    N'Dama 267
    zebu 107, 108
  small ruminants 351–2
tsetse fly, trypanosomosis and 197, 493
Tswana cattle, in Botswana 458
tukump, in ground contamination 452
tullway (*Trichocerus* sp.) 315
tumours/swellings 65, 132, 236
Tungus, reindeer herders 187
Tunisia 132–3, 551
  see also Ghrib Bedouin
Turkana 253–5, 540–1, 543–4
  livestock husbandry 256, 272, 403–4
    diseases 96, 326, 355, 379, 403
    scarification/bleeding techniques 51, 96
  sheep 98, 268
Turkana District (Kenya) 48

Turkey, EVK in 152–3
turkeys (poultry), in Mexico 321
Turkic peoples, Central Asia 368
Turkmenistan 282
turmeric 213, 449, 450
    cattle 260, 400, 508
    cows 129, 416–17, 507
    dogs 264
    fish diseases 192
    for wounds 340, 388, 452, 486
    pigs 161
    poultry 436
    see also Curcuma longa
turmeric powder 235, 281, 399, 400
    for fractures 234, 238
    for parasites 415, 458
    horses 127–8
turmeric (rhizome) 300, 401, 503
turpentine 132, 213, 461
turpentine oil 465
Tussilago farfara (coltsfoot) 485, 499
Twareg 157–8, 289, 471
    scarification/bleeding techniques 96, 157–8
    vaccination technique 96, 220
    see also Kel Adagh Twareg; Kel Ewey Twareg
Twareg (Mali/Algeria) 551
Twareg (Niger) 90, 496, 500, 555
Twareg (Sahara) 138
Twareg (Sahel) 90, 459, 498–9
Tylophora asthmatica leaves 231
Tylophora indica 455, 458
tympanites/tympany *see* bloat
Tzotzil Maya shepherdesses 193–4, 420–30

Uapaca togoensis Pax tree 513
Ubaye Valley (France) 396
udder inflation, milk fever treatment 75
udder problems 91, 198, 210, 416, 513
    swollen 238, 281, 415, 437
    see also mastitis
Uganda 48, 162, 201, 269
    insect pest control 14, 148
    poultry 148, 497–8
    see also Karamajong; Karamoja District; Sebei
ultrasound, physical therapy 434
Unani, traditional medicine 170, 172
Unani-Tibb, ethnoveterinary medicine 56
UNICEF, Operation Lifeline Sudan 44
United States, Book of Home Remedies 233
unthriftiness, in Africa 282, 472
Upper Volta *see* Burkina Faso
urban EVM 319, 340
urea, medicinal uses 211, 365–6, 514
urinary problems 198, 300, 485
    blockage 12, 132, 210, 212, 317, 416, 505
    in India 213, 234, 236, 415
    infections, cats/dogs 233
urine 8, 135, 159, 527
    for ectoparasites 189, 336, 386, 437–8, 480
    for FMD 201, 325, 531
    for liver fluke 126, 461
    for wounds 55, 334, 429–30, 507, 514
urine (barn) 514

urine (bloody) 481
urine (bulls') 539
urine (camels') 333, 386
urine (cattle) 189, 287, 429–30, 531
urine (cows') 400
urine (ewes') 90
urine (fermented, human) 381
urine (goats') 399
urine (human) 102, 111, 129, 133, 437–8, 536
    draught animals 77, 127, 400, 539
urine (llamas') 228
urine (own) 481, 507
urine smell, trypanosomosis diagnosis 245, 288, 293, 457
urine (spider's) 395
urine (young boy's) 465
Urospermum picioides 536
Urtica dioica 127, 207
Urtica spp. (stinging nettle) 201
USA 51, 120, 164, 462
    stockraising 14, 64–5, 281, 511–12
    therapies 233, 477–8, 549–50, 556–7
    see also American Indians; Amish; California; Texas Longhorn cattle
Usi (Peru) 356
USSR
    Central Asian Republics *see* Kazakstan; Turkmenistan
    Russian federation (former) 313
    Saami Lapps, reindeer-herding 52
utashayli (*Nicotiana paniculata* L.) 85
uterotonics evaluated, India 412
uterus 64, 138
    eversion 456
    prolapse 289, 292–3, 308
    in India 211, 230, 236, 237
Uttar Pradesh (India) 126, 127, 213, 381, 519, 522
    livestock treatments 213, 261, 492
    see also Bharud
Uttrakhand Himalayan region (India) 256

vaccination 11, 57, 197, 363, 504
    for braxy 483
    for duck plague 518
    indirect, calves 220
    rinderpest, new sustainable system 243, 558–9
    stress, poultry chicks 301
vaccination (modern) 108, 152, 312, 313
    in Africa 189, 223, 394, 560
vaccination (traditional)
    in Africa 39, 63–4, 96, 332, 366, 370
        Fulani 159, 219–20, 471
    in India 213
    in Turkey 152–3
    camels 229, 288, 289, 457
    cattle 106, 302, 332, 397
    for FMD 214–15
    for warts 148
    goats/sheep 78–9, 142
    technique 219–20, 332
vaccine (traditional) 8, 91, 101–2, 183, 333–4, 375

vaccine (*cont.*)
  advantages/disadvantages 164–5
vaginal problems 12, 282
vaginal route, for medicines 11
vaginal suturing 292–3
vakumba, tobacco plant parasite 238
Valeriana officialis 463–4
Valeriana sitchensis roots 499–500
Valeriana sylvatica roots 499–500, 507
validation, Conference working group 347
valo, cattle disease, in India 211
Valvis, Taluka (India), tribal people 528
vampire bats, predators 238, 240
Vasaves, Taluka (India), tribal people 528
vaseline, for teat damage, in cows 138
vatha madakki seeds 482
VBKVK (Krishi Vigyan Kendram Badgaon) 93–4
veeli leaf 402
vegetable oil, medicinal use 233, 322, 505
'vein pullers', healers 298, 300
venepuncture *see* bleeding
Venezuela, EVM of 433–4
Ventilago denticulata root 236
ventilation, health problems and 287
Verbascum thapsus 486, 526
Verbena litteralis 194
vermifuge *see* anthelmintic
verminous conditions, names for, Andes 245
Vernonia adoensis 270–1
Vernonia amygdalina 62, 517
Vernonia anthelmintica 127–8, 211, 486
Veterinary Anecdotes, Vetaid Book of 57
veterinary anthropology 357–8, 495–6, 546
veterinary auxiliaries 106–7
veterinary bioethics 187–8
veterinary botanicals, preparation 269
veterinary herbalist (*kaviraj*) 562
veterinary medicine 89, 233, 341–2, 454
  EVM and 123–4, 388–9, 554, 555
veterinary personnel, healers and 257–8
veterinary phytotherapy 143, 405
veterinary saints, France 310, 372, 531
veterinary scouts 466, 501
veterinary surgeons 99, 100, 124, 180, 187–8
  EVM and 146–7, 266, 297–8, 299
  healers and 291–2, 311
veterinary technicians, booklet for 412
vetiver grass, graze 551
Vetiveria zizanoides 127
Viburnum stellulatum 412
Vicos (Peru) 392
Vietnam 136, 430–1, 517–18
Vigna aconitifolia 236
Village Animal Health Workers, Nepal 376
vinegar 116–17, 138, 329, 410, 481
  horses 118, 465, 536
vinegar (apple) 303, 510
vinegar (wine) 536
vines round neck, placenta expulsion 399
violet tree root 303
viper (dried carcase) 111, 112, 513
viral encephalomyelitis 446
viral skin conditions 330–1
Visayas (Philippines) 527–8

Vitex negundo 197, 409, 458
Vitex negundo leaves 210, 411
Vitis adnata R. 102
vitriol (burnt) 367, 368
volcanic sulphur, for mange 410
Voluntary Service Overseas (VSO), website 173
vomiting, cats/dogs 166, 233
vows, medicinal use in Sri Lanka 264
VSF, workshop with *atet* 334–5
Vugusu Bantu (West Africa) 537

Wa-Nande, Great Lakes people 274
wagesha, orthopaedists, in Ethiopia 515
WaKamba 204, 257–8, 382, 394
walking in water, for hypomagnesia 334–5
walnut oil 465
WaMeru farmers 205
war, clean pasture after, in Sudan 136
warble flies 52–4, 482–3
warming ointments 228, 412
warts 148, 244
wasaidizi(paravets), in Kenya 542–3
WaSwahili (East Africa) 462
'water bag/necklace', in fasciolosis 423
water bathing, parasite removal 12–13
water buffalo *see* buffalo
water quality (poor), diarrhoea and 222
watering management 163–4, 324
  disease control 289, 394, 471, 521
  flukes 14, 257–8, 422–3
watermelon seed oil 505
watery dung (pitcalu) 232
wax 234, 295, 402, 523
weaning 18, 369, 376, 539
  camelids 126, 134
  camels 92, 165, 246, 479
  cattle 397, 515, 521
  pigs 116, 395
  sheep/goats 41, 392, 551
  yaks 312
Webebaueri sp. (*amaro*) 437–8
websites
  Arid Lands Information Network 419
  ethnobotany 32–3
  EVM 347
  New Agriculturalist On-line 387–8
  Voluntary Service Overseas 173
weeds, control by chickens 243
weight gain, approval by Fulani 49, 50
wells
  livestock disease and 381
  mineral source, for nomads 90
Wenchi District (Ghana) 234
West Africa 97, 303, 469–73
  breeding strategies 16, 255, 470, 471
  see also Peul; Vugusu Bantu; Yorubaland
West African Fellata (Sahel) sheep 550
West African Shorthorn cattle 155, 255, 294, 517, 552
West Java (Indonesia) 43, 281, 382–3, 538
  see also Pasir Gaok
Western Africa, *see also* Bantu
western medicine *see* allopathic medicine
western-centric management 241–2

whale fat, medicinal use of 138
wheat 236, 527
wheat (boiled) 235
wheat bran 64, 406
wheat bread 235
wheat (crushed wheat porridge) 132–3
wheat flour 127, 212, 376
wheat germ 210
wheat (roasted, ground) 290
wheat seed (sprouted) 401
wheel grease, for hoof disorders 536
whey 235, 288, 437
whey and salt feeding 262
white camels, status of 92
white Fulani cattle 80–2, 441
white hellebore 323
white lead powder 132
white reindeer 53
white rhinoceros fat, use of 138
white stone powder 281
whitewash 76, 77
whitlow 225, 226
wila wichhu, bloody diarrhoea 410
wild animals, wounds caused by 501–2, 529
wild coffee leaves 299–300
wild okra, *see also* okra
wild okra (*Hibiscus trionium*) 39
wild rice *see* rice
wild tomato (*Physalis alkekengi*) 50
wildebeest, malignant catarrhal fever 148, 326–7
wildlife, protection by Bedouin 42
willka willka seeds 317
willow bark 114
willow cream 536
wilsere (bush diseases) 494–6, 554
wind, cattle protection against 164
wine, medicinal use of 234
wine (distilled) 536
wine vinegar 132
witchcraft 304, 379
witchdoctor 183, 516
witches, diarrhoea caused by 222
Withania somnifera 231, 411, 468
withers, fistulous, pack horses/mules 157
WoDaaße (Fulani) 158–9, 199, 328, 494–5, 500
wolf's hair, for glanders 367
wolfsbane (aconite), toxic plant 87–8
wolves, sheep predators 334
'womb cleaner', Trinidad and Tobago 300
women 490–1, 501
    Afghan Pashtun pastoralists 142
    in Africa 100, 335, 496, 521, 554
        Kenya 164, 205, 253, 316, 385
    in India 448–51
    in South America 85, 125–6, 280
    as paravets 223–4
    as plant dealers 298
    as traditional healers 259
    in ANTHRA veterinary NGO 58–60
    livestock husbandry 215, 298–9
        guinea pigs 377–8
        pigs 395–6
        poultry 238, 240, 515
        sheep 193–4, 360–2, 420–30

    special worship by 449
    World Veterinary Association 251
wood chewing, prevention 118
wood from old rice-pounding mortars 285
woodapple juice 273
wool ball/bath treatment 214
wool production 422, 424–5, 427–8
Wopell, Aurvedic preparation 455
word magic, in cattle protection 159
working animals, limbering up 13
worldwide bibliography, husbandry 492–3
worms 81, 221, 254–5, 433
    prophylaxis 75, 169, 230, 264
    see also anthelmintic; endoparasites; nematode;
        tapeworms; trichinellosis
wormwood, in green ointment 132
worship, at shrine of local deities 288
wounds 8, 179, 330–1, 452
    in Africa 198, 388
        Chad 429–30, 521
        Ethiopia 209, 514
        Fulani 55, 108, 157, 158, 512–13, 517
        Kenya 306, 379, 459
        Nigeria 50
        Senegal 282
        South Africa 371–2
        Sudan 39, 334, 521, 539
        Tanzania 373
    in Chinese medicine 128
    in India 213, 236, 237, 401, 415, 448
        Kannada-speaking region 231, 507
        medicinemen, tribal 491
    in Mexico 406, 503
    in North America 501–2
    in Scotland 485
    in SE Asia 149, 162, 253, 307, 340, 441
    in South America 50, 173, 317, 380
    in Sri Lanka 429
    buffalo 143, 191
    camels 386–7, 502
    castration wounds 486, 537
    cattle 86–7, 396, 402, 512, 529
    dogs/cats 233, 277, 303
    elephants 488
    horses 132, 329, 501–2
    oxen 195
    pigs 321–2, 518, 525
    sheep 295
Wrightia tinctoria latex 399
Wrightia tinctoria leaves 400, 401
wry neck syndrome, firing for 453

Xanthium strumarium leaves 160–1

yak/cattle crossbreeding 312, 461–2, 556
yaks 14–15, 87–8, 224, 311–13
    Sichuan (China), husbandry 16, 556
    Tibetan husbandry 14–15, 134, 221, 223
Yakut horses, Siberia 16, 137
Yanadulu tibals (India) 507
yanawami leaves, for ectoparasites 317
yarita tea bath, for ticks 126

yarrow stalk implant, for wounds 501–2
yellow plants, in law of signatures 298
Yin and Yang, in TCVM 141–2, 309, 371, 558
yoghurt cultures, in feed 197–8
yoke galls 210, 212, 238, 415, 416, 507
Yorubaland (West Africa) 303
Yörüks (Turkey) 152–3
young stock
   rearing 17, 311
   see also animal species
yunani medicine 531
Yuracaré, forest people (Bolivia) 239–40

Zaghwa people (Sudan-Chad border) 520–1
Zaire 73, 276, 520
   'local research brigades' 330–1
   plants and prescriptions 273–4, 276–7
   PRELUDE databank 121–2
   see also Bushi region
Zambia 24, 115–16, 502, 537
   cattle 13, 86–7, 429
   poultry 50–1

   see also Lozi
Zaria (Nigeria) 251
Zea mays 207
zebra (wild), in mixed grazing 472
zebu cattle 92, 107–8, 133, 158–9, 310
   cross-breeding 355, 517
   see also azawak; bororoji
Zeetress, polyherbal formulation 411
Zehneria scabra, for wounds 373
Zimbabwe 14, 184, 209, 479
   see also Tonga
zinc, in holistic healthcare 456
Zingiber officinale see ginger
Ziziphus 335, 450
Ziziphus mauritiana ash 210
zoo animals, plant medicines for 461
zoonoses 18, 224–5, 326, 395, 473
   brucellosis 481
   hydatidosis 60, 116, 245, 326–7
   trichinellosis 194
zooprophylaxis, in Africa 206–7
zuela de zapato (toasted), in Peru 135
Zulu pastoralists *see* Kwazulu

www.ingramcontent.com/pod-product-compliance
Lightning Source LLC
Jackson TN
JSHW011350130125
77033JS00015B/545